FOUNDATIONS OF
CLINICAL PSYCHOLOGY

FOUNDATIONS OF CLINICAL PSYCHOLOGY

Edited by
Salvatore Cullari
Lebanon Valley College

Allyn and Bacon
Boston   London   Toronto   Sydney   Tokyo   Singapore

Series editor: Carla F. Daves
Series editorial assistant: Susan Hutchinson
Manufacturing buyer: Suzanne Lareau

Copyright © 1998 by Allyn & Bacon
A Viacom Company
Needham Heights, MA 02194

Internet: www.abacon.com
America Online: keyword: College Online

Library of Congress Cataloging-in-Publication Data

Foundations of clinical psychology / Salvatore Cullari, editor.
    p. cm.
  Includes bibliographical references and index.
  ISBN 0-205-26202-3
  1. Clinical psychology.   I. Cullari, Salvatore.
RC467.F685 1998   97-38141
616.89--dc21   CIP

Printed in the United States of America
10   9   8   7   6   5   4   3   2   1   02   01   00   99   98

CONTENTS

Preface and Acknowledgments   vii

About the Contributors   ix

PART I. FOUNDATIONS OF CLINICAL PSYCHOLOGY

1. History and Introduction to Clinical Psychology   *Bonnie R. Strickland*   1

2. Clinical Assessment and Diagnosis   *Robert J. Gregory*   26

3. Testing in Clinical Psychology   *Robert J. Gregory*   51

4. Ethics and Ethical Reasoning   *Mitchell M. Handelsman*   80

5. Evaluating What We Do   *David L. Streiner*   112

PART II. PSYCHOLOGICAL APPROACHES TO TREATMENT

6. Treating the Individual   *Jerold R. Gold* *George Stricker*   138

7. Psychotherapy in Groups   *Rae Dezettel Perls*   164

8. Brief Therapy in Clinical Psychology   *John F. Cooper*   185

9. Assessment and Treatment of Children and Adolescents   *Gary Geffken*   216

10. Treatment Resistance   *Salvatore Cullari*   249

PART III. BIOLOGICAL ISSUES IN CLINICAL PRACTICE

11. Biological Foundations of   *Clifford N. Lazarus*   272
Clinical Psychology

12. Psychopharmacology for   *Dan Egli*   305
Clinical Psychologists

13. Behavioral Medicine/Health   *Kathy Sexton-Radek*   331
Psychology

PART IV. SOCIAL, CULTURAL, AND LEGAL ISSUES IN CLINICAL PSYCHOLOGY

14. Community Psychology   *Karen Grover Duffy*   348

15. Transcultural Psychology and   *Juris G. Draguns*   375
the Delivery of Clinical
Psychological Services

16. Forensic Psychology   *Gerald Cooke*   403

Glossary   424

Name Index   437

Subject Index   457

PREFACE AND ACKNOWLEDGMENTS

TO THE INSTRUCTOR

Clinical psychology has come a long way since Lightner Witmer opened the first clinic at the University of Pennsylvania in 1896, and gave our discipline its name. Since that time, our primary professional activity has changed from psychological testing to treatment; the clients we treat have become mostly adults rather than children; and the scientist-practitioner model has perhaps become more practice-oriented and less scientific. Meanwhile, clinical psychology has become the single largest specialty area in the American Psychological Association.

Despite these significant changes, the next hundred years promise to be even more turbulent. Already in the last decade, managed care has dramatically changed the way some clinical psychologists run their practice. While psychotherapy itself has become briefer, paperwork and other non-treatment-related obligations have proliferated. For example, one of my colleagues only half in jest suggested that he spends more time talking to the Managed Care Organization than with his clients.

At the same time, biological aspects of behavior have assumed a much more prominent role in our field. It is rare these days to find a clinician who does not refer a large proportion of his or her clients to physicians or psychiatrists for medications. Correspondingly, it is becoming increasingly clear that many disorders such as schizophrenia and major depression have (at least in part) biological and genetic origins.

As many professionals have noted in the past, clinical psychology is in a unique position of trying to balance the rigors of a science with the demands of practice. Although we may not have reached a consensus as to whether we have been successful in this endeavor or not, this distinctive aspect is one of our greatest strengths and assets. It clearly sets us apart from other mental health professionals, and maintaining this balance is probably the only way we can hope to make significant progress in our field. Consequently, this model serves as the backbone of this book.

It is against this framework that this book is written. Despite the notable changes outlined here, many introductory texts for clinical psychology have remained essentially the same over the years. This book differs from the others in a number of ways. First, rather than being written by a single individual or a small number of authors, it brings together sixteen different specialists. The field of clinical psychology, like most other similar professions, has become so specialized that it is impossible for one or two authors to keep abreast of important changes and advances in all realms. As will become apparent from reading this book, each author has been able to compile the most up-to-date and concise description of his or her specialty area.

A second major way in which this book differs from others is that it is written by true practitioners. Almost half of the authors are in full-time private practice, and virtually all of the others have extensive real-world experience. It is no secret that many clinicians have a tendency to ignore current research findings. Part of the reason for this is that more than half of the clinical research articles published in our country are contributed by academicians. Often, the subjects, settings, and conditions in these studies are far removed from those of the real world. Thus, external validity tends to suffer, and generalization of results becomes a major problem. Many of the practicing psychologists with whom I interact report that these studies are often simply irrelevant for them. On the other hand, as I stated earlier, maintaining the scientist-practitioner model appears to be crucial for our field. This book is an attempt to bridge this gap.

In addition to the traditional topics found in introductory clinical psychology texts (e.g., history, testing and assessment, treatment methods, ethics, and statistics), this book presents chapters on brief psychotherapy, forensic psychology, psychopharmacology, biological aspects of behavior, transcultural psychology, behavioral and health psychology, child and adolescent psychology, and treatment resistance. It contains sixteen chapters and takes an integrative and eclectic approach to assessment and treatment.

This book is written primarily for senior-level undergraduates or first-year graduate students. It assumes that the reader has had basic preparation in statistics, personality theory, abnormal psychology, and testing and assessment. The book can also be used by students in related fields such as psychiatry, psychiatric nursing, social work, special education, and counseling psychology.

TO THE STUDENT

Those of you entering the field of clinical psychology are about to embark on a very exciting journey. Working with individuals who have emotional problems can be an exhilarating experience, and helping someone overcome a major life crisis can be very rewarding. At the same time, our field offers many challenges. You will be working with some clients whose problems may seem insurmountable and others whose suicidal tendencies may be difficult to overcome. In addition, clinicians face economic and political challenges that unfortunately have become a major concern of our field.

This book is designed to address these issues and help you take your first steps toward becoming a professional therapist. Perhaps you can consider this book as an appetizer to your main course of training that lies ahead. We have attempted to make this book as reader-friendly as possible. Each chapter contains a number of references and a list of recommended books for future reading that will allow you to explore further the given topic area. We have also provided a comprehensive glossary of terms at the end of the book.

This book is consistent with the scientist-practitioner model of clinical psychology, which we believe is the most appropriate course to follow. It also takes an integrative approach to treatment, which involves using the most effective aspects of many different orientations, while at the same time treating each client as a unique individual.

ACKNOWLEDGMENTS

I would like to take this opportunity to thank the many clients I have worked with throughout the years for providing me with an education that I could never receive in school. I would also like to thank all of the contributing authors of this book for their outstanding efforts in putting this book together.

I am indebted to the staff of Allyn and Bacon, especially Mylan Jaixen, Susan Hutchinson, and Carla Daves, for their suggestions and overall support of this project. Steve Specht and Mary Pettice of Lebanon Valley College reviewed several of the chapters and provided me with some very helpful suggestions.

My appreciation goes to the following reviewers for their comments on the manuscript: Bernie Jensen, University of Central Florida; Stephen Black, Millsaps College; Edward J. Yelinck, Wilson College; Robert W. Wildblood, Northern Virginia Community College; James P. Guinee, The University of Central Arkansas; and Diane L. Finley, Towson State University.

I would especially like to thank my wife, Kathi, and children, Dante and Catie, for putting up with another project that has kept me away from them for extended periods of time. Finally, I would like to thank the students of Lebanon Valley College for inspiring me to initiate and complete this project.

ABOUT THE CONTRIBUTORS

Gerald Cooke received his Ph.D. in clinical psychology from The University of Iowa in 1966. He is a diplomate of the American Board of Forensic Psychology/American Board of Professional Psychology and a Fellow of the American Academy of Forensic Psychologists. He has taught at a number of universities and has authored a book, book chapters, and journal articles on forensic psychology. He and his wife, Margaret, are in practice together in Plymouth Meeting, Pennsylvania. The practice is limited to forensic psychology.

John F. Cooper, Psy.D., L.P., is a practicing clinician and consultant in Minneapolis. Formerly president of the Minnesota Society of Brief Therapy, he is the author of *A Primer of Brief Psychotherapy* (1995, Norton) and an adjunct professor at the Minnesota School of Professional Psychology.

Salvatore Cullari received a Ph.D. in Psychology from Western Michigan University in 1981. Currently, he is a professor and chairman of the Psychology Department at Lebanon Valley College, where he teaches courses in the clinical/counseling concentration. Prior to his teaching career, he worked in several psychiatric hospitals and centers for developmental disabilities, and in private practice. He is the author of *Treatment Resistance: A Guide for Practitioners,* published by Allyn and Bacon in 1996.

Juris G. Draguns was born in Latvia in 1932 and completed his primary schooling there. He graduated from high school in Augsburg, Germany. In the United States, he obtained his bachelor's degree from Utica College of Syracuse University in 1954 and was awarded a Ph.D. in clinical psychology from the University of Rochester in 1962. After employment as clinical and research psychologist at the Rochester (NY) State Hospital and Worcester (MA) State Hospital, in 1967 he accepted a faculty appointment at The Pennsylvania State University, where he is professor of psychology. He also taught part time at Clark University, Leicester Junior College, University of Rochester, and Florida Institute of Technology. He held visiting faculty appointments at the Johannes Gutenberg University in Mainz, Germany; East–West Center in Honolulu; Flinders University in Bedford, South Australia; and National Taiwan University in Taipei.

Dr. Draguns's cross-cultural research interests have been focused on psychological disturbance. They have expanded to include personality characteristics, complex social behavior, and therapeutic and counseling relationships. At this time, he is especially interested in the role of cultural factors in mediating economic, political, and social change in Eastern and Central Europe. He is a member of the advisory board of the Multicultural Research Center in Daugavpils, Latvia. Dr. Draguns has published over 100 articles, chapters, and monographs in psychological, psychiatric, and interdisciplinary publications, many of which deal with cultural topics.

Karen Grover Duffy holds a Ph.D. in personality/social psychology from Michigan State University. She is currently chair and Distinguished Service Professor at Geneseo College of the State University of New York, where she teaches community psychology, social psychology, and psychology of personality. Karen is a certified family mediator for the Unified Court System of New York State, is a member of the executive board of the New York State Employee Assistance Program, and serves in several other community posts. In 1995 she won a Fulbright Fellowship to St. Petersburg, Russia, where she taught community psychology as well as family mediation. She continues to consult with community agencies and to teach in Russia when possible.

Dan Egli, Ph.D., is a licensed clinical psychologist who has been in full-time private practice in Williamsport, Pennsylvania, for 17 years. He specializes in psychopharmacology consultation, is a Fellow of APA, and was chair of the APA Task Force on Psychopharmacology.

Gary Geffken, Ph.D., is an associate professor of clinical psychology in the Department of Psychiatry, Pediatrics, and Clinical and Health Psychology at the University of Florida Health Science Center. His teaching, research, and clinical practice is with children and adolescents. He is the president of the Florida Psychological Association for 1997.

Jerold R. Gold, Ph.D., is professor of psychology at Long Island University and is clinical professor and supervisor in the postdoctoral program in psychoanalysis at Adelphi University. A frequent contributor to the literature in psychotherapy integration, he is the author of *Key Concepts in Psychotherapy Integration* (Plenum Press, 1996) and is on the editorial board of the *Journal of Psychotherapy Integration.*

Robert J. Gregory, Ph.D., currently professor of psychology at Wheaton College (Illinois), teaches graduate and undergraduate courses in research, statistics, and intellectual assessment. He was on the faculty of the University of Idaho for 23 years and served as chair from 1990 to 1995. He is the author of *Psychological Testing: History, Principles, and Applications* (2nd ed.), published in 1996 by Allyn and Bacon.

Mitchell M. Handelsman received his B.A. from Haverford College and his M.A. and Ph.D. from the University of Kansas. He is professor of psychology at the University of Colorado at Denver. In 1995 he received the Excellence in Teaching Award from the Society for the Teaching of Psychology.

Clifford N. Lazarus, Ph.D., is a licensed psychologist currently in full-time practice in Princeton, New Jersey, where he directs Comprehensive Psychological Services. In addition to general clinical practice, he specializes in health and neuropsychology.

Dr. Lazarus received his B.A., M.S., and Ph.D. degrees in psychology from Rutgers University, where he was a Henry Rutgers Research Scholar, and completed his clinical internship at Fairleigh Dickinson University–Division of Psychological Services. From 1989 to 1994 he was the associate director of Princeton Biomedical Research, P.A., a leading facility dedicated to evaluating new-generation psychiatric medications for pharmaceutical companies and the Food and Drug Administration.

Dr. Lazarus consults widely to corporations and industry on matters of health psychology, stress management, effective communication, and conflict resolution. He has published numerous professional papers, articles, and book chapters, and has co-authored two popular books, *Don't Believe It for a Minute—Forty Toxic Ideas That Are Driving You Crazy* and *The 60-Second Shrink—101 Strategies for Staying Sane in a Crazy World.*

A member of the American Psychological Association and the Association for the Advancement of Behavior Therapy, Dr. Lazarus is a regional director of The Prescribing Psychologists' Register and serves on its Curriculum Development Committee. In addition to his clinical and consultation work, Dr. Lazarus is co-host of a weekly listener call-in radio program, "Mental Health Matters."

Rae Dezettel Perls, Ph.D. (A.B., The University of Chicago; M.A. and Ph.D., The University of New Mexico) is a clinical psychologist practicing in Albuquerque, New Mexico; consulting school psychologist with the Albuquerque Public Schools; and clinical professor in the Department of Psychiatry, University of New Mexico School of Medicine. Dr. Perls is a Certified Group Psychotherapist and Fellow of the American Group Psychotherapy Association.

Kathy Sexton-Radek, Ph.D., is a full professor of psychology at Elmhurst College, Elmhurst, Illinois, where she has taught for the past ten years. She is also a licensed clinical psychologist in private practice part time. Her research and clinical expertise are in the areas of behavioral medicine/health psychology, sleep medicine, sport psychology, and teaching pedagogy. She is a member of the Society for Behavior Medicine, Association for the Advancement of Behavior Therapy, and American Psychological Association.

David L. Streiner graduated from Syracuse in 1968 with a Ph.D. in clinical psychology. Since then, he has been at McMaster University, where he is a full professor in the departments of clinical epidemiology and biostatistics and of psychiatry. Pre-

viously, he was chief psychologist at the McMaster University Medical Centre for 12 years. With colleagues, he has written four books in the areas of statistics, epidemiology, and measurement.

George Stricker, Ph.D., is Distinguished Research Professor at Adelphi University. He received APA awards for Distinguished Contributions to Applied Psychology in 1990 and for Distinguished Career Contributions to Education and Training in Psychology in 1995. He was president of APA's Division of Clinical Psychology and is on the board of directors of the National Register.

Bonnie R. Strickland, Ph.D. (Clinical Psychology, 1962, Ohio State University), has been on the faculties of Emory University and the University of Massachusetts at Amherst as teacher, researcher, administrator, and clinician. She has been president of the American Psychological Association, the Division of Clinical Psychology, the American Association of Applied and Preventive Psychology, and a Founder of the American Psychological Society.

CHAPTER 1

HISTORY AND INTRODUCTION TO CLINICAL PSYCHOLOGY

Bonnie R. Strickland

A young man comforts a grieving couple who have just learned that their 9-year-old child has an incurable illness. In the same teaching hospital, a middle-aged woman meets with a group of women with breast cancer to discuss their illness and ways they might improve the quality of their lives. At a nearby university, a young professor meets with her students, both graduate and undergraduate, to discuss their research on racial and gender stereotyping and psychopathology. Later that evening, in the same city, a minority male engages in heated negotiations with the leaders of two inner-city gangs who are angrily threatening violence over a turf dispute.

All of these activities are being conducted by doctoral-level clinical psychologists, although they could also be accomplished by members of other disciplines and professions. The grief counselor could be a physician or a member of the clergy. The group therapist could be a nurse or a lay person who has experienced breast cancer herself. The professor could be a social psychologist or represent a discipline other than psychology, such as education or sociology. The gang negotiator could be a social worker or a former gang member himself. But clinical psychology is the only field that trains students to do each, and all, of these activities. So what exactly is a clinical psychologist? What do they do? How do you know one when you meet one? Would you want to be one?

Psychology has become one of the most popular undergraduate majors for college students across the country. Graduate programs in psychology graduate about four thousand doctoral students every year, the large majority of whom are clinical psychologists. The American Psychological Association (APA), the largest national organization of psychologists in the world, has more than 87,000 members. It also has 59,000 student affiliates, 3,300 interntional affiliates, and 1,700 high school teacher affiliates. Almost 90% of APA members are clinical psychologists or other applied professionals such as school, counseling, and industrial/ organizational psychologists. How did clinical psychology become so attractive? What about it is so appealing?

WHAT IS CLINICAL PSYCHOLOGY?

Clinical psychology purports to be a field, a discipline, a science, and a profession that covers the range and totality of human behavior. The work of clinical psychologists covers events from brain cells through prison cells. After years of trying to define clinical psychology, the Division of Clinical Psychology of the APA published a pamphlet with this definition:

> The field of clinical psychology integrates science, theory, and practice to understand, predict, and alleviate maladjustment, disability, and discomfort as well as to promote human adaption, adjustment, and personal development. Clinical psychology focuses on the intellectual, emotional, biological, psychological, social, and behavioral aspects of human functioning across the life span in varying cultures, and at all socioeconomic levels.

Perhaps it is no wonder, then, that clinical psychology has appeal for people who are interested in science and curious about how human behavior is developed, maintained, and changed. Clinical psychology is also powerfully attractive to people who are drawn to a helping profession with its goals of alleviating distress and improving the human condition. But can any one field cover and contain all of these diverse interests in understanding and changing human behavior? Can a single field truly integrate science and practice? Has contemporary clinical psychology met its mission and risen to the challenge of its broad goals? For some of these answers, let's look at the historical development of clinical psychology, with its beginnings in medicine, philosophy, science, and theology.

THE ROOTS OF PSYCHOLOGY

Prehistoric people felt the heat and saw the light of the sun, tracked the moon and stars, counted the days, and marked the seasons. They built fires and shelters, used gravity for their benefit, developed tools, and sculpted vessels. Early humans could not escape the simple laws of science—cause and effect, observation and replication. They developed a rudimentary classification system in which they could place inanimate objects (rocks and mountains) versus animate objects (wild beasts and other people), food versus poisonous substances, heat versus cold. Although early science consisted only of mathematics and a search of the heavens (astronomy, astrology), primitive people had to be natural

psychologists, aware of emotions and dependent on their senses and their perception of the world and the people in it. Further, they evolved social norms and a sense of social justice within their families, groups, and communities, constantly alert to ensure their safety and security.

Our early citizens and scientists watched the skies and looked to the stars to determine how to describe the passage of time and life on earth. They developed mythical concepts to explain human behavior and magic rituals to relieve physical suffering. Five thousand years later, clinical psychologists, still curious about human behavior, look to people instead of planets. But they continue to develop theoretical notions about who we are and how we come to be, as well as psychotherapeutic techniques to relieve emotional suffering.

Although the earliest sciences and mathematics evolved from basic human need and the application of knowledge to problems of survival, the stresses between theoretical science and putting that scientific understanding into practice in Western history have been with us at least since Plato. For over two thousand years, science as a pure exercise of reason, divorced from the senses and from "the object of servile trades," was a hindrance to progress (Metraux & Crouzet, 1963). For example, pumps and a steam engine were invented before the Christian era but were never used for mechanically raising water or driving weights (perhaps because the widespread use of slaves as construction laborers made such inventions unnecessary). Science as reason continued until the early seventeenth century. Francis Bacon, with his emphasis on experimental proof, is credited as the founder of modern science in the 1600s. The nineteenth and twentieth centuries have seen the flourishing of scientific discoveries, technological advances, and, in many cases, a synergy between theory and application.

Like people today, our prehistoric forebears wanted to stay alive and live free of pain. But their lives were usually short, brutally cut down by natural disasters, accidents, and violent encounters— sometimes with wild animals but more often from their fellow humans. The soft tissues of our earliest ancestors have vanished, although some bone fragments and fossilized bacteria remain. Rickets and tooth wear attest to the scarcity of food; bone deformities suggest arthritis and rheumatism ("cave-gout"). To relieve suffering and cure illnesses, prehistoric people looked to nature. They could see animals licking their wounds and eating certain grasses and plants. Very likely, ancient people began to identify medicines from various plants they found soothing; early skeletons show that they were skilled in setting bone fractures. Still, buffeted by the powerful forces of nature, primitive people ascribed the power to harm (and to heal) to animals and spirits and looked to these totems for relief. Magic, religion, and medicine became intertwined; healers, or witch doctors, were thought to have magical powers to battle the demons of disease (Leff & Leff, 1958). When herbs or ritual failed to heal a disorder, the medicine man or woman resorted to other treatments such as blood-letting or even brain surgery (trephining). Using natural potions to protect the brain, these early surgeons cut through the skull with sharp flints, perhaps to release the evil spirits that afflicted the patient and caused such disorders as madness, epilepsy, blindness, or persistent painful headaches. Often, patients and their belongings were segregated to protect the community from the malevolent spirits, thereby inadvertently protecting others from infection as well.

The Egyptians developed a sophisticated approach to medicine and healing, at least for their rulers and soldiers. Slaves, working to build palaces and the pyramids, were easily replaced and not usually treated for the effects of the malnourishment and accidents that shortened their lives. Priest-physicians used a wide variety of drugs and herbs to treat diseases. They even wrote textbooks; one described remedies for over 260 diseases; another listed surgical techniques to be used for battlefield injuries (Leff & Leff, 1958).

The growth of medicine occurred across all of the developing cultures, and health knowledge was shared along with commerce and trade. Babylonia had a code of medical ethics and also a unique way of treating some individual ailments. The sick person would sit in the marketplace and talk with passers-by about whether or not they had a similar disorder and how they had treated it. China held state medical examinations and controlled physicians' salaries. The ancient Hindus trained medical students in surgery by having them practice on animals and plants, like the hollow stalks of water lilies or the large veins of leaves. Through their Talmudic law, the Jews taught other nations social hygiene, especially the importance of cleanliness (Leff & Leff, 1958).

Inoculation against smallpox was also practiced by widely separated cultures. Perhaps noting that people who recovered from smallpox were never afflicted again, healers would rub pus from an infected person into a prepared wound of the person they were trying to protect (Leff & Leff, 1958). Most early medicine, however, was based on beliefs that both physical diseases and mental disorders occurred because of demon possession or on notions that the ill had offended the deities in some way. From extravagant burial rituals to simple remedies of the blending of blood and dung from certain animals, early medicine was an attempt to appease the gods so that the patient might be restored to a healthy state. No doubt, the first practice of psychotherapy was by witch doctors and those recognized in the community as priests and healers, who would advise patients as to how to change their behavior to please the deities.

As the great empires of the Bronze Age began to decline, the Greeks, using iron for tools and blessed with abundant coastlines at the crossroads of civilization, became the dominant culture in agriculture, the arts, commerce, philosophy, science, and medicine. Greek philosophers and physicians replaced the ancient mystico-magical medical practices with a reasoned, empirical approach to sickness and healing. Carefully observing their patients, they analyzed patterns of pain, tracked the course of an illness, and thoughtfully recorded the outcome, even when the outcome was death. Some Greek clinical records and case descriptions for diseases such as tuberculosis, childbed fever, epilepsy, mumps, and malaria are classics, and we still use some of the medicinal prescriptions the Greeks derived from plants (Leff & Leff, 1958). Acclaiming the healing power of nature and the importance of adequate housing, clean water, diet, and exercise, the Greeks were also pioneers in public health.

Though impeccable in their observation and careful recording of symptoms and the disease process, the Greeks were woefully ignorant of physiological processes. They believed, for example, that the brain cooled the heart, which was the site of reason. Thinking the number "4" to be of special import, Greek philosophers described four basic elements—fire, earth, air, and water—with four corresponding qualities—hot, dry, cold, and moist. They then proposed that the human body was composed of four corresponding elements, or humours—blood, phlegm, and yellow and black bile. The balance of humours accounted for an individual's personality and well-being; excess of one would lead to psychological disorders (e.g., too much black bile caused depression). Greek physicians treated the person by attempting to restore the balance of humours through bleeding, enemas, and forced purging. Despite the rules of logic of the philosophers, many Greeks turned to religion for healing purification of the body and would visit certain temples, much as we might visit a spa today. In lovely settings, visitors were urged to relax from the stress of their daily lives. They were given special diets and opportunities for ritual baths. Priests offered advice and suggestions for improved well-being; sometimes they took the role of gods and appeared to residents as they slept.

Though lost to most history books, women played a major role as healers and physicians in early Greece. Helen of Troy is described in Homer's *Odyssey* as a particularly skilled healer who prescribed drugs to relieve pain and alter mood. Pythias, the wife of Aristotle, wrote some of the work attributed to him, especially about reproduction. Female healers were particularly knowledgeable about both preventing miscarriage and inducing abortion. One woman physician, Agnodice, wore men's clothes to disguise her sex and was put on trial when her ruse was discovered. The women of Athens rushed to her defense and threatened their husbands if she was not released. Agnodice was pardoned, resumed her practice, and thereafter dressed as she wished (Achterberg, 1990).

Greek medicine held sway through the rise of the Roman Empire because the Romans had little regard for medicine or its practitioners. The Alexan-dria library and medical school in Egypt, built by Alexander the Great, was the repository of Greek knowledge. Physicians there conducted research in anatomy, physiology, and pathology, sometimes using prisoners who were dissected alive. The Romans did, however, become particularly adept at surgery during their widespread military conquests. They set up sick-bays for the wounded on the battlefield; these "camp" hospitals occasionally became permanent and were used for civilians and slaves as well as soldiers. Both men and women practiced the full range of known medicine in these infirmaries. Public health also flourished in that public health officers, paid by the state, tested food and supervised the water and drainage systems of the elaborate aqueducts (Achterberg, 1990; Leff & Leff, 1958).

The fall of Rome and the Dark Ages ushered in a millennium of Western history almost bereft of great advances in science and medicine. The Christian Church, in conflict with the superstitious, violent, and primitive religious beliefs of the invaders from the north, eventually expressed itself in the unassailable dogma that happiness could only be found in life after death (assuming, of course, that one followed the teachings of Christianity). Religious monks did preserve the written knowledge of Greece and Rome, but Church dogma allowed no dissent from its rigid teaching nor any examination of science or early medicine. The great plagues that swept western Europe were thought to be punishment for sin, as all diseases were ascribed to demons. Only occasionally would Western culture be influenced by travelers from the East who had continued their advancements in the arts and sciences. The Arabs had translated earlier Greek and Roman manuscripts on healing and added their own important advancements in medicine. New perfumes and spices from Asia, along with the known herbal remedies, became the basis for the sciences of chemistry and pharmacy. The Arabs built hospitals in every major city; supposedly, they chose the sites by the freshness of the air. Baghdad, for example, had over 60 hospitals, including outpatient clinics and pharmacies (Leff & Leff, 1958).

The scientific revolution, however, begun so successfully by ancient civilizations, was denied for over a thousand years in western Europe. Medicine was a mixture of pagan and Christian rituals, and the careful observations of cause and effect in physical and mental illness all but disappeared.

Universities for the study of the arts and sciences had existed in China and Southeast Asia for centuries but did not develop in the West until about 1000 A.D. The most distinguished of these was at Salerno, Italy, a crossroads of the Mediterranean already famous for its healing baths. Arabs, Christians, Jews, and Latins, both male and female, made up the faculty and student body of this major medical school. Within the next 300 years, over eighty major centers of learning would be established in European cities. They would cover the sum of knowledge on all subjects from anatomy and surgery to law, philosophy, and theology. Practitioners of the healing arts, however, gained little knowledge from the basic arts and sciences. They were more likely to ply their craft of rudimentary medicine with techniques acquired through experience and apprenticeships. Professional practice, then as now, was based on accumulating knowledge from experienced practitioners and applying this practical knowledge to people who were suffering. To reserve professional activities to those experienced in the healing arts, various "guilds" were organized. In England, the Royal Physicians and Surgeons Guild was established in 1435 to license barbers who could perform "bleedings" and give enemas and executioners who could set bones. The authority to practice was controlled by the Church and the courts, which also determined the content of medical knowledge.

As the Church gained in influence, the clergy took over the treatment of hysteria and afflictions such as tremors or epilepsy, which were believed to occur when the hapless victims were possessed by the devil. Cures ranged from sprinkling holy water through exorcism to death. Because women were not made in God's image and were the source of original sin, any healing practices that they used were thought to originate with the devil. Women did practice midwifery but could be imprisoned or executed if they assisted at the birth of a stillborn or deformed child who was thought to be the spawn of the devil (Achterberg, 1990). Moreover, because of the alleged evil power of women, and especially the

nefarious influence she could wield through her knowledge of herbs and potions, the Church declared that if a woman involved herself in healing practices, she must be a witch. Her punishment for attempting to cure the sick was to be tortured and executed. Groups other than women were also persecuted for their beliefs when these differed from the dogma of the Christian church. The Jews, in particular, were vilified, exiled from their homelands, and sometimes expelled from whole countries.

In 1484 Pope Innocent VIII commissioned two inquisitors to organize trials and prosecute witches under the authority of the Church. These Dominican monks compiled a manual, *Malleus Maleficarum* (*The Witches' Hammer*), which first affirmed the existence of witches and then gave instructions for identifying them. Citizens believed it their civic and Christian duty to report neighbors, friends, and family; many made a lucrative living in finding, torturing, and executing "witches" (50 times as many female as male witches). Authorities were proud of their record of recognizing witches, and the Inquisition boasted of executing (usually by burning but also by beheading, crushing between stones, drowning, flogging, and hanging) 30,000 witches in 150 years. Seven thousand women were burned to death in Treves and 500 in a single month in Geneva, Switzerland. Some towns lost all of their women, and in Germany inquisitors built large ovens, of much the same design as was later used in the Holocaust, to handle the mass murders. Because pets, especially cats, were thought to be used in the shamanistic practices of the witches, they were also tortured and killed along with the women (sometimes the cats were burned in sacksful) leaving fewer defenses against plague-infested fleas on the rats that spread disease. Authorities estimate that about 1,000 witches were hanged in England and over 200 in New England (Achterberg, 1990). In seventeenth-century Boston, the only two women listed as physicians were denounced as witches; one was expelled from the city and the other executed. It would be almost 200 years before another female physician, Harriot Hunt, would open an office in 1835 (Walsh, 1977).

During the Dark Ages, calamities, misfortunes, natural disasters, and illness were assumed to result from the work of the devil and his followers—evil that was personified in the flesh through convulsive seizures, the rantings of the mentally ill, or even the use of drugs and potions to relieve pain. These beliefs continued well into the Renaissance, although gradually men of medicine began to embrace the Scientific Revolution so that the healing arts were to become something more than magic and religious beliefs. Science and medicine turned their attention to a physical reality when Descartes separated the mind and the body.

FOUNDATIONS OF CONTEMPORARY SCIENCE AND MEDICINE

The period of the Renaissance in western Europe, though bound by the dogma of the Church and the lure of magic and witchcraft, was marked by an unfolding of remarkable discoveries in science, ranging from the circling of the planets to the circulation of blood. Arguments still raged about the role of reason versus empiricism in the understanding of the natural world, but clearly a paradigm shift was occurring in which form and matter in nature were not only to be contemplated but controlled. Knowledge could not be acquired by mere contemplation of the physical world but must be learned through sensory observation and critical experiments, although it was difficult, especially for the clergy and the authorities, to think of human beings as a part of nature. It was also difficult for western Europeans to acknowledge any contributions to medicine from women or from any group other than their own. For example, a model of the circulation of blood in the body had been proposed by Hildegard of Bingen long before William Harvey was credited with the discovery. Women had also learned to use herbal remedies to reduce pain before the discovery of ether and chloroform. Surgeons, however, relied on almost lethal doses of ether and chloroform rather than the "devilish" drugs of women. In fact, women were not allowed to administer herbs to assuage the pains of childbirth, since women were supposed to suffer for their (and Eve's) sins. Lady Mary Montagu described how one might be inoculated against smallpox some 80 years before Edward Jenner was credited with the discovery of a smallpox vaccine.

The Royal College of Physicians and Surgeons, however, refused to allow a practice performed by "ignorant women" in the Muslim world into England, "one of the most Learned and Polite Nations in the World"—dooming thousands, perhaps millions, to death from smallpox (one in five victims).

Mathematics and astronomy, chemistry, and physics were easily considered basic sciences, but scientific understandings of the working of the human body and the make-up of consciousness would not emerge until the nineteenth century. Empirically based medicine also was a late arrival on the scientific scene. The growth of biology and an interest in human consciousness and sensory perception were influenced by changes in the conception of the merit of an individual being. Literature and the arts began to celebrate the worth of each person, and powerful political pressures brought reform and social liberation, at least for many men. The distinct boundaries between ruler and slave, rich and poor, and powerful and oppressed were to become more permeable as a romantic humanism recognized the value of human beings and human existence. Not only did the French Revolution mark the emergence of a middle class, but the humane interests of the revolutionaries also allowed attention to be given to the mentally ill. Philippe Pinel, appalled by the conditions of cruelty and filth in which the "insane" were housed, asked hospital administrators to give the "lunatics" the benefits of liberty and equality for which the Revolution was fought. Pinel removed the chains from the residents and made certain that they were well fed and treated with kindness. He believed that psychiatry should become more scientific, treating mental illnesses as one might treat physical disorders. Pinel believed that "To apply our principles of moral treatment, with undiscriminating uniformity, to maniacs of every character and condition in society, would be equally ridiculous and unadvisable" (Ehrenwald, 1991, p. 213). The first of the modern era to keep careful records of patient behavior, he began an attempt to classify mental illnesses.

In England, at about the same time, William Tuke, a wealthy Quaker, was told by friends of the death of a relative in the Lunatic Asylum in York. Like Pinel, Tuke, horrified by the conditions he found in the housing of the insane, raised money to open the York Retreat for the mentally ill. Respect, nourishing food, and exercise in a farmlike setting was a far cry from the usual treatment of chains, bleedings, and purges in other institutions.

In the United States, similar reform movements improved conditions of the "idiots, lunatics, and other persons of unsound mind" who earlier had been housed in workhouses and almshouses, and sometimes in dungeons. The first public institution for the mentally ill in the United States opened in 1773 in Williamsburg, Virginia, and 25 years later The Maryland Hospital was built. During the first half of the nineteenth century, almost every state established hospitals for "the insane," mostly in rural areas, to house large numbers of patients. A few private institutions such as The Friends' Asylum in Philadelphia and the Hartford Retreat, were modeled after the York Retreat, with patients in a homelike setting. Dorothea Dix, in particular, traveled throughout the country urging humane treatment for the mentally ill, and her suggested reforms were influential around the world (Reisman, 1966). A hundred years later, in 1908, an ex-patient, Clifford Beers, wrote a book, *A Mind That Found Itself*, documenting his abuse in a psychiatric hospital (Beers, 1908). He also established the National Committee for Mental Hygiene, a citizens' group that began to advocate for improved treatment for the mentally ill (and still does to this day as the National Mental Health Association). Abuses such as physically restraining some patients and "warehousing" many in back wards continued, however, until the 1960s and 1970s, when the advent of psychiatric medications allowed movement of patients from hospitals to less restrictive community settings. Today, most of the large mental hospitals, some of which once held 30,000 to 40,000 patients, sit empty and deserted. Still, in far too many instances the seriously mentally ill may be ill served by their "freedom." As in the days before mental health reforms in this country, psychotic individuals are again too often homeless or incarcerated in jails and prisons.

SCIENTIFIC PSYCHOLOGY

At the beginning of the nineteenth century, anthropology and sociology were founded and biology was marked by a number of major developments, including the theories of evolution and developmental history. In medicine, Pasteur formulated the law of biogenesis—that all life comes from preexisting life. A "germ" theory of disease was formulated and antiseptic surgery introduced. With the gains of science, "truth" became more relative; dogma and cherished beliefs were replaced with an optimistic skepticism. The discovery that micro-organisms caused disease was a particularly fortuitous advance. Scientists and physicians assumed that even those unfathomable disorders such as epilepsy and the "mental" illnesses would soon yield their secrets so that they too could be controlled.

In 1875 the Minister of Culture in Saxony offered Wilhelm Wundt, M.D., a chair at the University of Leipzig in philosophy, with a focus on the natural sciences. Wundt founded the first ongoing research facility devoted to psychology in 1879. During his forty-five-year tenure at Leipzig, Wundt awarded 186 Ph.D.'s in psychology to scholars who came to study with him from ten countries (Popplestone & McPherson, 1994). Wundt's laboratory was based on the scientific method, which was proving useful in understanding the physical world. Scientists would now attempt to understand the people who inhabited and influenced this world, beginning with sensory processes.

The early American psychologists were generally wealthy young men who had traveled to Germany to study with Wundt. These included William James, who had actually begun a laboratory at Harvard in 1875, four years before Wundt, and who would later popularize psychology with his *Principles of Psychology*; James McKeen Cattell, who emphasized the importance of individual differences and mental testing; and G. Stanley Hall, who founded the American Psychological Association (APA). The major universities in the United States had only recently initiated graduate studies, thus giving early psychologists the opportunity to shape graduate education and establish psychology as a discipline distinct from philosophy and/or physiology. Psychologists assumed that, like other scientists, they would hold the most advanced scholarly degree available, the Doctor of Philosophy. On July 8, 1892, Hall met at Clark University in Worcester, Massachusetts, with seven of his colleagues interested in this new field and founded the American Psychological Association. They elected 24 others (all men) to membership and held their first convention in December of that year in connection with the American Association for the Advancement of Science. Only a few members of this group had been trained as psychologists; the others were educators, philosophers, and physicians.

THE BEGINNING OF CLINICAL PSYCHOLOGY

The field of clinical psychology inherited not only a respect for the scientific method but also the clinical findings of physicians, especially in Europe, who were working with people who had symptoms of what we now call mental illness (see Table 1.1). In the late eighteenth century, an Aus-

Table 1.1 Highlights in the History of Clinical Psychology

CLINICAL PSYCHOLOGY		UNITED STATES HISTORY
1773	First public institution for mentally ill, Williamsburg, VA.	
1776		War of Independence.
1789		French Revolution.
1793	Pinel introduces humane reforms in mental hospitals.	
1848	Dix campaigns for improved mental health facilities. First state hospital built in New Jersey.	
1860	Fechner's *Elements of Psychology* published.	U.S. Civil War begins.
1865		U.S. Civil War ends.
1873	James begins informal laboratory at Harvard.	
1879	Wundt establishes first psychology laboratory at University of Leipzig.	
1885	Sir Francis Galton establishes first mental testing center, London.	Rise of graduate education.
1887	*American Journal of Psychology* published.	
1890	Cattell coins the term *mental test*. James's *Principles of Psychology* published.	
1892	American Psychological Association (APA) founded by G. Stanley Hall.	
1893	Exhibits of psychological tests seen at Columbian Exposition.	
1895	Breuer and Freud's *Studies in Hysteria* published.	
1896	Witmer establishes first psychological clinic at University of Pennsylvania, first uses term *clinical psychology* at fourth APA conference in Boston.	
1898		Spanish-American War.
1905	Binet-Simon intelligence test published in France. Vineland Training School opens for retarded children, eventually offers first internship.	
1907	Witmer edits first clinical journal, *Psychological Clinic*.	
1908	Beers's *A Mind That Found Itself* published.	
1909	Freud lectures at Clark University. Healey opens first child guidance clinic, attached to a juvenile court in Chicago; Fernald tests children brought before the court, performance tests are developed.	
1910	Goddard translates Binet-Simon test into English.	
1913	Kraepelin describes and classifies psychopathological states.	
1914		World War I begins in Europe.
1916	Terman translates Binet scale.	

Table 1.1 *Continued*

	CLINICAL PSYCHOLOGY	UNITED STATES HISTORY
1917	Scott develops proficiency tests; 3,500,000 men are classified for military jobs. American Association of Clinical Psychology (AACP) is formed by psychologists who break away from APA.	U.S. enters World War I.
1918	Alpha and Beta group intelligence tests are developed, millions of recruits are tested.	World War 1 ends.
1919	AACP rejoins APA as its Clinical Section.	
1920	Intelligence testing helps to determine immigration quotas.	
1921	The Rorschach Test published.	
1924	Levy introduces Rorschach to U.S.	Immigration Restriction Act passes.
1929		Stock market crashes, ushers in Great Depression.
1930s	Well-known psychoanalysts immigrate to U.S.	
1934		Hitler becomes German Führer.
1935	Thematic Apperception Test (TAT) published.	
1936	First clinical text, Lowitt's *Clinical Psychology,* is published.	
1937	American Association for Applied Psychology (AAAP) is formed for clinical psychologists unhappy with APA. *Journal of Consulting Psychology* founded.	
1939	Wechsler-Bellevue Intelligence Scale published.	World War II begins in Europe.
1940	Hathaway and McKinley report MMPI I data.	
1941		Pearl Harbor / U.S. enters World War II.
1942	Rogers's *Client-Centered Therapy* published.	
1943	Minnesota Multiphasic Personality Inventory (MMPI) is published.	
1945	APA is reorganized to support practice; AAAP becomes Division 12, Clinical Section of APA. Psychologists begin to treat veterans for mental health problems. Connecticut passes first certification law.	World War II ends.
1947	American Board of Examiners in Professional Psychology (ABPP) is established.	
1949	Clinical psychology education and training conference held in Boulder, Colorado, recommends science/practice model. Veterans' Administration begins to train and hire large number of clinical psychologists. Salter's *Conditional Reflex Therapy* published.	National Institute of Mental Health is established.
1950		Korean War begins.
1952	First *Diagnostic and Statistical Manual* (DSM-I) is published by American Psychiatric Association. Eysenck critique of psychotherapy appears.	
1953	APA publishes *Ethical Standards for Psychologists.*	Armistice in Korea.
1954	Rotter publishes his social learning theory. Rogers and Dymond present research on counseling process.	
1955		Bus boycott begins in Montgomery, Alabama.
1960s	Psychotropic drugs are developed for treatment of schizophrenia.	
1963		Community Mental Health Centers Act passes. John F. Kennedy assassinated.

Continued

Table 1.1 *Continued*

CLINICAL PSYCHOLOGY	UNITED STATES HISTORY
1964	Civil Rights Act passed.
1965	Voting Rights Act passed.
1968 Psy.D. progam is begun at University of Illinois. DSM-II published.	Robert Kennedy, Martin Luther King assassinated, 100,000+ march on Washington for civil rights.
1969 California School of Professional Psychology.	Upsurge in student demonstrations. Stonewall riots.
1970s Computer-based test interpretations proliferate. Rise of health psychology.	Kent State killings
1973 Vail Conference affirms Psy.D. and practitioner model.	
1974	Nixon resigns, U.S. abandons South Vietnam.
1975 National Register of Health Care Providers is published.	
1979 Model licensing bill passed by APA Council.	
1980 DSM-III published.	
1981 Revised *Ethical Standards for Psychologists* published.	
1987 DSM-III-R is published. Utah conference on graduate education. APA reorganizes into Science, Practice, and Public Interest directorates, eventually adds Education directorate.	
1988 APA members reject reorganization plan. American Psychological Society (APS) formed.	
1989	Berlin Wall topples, Cold War ends.
1990 American Association for Applied and Preventive Psychology is established, with close links to APS.	
1990s Psychotropic medications more specific for depression and schizophrenia are marketed. Clinical psychologists advocate for prescription privileges.	Health care revolution, advent of managed care.
1992 Most recent revision of *Ethical Standards* published.	
1994 DSM-IV published.	

trian physician, Anton Mesmer, believed that mental states were influenced by the movement of planets that controlled a universal magnetic force, or fluids. Mesmer designed elaborate ceremonies or seances in which people would sit around a large vat of fluid with iron rods protruding. In dim light, accompanied by music, Mesmer would appear, wearing spectacular robes and waving a wand. He would pass among the participants and touch them with his wand or his hands while suggesting, even commanding, that their neurotic symptoms disappear. Mesmer maintained that he was harnessing animal magnetism as a treatment, but we now know that he had basically discovered the power of suggestion

and hypnosis. Mesmer's techniques were effective in relieving some patients of their debilitating symptoms, but he was investigated by authorities, including Benjamin Franklin, who declared that he was a charlatan and that his cures resulted from "the excitement of the imagination." In his later years, a penniless Mesmer roamed the streets and eventually died a "madman" like the patients he had attempted to help. He never knew that history would credit him, as one of his students noted, a "wonder worker" by his demonstration that imagination and suggestion influenced emotional symptoms. Thus began the essence of the psychogenic theory of mental illness—the notion that emotional symptoms are not caused by organic or physical factors but result from unusual psychological reactions.

An English surgeon, James Baird, was the first to describe the phenomenon of hypnotism, which he believed was based on suggestion rather than "animal magnetism." Fascinated that "mesmerism" could relieve symptoms, a number of physicians in France began to use hypnotism with certain patients. Liebeault and Bernheim worked together in the town of Nancy to induce and then cure hysterical symptoms with hypnosis. Charcot, and later his student Janet, also noticed that hysterical symptoms did not follow the normal course of anatomical degeneration expected in physical disease. Some of their patients might unexpectedly sleepwalk, although in their waking states they appeared to be paralyzed. Patients would recover from "functional blindness" with no physical aftereffects. These neurologists, who used hypnosis to induce and relieve hysterical symptoms, also gave demonstrations of their techniques to other interested physicians, including Sigmund Freud, who came to study with them. Excited by what he had learned about hysteria, Freud returned to Vienna where he used hypnosis as a treatment tool. With Breuer, however, he determined that free association was a quicker method of eliciting a trancelike state in which emotional abreaction occurred, and he began to lecture and write about the role of the unconscious in people's lives.

In the 1890s, as North American clinical psychology was begun, Freud was developing his theory of psychoanalysis and working with neurotic patients in Vienna. In England and Germany, physicians were particularly interested in psychotic patients. Emil Kraepelin, a psychiatrist who also studied with Wundt, is credited with proposing an organic and medical model of mental illness. He believed that psychotic states and mental retardation were essentially physical diseases, with an etiology, a cluster of symptoms, a duration of illness, and a specific outcome. Such organic theories were particularly enhanced when syphilis was found to be a cause of general paresis, a degenerative brain disorder with severe neurological and psychological symptoms (such as "hearing voices" and wide shifts in mood). Krafft-Ebing and others discovered

that syphilitic spirochetes eventually move through the bloodstream to the central nervous system and the brain—usually after many years—causing dementia. Kraepelin assumed that it would be only a matter of time until the other "mental illnesses," including the two that he identified, manic-depressive psychosis and dementia praecox (schizophrenia), would be conquered by medicine.

Lightner Witmer, the father of clinical psychology, began his academic career as great debates were raging about the degree to which mental deficiencies resulted from either organic causes—the biogenic hypothesis—or from psychological processes—the psychogenic thesis. Witmer, who received his Ph.D. from Wundt and was a student of Cattell, also was immersed in the tradition of individual differences that marked so many psychologists of the late 1800s (Routh, 1996).

Astronomers had long been aware that individuals using telescopes to observe the movement of the stars differed in reaction times. A German astronomer, Friedrich Bessel, gathered systematic data on these differences, which he called "personal equations." Sir Francis Galton traveled throughout England giving thousands of people various tests of physical strength and mental agility (discovering at the same time that fingerprints were unique for each person, did not change, and could be used for identification purposes). Galton's interests were, no doubt, motivated by his boundless curiosity about people, but like many scientists of his era, he was a part of the political movements of his day that were "guiding" science. Galton was dedicated to improving the human gene pool and coined the term *eugenics*. With his faith in measurement, even as he walked the streets of English cities, Galton was classifying women as to beauty and everyone as to "good," "medium," and "bad." He hoped to develop individual difference measures so that people could be classified according to intelligence and physique for purposes of improving the superiority of the English race. Galton joined a long line of scientists who measured everything they could about people, including their heads (Gould, 1981). Assuming that brain size (and thus head size) reflected the capacity of intelligence, physicians and scientists had developed a theory of craniology. They used head measurements as evidence of the superiority of Caucasian western European males to women and other racial groups, despite the fact that many male criminals and men who were not French or English had large heads. Craniology was similar to phrenology in which bumps or depressions on the outer edge of the skull were thought to represent certain mental faculties. Measurement of head sizes across cultures was simpler, however, and craniology became a respected way of assessing intelligence. With its basis in biological determinism, craniology set the stage for the importance of intelligence tests for classifying people. In this country, Samuel George Morton, a Philadelphia scientist and physician, was much respected for his collection of more than a thousand skulls from all over the world. James McKeen Cattell was the earliest North American psychologist with major interests in individual differences and their measurements. In his travels to Europe, Cattell met Galton and was so impressed that he coined the term *mental testing* and tried to develop a standardized test battery that could be used routinely for everybody.

Lightner Witmer studied with Cattell at the University of Pennsylvania and translated his interest in individual differences into work with children. Witmer became the most influential figure at that time in moving psychology toward practical goals, such as identifying the reasons that students might be having difficulty learning in school. Before becoming a psychologist, Witmer had been a college preparatory school teacher of English and history, and he was well aware of the difficulties that some students had in school. He was particularly taken with one boy who, though planning to go to college, could not write a grammatically correct sentence. Five years later, Witmer found the student enrolled in a class that he was teaching at the University of Pennsylvania and noted the deficiency of his "articulation, written discourse, and verbal audition" and the fact that he eventually failed to graduate (Witmer, 1907, p. 2). Witmer discusses this student in a journal that he founded, *The Psychological Clinic,* along with his conviction that if the student had been given remedial tutoring during his very early school years, his serious academic deficits and subsequent failures could have been avoided.

Witmer established the first Psychological Clinic at Penn in 1896 to help children like this student improve their academic prowess. His first case was a 14-year-old boy, a chronically bad speller, referred by his teacher. Witmer wrote that he "could not find that the science of psychology had ever addressed itself to the ascertainment of the causes and treatment of a deficiency in spelling. Yet here was a simple defect of memory; and memory is a mental process of which the science of psychology is supposed to furnish the only authoritative knowledge. It appeared to me that if psychology was worth anything to me or to others it should be able to assist the efforts of a teacher in a retarded case of this kind" (Witmer, 1907, p. 3).

Witmer was absolutely clear in his assertions that "the pure and applied sciences advance in a single front ... and in the final analysis the progress of psychology, as of every other science, will be determined by the value and amount of its contributions to the advancement of the human race" (Witmer, 1907, p. 4). Witmer put his thoughtful policies into practice. Working closely with colleagues in the hospital and medical school at Penn, he routinely insisted that his "clients" have a complete physical examination. In fact, the youngster who was Witmer's first case could not see well. Witmer only began remedial work in reading and spelling after the visual difficulties were corrected (Routh, 1996).

Witmer was equally at home with lawyers, social workers, and teachers and considered the courts, schools, and streets to be psychology laboratories. He could be regarded as the father of community psychology in that over a hundred years ago he was calling for "preventive social action... [that] ... would offer the slum parent something better than a choice between race suicide and child murder" (Reisman, 1966, p. 81). School psychology also claims him as its founder, and counseling psychology could as well, given that he was concerned with enhancing the functioning of normal children and was the first to ask questions about vocational interests. In 1897 Witmer taught the first practical course in child psychology. In addition to lectures and laboratory assignments, classes included case presentations from the Psychological Clinic and observation of work with children in a training school. Fifty years later, when standards of education and training in clinical psychology were proposed at the Boulder Conference, recommendations would include much of Witmer's pedagogy, including the integration of science and practice and the need for both academic training and practical experience.

On the basis of Witmer's work, numerous psychological clinics were established over the next two decades. Most of these were associated with universities, where psychologists worked with children from the local schools. Numerous women were involved in the new psychological clinics but had been predominantly trained in education or social work. Graduate study in psychology was relatively new; university departments emphasized experimental psychology and did not offer clinically related courses. Responding to a need for clinical training, the psychological clinics began offering internships and practicum experiences. Clinics also moved beyond university venues and opened doors to new populations. In 1909 William Healy founded the Juvenile Psychopathic Institute in a Detention Home in Chicago and later moved to Boston to organize the Judge Baker Foundation. Along with Grace Fernald and Augusta Bronner, Healy proposed diagnosis (performed by psychologists) and treatment procedures (conducted by probation officers) for delinquents that ushered clinical psychology into a new arena of forensic work. It should be noted, however, that even with the outreach to delinquents, the early psychological clinics did not truly follow Witmer's recommendation of interdisciplinary interventions and deep involvement in community settings. Rather, they were usually insular in nature and focused on the alleged pathology of the individual client.

The other institutions in which clinical psychologists worked were facilities for the mentally retarded. Again, their major responsibilities were intelligence testing. In 1904 the Ministry of Public Instruction in France had appointed a commission to advise the schools about how best to educate retarded children. Alfred Binet, with a 15-year history of research on individual differences, was on the commission and recognized the need for an examination or testing instrument that would assess intellectual functioning. With Theodore Simon, Binet devised a series of scales with questions about everyday situations that children could be expected to answer at certain ages. Henry Goddard, director of the New Jersey Training School for Feeble-Minded Girls and Boys at Vineland, New Jersey, had been unsuccessfully using various laboratory equipment to try to assess intelligence. In 1908 he traveled to Paris to learn about the verbal IQ tests and returned with them to the States where he translated them and began validated studies at the Training School. The Binet-Simon revisions became enormously popular but could not be used to test children who did not speak English. This was particularly problematic for Healy and Grace Fernald, who were working with immigrant children at the Juvenile Psychopathic Institute. They then developed nonverbal performance tests to assess intelligence, adaptations of which were eventually used at Ellis Island to examine immigrants coming to the United States (Popplestone & McPherson, 1994).

Early clinical psychologists, working primarily with children, had little contact with seriously mentally ill adults. Generally, these patients were housed in large state mental hospitals or private retreats under the care of psychiatrists. Still, some academic psychologists were interested in adult psychopathology. Around 1900, Shepherd Franz began a cortical mapping of the brain and later applied his experimental results with animals to patients with brain damage. In 1909 G. Stanley Hall invited Freud to speak at Clark University, where his ideas were generally well received. Morton Prince, a neurologist, studied disassociative disorders and multiple personalities and concluded that unconscious mechanisms might "pervert" memory of past events, especially trauma. Believing that psychopathological symptoms were learned, Prince thought they could be unlearned through psychotherapy, which he considered a kind of education. In 1906 Prince founded and was the editor of the *Journal of Abnormal Psychology*. He also began the Harvard Psychological Clinic, where the faculty was sympathetic to psychoanalysis and eventually became involved in developing projective testing (Reisman, 1966).

When the United States entered World War I in 1917, psychologists with expertise in intelligence testing were asked to classify recruits according to their abilities. A small committee of five to seven experimental psychologists (all men) headed by Robert Yerkes developed a group intelligence test, the Army Alpha (a verbal test) and Army Beta (a nonverbal test). Over 2 million men were tested, and about one-fifth were found to be illiterate. Some 8,000 were discharged on the basis of low intelligence; the mental age of the nation's young recruits was said to be 13½ years. Inspired by their supposed "success" in identifying intelligence, psychologists used testing within a theory of biological determinism and ushered in perhaps the most shameful era of clinical psychology. Henry Goddard, basing his claims on "science," identified the cause of mental retardation, which could be assessed through intelligence testing, as lying within a single gene. The country now had a simple solution to its concerns about the feeble-minded: "... don't allow native morons to breed and keep foreign ones out" (Gould, 1981, pp. 164–165). Goddard, believing that women showed innately superior intuition, had two women go to Ellis Island and pick out the feeble-minded by sight so that they might be tested. Although conspicuously mentally handicapped individuals had already been culled by government officials, the women tested 35 Jews, 22 Hungarians, 50 Italians, and 45 Russians. They found 79% of the Italians, 80% of the Hungarians, 83% of the Jews, and 87% of the Russians to be "feeble-minded"—that is, less than age 12 on the Binet scale. Even Goddard had difficulty accepting the fact that some four-fifths of any nation were "morons"; he reconfigured the data and settled on 40% to 50%. Goddard's findings and, later, the similar work of Lewis M. Terman had enormous implications for social and legislative action. Hundreds of immigrants were deported, and immigration quotas kept large numbers (some say as many as 6 million) southern, central, and eastern Europeans from access to this country. This was particularly tragic in that these laws lasted into the 1930s, when so many European Jews were trying to escape the rise of the Nazis (Gould, 1981).

Psychologists were not only busy testing soldiers and immigrants. Following World War I they turned their attention to ordinary citizens, especially children with learning problems. "Mental testers" sprang up everywhere, and applied psychologists began busily building careers giving tests. Further, during the decade of the 1920s, psychology had become an increasingly fascinating topic in this country and was achieving considerable economic success. People wanted to "adjust" to a thriving society and seemed fascinated by opportunities for self-examination, especially through psychoanalysis. Psychology became something of a national mania; "even Sears Roebuck began retailing Freud; its catalog offered customers *Ten Thousand Dreams Interpreted* and *Sex Problems Solved* " (Napoli, 1981, p. 43). Applied psychologists were both pleased and perturbed about this turn of events—pleased because people obviously believed that psychology could be valuable in their lives and perturbed because they could not protect themselves from the mind readers and magicians who also held themselves out as mental healers. Clinical psychologists received no help from the academic psychologists, who were committed to psychology as a science and embarrassed by the excesses of pseudopsychology. One academic, Dorothy Yates, wrote a book called *Psychological Racketeers*, in which she felt compelled to keep repeating that there *is* a body of sound information in psychology that constitutes a science and that there *is* a genuine applied psychology (Yates, 1932). The American Psychological Association (APA), as well, was made up primarily of scientists and hoped to rise above what they considered petty professional issues. Even the APA, however, had recommended in 1915 that only qualified psychologists should administer mental tests for purposes of psychological diagnosis, its first attempt to regulate psychological practice. But few clinical psychologists were members of the APA, which had been steadily raising its membership requirements so that members had to hold a full-time professorial position in psychology and publish acceptable psychological research. Concerned with a need for identifying appropriately trained, qualified applied psychologists, William Wallin and Leta Hollingsworth, with others, formed the American Association of Clinical Psychologists in 1917. This group was short-lived; in 1919, the APA created a Clinical

Section, which incorporated the association's members and in 1924 provided associate membership for professionals. Although associates could not hold office, vote, or speak at business meetings, so many joined the APA that by 1929 they outnumbered full members. During this time, the APA, at the urging of the Clinical Section, made some attempts at certifying practitioners, but standards were so high that in 1925 only 25 psychologists were certified; two years later the APA ended its certification program (Napoli, 1981; Routh, 1996).

Although many clinical psychologists had joined the APA, likely for the prestige and respect associated with a scientific society, the great majority (80%) were not members. During the 1920s, students had flocked to graduate programs in psychology and emerged to take their place testing and working in child guidance centers (which numbered 232 in 1932). No opportunities existed for private practice and although psychologists might do testing in the large mental hospitals, psychiatry basically controlled admissions, treatment, and release of patients. Clinical psychologists struggled to establish themselves as respected professionals but, aside from the educational and child guidance clinics, were usually subservient to medicine. Moreover, by 1932, 63% of this country's clinical psychologists were women, whereas only a few women were represented in academic, scientific psychology. Napoli (1981) speculates that academics and scientists did not take clinical psychology seriously because they, like so many others in the United States, did not take women seriously. At that time, women had only had the vote for a little over a decade.

With the advent of the Great Depression of the 1930s, citizens and psychologists alike would find their livelihoods threatened and their lives abruptly changed. But, at a time when psychologists might have been expected to rally themselves to develop theories about the impact of economic devastation and propose social programs to improve citizen well-being, psychology was strangely silent. President Franklin D. Roosevelt did not recruit psychologists as advisors in the government, nor were they appointed to his Science Advisory Board. Psychology had no role in shaping the most sweeping social changes ever effected in this country such as Social Security, unemployment insurance, and government programs that put people back to work. Psychologists were out of work as well. In 1932 a hundred new doctoral psychologists competed for only 32 newly created positions, and in 1933 the situation was even worse; 736 master's-level psychologists graduated and found *no* academic jobs at all (Napoli, 1981).

Among those who could afford to go to college, psychology was a particularly popular subject. Then, as now, students were interested in human services (as evidenced by the large numbers going into the master's program), but then, as now, academic psychologists remained committed to psychology as a science based on experimental methods. Their interests were, for example, understanding "feeble-mindedness" in order to better comprehend the inheritability of intelligence; they believed that actually working with mentally retarded individuals was best left to clinical technicians. Still, even for academics, there was no escaping a continued interest in personality development and dynamics that would have a profound effect on the profession of clinical psychology. At Yale, a group of young men (including the sociologist John Dollard, Neal Miller, O. H. Mowrer, and Robert Sears) tried to integrate Clarke Hull's learning theory and psychoanalysis. They believed that aggression resulted from frustration and was expressed and/or inhibited in many different ways. Similarly, Henry Murray at the Harvard Psychological Clinic was developing a theory in which a "need," such as to hurt another, might arise as a result of frustration. But for Murray, frustration and aggression were simply part of a complex of personal needs and environmental pressures. Eventually Christiana Morgan, working with Murray, would develop the Thematic Apperception Test (TAT) to assess these needs and how people respond to situational pressures.

Perhaps the greatest influence on clinical psychology during this era, however, was the influx of psychologists from Europe who were fleeing the Nazis. In this country, psychology and psychiatry were trying to understand and treat the seriously mentally ill and profoundly retarded. In Germany,

Adolph Hitler simply enacted sterilization laws that covered not only mental deficiency, schizophrenia, and epilepsy, but also blindness, deafness, and deformity. Physicians, aided by psychiatry, performed over 400,000 sterilizations and murdered over 300,000 mentally ill and retarded individuals. While Freud's theories on the unconscious were being discussed at the most respected academic programs in this country, the Nazis burned Freud's books and "abolished" Jewish-founded psychoanalysis. They took over the German Society for Psychotherapy and installed Carl Jung as president, his chief function being to discriminate between Aryan and Jewish psychology. Almost all of the centers of psychological research were closed, and Jewish psychoanalysts and psychologists, including Anna and Sigmund Freud, were forced to flee their homes (Reisman, 1966). Many immigrated to the United States, where the work of people like Alfred Adler, Erich Fromm, Kurt Lewin, and Otto Rank would have an enormous impact on every aspect of the science and practice of clinical psychology. Other notable figures who immigrated, such as Karen Horney, also brought a rich legacy of a concern for the impact of culture and the environment on one's being. The emphasis on intrapsychic conflicts which characterized psychoanalysis was tempered somewhat by a consideration of context.

The influx of European psychologists also had an impact on job opportunities as well. At the height of the Great Depression, about 40% of U. S. psychologists were unemployed. The APA tried to find both academic and applied positions for American and displaced European psychologists, but their efforts were not particularly successful. Scientific psychologists began to organize outside of the APA in efforts to find jobs. The Society for the Psychological Study of Social Issues (SPSSI) was founded in 1936 with the goals of promoting research on social issues with an aim toward eliminating poverty and prejudice and promoting peace; these worthy aspirations would also include jobs and activities for psychologists. The SPSSI became an affiliate of the APA, and so did the Psychonomics Society, begun in 1935 with a focus on the use of mathematics in psychology. Professional psychologists also began to organize and advocate for jobs. In 1937 the

Psychologists League of New York City proposed to examine "the social roots of and implications of psychology as a service, a science, and a profession" and to provide secure clinical jobs for psychologists. Joining New York City's annual May Day parade, some 70 league members marched with placards that psychologists might still carry today: "Build More Clinics—You'll Need Less Prisons!" and "Adjustment Comes with Jobs!"

Although the Clinical Section of the American Psychological Association had become more active during the 1930s, the APA was resolved, especially after the early failure of certification, not to become involved in professional activities such as designation of who could practice psychology. The Association of Consulting Psychologists (ACP), originally a statewide organization of New York psychologists, had no such qualms, however. The group joined other state associations and reorganized nationally to propose and protect professional interests with the introduction of an ethical code, standardized clinical training, and state licensing. Hampered by APA's refusal to meet practitioner concerns, the Clinical Section dissolved itself and gave its assets to the new American Association of Applied Psychology (AAAP), made up of members "actively engaged in the application of psychology as their primary profession" (Napoli, 1981).

The long battle between the science and practice of psychology was soon overshadowed by the more devastating battles of World War II. Psychologists rallied to the war effort and once again brought their talent for testing to bear on the need of the military to assigning troops, not only to combat but also to the myriad tasks of leadership and logistics. By the end of the war, some 9 million men (one-seventh of the male population of this country) had taken the general classification test (Napoli, 1981). World War II, however, also involved psychologists in activities that went well beyond testing. Psychologists in sensation and perception became human factor engineers and helped design airplane cockpits and landing fields. Psychologists in learning taught pigeons and monkeys to guide missiles. Academic psychologists from 30 universities helped select and train pilots. The Office of Strategic Services, later the CIA, was staffed by psychologists. The executive secretary of the American Association of Applied Psychologists, C. M. Loutitt, recruited naval officers from the association. Although clinical psychologists (or psychiatrists) did not initially work in military hospitals, they became "personnel consultants" who provided personal counseling to soldiers and conducted group psychotherapy. As psychiatric casualties from combat increased, however, psychologists were called upon to join psychiatry in treatment. By the end of the war, some 450 clinical psychologists were serving in the Army. Female psychologists wanted to serve as well, but few opportunities were available to them. In 1941 they founded the National Council of Women Psychologists, with their activities primarily aimed at helping civilians, mostly women and children, cope with the vagaries of war.

World War II brought unprecedented opportunities to psychology. Praised by military leaders for their contributions to selecting and training personnel as well as fitting the weapons of war to the men using them, both research and applied psychologists had worked together on practical problems, eased the tensions among themselves, and came to appreciate the importance of applying psychology to major social tasks. Government policymakers and the public also forged a new awareness of psychology's potential contributions to the public good. At this time, however, APA continued as a scientific society, and professional interests were handled almost exclusively within the American Association of Applied Psychologists. Feeling a need for more cooperation, representatives from disparate groups in psychology began to meet together when they could during the war. In 1945–1946, acting on recommendations from a committee headed by Robert Yerkes, APA revised its bylaws to "advance psychology as a science, a profession, and as a means of promoting human welfare." Although suspicion ranged on all sides, APA and AAAP agreed to merge, and a newly organized APA governance structure was constituted of representatives from state associations and specialized interest groups such as the SPSSI. The American Association of Applied Psychology became the Clinical Division of APA (Division 12). A Division 11 (Abnormal Psychology and Psychotherapy) had been proposed but merged with Division 12. Thus, from its beginning, Division 12 represented both clinical science and practice, with a strong and steady presence in APA governance, and was the largest division in APA until the establishment of the Division of Independent Practice (42) in the late 1970s. The National Council of Women Psychologists also asked to be recognized as an entity of APA but was told that no single-sex groups could be acknowledged. In fact, John Anderson, the 1943 APA president, said that psychology had been remiss in training intellectually talented women for high-level jobs that did not exist. He recommended taking more moderately intellectual women into degree programs so that when they graduated, they would be satisfied with the opportunities to work with women and children for which they were fit. It would be three decades before the Division for Women in Psychology would become a reality in APA and more than forty years before gay and lesbian psychologists and psychologists of color would have a representative voice in the governance structure.

EDUCATION AND TRAINING IN CLINICAL PSYCHOLOGY

The end of World War II marked the beginning of psychology's second half-century which was to be one of unprecedented growth and influence. In 1945 the newly reorganized American Psychological Association had about 4,000 members, a central administrative office, and a new willingness to support applied and clinical psychologists. The Veterans' Administration (VA) in particular saw a need for trained professionals to deal with veterans who had returned from the war with psychological and emotional problems. The VA and the National Institute of Mental Health (NIMH) planned to subsidize clinical psychology training, along with training in other health professions, if universities capable of such training could be identified. A committee of APA supplied the government with a list of such graduate programs (22) and thus entered the accreditation process. Carl Rogers, the president of APA at that time, appointed David Shakow to chair a Committee on Training in Clinical Psychology

(Committee, 1947). Their report became the basis for an NIMH-sponsored conference in Boulder, Colorado, in 1949. Some 70 university faculty involved in the accredited programs met with interested others to develop consensual standards for education and training in clinical psychology. Most of these participants were psychologists of a new generation, interested in and involved in the application of psychology to clinical problems. Often the children of immigrants, well acquainted with the Great Depression, tempered by the war, and educated and trained in public schools and universities, these newly emerging clinical psychologists were called upon to define their field and propose standards of education and training for the students that would follow them.

The importance of the Boulder Conference in shaping clinical psychology cannot be overemphasized. The decision that clinical psychologists should be trained as doctors of philosophy in general psychology assured that clinical psychology would fall squarely in the sciences, marked by an empirical base, and generating knowledge via the scientific method. The demand for practical experience and a predoctoral internship meant that clinical psychologists would be continually reminded of the complexity of human needs and problems and trained in assessment and treatment (Raimy, 1950). The fact that clinical psychologists were educated and trained to be *both* scientists and practitioners created a model not previously known in either the sciences or the professions, namely a bold attempt to integrate science and practice for an evolving field.

The Boulder model of clinical training continues in most university-based, Ph.D.-granting programs. The curriculum usually includes two years of academic requirements in general areas of psychology, such as cognitive, developmental, experimental, history and systems, personality, physiological, and social psychology. Psychopathology and methods of assessment and intervention are covered and include supervised practical training and a one-year predoctoral internship. In addition to academic instruction and clinical supervision, students are expected to learn to conduct research and be familiar with the various statistical methods nec-

essary to evaluate results. Most programs require a research project at the master's level and an original research dissertation for the doctoral degree. The time to complete a degree in clinical psychology ranges from four to six or seven years, and a year of post-doctoral supervision is required in most states for licensing.

In the early years of the Boulder model, graduates took jobs in the public sector or became faculty in colleges and universities. As large numbers of students became interested in clinical psychology, however, more turned their attention to professional activities, and questions were raised about the Boulder model for training. Some had already noted the shortcomings of clinical psychology as it was developing. Seymour Sarason, one of the Boulder participants, wrote thoughtfully of his disappointment that clinical psychology had largely abandoned its legacy of work with children in educational and community settings (Sarason, 1988).

Many noted that clinical psychologists were working in "other people's houses" (i.e., in psychiatry) and had too readily embraced a pathology model rather than considering the adaptability and resilience of people faced with adversity. George Albee reminded clinical psychologists that the occurrence of a disease or disorder had never been altered by treating individuals one at a time, as occurs in psychotherapy. He urged clinical psychologists to turn their talents to prevention and attack the social problems of poverty, violence, and discrimination that lead to individual difficulties (Albee, 1968, 1970). The major concerns, however, were raised by practitioners who thought that clinical psychologists and the public they served would be better prepared by more training in clinical activities and less emphasis on *doing* science. As early as 1951 (two years after the Boulder conference), Gordon Derner began a Ph.D. "scholar-practitioner" program at Adelphi University that allowed students to complete nonempirical dissertations such as psychohistories or theoretical formulations. The program was accredited in 1957, but it would be another decade until a second professional clinical program was introduced by Donald Peterson, offering a Doctor of Psychology (Psy.D.) degree at the University of Illinois. Students completed the regular clinical program but opted for more practicum experience and substituted a clinical project for the research dissertation.

A skeptical questioning of the Boulder model was exactly what a scientist would expect. Most were pleased that the model of scientific training, even if clinical psychologists did not do research, led to a spirit of experimentation, a continued questioning of assumptions, a willingness to consider alternative explanations, and a resistance to accept dogmatic or authoritative theories without empirical support. In addition to the benefits of research findings, an openness to new ideas and a respect for objective evidence were clearly necessary as clinical psychologists struggled to define and develop an evolving discipline.

Practicing psychologists, however, faced with the immediate demands of clients in emotional pain could not wait for years of empirical investigation and research findings. Moreover, mental health services were not available to people in underserved areas such as rural locations and inner cities. University-based Ph.D. clinical programs had deliberately kept their acceptances low in order to support students financially and offer them the individual research mentoring typical in the sciences. In the late 1960s, noting that the two accredited clinical programs in the state of California, at Berkeley and Los Angeles, together graduated less than a dozen clinical students each year, practitioners began their own training programs. The California School of Professional Psychology, offering a Ph.D. in clinical psychology, with free-standing campuses in Berkeley, Fresno, Los Angeles, and San Diego, was founded by Nicholas Cummings in 1969 with the enthusiastic support of the California State Psychological Association. A second conference, held in Vail, Colorado, some twenty years after Boulder, embraced a model of professional training (Korman, 1974). Clinical psychologists would continue to learn general psychology and be "consumers" of the science of psychology, but their major education and training would be in clinical process and practice. These programs were enormously attractive to students, and within the next two decades over forty professional schools and programs, some offering the Ph.D., some the Psy.D., some in univer-

sities and some free-standing, were established and accredited.

The professional school model is quite different from the Boulder model in ways that go far beyond the emphasis on science training. Like other professional schools, such as law or medicine, most programs are not housed within the traditional arts and sciences in a graduate school. Even when located within the academy, professional units are independent, with their own dean and administrative structure. Larger numbers of students are admitted than to graduate programs; faculties are smaller and are often practitioners who teach in the program part time. Classes are large, and students generally follow a set curriculum. Financial aid through assistantships is not generally available, and tuition costs are rarely deferred. Students are four times more likely to gain admission but six times less likely to receive full funding at professional versus research-oriented programs (Mayne, Norcross, & Sayette, 1994).

Many students still train for clinical positions in master's programs, but APA recognizes the independent practice of clinical psychology only at the doctoral level. Nonetheless, about 8,000 master's degrees in psychology are awarded each year, and large numbers of this group are providing clinical services, especially in public institutions. Employment figures for master's-level psychologists and job satisfaction are similar for both master's- and doctoral-level psychologists. Master's psychologists are organized nationally and are recognized by legal statute in 27 states.

As professional psychology was growing rapidly, doctoral practitioners began organizing to advocate for legislative support. A *National Register of Health Care Providers in Psychology* was published in 1975, and the American Board of Examiners in Professional Psychology reemphasized the diplomate recognizing professional competence in Clinical Psychology (as well as other specialty areas such as Counseling, Industrial/Organization, and School Psychology). The APA undertook a number of initiatives to support professional psychology. Accreditation standards were expanded to include professional programs. A model licensing bill was adopted, and assistance was offered to the state associations in their efforts to gain certification or licensing for practitioners and parity with other health professionals. Battles were fought for psychologists to be reimbursed by third-party payers (insurance companies) and to gain hospital privileges. The APA ethical code was revised to clarify standards of treatment. Psychologists developed their own insurance plans to provide protection against malpractice suits. Perhaps of most importance to practitioners, APA took steps to develop a Practice Directorate supported by additional dues paid by practitioners to advance and protect professional activities. A College of Professional Psychology was established by the APA in 1995 to help psychologists gain certification in competency areas such as substance abuse counseling. Practicing psychologists supported by the APA Practice Directorate began to advocate for prescription privileges, and training programs were developed for selected psychologists to gain competence in prescribing certain psychotropic drugs.

The growth of APA and the emphasis on professional issues exacerbated the long-standing conflicts between scientific and professional psychologists. As the discipline of psychology matured, many scientific psychologists, especially, found themselves drawn to more specialized societies (such as Neuroscience or the Society for Research in Child Development) rather than a general psychology association, especially one that seemed to be so focused on guild issues. Some academic psychologists became so concerned about psychology's "clinical" image that they began to identify themselves by terms other than *psychologist*—such as "neuroscientist" or "psycholinguist." A few academic departments actually changed their names from Psychology to terms such as Cognitive Sciences. APA created a number of commissions and task forces charged with recommending a possible reorganization of APA to streamline its governance and meet the needs of scientists, who were by now a minority of membership. In 1988 the APA Council of Representatives recommended such a plan to the membership for approval. Considerable controversy surrounded the reorganization proposal, which was favored by scientists but not professionals. Scientists had already begun to reorganize

within APA to form an Association of Scientific and Applied Psychology (ASAP). Fearful that reorganization would fail, another small group of six psychologists (half of them women) met on another summer day in Belchertown, Massachusetts, some 95 years and 45 miles from Hall's founding of APA. They (Kathleen Grady, Milton Hakel, Virginia O'Leary, Steve Hays, Bonnie Strickland, and Logan Wright) wrote by-laws for a new independent scientific society for psychologists, the American Psychological Society (APS).

When the reorganization plan was defeated by the APA membership, the 1,200 members of ASAP voted to become APS. Janet Spence, the president of ASAP became President of ASP and Charles Kiesler its past president. Alan Kraut was hired as the first executive director. In 1990 clinical scientists established the American Association of Applied and Preventive Psychology (AAAPP), closely tied to APS, to represent and advocate for their interests. Within less than a decade, APS had over 16,000 members, including students, published several journals, and was a strong voice, especially in the Congress, for the discipline and science of psychology. AAAPP had close to 2,000 members, a newsletter, and a journal. Once again the strains between the scientists and practitioners had become such a force that U.S. psychology was represented by several national organizations. Fifty years after the American Association of Applied Psychologists, comprising predominantly practitioners, broke away from the APA, the American Psychological Society, with a majority of basic and applied scientists, came into being. Once again, scientist/practitioners, in much greater numbers this time, were torn in their loyalties across national associations.

WHAT DO CLINICAL PSYCHOLOGISTS DO?

Psychologists who graduated from the early clinical training programs, like other general psychologists, were likely to take faculty positions in colleges and universities. Their other major placement was within the Veterans' Administration, which is still the largest single employer of psychologists. As clinical psychology flourished, more opportunities became available for clinicians to work independently, often as consultants to community mental health agencies, and increasingly with individuals. Credentialing and/or licensing laws were eventually enacted in all fifty states (and the Canadian provinces), third-party reimbursement became available, and hospital privileges were awarded in some locales.

The World Federation for Mental Health reports that mental health issues continue to be critical problems for millions of people all over the world. Depression and anxiety disorders account for between one-quarter and one-third of all primary health care visits worldwide. Suicide is among the top ten causes of death and among the top two or three causes for youth. Around the world, more than 52 million children labor daily, subjected to mental and physical health risks, limited intellectual and social development, and intense mental trauma including severe depression, withdrawal, and inferior status identity. Millions of children suffer the devastating effects of child prostitution. Rates of domestic violence against women vary from 20% to 75% in developing nations. Alcohol-related diseases affect as much as 10% of the world's population, and drug abuse is a rapidly growing source of violence and death. Political violence has created more than 40 million refugees and internally displaced persons who are at high risk of depression, anxiety disorder, and post-traumatic stress disorders.

Clinical psychologists and other mental health professions have much to do and innumerable venues within which to work. In the United States, most clinical psychologists (with almost 90% accounting for about one-third of their time in this way) are involved in some aspect of providing psychotherapy. Three-quarters are engaged in assessment and diagnosis, and two-thirds are consultants or clinical supervisors. Over half are in teaching and in administration, but these activities, aside from psychotherapy, account for only 10% to 15% of their time. The proportion of clinical psychology graduates who take university positions has dropped steadily and is now less than one in five. About one-third of clinical psychologists are in private practice, and

one-quarter work in hospital and medical school settings. Over half report themselves to be engaged in research but the modal number of research papers published by clinical psychologists is zero. Ten to fifteen percent of clinicians produce about half of the research (Norcross, Prochaska, & Gallagher, 1989; Phares, 1991). Clinical psychologists also have become specialists in providing mental health services to specific populations, such as children or the elderly. Others have branched out into newly emerging areas such as forensic and health psychology. Neuropsychology is another appealing area in that clinical psychologists are especially well trained in assessment and diagnosis, a crucial need in understanding and treating brain disorders and head injuries. The statistical skills offered to clinical students also serve them in good stead for positions in program and systems evaluation.

CONTEMPORARY CLINICAL PSYCHOLOGY

A hundred years after its founding, the field of clinical psychology is a vibrant, powerful influence, still seeking answers to the most basic questions about human behavior and behavior change. Clinical psychologists are engaged in careers across the spectrum of science and practice; they provide services to diverse populations in almost every conceivable situation. Students are trained in almost 200 accredited graduate programs and over 400 predoctoral internships; they join the largest doctoral-level health care profession in this country. Women have been well incorporated into psychology, especially clinical psychology, and now receive more doctoral degrees relative to men (61% in 1991) than in any other major field (ranging from Education, 58%; through Law, 49%, Medicine, 36%, to Engineering, 9%) (Pion et al., 1996).

Clinical psychologists have brought unique talents and skills to the understanding and treatment of people's problems in living. First, clinical psychologists are (or should be) well trained in general psychology and the scientific method. The burgeoning knowledge base in cognitive, developmental, experimental, personality, physiological, and social psychology has given us a deeper and clearer understanding of people's behavior and behavior change. We know many of the boundaries of "normal" functioning and the differences in ways that individuals respond to challenges in their lives. We are also taught the crucial importance of using such knowledge in our clinical activities, always with a spirit of openness and questioning about the value of our services. Clinical psychology and counseling and school psychology are the only health-related professions that evolved from the academy. Barbers left their shops to study in the medieval universities; women healers went to nursing schools. Social workers studied in professional schools and then returned to their settlement houses. Only psychologists, with their own science base, built their discipline in a scholarly tradition within the arts and sciences.

Clinical psychologists have been especially focused and trained in psychopathology—how to understand, assess, and treat "abnormal" behavior. Historically, clinical psychology's unique contributions in this area have been in assessment and psychological testing, including research on tests. Psychologists have developed intelligence tests that also become important in assessing organicity and neurological functioning. Although psychologists use and have developed projective techniques like the Thematic Apperception Test, their contributions here have probably been most marked by their investigation of the reliability and validity of such measures and their development of more objective instruments.

The major activity of clinical psychologists, however, is psychotherapy, a service that we share with a number of other fields and even with lay people. The term *psychotherapy* is not owned by any group. Clergy, counseling psychologists, marriage and family counselors, mental health counselors, psychiatric nurses, psychiatrists, social workers, school psychologists, and many others provide psychotherapy to individuals, families, and groups. We have little or no evidence that one's discipline or years of experience make a significant difference in one's effectiveness as a psychotherapist with the moderately disturbed (Dawes, 1994; Christensen & Jacobson, 1994) although research on psychotherapy does suggest that some approaches are more ef-

fective for some particular disorders. The treatment of the anxiety and panic disorders (Barlow, 1988, 1990), depression (Butler & Beck, 1996), and pain management (Keefe, 1996) through cognitive behavioral therapy has been particularly impressive.

CRUCIAL ISSUES IN CLINICAL PSYCHOLOGY

In any science or profession, perhaps the most crucial goal is the development and application of knowledge. Theoretical approaches and clinical techniques must be based on sound, reliable principles that represent the best understanding of the discipline and profession. Also implicit in the helping professions is a clear sense of integrity and ethics that guides our actions for the benefit of humankind.

Clinical psychologists have sometimes been remiss in their reliance on traditional methods that may not represent the state of the art in clinical practice. Projective techniques, for example, are still widely used psychological tests although the "theory" of projection on which they are based has little or no empirical support (Dawes, 1994). Evidence for the reliability and validity of the Rorschach Inkblot Method is only slowly accumulating (Weiner, 1997). Likewise, clinicians may have engaged in outmoded and ineffective kinds of treatment modalities without keeping abreast of the contemporary literature describing more effective techniques. We continue to depend on clinical intuition when statistical prediction might serve us better. Despite our training in science, we often engage in a fundamental attribution bias in which we ascribe our own maladaptive behaviors as responses to the environment but our client's as pathology. In fact, we have embraced a "disease" and diagnostic model that may distort our understanding of behavior and behavior change and does not do justice to the resilience, strength, and adaptive coping with which many people meet adversity. We have also, in the main, adopted a medical model that treats individuals, usually at a fee for service, and focuses less on those social problems and community systems that demand change so that people may have opportunities to make healthy choices. Within the medical model, government and business have stepped in to control the spiraling costs of health care, sometimes by eliminating our jobs. We will be continually called on to evaluate health services, including our own, to demonstrate efficacy and cost savings. In that regard, we are fortunate to have an empirically based science and experimental methods that allow us to do just that. We would also do well to use these methods to assess and evaluate our own field.

FUTURE TRENDS

Historically, clinical psychology has arisen in response to marketplace pressures. When a need for clinical services became obvious at the beginnings of organized psychology, Witmer and others responded by developing a new profession. Following World War II, encouraged by the government and supported by the Veterans' Administration, graduate programs began to educate and train clinical psychologists in a scientist/practitioner model. In the 1960s, when a need for more practitioners was noted, professional schools were established. This means, however, that the growth and development of clinical psychology has not always followed a carefully planned trajectory. For example, the number of students in clinical graduate programs at this time is problematic. Predoctoral internships, required for graduation and licensing, are not available for all of our deserving students. The demand for clinical practica hours imposed on students anxious to find internships has also, perhaps, outstripped our equally important requirements of other aspects of clinical education and training, such as knowledge about general psychology and research. The advent of managed care means that fewer positions are available for new graduates and the possibility of successfully beginning a private practice is practically nonexistent. Positions in academia are also increasingly difficult to obtain. Still, as was true in our beginning, jobs remain available in underserved areas and with disadvantaged populations. Clinical graduates can be assured that their commitment to the public interest allows them exceptional opportunities. And clinical psychology is still the only major science and profession for stu-

dents who wish to combine their scientific and practice interests.

Future trends are always difficult to predict, particularly in an area of such volatility as the enormous upheaval in demographics and health care now occurring in this country. This is also accompanied by economic pressures that corrections be made to secure our nation's financial future. Politicians and policymakers have determined that the high cost of specialists in medicine and health-related fields, like clinical psychology, must be reined in. People in need of either physical or mental health care are referred to general practitioners or gatekeepers and are not likely to make their way easily to clinical psychologists, especially those invested in providing long-term treatment. The provision of psychotherapy, which most clinical psychologists note as their most predominant activity, will increasingly be offered by other mental health professionals for shorter times and at lower costs. Clinical psychologists may continue to be a part of this cadre but will also likely be more drawn into research and evaluation of psychotherapy, a skill for which many other mental health practitioners are not trained. Clinical psychologists are also uniquely trained in psychological assessment and testing, an expertise that increasingly may be used in areas beyond mental health assessment. Especially with an aging population, neuropsychological assessment will become an even more important domain of clinical psychologists for both research and treatment. Psychological testing is also a mainstay of forensic psychology, ranging across almost all aspects of the law, from custody battles to competency to stand trial. Within the legal system, psychologists also might do well to turn their attention to understanding and treating special populations. Again, the range of opportunities is broad, extending from victims such as abused children to perpetrators of violent crimes.

Some expect that the greatest growth of clinical psychology will occur within the physical health realm. This prediction is based not only on the fact that emotional distress and disorders accompany many disease processes and responses to illness, but also on the knowledge that psychological treatment may improve functioning across a spectrum of illnesses, diseases, and health problems through activities such as biofeedback, conditioning, compliance, relaxation, and stress reduction. Clinical psychologists may find themselves working more closely with physicians, in hospitals, and with the chronically ill as they bring their knowledge and skills to physical as well as mental health. These activities may also be extended to prevention and especially to work with children.

No doubt, clinical psychologists will continue to expand their scope of practice and "reexamine the question of what should be the central activity or activities of a field in which the purpose is to use psychological knowledge to promote human welfare" (Humphreys, 1996, p. 191). It is hoped that we will return to and continue those lofty aims of Witmer and others who envisioned psychologists as attempting to alleviate our chronic social problems and improve the social institutions that affect the lives of our citizens. We do this through the advancement of knowledge and the application of that knowledge for the public good.

REFERENCES

Achterberg, J. (1990). *Woman as healer*. Boston: Shambhala.

Albee, G. W. (1968). Conceptual models and manpower requirements in psychology. *American Psychologist*, *23*, 317–320.

Albee, G. W. (1970). The uncertain future of clinical psychology. *American Psychologist*, *25*, 1071–1080.

Barlow, D. H. (1988). *Anxiety and its disorders: The nature and treatment of anxiety and panic*. New York: Guilford Press.

Barlow, D. H. (1990). Long-term outcome for patients with panic disorder treated with cognitive-behavior therapy. *Journal of Clinical Psychiatry*, *51*, 17–23.

Beers, C. (1908). *A mind that found itself*. New York: Longmans, Green.

Butler, A. C., & Beck, A. T. (1996). Cognitive therapy for depression. *The Clinical Psychologist*, *49*, 6–7.

Christensen, A., & Jacobson, N. S. (1994). Who (or what) can do psychotherapy: The status and challenge of nonprofessional therapies. *Psychological Science*, *5*, 8–14.

Committee on Training in Clinical Psychology. (1947). Recommended graduate training program in clinical psychology. *American Psychologist*, *2*, 539–558.

Dawes, R. (1994). *House of cards: Psychology and psychotherapy built on myth*. New York: The Free Press.

Ehrenwald, J. (Ed.). (1991). *The history of psychotherapy*. Northvale, NJ: Jason Aronson.

Gould, S. (1981). *The mismeasure of man*. New York: W. W. Norton.

Humphreys, K. (1996). Clinical psychologists as psychotherapists: History, future, and alternatives. *American Psychologist*, *51*, 190–206.

James, W. (1890). *Principles of psychology* (Vols. 1–2). New York: Holt.

Keefe, F. J. (1996). *Cognitive behavioral therapy for managing pain*, *49*, 4–5.

Korman, M. (1974). National conference on levels and patterns of professional patterns in psychology: The major themes. *American Psychologist*, *29*, 441–449.

Leff, S., & Leff, V. (1958). *From witchcraft to world health*. New York: Macmillan.

Mayne, T. J., Norcross, J. C., & Sayette, M. A. (1994). Admission requirements, acceptance rates, and financial assistance in clinical psychology programs. *American Psychologist*, *49*, 605–611.

Metraux, G. S., & Crouzet, F. (1963). *The evolution of science*. New York: New American Library.

Napoli, D. (1981). *Architects of adjustment*. Port Washington, NY: Kennikat Press.

Norcross, J. C., Prochaska, J. O., & Gallagher, K. M. (1989). Clinical psychologists in the 1980s: II. Theory, research, and practice. *The Clinical Psychologist*, *42*, 45–53.

Phares, E. J. (1991). *Clinical psychology: Concepts, methods, and profession*. Pacific Grove, CA: Brooks/Cole.

Pion, G. M., Mednick, M. T., Astin, H. S., Hall, C. C. I., Kenkel, M. B., Keita, G. P., Kohout, J. L., & Kelleher, J. C. (1996). The shifting gender composition of psychology. *American Psychologist*, *51*, 509–528.

Popplestone, J. A., & McPherson, M. W. (1994). *An illustrated history of American psychology*. Madison, WI: Browne and Benchmark.

Raimy, V. C. (Ed.) (1950). *Training in clinical psychology*. Englewood Cliffs, NJ: Prentice-Hall.

Reisman, J. (1966). *The development of clinical psychology*. New York: Appleton-Century-Crofts.

Routh, D. (1996). Lightner Witmer and the first 100 years of clinical psychology. *American Psychologist*, *51*, 244–247.

Sarason, S. (1988). *The making of an American psychologist: An autobiography*. San Francisco: Jossey-Bass.

Walsh, M. R. (1977). *Doctors wanted, no women need apply*. New Haven: Yale University Press.

Weiner, I. B. (1997). Current Status of the Rorschach Inkblot Method. *Journal of Personality Assessment, 68*(1), 5–19.

Witmer, L. (1907). *The psychological clinic, 1*, 1–9.

Yates, D. (1932). *Psychological racketeers*. Boston: Richard G. Badger.

FOR FURTHER READING

For students interested in a history of general psychology that includes detailed descriptions of the long-time tensions between academic and professional psychologists, see *A History of Modern Psychology* by Thomas H. Leahey (1994, second edition). Donald Napoli gives a fascinating description of the development of clinical psychology from a historian's point of view in *Architects of Adjustment* (1981). Though not precisely linked to clinical psychology, Jeanne Achterberg's *Woman as Healer* (1990) is a carefully crafted history of the role of women in the healing arts and medicine. Students interested in a contemporary critique of modern clinical psychology should read Robin Dawes's book *House of Cards: Psychology and Psychotherapy Built on Myth* (1994).

CHAPTER 2

CLINICAL ASSESSMENT AND DIAGNOSIS

Robert J. Gregory

In this chapter and the next, we explore the contributions of assessment and testing to the practice of clinical psychology. Whereas testing entails limited inferences about particular test scores, assessment embraces the larger question of meaning: What does information from all relevant sources (including tests) *mean* about the client? Testing is relatively objective, so that well-trained clinicians usually agree on the interpretation of individual test results. In contrast, assessment embodies a subjective component. Clinicians who appraise the same information about a client typically arrive at slightly different assessments of that individual. Put simply, assessment is both science and art (Matarazzo, 1990; Tallent, 1992).

Formal diagnosis of a patient's disorder is often an essential goal of assessment. Although several approaches to diagnosis are feasible, the *Diagnostic and Statistical Manual of Mental Disorders*, now in its fourth edition (DSM-IV), dominates practice in clinical psychology and related fields (American Psychiatric Association, 1994). For this reason, we examine the nature, purposes, strengths, and weaknesses of the DSM-IV in this chapter. First, we provide a brief survey of historical trends to help place contemporary assessment in perspective.

BRIEF HISTORY OF ASSESSMENT

Assessment involves the appraisal of individuals as a basis for decision making. The decisions involved in assessment are varied and depend on the setting. For example, a psychotherapist typically uses assessment as a basis for choosing an effective treatment approach with a new client. In contrast, a psychologist in the armed forces might use assessment to select individuals for specialized assignments. In fact, the term *assessment* was invented during World War II to describe a program to select trainees for secret service assignment in the Office of Strategic Services (OSS Assessment Staff, 1948). The first application of assessment was to choose military personnel for sensitive, high-risk overseas assignments. Candidates for the secret service underwent four days of written exams, interviews, and personality tests under the scrutiny of OSS psychologists and psychiatrists. The OSS staff collected a huge amount of information on candidates, including interview impressions, test data, checklists, and ratings of the candidates by one another. In addition, the assessment process included a variety of situational tests designed to evaluate the behavior of applicants under stressful, frustrating, and anxiety-inducing conditions. In one test, each candidate was told to perform a task such as building a bridge over a small stream with two "helpers," who were intentionally obstructive. Another situational test used a leaderless group as a method for appraising personal characteristics such as leadership, initiative, and cooperation. On the basis of information from all sources, the OSS staff rated each candidate on dozens of specific traits in such broad categories as emotional stability, physical ability, social relationships, and leadership. These ratings served as the basis for the selection of OSS military personnel.

After World War II, a serious shortage was observed in the number of persons qualified to help returning veterans and other individuals with psychiatric problems (Peterson, 1987). In response to this problem, the Veterans' Administration created modern clinical psychology by providing stipends for thousands of trainees. Doctoral-level programs in clinical psychology arose at most major universities. Clinical psychology became a recognized profession with duties that included psychodiagnosis and individual psychotherapy.

Initially, psychologists functioned under the supervision of psychiatrists. For this reason, assessment was oriented toward the identification and treatment of psychiatric disorders within the framework of the *Diagnostic and Statistical Manual of Mental Disorders*, first released in 1952 and revised several times thereafter. Thus, an early purpose of assessment was detailed psychiatric diagnosis based on a codified system. Psychiatric diagnosis is still one important function of assessment, particularly insofar as it may provide a basis for treatment planning. However, as will be discussed, assessment typically involves much more than traditional diagnosis.

OVERVIEW OF THE ASSESSMENT PROCESS

Assessment: A Definition

Assessment can be defined as the process of evaluating the characteristics, strengths, and weaknesses of an individual as a basis for informed decision making. The term incorporates a wide variety of activities, ranging from descriptive assessment (describing the symptoms of a client as an aid to diagnosis) to functional assessment (determining situational and characterological features that serve to maintain maladaptive behaviors) to prescriptive assessment (recommending types of intervention most likely to be beneficial). For example, descriptive assessment might proceed by means of an interview in which the clinician seeks to determine whether a patient exhibits the symptoms indicative of major depression (sad mood, loss of interest, sense of guilt, sleep disturbance, loss of energy, concentration problems, appetite disturbance, motor slowing, suicidal preoccupation). A functional assessment would be depicted by a psychologist's conclusion that the refusal of a third-grader to attend school was fueled, in part, by the solicitous overprotection of a doting mother. A prescriptive assessment is illustrated by a practitioner's sensible choice of cognitive-behavioral therapy to treat a lawyer plagued by panic attacks when faced with delivering the opening argument in court cases.

Assessment is *problem solving*. Implicitly or explicitly, assessment serves to answer questions about persons referred to a psychologist. The questions encountered in assessment can be relatively straightforward (e.g., "Is this client suicidal at this time?") or more complex and multilayered (e.g., "Why does this child refuse to attend school and how should we respond to this problem?"). It is characteristic of assessment that many sources of information are needed to answer the relevant referral questions.

Assessment is a *process* in which the clinician integrates three components: (1) the reason for assessment, (2) a preferred theoretical orientation, and (3) relevant sources of information (Tallent, 1992). Although the practitioner always serves as the chief evaluative instrument, he or she must continually integrate these three elements to perform a successful assessment. The result is a meaningful case conceptualization, which may include formal diagnosis and recommendations for treatment. The elements of assessment are depicted in Figure 2.1 and discussed in more detail in the remainder of this chapter.

Figure 2.1. Overview of the assessment process

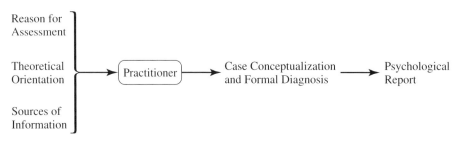

Source: Based on Tallent, N. (1992). *The practice of psychological assessment.* Englewood Cliffs, NJ: Prentice Hall.

Assessment is also a *result* in which the practitioner expresses conclusions, recommendations, or decisions in a written report. The assessment report can make a substantial difference in the life of the client and therefore should be written with great care. For example, an assessment report might involve conclusions, recommendations, or decisions about the following concerns:

- Does an elderly patient complaining of memory loss suffer from dementia?
- Will a ruminative and depressed adolescent improve with psychotherapy alone?
- Is an eccentric old man accused of shoplifting competent to stand trial?
- Does a young patient with a history of drug abuse display subtle brain damage?
- Does a depressed and possibly suicidal housewife require hospitalization?
- Is a person with mildly deviant personality test scores a good bet for the job of police officer?

These examples illustrate a few of the many situations in which psychologists are asked to provide an assessment. The conclusions of the clinician can have a major impact on both the examinee and society at large. For example, based, in part, on the assessment findings, elderly patients will (or will not) be institutionalized, eccentric old men will (or will not) proceed to trial, depressed housewives will (or will not) be hospitalized, and law enforcement candidates will (or will not) be hired.

Phases of Assessment

Assessment proceeds through four phases: planning, data collection, inference, and communication. In *planning*, the clinician determines the purposes of the assessment. This can be a considerable venture, especially within institutional settings. The challenge is that referral sources do not always specify the problem that prompted the request for an assessment. A hospital physician might ask, "Psychological evaluation, please," when what she really wants to know is whether her patient's experience of chronic pain is maintained, in part, by psychological factors. In this case, the clinician's job is not only to determine the underlying referral issue, but also to educate the physician as to the need for explicit referral questions.

Data collection involves the selection of the best sources of information in light of the purposes of the assessment. Clinical interview is almost always one component of data collection, and this may include a specialized form of interview known as the *mental status examination*. Structured interview schedules, observation, behavioral assessment, and psychological testing also provide information relevant to assessment. Each of these approaches is discussed next.

The *inference* stage is pivotal, for here the practitioner must decide whether to trust personal judgment or rely on research-based formulas in the interpretation of data. The quandary is illustrated by the hypothetical (but realistic) case in which a clinician intuitively senses that a hospitalized psychiatric patient is at risk for suicide but the patient exhibits none of the research-based characteristics suggestive of suicide risk, e.g., depressive illness, alcoholism, prior attempts, talk of suicide, social isolation (Motto, 1985). Should the clinician trust personal judgment and deny the patient's request for a weekend pass, or believe the formula and grant the request? This example illustrates the clinical versus actuarial debate which is at the heart of psychological decision making. In **clinical judgment**, the practitioner uses personal judgment to diagnose, classify, or predict behavior. In **actuarial judgment**, the practitioner uses a research-based formula to diagnose, classify, or predict behavior. Although actuarial judgment is usually superior, clinicians still rely heavily on clinical judgment. We will discuss the strengths and weaknesses of each approach.

Finally, assessment involves the transmission of results and the *communication* of recommendations. Although the conclusions from an assessment are often conveyed in person (i.e., the psychologist makes a verbal report to the referral source or the client), the written report is also important and should not be viewed as obligatory only for administrative requirements. An effectively written report functions as a permanent and positive guide for the referral source and others who might work with a client. However, if the report is slipshod, vague, or inconclusive, it will have no impact (or worse, a negative impact) on the welfare of the client. Furthermore, reports have an annoying habit of showing up years later because of litigation involving clients. The wise clinician anticipates the possibility that he or she might be asked to explain and justify every sentence in a report. Careful attention to the assessment report not only advances the welfare of the client but also averts future professional embarrassment for the clinician.

REASON FOR ASSESSMENT

The most common referral milieus are school systems, psychiatric clinics, medical settings, the forensic context, industrial companies, and psychological clinics. The specific reasons for assessment will differ from one setting to another, so we begin by highlighting prominent issues and concerns pertinent to each referral environment. For example, psychologists who work within school systems will receive many referrals for learning disability assessment. Because a common referral question is whether a student qualifies for federally funded services, the practitioner must understand published guidelines and respond in language and terms acceptable to auditors who approve funding. An otherwise superlative assessment with highly detailed recommendations for remediation will be wasted if a learning-disabled student is deemed ineligible for services. In this example, sensitivity to the context of the assessment would dictate the use of specific tests (nationally normed tests of general intelligence and specific academic achievement) combined with a focus on particular aspects of the results (e.g., existence of a 15-point discrepancy between IQ and achievement scores).

Referral from a psychiatric clinic may portend unresolved questions about case conceptualization. Implicitly, the referring psychiatrist may be asking whether a patient's maladaptive behavior represents a serious thought disorder (which would indicate the need for psychotropic medications), or a long-standing problem with character (which might mandate a strict behavioral program), or a manifestation of unrecognized brain damage (which would justify further assessment). Another reason for psychiatric referral is decision making, such as determining whether a patient is suited for individual therapy. Clarification of the underlying referral question(s) is essential when working with psychiatric referrals.

Medical referrals raise a number of interesting issues because of the mutual interplay between physical health and psychological functioning. One common (and understandable) trend is that physicians excel at identifying medical illness but overlook psychological contributions and consequences. A patient with documented heart disease might also experience serious depression, which is not only a consequence of this health problem but also contributory to it. In one study of 150 elderly medical inpatients seen in general medicine and surgery units, attending physicians failed to detect and diagnose major depression in 21 of the 23 patients suffering from this life-threatening disorder (Rapp, Parisi, Walsh, & Wallace, 1988). Psychologists who work with medical referrals are well advised to screen for depression when the patient suffers from a chronic physical illness such as heart disease. Another area of convergence between medicine and psychology is understanding the patient with chronic pain. In most cases, chronic pain includes a substantial psychological component—which is not to deny or dismiss the reality of the pain. The clinical psychologist has much to offer the medical practitioner by way of assessing and understanding the phenomena of chronic pain (Turk & Rudy, 1990).

Psychologists who work within the court system must have a firm grasp of the legal issues pertaining to forensic assessment. Consider one type of forensic assessment, advising a trial judge whether an accused person is competent to stand trial. The judge is not interested in the personal view of the psychologist but instead expects the consultant to offer an opinion within the framework of case law, which specifies that the defendant must understand the charges against him and be able to assist in his defense (Wrightsman, Nietzel, & Fortune, 1994). Increasingly, the practice of forensic psychology requires a technical expertise available only through specialized training (see Chapter 16, "Forensic Psychology").

A special concern encountered with industrial assessment is that employment-related consultation is highly constrained by legal guidelines. One example: Testing practices must have a demonstrable link to job performance or else the consultant psychologist (and the employer) can be found legally liable. It does not matter that a prospective employee produces an extremely elevated antisocial scale on a personality test. What matters is whether that specific test (and in particular the antisocial scale) has been validated for use in employee selection. In employment-related testing, the judgment of psychologists is held to be irrelevant (Lowman, 1989). Industrial assessment is a highly technical enterprise for which the examiner needs specialized training.

The most common clients in a psychological clinic are self-referred individuals seeking relief from psychological turmoil. The crucial assessment-related question for these persons is whether formal testing should play any significant role at all:

> For most of these individuals, psychological testing is not relevant and, in fact, may be contraindicated because the delay between the time of testing and the feedback of the results is usually time that could best be applied toward treatment. (Groth-Marnat, 1997)

This example argues against the practice of requiring every client to take a common battery of tests at intake. Unless assessment benefits the examinee, there is no justification for it.

THEORETICAL ORIENTATION

Theoretical orientation refers to the views of the practitioner on personality, psychopathology, and approaches to assessment (Tallent, 1992). The range of theoretical orientations embraced by clinicians is substantial. The most obvious disparity is between clinicians who focus on overt behaviors (the behaviorist approach) and those who seek to understand unconscious motivations (the psychodynamic outlook). But many other theoretical orientations are also observed. Some practitioners seek to understand current behavior by delving into its developmental context (the developmentalist perspective), whereas others focus on identifying the psychopathological syndrome that best fits the behaviors of the client (the psychodiagnostic viewpoint). Practitioners from each of these camps will likely choose different instruments for an assessment and invoke contrasting assumptions in making sense out of the data.

The same presenting complaint can be viewed from several theoretical orientations, each stipulating a different approach to assessment. A case in point is the phobic client whose fear of driving over bridges has wrought havoc with her life, mandating a two-hour, roundabout drive to get to work. Depending on the theoretical orientation of the clinician, assessment for this client would proceed along different lines. Those of psychodynamic persuasion might see the behavior as symbolic of the client's need for nurturance. As part of the assessment they might administer a projective technique such as the Rorschach, which could reveal unconscious dependency needs. The behaviorally oriented practitioner could evaluate the client's history of learned fears by administering a fear survey schedule. This practitioner might also assess the level of fear with a behavioral avoidance test in which the client rates the level of fear approaching a bridge, driving onto it, getting stuck in traffic on a bridge, and so on. The practitioner with a strong belief in the reality of psychopathological syndromes would wonder about the "big picture," such as whether the client exhibits depression or disordered thinking alongside the phobia. This practitioner might administer a multiphasic personality inventory. In sum, theoretical orientation dictates the approach taken in psychological assessment.

SOURCES OF INFORMATION

The sources of information for assessment range from unstructured interviews guided only by the intuitions of the examiner to standardized tests governed by formal procedures and scoring principles. Somewhere in between are procedures with moderate structure such as the mental status examination, behavioral assessment, and interview schedules. In this section we review the promise and pitfalls of gathering information for assessment.

The Assessment Interview

An **interview** is a face-to-face verbal exchange in which the interviewer attempts to elicit information or expressions of opinion or belief from a client (Wiens, 1990). The clinician usually begins an assessment interview with one or more explicit goals in mind, for example, arriving at a diagnosis, identifying the client's problems, or formulating a treatment plan. Beutler and Harwood (1995) list the five most common referral questions that prompt an assessment:

1. What diagnosis fits this person's current presentation?

2. What is the prognosis for this person's condition?
3. How impaired is this person's current functioning?
4. What treatment will be most likely to yield positive effects?
5. What factors are contributing to or causing this client's disturbance?

Even though psychological assessment is a method for obtaining answers to one or more of these questions, this does not mean that the practitioner should jump right in with a detective-like interrogation. Effective interviews are facilitated by the development of trust and rapport so that the client feels comfortable revealing personal information. In the beginning phases of the interview, the clinician typically responds to misgivings, discusses openly the goals of the interview, and indicates how the process will benefit the client.

The assessment interview is not a conversation and the roles and responsibilities of the two parties are not equal. The interviewee typically does most of the talking, using perhaps 80% of the talking time. The task of the clinician is to ask the right questions and keep the interview focused on the original purposes. The assessment interview also has continuity, as themes and subthemes are explored. For example, the mention of a melancholic mood by the client might elicit questions about sleep disturbance, loss of interest, and feelings of guilt, as the practitioner explores a particular diagnosis (depression in this example).

A vital purpose of the assessment interview is to *rule things out*. Consider the use of illicit drugs and the abuse of alcohol, both of which can mimic a variety of psychological disorders. A key purpose of the assessment interview is to rule out (or to rule in) the contributory role of drug and/or alcohol abuse. Another common practice in the assessment interview is to rule out suicide risk by asking explicitly (after rapport has been established) whether the client has any thoughts of self-harm.

The interview has been the subject of substantial research, and it is not exaggerating to say that several volumes would be needed to review the vast literature on this topic. We can only highlight a few key trends and findings here. One line of research that began with Carl Rogers (1957) has investigated the qualities of the therapist and the nature of the interactions within the interview that promote the development of rapport. The capacity to listen empathically and then the ability to reflect back accurately in a sentence or two the personal meaning of what the client is expressing appear to be important ingredients in a successful interview (Goldfried, Greenberg, & Marmar, 1990).

Another line of research has partitioned the complex interactions of the interview into discrete microskills as a basis for understanding the conditions of successful assessment. For example, the basic listening sequence has been divided into five steps: questioning, encouraging, paraphrasing, reflecting, and summarization (Ivey, Ivey, & Simek-Morgan, 1993). Examples of these steps with a patient who experiences a disabling fear of going out in public—a condition known as *agoraphobia*—might be as follows:

1. Could you tell me about your husband and how he responds to your fear of going out in public? [questioning]
2. You say that he seems to want to protect you? [encouraging]
3. So, when you indicate you don't want to leave the house, your husband goes out for you? [paraphrasing]
4. And that makes you feel safe but also sad and inadequate. [reflecting]
5. What I hear you saying, then, is that... [summarization]

Another approach to research on the interview is the exploration of thematic content. Clients and therapists can choose to talk about an essentially infinite variety of topics, but in actual practice a few themes tend to dominate interview sessions. But what are these themes, and how can we summarize them? Richards and Lonborg (1996) developed the Counseling Topic Classification System (CTCS) for this purpose. Their coding system consists of 28 topics (e.g., Abuse, Finances, Interpersonal Concerns, Performance Concerns, Relationships, Sleep Disturbance) and various subtopics (Table 2.1).

The CTCS has proved useful in identifying differences between clinicians in eliciting preferred topics; that is, some clinicians appear to direct clients toward some topics and away from others. The approach shows promise in the study of how the process of the interview affects its content.

The analysis of **nonverbal behavior** within the interview is yet another approach to understanding the dynamics of successful assessment. Gesture, body language, tone of voice, and facial expression constitute subtle but powerful forms of human communication (Siegman & Feldstein, 1987). In some cases, *how* a verbalization is expressed is more important than its content. A client's denial of marital conflict might indicate just the opposite when accompanied by a stiffening of posture and a quick change of topic. Of course, nonverbal communication works in both directions, and the counselor may also convey unwitting messages. A hint of anger when paraphrasing the client's expressed worry about a minor health problem might close off an important avenue of inquiry. Sensitivity to nonverbal cues—whether they arise from the interviewer or the client—is an essential skill for effective interviewing.

Reliability of the Interview

Research within the context of industrial and organizational psychology has provided a wealth of information relevant to clinical assessment by means of interview. Beginning in the 1940s, the reliability of the interview was assessed by correlating the personality impressions of different interviewers who had access to the same clients. If the interview is a reliable source of information, then interviewers should form similar impressions of clients. Unfortunately, the interrater reliability from dozens of early studies was typically in the mid-.50s, much too low to provide a reliable basis for making decisions about individuals.

Recent research using *structured* interviews provides a much more positive picture of interview reliability (Schmitt & Robertson, 1990). In a **structured interview**, clients are asked the same questions in the same order, and discretionary probing questions are specified in a lengthy and detailed

Table 2.1 The Counseling Topic Classification System: A Method for
Coding Interview Content

1. Abuse	17. Problem management
(a) physical	(a) coping
(b) sexual	(b) decision making
(c) emotional	(c) problem solving
2. Academics (school)	18. Relationships
3. Alcohol—other drug use	(a) parents
(a) alcohol use	(b) siblings
(b) drug use	(c) children
4. Career/life planning	(d) other relative
(a) decision making	(e) family (other)
(b) employment/job issues	(f) romantic/dating
(c) avocational/leisure	(g) friends
5. Child rearing/parenting issues	(h) marriage/partnership
6. Discrimination	(i) roommate
7. Eating behavior	(j) teacher
8. Finances	(k) supervisor/boss
9. Individual differences	(l) colleagues/co-workers
(a) age	(m) counselor
(b) disability	(n) client
(c) gender	19. Self-esteem/inferiority
(d) racial-ethnic	20. Self-injury/suicide
(e) religious	21. Sexuality
(f) spiritual	22. Sleep disturbances
(g) sexual orientation	23. Social issues
10. Interpersonal concerns	24. Stress
(a) alienation/loneliness	25. Emotions
(b) conflict	(a) affiliation (love, liking)
(c) loss	(b) rejection (disgust, dislike)
(d) shyness	(c) destruction (rage, anger)
11. Legal issues	(d) protection (panic, anxiety)
12. Living conditions	(e) self-affirmation (joy, serenity)
13. Moral/ethical issues	(f) reintegration (grief, depression)
14. Performance concerns	(g) orientation (surprise, confusion)
(a) speech anxiety	(h) exploration (anticipation, curiosity)
(b) test anxiety	26. Ambiguous topic
(c) perfectionism	27. No topic
15. Physical health	28. Other topic (A–Z)
16. Political issues	

Source: Reprinted with permission from P. Richards & S. Lonborg, "Development of a Method for Study-ing Thematic Content of Psychotherapy Sessions," *Journal of Consulting and Clinical Psychology*, 1996, Vol. 64, pp. 701–711.

manual. Interviewers also receive standardized training. Clients are then rated on scales anchored with behavioral illustrations. For studies employing structured interviews, reliabilities are substantially stronger, with interrater agreement typically in the .70s and .80s.

The success of the structured interview approach has prompted clinical psychologists to develop a variety of interview schedules. These devices require substantial training and are cumbersome in application. Many clinicians, therefore, prefer to rely on the relatively unstructured approach of the clinical interview. Yet, the evidence is strong that for well-defined purposes such as arriving at an accurate diagnosis, a structured interview schedule is the preferred approach.

Structured Interview Schedules

Structured interview schedules typically embody several common features. For example, the precise phrasing of each question is specified in the interview schedule. The use of follow-up questions is clarified in the accompanying manual and, in addition, the manual provides objective rules for the flow of questions, decision making, and overall scoring. The obvious advantage of this approach is that variations between interviewers are minimized, which tends to improve the reliability of the evaluations. The most significant drawback of the structured approach is lack of efficiency: the process takes substantially longer than a traditional diagnostic interview, and patients often end up responding to questions for which the answers are almost foregone conclusions. In addition, the lack of flexibility may cause the examiner to overlook promising avenues of inquiry not covered in the schedule. In spite of these problems, structured interview schedules have become highly popular, especially for purposes of formal diagnosis.

The best known structured interview schedules are those that allow the examiner to determine a formal diagnosis within the framework of the *Diagnostic and Statistical Manual of Mental Disorders* (DSM), an important guide to mental disorders, discussed below. The DSM is now in its fourth edition (DSM-IV), but published research on relevant interview schedules pertains mainly to the third and revised edition (DSM-III-R), which is substantially similar to the current version. The Structured Clinical Interview for DSM-III-R (SCID) provides a basis for diagnostic decision making (Spitzer, Williams, Gibbon, & First, 1988). SCID is essentially a flowchart of questions and decision points from which the clinician can determine the diagnostic classifications that apply to a client. For example, one very small portion of the section relevant to major depressive disorder requires the examiner to ask: "During that time, were you a lot less interested in most things or unable to enjoy the things you used to enjoy?" According to the decision tree in the interview schedule, an answer of "yes" then prompts the examiner to ask a series of nine questions about weight loss, sleep problems, loss of energy, and the like. If at least five symptoms are coded "true" and certain other conditions are ruled out, the client receives a diagnosis of major depressive disorder. When used by trained clinicians, the SCID yields levels of interrater agreement that are significantly higher than found for clinicians who make diagnoses from traditional unstructured interviews. Table 2.2 provides a diverse list of additional interview schedules.

Mental Status Examination

The **mental status examination** (MSE) is a semistructured interview designed to assess the patient's current intellectual and emotional functioning. The scope of the MSE is broad, but relatively

---

Table 2.2 A Sampling of Structured Interview Schedules

Schedule for Affective Disorders and Schizophrenia (SADS): Provides a differential diagnosis of affective disorders (e.g., major depression, bipolar disorder), schizophrenia, and related disorders (Endicott & Spitzer, 1978).

Giannetti On-Line Psychosocial History (GOLPH): A computerized clinical history that produces a narrative report on demographics, educational history, physical illnesses, and presenting complaints (Giannetti, 1985).

Anxiety Disorders Interview Schedule—Revised (ADIS-R): A structured clinical interview that evaluates the presence of DSM-III-R anxiety disorders and accompanying mood disorders (DiNardo & Barlow, 1988).

Yale–Brown Obsessive Compulsive Scale (Y-BOCS): An interview schedule that allows the clinician to assess the amount of time occupied by obsessions and compulsions, the level of distress, the degree of impairment, and the level of control over the symptoms (Goodman, Price, Rasmussen, et al., 1989a, 1989b).

Clinician Administered PTSD Scale (CAPS): A systematic interview that assesses the severity and frequency of PTSD symptoms and evaluates behavior change after the traumatic experience (Blake, Weathers, Nagy, et al., 1990).

Multicenter Panic Anxiety Scale (MC-PAS): A scale used to rate the frequency and distress of panic symptoms, the severity of anticipatory anxiety, situational avoidance, and impairment in functioning (Shear, Sholomskas, Cloitre, et al., 1992).

Structured Interview of Reported Symptoms (SIRS): An objective, interview-based method for the identification of malingering in a variety of populations including inmates and psychiatric patients (Rogers, Bagby, & Dickens, 1992).

Structured Clinical Interview for DSM-IV Dissociative Disorders (SCID-D): A systematic interview protocol that helps diagnose dissociative disorders and assess the severity of symptoms (Steinberg, 1993).

shallow, including assessment of memory, thought, language, feelings, and judgment. In addition, the clinician describes the physical appearance of the patient and records any unusual mannerisms or other behaviors. The purpose of the MSE is to provide a guide for further assessment (such as which areas need more detailed scrutiny). The MSE is also helpful in formal diagnosis, as will be discussed.

Over the last hundred years or so, practitioners have evolved a list of functional areas covered in a typical mental status examination (Trzepacz & Baker, 1993). Although the list might differ slightly from one textbook to another, most sources recommend assessment of the categories displayed in Table 2.3. Clinicians often use semistructured inventories such as the Mini-Mental Status Examination (Tombaugh, McDowell, Kristjansson, & Hubley, 1996) as part of the mental status evaluation. These instruments are helpful as ancillary measures, but they cannot substitute for a thorough assessment. Aspects of the MSE such as speech quality, thought processes, and adequacy of judgment cannot be reduced to simple inventory items. Competent evaluation is a clinical skill learned through training, experience, and supervision.

The nature and purpose of the mental status examination are best illustrated through example. Reprinted here is a report on the examination of a 71-year-old widow living alone in a housing complex for the elderly. Certain peculiarities in her behavior had elicited a request for evaluation. In particular, the client's adult children had noticed that on two occasions she had forgotten to turn her range off, leaving it on "high" for hours at a time. Also, she had become lost one afternoon when walking in the neighborhood. On the basis of a brief MSE, here is what the consulting psychologist wrote:

The client was well dressed and neat in appearance, in a good mood, and conversed eagerly about superficial matters. She maintained good eye contact and sat in a still, upright position on a couch while conversing with the examiner. Although her rate, tone, and volume of speech were appropriate, the content was occasionally a little bizarre. For example, at one point she talked about pushing the blood out of her fingers so that it could go up her arms. No delusions or loose associations were noticed.

Cognitive and memory functioning showed a number of noteworthy failures. Initially, she refused to do serial 3s from 20, claiming that it was too easy. However, it became clear that this was part of a generalized strategy for covering up her many impairments by making a joke out of questions and requests. For example, she was totally uncertain as to her age and turned this question back upon the examiner ("Well, how old do you think I am?"). Her social judgment appeared to be severely impaired as well. She judged the examiner's age to be 71, then 64. In fact, the examiner is a youthful-looking 42. The client evidenced memory disturbance as well. At one point she insisted that she needed to return to her private home (she has not lived there for two years) to prepare dinner.

The client's emotional functioning seemed surprisingly good, given the apparent degree of her impaired intellectual functions. Even though this probably indicated a great deal of denial and lack of insight, it was adaptive in the short run. Orientation to day, date, time, and location was grossly impaired. For example, she was off by two months and two years for date.

All of these symptoms point to intellectual deterioration based upon brain impairment. Some form of organic brain syndrome is strongly indicated. Because certain forms of dementia are treatable, it is imperative that the client see a neurologist for a complete workup at the earliest possible date. Based upon the results of that evaluation, additional intellectual testing may be appropriate to determine the extent of impairment. In the mean-

---

Table 2.3 Categories of a Typical Mental Status Examination

Appearance, Attitude, and Behavior
  Appearance (e.g., clothing, cleanliness, eye contact)
  Attitude toward examiner (e.g., hostile, indifferent, suspicious)
  Activity and motor abnormalities (e.g., odd mannerisms)

Speech and Language Functioning
  Speech quality (e.g., rate, tone, volume, fluency)
  Language skill (e.g., naming, confusion, misuse, repetition)
  Language comprehension (e.g., writing, reading)

Thought Process and Content
  Thought process (e.g., logic, clarity, connectedness, appropriateness)
  Thought content (e.g., delusions or hallucinations)

Emotional Functioning
  Predominant mood, variability of affect, etc.

Insight and Judgment
  Awareness of problems, adequacy of judgment, etc.

Cognitive Functioning
  Memory, attention, orientation, computation, etc.

time, the client should receive close supervision in order to prevent accidental self-harm. (Gregory, 1987)

Behavioral Assessment

Behavioral assessment encompasses a variety of straightforward approaches to evaluation that concentrate on obvious and identifiable target behaviors. Proponents of this approach prefer to steer clear of hypothetical constructs such as underlying traits or presumed dimensions of personality. Instead, the focus is directly on behavior: What is the undesired behavior? How often does it occur? In what settings? What is its intensity? What kinds of self-talk accompany it? What are the consequences that appear to maintain the behavior?

Haynes (1990) has identified seven stages or components of behavioral assessment:

1. Identification of target behaviors
2. Identification of alternative behaviors
3. Identification of causal variables
4. Development of a functional analysis
5. Design of intervention strategies
6. Evaluation and modification of intervention strategies
7. Facilitation of client–therapist interactions

The first and second steps are to identify the behaviors that constitute the focus of intervention efforts. These behaviors can be both undesirable (seek to decrease the frequency) *and* desirable (seek to increase the frequency). A key principle in choosing target behaviors is that of *shared variance*: Those behaviors whose modification would produce the greatest positive impact on other behaviors are the best targets for intervention. An example would be intervention with a client's marital communication deficits because this would also reduce his tendency to make inappropriate causal attributions (Haynes, 1990). This first step is intimately linked with the second step in behavioral assessment, which is the identification of positive behavioral goals (alternative behaviors).

Behavioral assessment also seeks to identify the causal variables that maintain undesirable behaviors and to arrive at a functional analysis of the identified target behaviors. For example, consider a client who repeatedly becomes angry and berates his teenage son whenever they disagree about curfew. A behavioral analysis might reveal that the causal variable is the client's self-talk ("This conflict is intolerable"). The analysis might also reveal that, functionally, the angry and berating behaviors produce a positive outcome, at least temporarily (the son leaves the room, terminating the conflict). These conceptualizations suggest certain intervention strategies (changing the self-talk and eliminating the berating verbalizations).

Once implemented, intervention strategies should be evaluated and modified if necessary. The evaluation of intervention most frequently occurs through serial assessment of the target behaviors. In the case of the phobic client referred to earlier (whose fear of driving over bridges necessitated a two-hour detour to work), an essential target behavior would be bridge avoidance, which could be measured precisely as a weekly percentage. With successful intervention, the weekly avoidance score should approach zero; otherwise, it would be wise to modify the intervention strategy. Ancillary measures might include a personal rating of anxiety (from zero to 100) for each successful trip over the bridge. The long-term goal would be to eliminate the avoidance and also reduce the anxiety score to near zero.

The behavioral approach to assessment also provides a basis for improving client–therapist interaction. Behavioral assessment is relatively objective and straightforward, which makes it easy to inform clients about the methods, intentions, and rationale of this approach. This helps facilitate a positive relationship between the client and the clinician which, in turn, boosts the likelihood of successful intervention (Haynes, 1990).

Some forms of behavioral assessment involve self-monitoring, which has the clear advantage of actively drawing the client into the assessment process. A case in point is the Pleasant Events Schedule (PES), an intriguing instrument that illustrates the subtle blending of evaluation and treatment that is so common in behavioral assessment (Lewinsohn, Munoz, Youngren, & Zeiss, 1986). The PES was predicated on the assumption that clinical depression goes hand in hand with a marked reduction in the experiencing of pleasant events. In the end, it becomes difficult to disentangle cause and effect: Depressed persons retreat from taking part in pleasant activities, which intensifies the depression, which in turn leads to further retreat. Fortunately, it is possible to reverse this downward spiral.

The purpose of the PES is to use self-monitoring of common everyday activities as a basis for reversing the downward spiral of depression. In the baseline assessment phase, clients use the PES to self-monitor the frequency and pleasantness of 320 largely ordinary everyday events. Examples of the rated activities include:

Reading magazines
Going for a walk
Being with pets
Listening to the radio
Reading poetry
Attending a church service
Playing catch with a friend

The frequency (F) of these everyday activities is rated on a three-point scale from 0 (has not happened in past month) to 2 (happened often in past month). In similar manner, the pleasantness (P) is also rated from 0 (not pleasant) to 2 (very pleasant). The mean rate of pleasant activities is then calculated as the sum of the F×P scores. The purpose of therapy, of course, is to increase the average rate of pleasant activities as a basis for reducing depression. Since participants also monitor their daily mood on a simple nine-point scale (1 = worst, 9 = best), clinicians can demonstrate the ongoing relationship between an increase in self-monitored pleasant activities and a reduction in depression.

Behavioral Ratings and Checklists

A major challenge in assessment is to summarize huge amounts of information in a succinct and useful manner. The clinician typically spends one or two hours interviewing the client and observing his or her behavior. Family members (e.g., parent or spouse) often contribute additional useful information. Even before a single test is administered, liter-

ally hundreds of data points (facts, impressions, behavioral vignettes) must be sorted, culled, and combined as the practitioner seeks to make sense of the client's behavior.

One approach to simplifying the results of initial interview and observation is to summarize the findings in a **behavioral rating scale** or checklist. Rating scales require the examiner to respond on a continuum regarding the behaviors of the client (e.g., child fails to wait his turn, rated on a scale from 1 or "almost never" to 5 or "almost always"), whereas checklists specify a yes–no style of rating (e.g., client is assertive, checked "yes" or "no"). What all of these approaches share in common is that the instruments provide a structured basis for the clinician to summarize impressions from interview and observation. Many rating devices also permit parents, guardians, teachers, or hospital personnel to perform a similar function.

The importance of rating scales and checklists is attested to by the huge number of forms currently available. In one specialized area alone—the assessment of mental retardation—over 100 rating scales were published prior to 1990 (Reschly, 1990). Literally thousands of behavioral rating scales and checklists are now available for a wide variety of applications. Test developers have been particularly fruitful in devising instruments for the assessment of children, mentally retarded persons, hospitalized psychiatric patients, and other client groups who are incapable of providing useful self-report information. Two widely used devices are described here.

Conners (1990) has published a group of rating scales that are helpful in identifying hyperactivity and other behavioral problems in children. The format of the various instruments is similar to the following:

	NOT AT ALL	JUST A LITTLE	PRETTY MUCH	VERY MUCH
Cries easily				
Restless and fidgety				
Daydreams				
Disobeys adults				

Two forms are available for teachers (one with 28 items, the other with 39 items), and two forms are also available for parents (48 items and 93 items). The most widely used is the Conners Parent Rating Scale—93 (CPRS-93), which is normed on children between 3 and 17 years of age. The scale yields summary ratings on eight dimensions: Conduct Disorder, Restless Disorganized, Psychosomatic, Antisocial, Fearful Anxious, Learning Problem–Immature, Obsessional, and Hyperactive-Immature. This instrument helps define problem areas in school-based referrals and also provides an objective basis for monitoring the effects of interventions such as drug treatment for hyperactivity.

The Brief Psychiatric Rating Scale (BPRS) is a simple instrument often used to monitor improvement of hospitalized psychiatric patients (Overall, 1988; Overall & Gorham, 1962). The scale consists of a seven-point rating scale (not present, very mild, mild, moderate, moderately severe, severe, and extremely severe) for 18 relatively independent categories of behavior. The categories are similar to the following:

Somatic preoccupation: Unwarranted concern with physical health, fear of physical illness, hypochondriasis

Suspiciousness: Distrust, belief that others are out to harm the patient

Depressed mood: Sad, tearful, despondent, pessimistic

Abnormal thought content: Peculiar, odd, strange, or bizarre thought content

By analyzing the patterning of scores (from 1 to 7) for hospitalized patients on the eighteen subscales, Overall and Hollister (1982) identified eight distinct BPRS profile patterns that represent different phenomenological types. Four of the patterns involved depression (anxious, retarded, agitated, hostile), and four concerned syndromes of disturbed thinking (florid, withdrawn, excited, suspicious). These turned out to be clinically significant assessment patterns, in that patients so classified were found to respond optimally to different types

of drug treatment. The BPRS is an outstanding example of an instrument that provides clinically relevant results that translate directly to specific treatment recommendations.

CLINICAL VERSUS ACTUARIAL DECISION MAKING

Assessment often involves formal judgment or decision making. Examples include recommending whether to hire a job candidate, deciding whether a patient is suicidal, and determining whether an alleged criminal is competent to stand trial. Psychologists have recognized for some time that decision making can proceed on one of two paths: clinical or actuarial (Meehl, 1954). In **clinical judgment**, the practitioner processes information in his or her head to diagnose, classify, or predict behavior. Clinical judgment is based on experience, intuition, textbook knowledge, or a combination of these. Often it is rooted in clinical lore or commonly accepted guidelines. An example of clinical judgment is a psychologist recommending not to hire a candidate for police officer because his personality test scores indicate impulsiveness, which is widely believed to be a negative quality in law enforcement.

In contrast, **actuarial judgment** is always founded on *empirically derived* formulas to diagnose, classify, or predict behavior. Actuarial judgment is objective and rule-based. More important, actuarial judgment always flows from the careful development and use of research-based formulas. The essence of the actuarial approach, then, is that "the human judge is eliminated and conclusions rest solely on empirically established relations between data and the condition or event of interest" (Dawes, Faust, & Meehl, 1989). For example, an actuarial approach to using personality test scores in the selection of law enforcement candidates would consist initially of collecting information regarding test scores and subsequent job performance. Once this information was obtained, objective formulas would be developed to identify the relationship between test scores and aspects of job performance. Perhaps supervisor evaluations or the probability of disciplinary action would be factored into the equation. Future job candidates would then be recommended (or not recommended) for employment on the basis of the overall score they received on the objective formula.

Which is the superior method for decision making, clinical or actuarial? On the basis of over 100 comparative studies in the social sciences, Dawes, Faust, and Meehl (1989) concluded that when conditions permit a fair comparison of the two approaches, the actuarial method is superior in virtually every case. A study by Leli and Filskov (1984) is typical of the findings that compare clinical versus actuarial decision making. The raw material for their study consisted of 24 Wechsler intelligence test protocols from adults, including 12 from normal individuals and 12 from persons with documented brain damage. A rich clinical lore surrounds the Wechsler tests, and certain patterns of subtest scores—especially a high degree of subtest scatter—are widely believed to indicate the presence of cerebral pathology. But do the patterns really convey impairment, and can human judges accurately decipher the presence of brain damage from the test data? Using a previously derived *empirical* formula (Leli & Filskov, 1979), the authors were able to classify correctly 83% of the protocols with a simple formula known as a linear stepwise discriminant function. In this approach, a weighted linear sum of the subscale scores is computed (e.g., .17 × Information + .08 × Picture Completion − .22 × Digit Symbol...). If the sum exceeds a certain cutoff value (typically 1.0), the protocol is classified as indicating brain damage; otherwise, it is considered normal. Using this simple approach, the authors achieved correct classification for 20 of the 24 cases, a hit rate of 83%.

On the basis of the same test protocols, how did the clinical judgment of humans compare to the statistical formula? The researchers used two groups of clinical raters, experienced and inexperienced. The experienced group consisted of five licensed psychologists working in medical settings. These individuals included three clinicians who had earned ABPP certification (American Board of Professional Psychology) which signifies a high level of clinical expertise as judged by colleagues. The inexperienced group consisted of five predoctoral interns in clinical psychology who had completed a graduate-level assessment course but otherwise had received limited clinical training.

Ironically, the inexperienced graduate students outperformed the experienced clinicians, correctly classifying 63% of the cases compared to 58% for the licensed psychologists. Of course, the performance of both groups was well below the 83% accuracy of the formula. The lesson to be learned from this and hundreds of other studies is that a good formula is almost always superior to human judgment when it comes to clinical decision making.

The reasons for the superiority of the actuarial approach shed light on certain foibles of human character and cognition. For example, practitioners are likely to notice confirming instances in their predictions and diagnoses, but to ignore the more numerous findings that contradict expectations (Chapman & Chapman, 1967). Clinicians, thereby, develop a false sense of their predictive accuracy and are likely to continue offering erroneous judgments with high levels of confidence. In one study, a sample of 42 clinical neuropsychologists overwhelmingly concluded with moderate to high levels of confidence that test batteries from three young children indicated brain damage. In fact, all the children were normal but had been instructed to fake bad—an outcome detected by none of the experienced neuropsychologists even though it was explicitly offered as one of the choices (Faust, Hart, & Guilmette, 1988). Pride goeth before a fall, and practitioners resist learning about the limits of clinical judgment.

As a final note on the clinical versus actuarial discussion, we need to acknowledge that for most decisions, inferences, or judgments, empirically confirmed formulas are not yet available—and perhaps they never will be (Kleinmuntz, 1990). In most areas of assessment and clinical practice, the clinician has no choice but to rely on his or her best judgment. Yet the clear message from decades of research is that practitioners should seek to develop and use a good formula whenever that is feasible.

DIAGNOSTIC CLASSIFICATION AND DSM-IV

The classification of mental disorders can serve many purposes, ranging from decision making about treatment to efficiency of communication with other professionals. Andreasen & Black (1995) have catalogued the following purposes of **clinical diagnosis**:

- Reduce the complexity of clinical phenomena.
- Facilitate communication between clinicians.
- Predict the outcome of disorders.
- Decide on appropriate treatment.
- Assist in the search for etiology.
- Monitor treatment.
- Make decisions about reimbursement.
- Play a role in malpractice suits and other litigation.
- Determine the incidence and prevalence of mental disorders.
- Aid in decision making about insurance coverage.

Making a careful diagnosis is fundamental to the practice of clinical psychology. The preferred approach to classification is known as the *Diagnostic and Statistical Manual of Mental Disorders*, now in its fourth edition (DSM-IV; American Psychiatric Association, 1994). The first edition appeared in 1952, with revisions in 1968 (DSM-II), 1980 (DSM-III), and 1987 (DSM-III-R).

Overview of DSM-IV

DSM-IV is a vast improvement over its predecessors. One major innovation has been the implementation of reasonably objective criteria for defining the disorders included in the classification system. DSM-IV specifies the type, number, and duration of behaviors needed before a particular diagnostic classification can be applied to a patient. An example of this approach is shown in Table 2.4, which lists the diagnostic criteria for Attention-Deficit/Hyperactivity Disorder. In theory, this approach should improve the reliability (interrater agreement) and validity (usefulness) of the classification scheme, although whether these goals have

Table 2.4 Diagnostic Symptoms of Attention-Deficit/Hyperactivity Disorder

Inattentive Type (6 or more symptoms)
Lack of attention to details
Difficulty sustaining attention
Does not seem to listen
Failure to follow through
Difficulty organizing tasks
Avoids sustained mental effort
Loses things
Easily distracted
Forgetful in daily activities

Hyperactive-Impulsive Type (6 or more symptoms)
Fidgets and/or squirms
Leaves seat in classroom
Inappropriate running or climbing
Difficulty playing quietly
Seems driven, always on the go
Talks excessively
Blurts out answers
Difficulty waiting turn
Interrupts or intrudes on others

Combined Type (meets both criteria above)

Source: Based on American Psychiatric Association, *Diagnostic and Statistical Manual of Mental Disorders* (4th ed.) (Washington, DC: Author, 1994).

been achieved is open to question, as will be discussed.

Classification within DSM-IV extends beyond the mere labeling of patients and includes a multiaxial approach that conveys substantial information. The patient is evaluated according to five axes:

Axis I   Clinical Disorders and Related Conditions

Axis II   Personality Disorders and Mental Retardation

Axis III   General Medical Conditions (Relevant to Mental Disorder)

Axis IV   Psychosocial and Environmental Problems

Axis V   Global Assessment of Functioning (GAF)

The patient must receive a principal diagnosis on Axis I or Axis II, but it is also possible to assign more than one classification from each of the axes. The major categories for these axes are listed in Table 2.5. Axis III pertains to a wide range of medical problems that might have an impact on psycho-

Table 2.5 Major Categories and Specific Classifications from the DSM-IV

Axis I: Clinical Disorders

Disorders Usually First Diagnosed in Infancy, Childhood, or Adolescence

Mental Retardation (Mild, Moderate, Severe, Profound)

Learning Disorders (Reading, Mathematics, Written Expression)

Pervasive Developmental Disorders (e.g., Autistic Disorder)

Attention-Deficit/Hyperactivity Disorder

Disruptive Behavior Disorders (e.g., Conduct Disorder)

Other Disorders (e.g., Separation Anxiety Disorder)

Delirium, Dementia, and Amnestic and Other Cognitive Disorders

Substance-Related Disorders

Alcohol Use Disorders (Alcohol Dependence, Alcohol Abuse)

Alcohol-Induced Disorders (e.g., Alcohol Withdrawal)

Schizophrenia and Other Psychotic Disorders (e.g., Schizophrenia, Schizoaffective Disorder, Delusional Disorder)

Mood Disorders

Depressive Disorders (Major Depressive Disorder, Dysthymic Disorder)

Bipolar Disorders (e.g., Single Manic Episode, Cyclothymic Disorder)

Anxiety Disorders (e.g., Social Phobia, Posttraumatic Stress Disorder)

Somatoform Disorders (e.g., Conversion Disorder, Pain Disorder, Hypochondriasis)

Factitious Disorders [Symptoms intentionally produced or feigned]

Dissociative Disorders (e.g., Dissociative Fugue, Dissociative Identity Disorder)

Sexual and Gender Identity Disorders

Eating Disorders

Sleep Disorders

Impulse-Control Disorders (e.g., Kleptomania, Pathological Gambling)

Adjustment Disorders

Axis II: Personality Disorders

Paranoid Personality Disorder

Schizoid Personality Disorder

Schizotypal Personality Disorder

Antisocial Personality Disorder

Borderline Personality Disorder

Histrionic Personality Disorder

Narcissistic Personality Disorder

Avoidant Personality Disorder

Dependent Personality Disorder

Obsessive-Compulsive Personality Disorder

Note: A few low-frequency classifications have been omitted from this list.

---

logical functioning (e.g., infectious diseases, cancer, heart disease, endocrine disorders). Axis IV is direct acknowledgment that environmental stressors are highly relevant to the understanding of mental disorders. Contributory factors such as divorce, death of a friend, academic problems, stressful work schedule, inadequate finances, and interaction with the legal system are listed here. Axis V is for reporting the clinician's judgment of the patient's overall level of functioning on a scale of 1 to 100. A low score of 1 corresponds to imminent suicide threat, while a high score of 100 indicates many positive qualities and superior functioning.

Here is an example of how the results from a DSM-IV multiaxial evaluation would be reported for a typical case:

Axis I	296.23	Major Depressive Disorder, Single Episode, Severe Without Psychotic Features
Axis II	301.6	Dependent Personality Disorder Frequent use of denial
Axis III		Ischemic Heart Disease
Axis IV		Threat of Job Loss
Axis V		GAF = 10 (on admission) GAF = 85 (on discharge)

The reader will notice that a substantial amount of information is contained in this simple capsule summary of the patient's DSM-IV assessment. The individual depicted here experienced a very disabling depression (Axis I diagnosis of Major Depressive Disorder and GAF of 10 on admission). Most likely, an impoverishment of individual resources contributed to his mental disorder (Axis II features of Dependent Personality Disorder with frequent use of denial). Furthermore, adverse health factors (Axis III diagnosis of Ischemic Heart Disease) and severe environmental stress (Threat of Job Loss) also contributed to his disabling depression. Despite these problems, his functioning was reasonably good upon discharge (GAF of 85).

Reliability and Validity of the DSM-IV

Evaluating the reliability of DSM-IV diagnosis is a straightforward matter of computing the inter-rater agreement for the classification of patients. In a typical reliability study, two or more clinicians independently interview and diagnose the same patients. The researcher then tallies the average rate of agreement for each diagnostic category. Diagnostic agreement can be expressed as a percentage, a correlation coefficient, or the kappa statistic, which corrects for chance agreement. Kappa can vary from 0.0 (no agreement) to 1.0 (perfect agreement). Values of .5 and above are considered acceptable and .8 or higher is considered very good.

Although published research with DSM-IV is scant at this time, on the basis of its similarity to previous editions we can expect that some classifications will possess excellent reliability, whereas others will reveal dismal levels of agreement. Reliability of the major categories (e.g., mood disorders) will be generally strong, whereas the level of agreement for specific classifications (e.g., dysthymic disorder) will be weaker, seldom exceeding 50% agreement between clinicians. In Table 2.6 we have reproduced data from an earlier field study that confirms these trends (Andreasen & Black, 1995).

The validity of DSM-IV hinges substantially on the meaningfulness and usefulness of the information provided by its diagnostic classifications. For example, of what value is it to know that a patient has received an Axis I diagnosis of Major Depressive Disorder, Single Episode, Severe Without Psychotic Features? Particularly relevant is the predictive validity of this or any diagnosis. Specifically, what does the diagnosis indicate about the typical course of the mental disorder? What kinds of coexisting symptoms (such as an excessive preoccupation with imagined health problems) might the clinician expect? Which treatments are likely to be effective? If a diagnosis provides nothing more than a shorthand description of the current condition, its value in clinical practice is limited. Validity is not just a theoretical issue, it is also a highly practical matter.

Viewed from this perspective, the validity of DSM-IV has been established for some disorders but not for others. The natural history of several

Table 2.6 Kappa Coefficients of Agreement for DSM-III Axis I and Axis II Diagnostic Classifications of 670 Adults

	AVERAGE KAPPA	PERCENT OF SAMPLE
Axis I		
Disorders usually first evident in infancy, childhood, or adolescence	.69	4.5
Organic mental disorders	.78	10.9
Substance use disorders	.83	21.2
Schizophrenic disorders	.81	20.5
Paranoid disorders	.71	1.4
Psychotic disorders not elsewhere classified	.67	9.0
Mood disorders	.76	41.4
Anxiety disorders	.68	9.0
Somatoform disorders	.48	3.6
Dissociative disorders	.40	.8
Psychosexual disorders	.84	1.8
Factitious disorders	.33	1.1
Disorders of impulse control not elsewhere classified	.54	1.8
Adjustment disorder	.68	10.3
Psychological factors affecting physical condition	.53	2.7
Overall kappa for Axis I	.70	
Axis II		
Personality disorders	.61	54.9

Note: The total for column 2 exceeds 100% because patients could receive more than one diagnosis.
Source: Based on data in N. C. Andreasen & D. W. Black, *Introductory Textbook of Psychiatry* (2nd ed.) (Washington, DC: American Psychiatric Press, 1995).

Axis I classifications has been fairly well mapped out, including the likelihood of future episodes and response to alternative treatment modalities. Consider one common diagnosis, Major Depressive Disorder. This classification reveals a lifetime risk of 7% to 12% for men and 20% to 25% for women; remits in 6 to 24 months without treatment; shows a 50% risk of recurrence after one episode and a 70% risk after two episodes; responds to antidepressant medication in 60% of the cases and psychotherapy in 50% of the cases; and commonly co-occurs with alcoholism and medical disorders such as stroke, dementia, diabetes, and heart disease (U.S. Department of Health and Human Services, 1993a, 1993b). Clearly, the diagnostic category of Major Depressive Disorder is both meaningful and useful—which is to say, highly valid.

Yet the practical validity of many other DSM-IV diagnoses is simply unknown. This is particularly true for the Axis II classifications (personality disorders), for which the validity evidence is meager at this time. With the possible exception of Antisocial Personality Disorder (which has been the topic of substantial empirical research), the associated characteristics, responses to treatment, and other features of most Axis II classifications have not been identified. In part this is due to the lower diagnostic reliability of these categories, which means that clinicians often disagree as to whether a patient meets the criteria for a specific personality disorder. Reliability constrains validity. When the reliability of a diagnosis is low, it becomes difficult to demonstrate its validity.

REPORTING ASSESSMENT RESULTS

Although there is no single way to report assessment results, a number of guidelines are worth mentioning (Gregory, 1987; Tallent, 1993; Wolber & Carne, 1993). Perhaps the most important point is that psychological reports should not be relegated to the inconsequential "caboose" that tags along at the end of the train. Assessment is only as effective as the report that summarizes the examiner's response to the uncertainties posed by the referral question(s). From this perspective, the report is more like the "engine" that pulls the entire assessment forward (Tallent, 1993).

Two general guidelines that pertain to all reports are those of responsibility and efficacy. **Responsibility** refers to a variety of ethical, professional, and legal concerns that exert powerful influences on how assessment results are reported. For example, clinicians are generally aware that psychological reports can become involved in legal proceedings even when they were not written for that purpose and regardless of any prior agreement that the results are "confidential" and for certain eyes only. The best interests of the client (and of the psychologist!) are well served by anticipating the future life of a psychological report. Consider this true case of a seriously head-injured young adult who was tested by a graduate trainee:

The graduate student wrote a very optimistic report that ignored and downplayed the many deficiencies revealed by a comprehensive test battery. The report was accurate in the sense that error scores were correctly reported, but the examiner cast the findings in the most positive light possible by dwelling on numerous extenuating circumstances that might explain the poor performance of the subject. At the time, the supervising psychologist saw no harm in this positive approach insofar as it seemed to be what the client and his parents wanted to hear. The client left the office after the feedback session with high motivation to regain the many cognitive skills he had lost from the head injury.

Two years later the report was subpoenaed in a lawsuit filed by the head-injured subject against the person who had caused the injury. Although he won a substantial settlement, it seems likely that the overly optimistic report only muddled the compensation issues raised in the lawsuit. Perhaps his interests would have been better served by a more realistic summary of his test results. (Gregory, 1987)

Many assessment specialists now write reports based on the expectation that outside parties—even hostile lawyers—will eventually read them. This is not altogether a negative trend, although it may lead to excessively cautious reports that overlook creative recommendations.

Another component of responsibility is assuring that the *client* receives accurate and constructive feedback about the assessment results. This is accomplished in large measure by careful attention to **informed consent,** whereby the client agrees, in writing, to the entire package of the assessment. As part of this agreement, the psychologist typically clarifies when, where, and how feedback to the client will be accomplished. The ethical principles of the American Psychological Association (APA) further emphasize that:

... psychologists ensure that an explanation of the results is provided using language that is reasonably understandable to the person assessed or to another legally authorized person on behalf of the client. (APA, 1992)

Pope (1992) has outlined several useful guidelines for providing assessment feedback to clients. For example, the clinician must guard against countertransference in which personal reactions can in-fluence, distort, and derail the feedback process. The practitioner who is angry with a client can un-wittingly use the feedback session as an opportunity to focus on negative aspects of the assessment re-sults rather than providing an accurate and balanced picture. Another important principle is that of *acknowledging fallibility*:

> The feedback process best focuses on hypotheses for which there are varying degrees of evidence in the test findings rather than on any sort of infalli-ble, unchallengeable pronouncements. The clini-cian has the responsibility to ensure that the client not only understands this general lack of infallibil-ity but also is aware of any specific reservations the clinician has about the validity, reliability, mean-ing, and implications of specific tests, findings, and so forth. (Pope, 1992)

In sum, feedback must occur in the context of clear communication, relatively unhindered by the per-sonal foibles of the clinician.

Efficacy in report writing has to do with whether the report produces the intended effect in the life of the client which, in turn, hinges especially on clear, direct writing. A 12-page magnum opus might never reach the eyes of the referral source and so can have no impact at all. The best reports tend to be shorter rather than longer. But a brief report can be pointless, too, if it contains a bog of jargonistic speculation that leaves the reader angry and con-fused. In general, reports should be short, clear, and direct if they are to yield a positive impact in the life of the client.

Nonetheless, admirable qualities of writing such as brevity and clarity do not guarantee a construc-tive outcome. The recommendations in the report must also embody *wisdom*, which has to do with training, experience, and additional factors that are beyond explanation. We remind the reader that as-sessment is both science and art. The scientific ele-ment in report writing can be taught directly by way of rules and directives, but the creative component is more difficult to convey.

Pitfalls in Effective Report Writing

One approach to the study of report writing is to ask professionals what they like and dislike about psychological assessment reports. Tallent (1993) provides a catalogue of responses from 1,400 clini-cal workers, including psychiatrists, social work-ers, and psychologists. Although many responses were favorable, hundreds of negative comments were received. The major criticisms included the following:

1. *Excessive raw data:* A very common com-plaint is that examiners refer to specific scores and scale names that have little or no meaning to non-psychologists. A typical example of this pitfall is a report based on the Rorschach that states "The F+ % of 40 indicates that the client has a poor grasp of reality." To the uninitiated, the cryptic reference to F+ % makes it appear that the report writer is swear-ing about the test data!

2. *Improper emphasis:* Another recurring criti-cism is that reports focus on inconsequential aspects of the test results that have no bearing on the referral questions. This is especially common in settings where lengthy test batteries are used. The examiner often feels compelled to discuss the implications of each and every subtest when, in fact, the essential information often resides in a few global scores. For example, a child referred for possible learning disability might be administered the 13 subtest Wechsler Intelligence Scale for Children—III, but it is rarely necessary or helpful to proceed with a subtest-by-subtest report of the results.

3. *Recommendations exceeding expertise:* Nothing is more offensive to practitioners in allied professions than to have psychologists wander into their backyard and offer advice beyond the psy-chologists' expertise. This is particularly a prob-lem with medical fields such as psychiatry and neurology. Clinical psychologists typically know just enough about these specialty areas to be dan-gerous. It is never appropriate for a psychologist to recommend that a patient undergo a specific medi-cal procedure (e.g., computerized tomography or CT scan of the brain) or receive a particular drug (e.g., an antidepressant or other psychotropic drug). Even when the need for a specific procedure or drug appears to be obvious, the prudent course

of action is to recommend consultation with the appropriate medical profession for further evaluation.

4. *Irresponsible interpretation:* Some psychologists make sweeping pronouncements in their reports that are not supported by test results or interview impressions. Although it is a rare occurrence, it is always unfortunate when the examiner speculates about latent homosexual tendencies in a client or simply gets the diagnosis wrong because of a pet theory about psychopathology. A more subtle error occurs when the psychologist does not consider racial and ethnic differences in the interpretation of test results. Eyde, Robertson, Krug, and collleagues (1993) describe a clinician who diagnosed a language disorder in an inner-city African American preschooler on the basis of a test devised with predominantly Caucasian subjects. The child's language skills departed from standard English but were nonetheless perfectly adequate.

5. *Exhibitionism:* Occasionally, report writers attempt to impress the reader with their erudition rather than offering helpful perspectives on the client. One respondent in Tallent (1993) refers to psychologists whose reports "reflect their needs to shine as a psychoanalytic beacon in revealing the dark, deep secrets they have observed." Other reports are "written in stilted psychological terms to boost the ego of the psychologist."

6. *Excessive abstraction and theory:* The assessment specialist who leans toward abstract and theoretical formulations is another target of criticism. For example, reference to oral-sadistic tendencies in the client is generally not helpful unless this abstract concept is anchored in typical behaviors. Fischer (1985) has proposed a useful antidote to excessive abstraction and theory—namely, reports should be written so that they can be understood by an intelligent 12-year-old!

7. *Poor writing:* Some reports are written in psychologese rather than English. The client is said to "manifest overt aggressive hostility in an impulsive manner" when, in fact, it would be more accurate to say that he "tends to punch people in the face when provoked." Other examples of poor writing include the following:

    a. The use of meaningless and imprecise words such as *viable*, *input*, *interface*, *orient*, *parameter*, and *finalize*.

    b. Confusion of *affect* and *effect* (e.g., "The timed tests had a negative *affect* [should be *effect*] on John");

    c. Reliance on vague language (e.g., "It is recommended that he be tested again after a year to determine whether or not maturation will outstrip environmental inputs," which, translated, means "Retesting in a year is recommended in order to assess developmental changes") (Gregory, 1987).

Approaches to Report Writing

The "flavor" of an assessment report depends on the framework from which it is written, the audience to whom it is addressed, the particulars of the referral issues, and the idiosyncrasies of the report writer. Reports come in more varieties than the recipes in an all-purpose cookbook (Tallent, 1992; Wolber & Carne, 1993). We can highlight only a few approaches here. Table 2.7 provides the outlines for several common styles of report writing. The remainder of this chapter is devoted to an annotated assessment report written from a generalist perspective.

ANNOTATED ASSESSMENT REPORT

The following report is based on an assessment of a college student referred because of academic difficulty. A few inessential details have been altered to protect the privacy of the student, but the essential facts of the case and the test results are authentic. The italicized material is commentary and was not included in the report.

Intellectual and Psychological Assessment

Date: October 14, 1997

Demographic Information
Client: Jane Edwards, female

Table 2.7 Outlines for Assessment Reports Written from Four Perspectives

(a) Traditional	VI. Defenses
I. Title and Demographics	A. Immature
II. Source and Reason for Referral	B. Neurotic
III. Tests and Procedures	C. Mature
IV. Relevant Background	VII. Recommendations for Psychotherapy
A. Medical History	**(c) Behavioral**
B. Educational History	I. Title and Demographics
C. Prior Test Results	II. Behavior During Assessment
V. Behavioral Observations	III. Presenting Problem
VI. Assessment Results	A. Nature of Problem
A. Intellectual Functioning	B. Relevant History
B. Personality Functioning	C. Current Situational Determinants
C. Diagnostic Impressions	D. Relevant Personal Variables
VI. Summary and Recommendations	E. Extent of Problem
	F. Consequences of Problem
(b) Psychodynamic	IV. Personal Assets
I. Title and Demographics	V. Targets for Modification
II. Reason for Assessment	VI. Motivation for Treatment
III. Psychological Conflicts	VII. Recommended Treatment Approaches
A. Self-Perception	**(d) Phenomenological**
B. Perception of Environment	I. Title and Demographics
C. Interpersonal Relations	II. Reason for Assessment
D. Drives and Dynamics	III. Client's View of the Problem
E. Emotional Cathexes and Controls	IV. Tests Administered and Results
IV. Social Stimulus Value	V. Client as Reflected in Test Results
A. Cognitive Skills	VI. Summary and Impressions
B. Goals	
C. Social Roles	
V. Cognitive Functioning	
A. Strengths	
B. Deficits	
C. Psychopathologies	

Age: 19 years, 10 months
Date of birth: December 10, 1977
Date of tests: October 12, 1997

The demographic information contains suffi-cient data for readers to check the accuracy of the age—which will affect scoring norms for certain tests. Notice also that the date of the report is listed separately from the date of testing. This practice promotes efficiency on the part of the examiner—a delay of weeks or months is embarrassing! Further-more, readers have a right to know whether diag-nostic impressions and other interpretations are based on fresh memories or delayed recall.

Reason for Referral
Ms. Edwards was referred by the Student Counsel-ing Center for intellectual and psychological eval-uation. The primary referral question is whether enrollment in college is realistic for her at this time. She attended briefly last year but withdrew from

school after a serious automobile accident on Oc-tober 5, 1996. She is just now returning to college as a first-semester freshman and is experiencing major difficulty in several courses.

Notice that the reason for assessment is ex-pressed as a prognostic question: Can this student succeed in college at this time? Assessment is prob-lem solving. The best writeups state the problem ex-plicitly in the beginning and then offer an answer later in the report.

Relevant Background
When Ms. Edwards graduated from high school in 1996, she ranked 27th in a class of 283 students. In the fall of 1996 she earned A's and B's on her first tests in college before the automobile acci-dent in October that necessitated a withdrawal. According to the medical records of 10/27/96 from her attending neurosurgeon, Dr. Manfred Attela, Ms. Edwards experienced a closed-head injury with a small subdural hematoma in the area

of the left frontal lobe. The hematoma was surgically removed, but Ms. Edwards remained unconscious for two days. From that point onward she made an excellent recovery of her physical functions and was released from the hospital after two weeks. However, her parents reported that she was more irritable than before and was prone to emotional outbursts. Apparently, there was no additional assessment. According to the parents, medical follow-up consisted of a brief neurological examination on January 7, 1997, which was unremarkable. Since that time Ms. Edwards has been employed as a cashier in a fast-food restaurant while awaiting the opportunity to return to school this fall.

A wealth of background information is usually available and might include circumstances of birth, developmental history, medical illnesses, educational history, parental demographics such as education and occupation, and so on. However, the task of the report writer is to select the relevant information, not to report every extraneous detail in encyclopedic fashion. In the case of Ms. Edwards, the most important background information has to do with (1) her prior success, which is documented in objective terms, and (2) her accident, which is described in pertinent detail. For example, length of coma is very important in predicting recovery from neurological impairment, so this information is mentioned prominently. Notice also that the source of factual statements is indicated (e.g., dated medical reports, parental feedback).

Behavior in Testing

Ms. Edwards was cooperative during testing and appeared highly motivated to do her best. She expressed concern that her test scores might be low and therefore substantiate that college was beyond her abilities. Whenever she failed a test item, she berated herself ("Oh, I just feel so stupid!"). The results are considered to be a valid index of her current intellectual functioning.

Any behavior that bears upon the validity of the test results is mentioned here. In addition, any behavior that is relevant to the referral issue is discussed. In the case of Ms. Edwards whose test results turned out to be indicative of brain impairment (see below) it was important to emphasize that her motivation appeared to be strong—which bolsters

the validity of the findings. In addition, her self-berating behavior was relevant to the diagnostic impression and so is featured prominently in this section.

Tests Administered and Results

Wechsler Adult Intelligence Scale—Revised (WAIS-R)

Information	7	Picture Completion	11
Digit Span	2	Picture Arrangement	9
Vocabulary	10	Block Design	4
Arithmetic	7	Object Assembly	9
Comprehension	8	Digit Symbol	7
Similarities	9		

Verbal IQ:	84	Performance IQ:	88

Full Scale IQ: 86

Short Category Test, Booklet Form: 56 errors/100

Trail-Making Test

Part A	93 seconds, 0 errors
Part B	178 seconds, 2 errors

Interpretation of Test Results

On the WAIS-R Ms. Edwards obtained a Full Scale IQ of 86, which is below the average of 100 for the general population and significantly lower than the average for college students, which is about 110–115. Given her previous levels of educational attainment, this score almost certainly represents a significant decline as a consequence of her head injury.

Ms. Edwards displayed an unusually high degree of variability on the subtests, with scaled scores as low as 2 but as high as 11 (the average score in the general population for the subtests is 10). The relatively high score of 10 on Vocabulary indicates good facility with words, and the score of 11 on Picture Completion indicates good capacity for visual details. However, the low score of 2 on Digit Span portends a serious degree of distractibility for orally presented stimuli, and the low score of 4 on Block Design indicates a weakness in visual-perceptual problem solving. These areas of weakness are especially problematic for a college student, who must learn by listening to lectures and must also solve practical problems in the course of her studies.

The Short Category Test, Booklet Form, is a measure of abstract reasoning that requires the examinee to learn from ongoing feedback from prior responses. A typical error score for young adults is 19 wrong from the 100 stimuli. Ms. Edwards made 56 errors in the course of the test, which indicates a substantial impairment of high-level abstract reasoning—most likely as a consequence of her closed-head injury.

On the Trail-Making Test, the examinee is asked to draw a line connecting numbers in sequential order (Part A) and then connecting numbers and letters in alternating, sequential order (Part B) under pressure of time. This screening instrument is sensitive to disruptions in the cognitive processes of attention, visual search, and mental flexibility. Ms. Edwards experienced major difficulty on this screening test of brain impairment. For example, on part B, a time of more than 90 seconds is considered indicative of impairment. Ms. Edwards needed 178 seconds to complete this task.

The results are interpreted succinctly and in reasonably nontechnical terms. Notice that test scores are placed in context of national averages and normative data. Of course, what stands out for this examinee is the apparent decline in functioning. Nonetheless, areas of strength are also mentioned. The relevance of the results for the referral issue is highlighted.

Interview Impressions

In one-to-one social conversation, Ms. Edwards is very sharp, even cleverly argumentative. She comes across as verbally facile, which is both a blessing and a detriment. It is a blessing because verbal skills are important for educational attainment and work advancement. But her verbal facility also works against her by giving others a reason to conclude that her brain impairment is inconsequential (or even nonexistent). In fact, these preliminary test results indicate otherwise.

During our interview Ms. Edwards displayed a "smiling depression" and shared prominent suicidal ruminations. Her planning is relatively specific, and she should be considered a high risk for suicide at this time. Personnel at the Student Counseling Center have been informed of this concern and appropriate preventive measures have been taken. In addition to her closed-head injury, Ms. Edwards presents a diagnostic impression of Major Depressive Disorder.

Psychological reports need not be formal, stilted, and jargonistic, as indicated by the use of an unofficial diagnostic term here ("smiling depression"). It is also permissible for the examiner to interpret the client's behavior within any framework that appears to be relevant. In this case, the exam-

iner has focused upon a social-psychological analysis, pointing out how others might be misled by the client's strong verbal skills.

Summary and Recommendations

Ms. Jane Edwards is a 19-year-old college freshman who experienced a closed-head injury one year ago in an automobile accident. As a consequence of this injury, Ms. Edwards has sustained a diffuse impairment of brain functions. The testing completed here was not designed to assess the details of her impairment, but it is clear that college coursework will be very difficult for her. I recommend that she discontinue her college studies at this time.

Ms. Edwards is currently experiencing a severe depression with suicidal ruminations. The first priority should be management of the suicidal crisis, including treatment of the depression. Referral to a psychiatrist is strongly recommended. At a later point it would be advisable for Ms. Edwards to obtain a comprehensive neuropsychological assessment. Results of this evaluation would provide a basis for educational and vocational planning.

Robert J. Gregory, Ph.D.
Licensed Psychologist

The examiner gets right to the point in the last sentence of the first paragraph by stating: "I recommend that she discontinue her college studies at this time." This is a direct response to the referral question. In addition, the examiner introduces an issue not mentioned by the referral source but which is nonetheless crucial for the welfare of the client—namely, future assessment for educational and vocational guidance.

REFERENCES

American Psychiatric Association. (1994). *Diagnostic and statistical manual of mental disorders* (4th ed.). Washington, DC: Author.

American Psychological Association. (1992). Ethical principles of psychologists and code of conduct. *American Psychologist, 47,* 1597–1611.

Andreasen, N. C., & Black, D. W. (1995). *Introductory textbook of psychiatry* (2nd ed.). Washington, DC: American Psychiatric Press.

Beutler, L., & Harwood, T. (1995). How to assess clients in pretreatment planning. In J. N. Butcher (Ed.), *Clinical personality assessment: practical approaches* (pp. 59–77). New York: Oxford University Press.

Blake, D., Weathers, F., Nagy, L., et al. (1990). A clinician rating scale for assessing current and lifetime PTSD: The CAPS-1. *The Behavior Therapist, 13,* 187–188.

Chapman, L. J., & Chapman, J. P. (1967). Genesis of popular but erroneous psychodiagnostic observations. *Journal of Abnormal Psychology, 74,* 271–280.

Conners, C. K. (1990). Conners Rating Scales manual. Willowdale, Ontario: Multi-Health Systems.

Dawes, R., Faust, D., & Meehl, P. (1989). Clinical versus actuarial judgment. *Science, 242,* 1668–1674.

DiNardo, P., & Barlow, D. (1988). *Anxiety Disorders Interview Schedule—Revised (ADIS-R).* Albany, NY: Graywind Publications.

Endicott, J., & Spitzer, R. (1978). A diagnostic interview: The schedule for affective disorders and schizophrenia. *Archives of General Psychiatry, 35,* 837–844.

Eyde, L., Robertson, G., Krug, S., et al. (1993). *Responsible test use: Case studies for assessing human behavior.* Washington, DC: American Psychological Association.

Faust, D., Hart, K., & Guilmette, T. (1988). Pediatric malingering: The capacity of children to fake believable deficits on neuropsychological testing. *Journal of Consulting and Clinical Psychology, 56,* 578–582.

Fischer, C. T. (1985). *Individualizing psychological assessment.* Monterey, CA: Brooks/Cole.

Giannetti, R. (1985). *Giannetti on-line psychosocial history: GOLPH (Version 2.0).* Unpublished manuscript.

Goldfried, M., Greenberg, L., & Marmar, C. (1990). Individual psychotherapy: Process and outcome. In M. Rosenzweig & L. Porter (Eds.), *Annual review of psychology* (pp. 659–688). Palo Alto, CA: Annual Reviews.

Goodman, W., Price, L., Rasmussen, S., et al. (1989a). The Yale–Brown Obsessive Compulsive Scale: I. Development, use, and reliability. *Archives of General Psychiatry, 46,* 1006–1011.

Goodman, W., Price, L., Rasmussen, S., et al. (1989b). The Yale–Brown Obsessive Compulsive Scale: II. Validity. *Archives of General Psychiatry, 46,* 1012–1016.

Gregory, R. J. (1987). *Adult intellectual assessment.* Boston: Allyn and Bacon.

Groth-Marnat, G. (1997). *Handbook of psychological assessment* (3rd ed.). New York: Wiley.

Haynes, S. N. (1990). Behavioral assessment of adults. In G. Goldstein & M. Hersen (Eds.), *Handbook of psychological assessment* (2nd ed., pp. 423–466). New York: Pergamon Press.

Ivey, A., Ivey, M., & Simek-Morgan, L. (1993). *Counseling and psychotherapy: A multicultural perspective* (3rd ed.). Boston: Allyn and Bacon.

Kleinmuntz, B. (1990). Why we still use our heads instead of formulas: Toward an integrative approach. *Psychological Bulletin, 107,* 296–310.

Leli, D., & Filskov, S. (1979). The relationship of intelligence with education and occupation as signs of intellectual deterioration. *Journal of Consulting and Clinical Psychology, 47,* 702–707.

Leli, D., & Filskov, S. (1984). Clinical detection of intellectual deterioration associated with brain damage. *Journal of Clinical Psychology, 40,* 1435–1441.

Lewinsohn, P. M., Munoz, R., Youngren, M., & Zeiss, A. (1986). *Control your depression: Reducing depression through learning self-control techniques, relaxation training, pleasant activities, social skills, constructed thinking, planning ahead, and more* (rev. ed.). New York: Prentice-Hall.

Lowman, R. L. (1989). *Pre-employment screening for psychopathology: A guide to professional practice.* Saratoga, FL: Professional Resource Exchange.

Matarazzo, J. (1990). Psychological assessment versus psychological testing. *American Psychologist, 45,* 999–1017.

Meehl, P. (1954). *Clinical versus statistical prediction.* Minneapolis: University of Minnesota Press.

Motto, J. (1985). Preliminary field-testing of a risk estimator for suicide. *Suicide and Life-Threatening Behavior, 15,* 139–150.

OSS Assessment Staff. (1948). *Assessment of men: Selection of personnel for the Office of Strategic Services.* New York: Rinehart.

Overall, J. E. (1988). The Brief Psychiatric Rating Scale (BPRS): Recent developments in ascertainment and scaling. *Psychopharmacology Bulletin, 24,* 97–99.

Overall, J. E., & Gorham, D. (1962). The Brief Psychiatric Rating Scale. *Psychological Reports, 10,* 799–812.

Overall, J. E., & Hollister, L. (1982). Decision rules for phenomenological classification of psychiatric patients. *Journal of Consulting and Clinical Psychology, 50,* 535–545.

Peterson, D. R. (1987). The role of assessment in professional psychology. In D. R. Peterson & D. B. Fishman (Eds.), *Assessment for decision* (pp. 5–43). New Brunswick, NJ: Rutgers University Press.

Pope, K. S. (1992). Responsibilities in providing psychological test feedback to clients. *Psychological Assessment, 4,* 268–271.

Rapp, S., Parisi, S., Walsh, D., & Wallace, C. (1988). Detecting depression in elderly medical inpatients. *Journal of Consulting and Clinical Psychology, 56,* 509–513.

Reschly, D. J. (1990). Adaptive behavior. In A. Thomas

& J. Grimes (Eds.), *Best practices in school psychology* (2nd ed., pp. 29–42). Washington, DC: National Association of School Psychologists.

Richards, P., & Lonborg, S. (1996). Development of a method for studying thematic content of psychotherapy sessions. *Journal of Consulting and Clinical Psychology, 64,* 701–711.

Rogers, C. (1957). The necessary and sufficient conditions of therapeutic personality change. *Journal of Consulting Psychology, 21,* 95–103.

Rogers, R., Bagby, R., & Dickens, S. (1992). *Structured Interview of Reported Symptoms (SIRS) and test manual.* Odessa, FL: Psychological Assessment Resources.

Schmitt, N., & Robertson, I. (1990). Personnel selection. *Annual Review of Psychology, 41,* 289–320.

Shear, M., Sholomskas, D., Cloitre, M., et al. (1992). *The Multicenter Panic Anxiety Scale (MC-PAC).* Unpublished manuscript.

Siegman, A., & Feldstein, S. (Eds.). (1987*). Nonverbal behavior and communication.* Hillsdale, NJ: Erlbaum.

Spitzer, R. , Williams, J., Gibbon, M., & First, M. (1988). *Instructional manual for the structured clinical interview for DSM-III-R* (SCID, 6/1/88 Revision). (Biometrics Research Department, New York State Psychiatric Institute, 722 West 168th Street, New York, NY 10032.)

Steinberg, M. (1993). *Interviewer's guide to the Structured Clinical Interview for DSM-IV Dissociative Disorders.* Washington, DC: American Psychiatric Press.

Tallent, N. (1992). *The practice of psychological assessment.* Englewood Cliffs, NJ: Prentice-Hall.

Tallent, N. (1993). *Psychological report writing* (4th ed.). Englewood Cliffs, NJ: Prentice-Hall.

Tombaugh, T., McDowell, I., Kristjansson, B., & Hubley, A. (1996). Mini-Mental State Examination (MMSE) and the Modified MMSE (3MS): A psychometric comparison and normative data. *Psychological Assessment, 8,* 48–59.

Trzepacz, P. T., & Baker, R. W. (1993). *The psychiatric mental status examination.* New York: Oxford University Press.

Turk, D., & Rudy, T. (1990). Pain. In A. Bellack, M. Hersen, & A. Kazdin (Eds.), *International handbook of behavior modification and therapy* (2nd ed., pp. 399–413). New York: Plenum Press.

U.S. Department of Health and Human Services. (1993a)*. Depression in primary care: Vol. 1. Detection and diagnosis.* Rockville, MD: Author.

U.S. Department of Health and Human Services. (1993b)*. Depression in primary care: Vol. 2. Treatment of major depression.* Rockville, MD: Author.

Wiens, A. N. (1990). Structured clinical interviews for adults. In G. Goldstein & M. Hersen (Eds.), *Handbook of psychological assessment* (2nd ed., pp. 324–344). New York: Pergamon.

Wolber, G. J., & Carne, W. F. (1993). *Writing psychological reports: A guide for clinicians.* Sarasota, FL: Professional Resource Exchange.

Wrightsman, L., Nietzel, M., & Fortune, W. (1994). *Psychology and the legal system* (3rd ed.). Pacific Grove, CA: Brooks/Cole.

FOR FURTHER READING

American Psychiatric Association. (1994). *Diagnostic and statistical manual of mental disorders* (4th ed.). Washington, DC: Author. *This compendium contains the official nomenclature and diagnostic criteria for mental disorders. Though somewhat technical and dry in its presentation, DSM-IV does summarize research-based findings as to clinical features, prevalence, course, cultural patterns, familial patterns, and other aspects of almost every conceivable mental disorder.*

Goldstein, G., & Hersen, M. (Eds.). (1990). *Handbook of psychological assessment* (2nd ed.). New York: Pergamon Press. *This is a relatively high level textbook that summarizes the state of the art of psychological assessment. The 23 chapters include summaries of test construction, different types of tests, interviewing, and specialized applications (e.g., assessment of minorities, computer-assisted psychological assessment).*

Groth-Marnat, G. (1990). *Handbook of psychological assessment* (2nd ed.). New York: Wiley. *This is a practitioner's handbook that provides guidelines and summaries for the application of major instruments such as the Wechsler scales, the Rorschach, MMPI-2, and so forth.*

Matarazzo, J. (1990). Psychological assessment versus psychological testing. *American Psychologist, 45,* 999–1017. *This short article effectively argues the point that assessment involves clinical judgment based on training and experience.*

Wetzler, S., & Katz, M. (Eds.). (1989). *Contemporary approaches to psychological assessment.* New York: Brunner/Mazel. *The 17 chapters in this book include several contributions not found elsewhere (e.g., assessment of the medically ill, scales for formal thought disorder, measurement of emotions).*

CHAPTER 3

TESTING IN CLINICAL PSYCHOLOGY

Robert J. Gregory

The profession of clinical psychology first earned its respectability through the successful application of psychological tests to pressing social issues. The classic example is the individual intelligence test invented by Alfred Binet in 1905 and used to identify children in need of special schooling. A less well known example is the Personal Data Sheet devised by Robert Woodworth in 1917 and used to screen army recruits susceptible to emotional disturbance. Many other instances could be cited to illustrate this essential point: In the early 1900s clinical psychology was synonymous with applied psychological testing. Only later did the profession branch off into other areas such as individual therapy, group therapy, community psychology, and forensic applications.

Of course, clinical psychologists now perform many functions in addition to psychological testing. Nonetheless, testing remains central to the profession and still ranks as one of its greatest achievements. Psychological tests assist in treatment planning and provide a basis for the evaluation of therapeutic efficacy—to cite just a few of their many applications. We consider here the nature of psychological tests, their uses and occasional abuses, approaches to test construction, and the

value of tests in the practice of clinical psychology. The starting point is a brief historical review.

ORIGINS OF PSYCHOLOGICAL TESTING

The term *mental test* was first used by James McKeen Cattell (1890), the preeminent American psychologist who studied with Wilhelm Wundt in Germany and Francis Galton in Great Britain. Cattell was a champion of what is now known as the "brass instruments" approach to psychological testing, so named because of its reliance on the use of brass equipment to measure sensory thresholds and reaction times. This approach was based on the reasonable (but incomplete) assumption that keen sensory abilities were essential to intelligence. In 1901, Clark Wissler, a student of Cattell, demonstrated that sensory test results (e.g., reaction time, naming of colors) bore no relationship to college grades. With these discouraging results, psychologists abandoned the use of reaction time and sensory measures as indices of intelligence.

The first modern intelligence test was invented by Alfred Binet (1857–1911) in 1905. The 1905 Binet-Simon Scale (Binet & Simon, 1905) developed in collaboration with Theophile Simon was highly successful in identifying children who could not benefit from regular instruction in the Paris school system. Rather than relying on elementary sensory processes, their simple scale consisted of 30 items of increasing difficulty that tested higher mental processes such as abstraction and comprehension. The Binet-Simon was revised in 1908 and again in 1911.

An intriguing footnote to history is that the original Binet-Simon scale did not yield a formal score and most certainly did not provide an IQ score. The IQ concept was a joint product of the German psychologist Wilhelm Stern (1912/1914) and the American psychologist Lewis Terman (1916). Terman was a professor at Stanford University where the Binet-Simon was translated, revised, and renormed for use with American subjects. That test has survived to the current day as the Stanford-Binet, now in its fourth edition (Thorndike, Hagen, & Sattler, 1986).

In addition to the Binet-Simon, the other major influence on modern intelligence testing was the Army testing program spearheaded by Robert Yerkes (1919). Yerkes and several other well-known psychologists devised two group tests of ability for screening and placement of Army recruits during World War I. The Army Alpha test consisted of eight verbally loaded tests for average and high-functioning recruits. The Army Beta test was a nonverbal group test designed for use with the less educated, the illiterate, and recruits whose first language was not English.

It would be difficult to overestimate the influence of the Binet-Simon and the Army tests on subsequent intelligence tests. The items in these tests inspired the development of virtually every individual intelligence test now in existence. In particular, the Wechsler intelligence tests (to be discussed) owe a large debt to these predecessors. David Wechsler borrowed not just the format but many exact test items directly from these earlier contributions.

Contemporary testing in clinical psychology also has roots in early personality tests such as the Personal Data Sheet developed by Robert Woodworth to screen World War I Army recruits who might be prone to emotional breakdown. This test consisted of 116 yes–no questions probing for serious psychopathology—for example, "Are you bothered by a feeling that things are not real?" The yes–no approach to personality measurement survives in the many popular true–false inventories, including the most widely used test of all time, the Minnesota Multiphasic Personality Inventory, now in its second version (MMPI-2). Of course, many present-day tests also originated from the depth psychology tradition embodied in the familiar inkblot technique invented just after World War I by Hermann Rorschach (1921).

The early history of testing is a fascinating topic with continuing relevance to present-day practices. One thing we learn is caution about the overzealous application of tests. For example, in a sad and regrettable chapter of American psychology, early testing pioneers, such as Henry H. Goddard, championed the use of individual intelligence tests for the screening of immigrants (Gelb, 1986). Goddard and his assistants used translators to administer the original Binet-Simon tests shortly after the immigrants walked ashore:

> Thus, a test devised in French, then translated to English was, in turn, retranslated to Yiddish, Hungarian, Italian, or Russian; administered to bewildered farmers and laborers who had just endured an Atlantic crossing; and interpreted according to the original French norms. (Gregory, 1996)

Surely this must rank as one of the most inappropriate uses of psychological testing ever recorded.

NATURE AND USES OF PSYCHOLOGICAL TESTS

Definition of a Test

A **test** is a standardized procedure for sampling behavior and describing it with scores or categories. In most cases, a test is perceived as an evaluation; that is, the examinee knows that he or she is being tested. This raises important issues with respect to test validity, particularly for the evaluation of personality, attitudes, aspirations, and the like. The essential problem is that of **social desirability**, the natural tendency for persons to answer questions in a socially desirable manner rather than being completely truthful. As discussed next, many tests utilize validity scales to ascertain such tendencies in the test-taker.

The crucial hallmarks of a psychological test include the following:

- The use of standardized procedures
- The sampling of behavior
- The production of scores or categories
- The interpretation by means of norms or standards
- The prediction of nontest behavior

These characteristics are reviewed next.

Standardized procedures are essential to ensure that testing procedures remain uniform for different examiners in varied settings. Lack of standardization in such elements as reading instructions or presenting stimuli can change not just the character of the test but its difficulty level as well, which reduces the validity of the enterprise. For example, recalling orally presented digits is much easier if they are presented rapidly. This is why test manuals usually specify that digits must be spoken at the rate of precisely one per second.

A psychological test is also based on a limited sample of behavior. When testing vocabulary, for example, it is not realistic to determine the totality of a person's word knowledge. The examiner must settle for a sample of 30 or 40 words and predict general word knowledge from this (much) smaller sample. The most important implication of the test-as-sample concept is that test results invariably contain some degree of error. For instance, the totality of a person's word knowledge might be stronger or weaker than conveyed by his or her responses to a 30-word vocabulary test. An individual of below-average ability might obtain a very high score as a result of lucky guessing, or, conversely, a person of superior ability could receive a low score because the test included a disproportionate number of colloquial terms. Although measurement error can be minimized by means of careful test design, it can never be eliminated.

Tests usually provide scores or categories which are then interpreted in reference to a standardization sample. The **standardization sample** (also called a norm group) must be representative of the population for whom the test is intended so that it is possible to evaluate each person's test results in comparison to a reference group. For example, knowing that an examinee scored 137 on a test of abstract reasoning conveys little information. But, if we learn that the average score for college-bound seniors was 103 and that only 1 percent of these students scored 135 or higher, we have a basis for making a nontest prediction, namely, that the examinee is a good bet for succeeding in college. This last point illustrates that it is not the result per se that is valuable. Rather, it is what the test result signifies in relation to *nontest* behaviors that is of primary interest.

The vast majority of tests are **norm-referenced**, which means that results from them are interpreted in reference to the standardization sample. But not all tests follow this model. In particular, **criterion-referenced** tests are used to determine where an examinee stands with respect to very tightly defined educational objectives. For these instruments, the comparison is with an objective standard rather than with the performance of other examinees. Results of a criterion-referenced arithmetic test might report that a student adds two three-digit numbers with 78% accuracy whereas the goal for the school system is 95%. Notice here that the performance of other students is irrelevant—what matters is whether this student meets the accepted criterion.

Another important distinction is between group tests and individual tests. A group test can be administered to many examinees at the same time, which is highly economical. The disadvantage is that the test-giver has no idea whether every test-taker put forth a good effort, answered in the correct columns, and so forth. An individual test has the advantage that the test-giver can keep the examinee on task and observe responses to success or failure and other clinical details of test-taking. In addition, an individual test permits a wider latitude as to the kinds of stimuli that can be presented (e.g., manipulating blocks or arranging puzzles).

Finally, we should distinguish testing from assessment. *Testing* is the more limited venture, which consists of administering, scoring, and interpreting individual tests. *Assessment* is the more comprehensive term that refers to the entire process of compiling information and synthesizing it to make predictions about the person. Assessment was discussed in the previous chapter. Here we restrict discussion to the more limited enterprise of testing.

Types of Tests

Clinical psychologists have access to literally thousands of different tests and the number of useful instruments continues to grow each year. For example, a recent issue of the *Mental Measurements Yearbook* contains descriptive information and critical reviews on 418 *new* or revised tests (Conoley & Impara, 1995). The *Yearbook* is published every few years; each issue surveys only a small fraction of the available instruments.

Even though the diversity of tests would appear to defy simple classification, most instruments fit within a few categories. The most widely used tests are those that evaluate intelligence, neuropsychological functioning, personality, and individual interests or values. Instruments for specialized purposes also receive significant usage by clinical psychologists. These categories are reviewed next.

Intelligence and Related Tests

Intelligence tests typically sample a broad assortment of skills in order to evaluate the examinee's general level of mental ability. These tests usually provide a profile of subtest scores as well, but it is generally the overall score that is of greatest utility. Intelligence tests might also be called ability tests in that they assess current ability.

The distinction between ability, aptitude, and achievement tests is important in this context. In truth, the correlations among scores on these three kinds of tests can be substantial, and items from all of them may be highly similar in style and content. The difference between them turns out to be largely a matter of how they are used. Intelligence or **ability tests** are used to evaluate an individual's general intellectual level for such purposes as identifying the sources of academic problems. An intelligence test would be an essential component in the diagnosis of a learning disability. In contrast, **aptitude tests** are

used to forecast future success in school, training, or a career. These tests often perform a gatekeeping function, including school admission, military entry, and corporate employment. Finally, **achievement tests** measure current skills in relation to identified educational goals of a school or training program. Their function is not only to assess the performance of examinees but also to evaluate the success of educational programs.

Neuropsychological Tests and Batteries

Neuropsychological tests and batteries are used in the assessment of persons with known or suspected brain impairment such as from head injury, stroke, or neurological disease. These procedures include a wide spectrum of approaches, ranging from 10-minute screening tests to six-hour comprehensive batteries. Common to all forms of neuropsychological assessment is the use of specialized instruments sensitive to the effects of brain impairment. These tests assess sensory, motor, cognitive, and behavioral strengths and weaknesses for purposes of treatment planning and documentation of improvement.

Personality Tests

Personality tests measure the traits, qualities, or behaviors that determine a person's individuality. These instruments include checklists, self-report inventories, and projective approaches such as sentence completion and inkblot techniques. Personality tests are used to determine functioning within the normal range of behavior (e.g., rating the assertiveness of a sales candidate) and also to evaluate abnormal behavior (e.g., assessing the degree of depression in a hospitalized patient). In most cases, the evaluation of personality aids in the prediction of behavior.

Tests of Interests and Values

Tests of interests and values assess an individual's preference for certain activities or values. These tests are based on the explicit assumption that interest patterns and personal values can be used to predict satisfaction within specific occupations. This kind of information has many uses, but a prominent application is to help examinees find a suitable occupation. For example, the Campbell Interest and Skill Survey (CISS; Campbell, Hyne, & Nilson, 1992) consists of 200 interest items, which the examinee rates on a six-point scale from "strongly like" to "strongly dislike." The items resemble the following:

A pilot, flying commercial aircraft
A biologist, working in a research lab
A police detective, solving crimes

The test also includes 120 skill items, also rated on a six-point scale from "expert" (widely recognized as excellent in this area) to "none" (have no skills in this area). The skill items resemble the following:

Helping a family resolve its conflicts
Making furniture, using woodworking tools
Writing a magazine story

Answers to the interest and skill items are compared to those provided by persons successfully employed within specific occupations to determine a respondent's fit for various lines of work.

Specialized Tests

Many tests are designed for highly specialized applications or intended for use within specific subpopulations. The well-read clinician might then recognize an appropriate application for tests such as these, selected at random from Conoley and Impara (1995):

Arizona Battery for Communication Disorders of Dementia
Children's Depression Scale
Multifactor Leadership Questionnaire
Substance Abuse Questionnaire—Adult Probation
Test of Early Reading Ability—Deaf or Hard of Hearing
Visual Search and Attention Test

This list is exemplary only, intended to illustrate the incredible range and diversity of tests available within the field of clinical psychology. The existence of these and thousands of other tests raises an important point about the practice of testing within clinical psychology: How is the practitioner to know if a new test is any good? As discussed in the next section, the psychological examiner must be conversant with standards of test construction and evaluation.

Test Construction and Evaluation

Tests are invented and assembled by psychologists and other specialists on the basis of one or more philosophies of test construction. The most common philosophies of test construction include theory-guided approaches, empirical procedures, and the application of factor analysis to preliminary data. Each of these methods is described next. Of course, some tests are constructed by means of interplay between two or all three approaches.

Theory-Guided Tests

The theory-guided approach begins with a listing of the qualities that the test specialist seeks to measure. Suppose the developer desires to construct a new self-report scale for leadership potential. Test development would begin with a review of relevant theory, which might reveal that leadership potential is characterized by self-confidence, resilience under pressure, high intelligence, persuasiveness, assertiveness, and the ability to sense what others are thinking and feeling. On the basis of this theory-derived list, the test developer might then construct a series of true–false questions which appear, on a rational basis, to tap these qualities (Gough & Bradley, 1992):

- I generally feel sure of myself and self-confident. (T)
- When others disagree with me, I usually just keep quiet or else give in. (F)
- I believe that I am distinctly above average in intellectual ability. (T)
- I often feel that I have a poor understanding of how other people will react to things. (F)
- My friends would probably describe me as a strong, forceful person. (T)

The T or F after each statement shows the keyed direction for leadership potential. For obvious reasons, this method of test development is also known as the method of rational scaling.

An important characteristic of a theory-guided test is that the scales should possess internal consistency. *Internal consistency* refers to the quality whereby individual scale items correlate positively with each other and also with the total score for the scale. In fact, this necessary characteristic can be used to select good items and eliminate poor ones early in test development. The statistic known as *coefficient alpha* is used to evaluate internal consistency. Coefficient alpha is calculated from the test data for hundreds of examinees and can vary from near zero to a perfect 1.0 (never achieved). The closer the score to 1.0, the greater the internal consistency of the scale. For tests constructed by means of the theory-guided method described here, coefficient alpha is usually .8 to .9 or higher. A good example of a theory-guided test is the Millon Clinical Multiaxial Inventory—III, discussed below.

Empirical-Criterion Tests

In the empirical approach, test items are selected for inclusion almost entirely on the basis of their capacity to separate a criterion group from a normative sample. This method is therefore less dependent on theoretical considerations, rational judgment, and the guidance of experts. What matters is the real-world performance of the individual items.

The empirical-criterion approach is best illustrated through example. Suppose a test designer wanted to derive a new Depression scale based on a preexisting, large pool of true–false personality questions. The following procedures would be used (Gregory, 1996):

1. A carefully selected, homogeneous group of persons experiencing major depression is gathered to answer the pool of true–false questions.
2. For each item, the endorsement frequency of the depression group is compared to the endorsement frequency of the normative sample.
3. Items that show a large difference in endorsement frequency between the depression and normative samples are selected for the Depression scale, keyed in the direction favored by depression subjects (true or false, as appropriate).
4. Raw score on the Depression scale is then simply the number of items answered in the keyed direction.

The most prominent example of a test developed by means of the empirical-criterion approach is the MMPI-2. For most of the clinical scales, item membership was determined by means of contrasting the endorsement frequencies of selected clinical groups (e.g., hypochondriasis, depression, antisocial personality, schizophrenia) versus a normative sample of adults. One unavoidable by-product of this method of scale construction is that many test items will serve on more than one scale. For example, an item that discriminates persons with depression from normal subjects might also discriminate persons with hypochondriasis from normal subjects and consequently end up being assigned to both scales. Item overlap between scales is an unavoidable consequence of this test development strategy.

Factor-Analytic Tests

Factor analysis is a statistical technique that is useful in summarizing the interrelationships among a large number of test items in a concise and accurate manner as a prelude to scale development. It is beyond the scope of this book to delve into the details of factor analysis, but a few notes and an example can be used to illustrate this approach. For instance, factor analysis might help a test developer discover that a collection of 200 true–false questions represents only five underlying variables, called factors. Factor analysis would also identify the specific items that best represent each of the five variables—information that can be used in scale construction. From this point, the content of the items on each scale could be used to identify what is being measured. A prominent example of a test developed by means of factor analysis is the Sixteen Personality Factor Test (16PF), to be discussed.

Of course, with all of the techniques discussed here, ongoing research is needed to identify the psychometric properties of a test. In particular, regardless of the manner in which a test is developed, further research will be needed to prove its reliability and validity. We discuss the evaluation of psychological tests in the next section.

EVALUATION OF PSYCHOLOGICAL TESTS

Reliability of Tests

Reliability refers to the attribute of consistency in what a test measures. When all other factors are held constant, a reliable test is one that produces identical (or at least highly similar) results for an examinee from one occasion to the next. Psychometricians have invented several ways to evaluate test reliability, which we review here.

The most straightforward approach to measuring reliability is to administer a test twice to the same group of subjects and then calculate a correlation coefficient between the two sets of scores. This is known as **test–retest reliability**, and results can vary from a dismal 0.0 (absolutely no reliability) to a theoretically possible 1.0 (perfect reliability). When test results are used to make decisions about individuals, an accepted guideline is that this form of reliability should be .90 or higher. Guilford and Fruchter (1978) offer the following advice:

> There has been some consensus that to be a very accurate measure of individual differences in some characteristic, the reliability should be above .90. The truth is, however, that many standard tests with reliabilities as low as .70 prove to be very useful. And tests with reliabilities lower than that can be useful in research. (p. 87)

Many other approaches can be used to evaluate the reliability of a test or scale. One popular method is to administer the instrument a single time to a large group of subjects and then correlate scores on one half of the scale (e.g., the even items) with scores on the other half of the scale (e.g., the odd items). This is known as the split-half approach. Since the initial correlation is derived on only one-half the total number of items, a minor statistical adjustment (the Spearman-Brown formula) is needed to estimate the reliability for the entire scale. A related method mentioned earlier is the internal consistency approach in which a specialized reliability index, **coefficient alpha**, is calculated. The split-half approach and coefficient alpha are related. In fact, it can be shown that coefficient alpha is the average of all possible split-half reliability coefficients.

For tests in which examiner judgment is needed to obtain the scores, the computation of interrater reliability is also necessary. This is a straightforward procedure in which a large sample of tests is independently scored by two or more examiners and then scores for pairs of examiners are correlated. Interrater reliability supplements other reliability estimates, but does not replace them.

A few cautions need to be observed when evaluating the reliability of psychological tests. Test–retest reliability will be spuriously low if it is based on a sample of subjects for whom there is a restriction of range on the characteristic being measured. Thus, it would be unwise to evaluate the test–retest reliability of an intelligence test on the basis of results for students in a gifted and talented program. Another situation that calls for caution is the evaluation of speeded tests in which the score is based primarily on the number of items completed. In this case, the odd–even approach to split-half reliability will yield a spuriously high result for test reliability.

Evaluation of Test Validity

The **validity** of a test is the extent to which it measures what it claims to measure. Although to some extent validity can be evaluated by means of statistical criteria, the validity of a test ultimately hinges on the accumulation of research findings. As Anastasi (1986) has noted, "validity is a living thing; it is not dead and embalmed when the test is released." The validation of a test is therefore a developmental process that begins with test construction and continues throughout the life of the test.

Traditionally, the different ways of accumulating validity evidence have been categorized into the "three C's":

- Content validity
- Criterion-related validity
- Construct validity

Another concept that requires brief mention is face validity, which is not really a technical form of validity but is nonetheless an essential matter of public relations. A test has face validity if it looks valid to test-users, test-givers and, especially, test-takers. Face validity is important because it helps ensure that a test will be accepted and used.

Content validity refers to the degree to which the questions, items, or tasks on a test are representative of the class of behaviors the test was designed to sample. One approach to content validity is the prior construction of a domain specification table that clearly identifies the subareas of content that the test developer hopes to measure. For example, in devising an achievement test of early American history, the developer might specify four domains: the colonial period, the American revolution, westward expansion, and Civil War events. Content validity would be ensured by designing questions that tap these four domains. Content validity is mainly a judgment call by the test developer and usually is not reduced to a single number. Often a panel of experts is assembled to confirm that the items do, in fact, pertain to the predetermined domains.

Criterion-related validity is demonstrated when a test is effective in estimating a subject's performance on a relevant outcome measure. In one approach to criterion-related validity known as **concurrent validity**, test scores are compared to a relevant external criterion. For example, results from a paper-and-pencil test of psychiatric diagnosis might be compared to the actual diagnosis received from clinicians. Of course, the clinicians must not have access to the test results; otherwise an error known as criterion contamination has been committed. Another example of concurrent validity is to correlate results for a new test with an existing

test administered at the same time. In this case, the relationship should be substantial, on the order of $r = .7$ or higher, to establish the concurrent validity of the new instrument.

Another approach to criterion-related validity is **predictive validity**. In this case the criterion measures are obtained in the future, often months or years after the original test scores are obtained. Many college entrance tests follow this model in which test scores obtained in high school are later correlated with college grade point average for purposes of validating the instruments. Confirmatory results for predictive validity are often lower than for concurrent validity, in the range of .3 to .7.

The final type of validity is **construct validity**. A construct is a theoretical, intangible quality or trait in which persons differ (Messick, 1989). Most psychological tests are designed to measure constructs, examples of which include depression, intelligence, leadership ability, and overcontrolled hostility. Construct validity refers to whether test results from several sources obey a theoretically sensible pattern. There is no single method for evaluating construct validity. Instead, the evidence of construct validity always rests on a program of research. Here are some examples of the kinds of findings that would indicate that a new scale possesses construct validity (Gregory, 1996):

- The scale appears to be homogeneous and therefore measures a single construct.
- Developmental changes over time or across subjects of different ages are consistent with the theory of the construct being measured.
- Differences between well-defined groups on the test are theory-consistent.
- Intervention effects produce changes on test scores that are theory-consistent.
- The scale correlates more strongly with related instruments than with unrelated instruments.
- The factor analysis of test scores yields results that are sensible in light of the theory by which the scale was produced.

The reader will notice that some of the criteria listed here were also discussed under content and criterion-related validity. This is because construct validity subsumes these other kinds of validity. Construct validity is the unifying concept by which test results are shown to be meaningful and is therefore considered the most important of the approaches to test validation.

INTELLIGENCE TESTS

Although there are hundreds of *group* tests of intelligence available for clinical practice, the number of *individual* tests is much, much smaller—less than a dozen at this time (Table 3.1). Of this number, practitioners substantially favor the Wechsler scales and the Stanford-Binet: Fourth Edition. We focus on these instruments but also mention other innovative and useful tests of intelligence.

Wechsler Scales: WPPSI-R, WISC-III, and WAIS-R/III

Although David Wechsler was not the first American to author an intelligence scale, his family

of related tests has dominated the clinical testing scene since the 1950s. When he began work on his first instrument in 1932, he conceived an elegantly simple methodology consisting of about a dozen subtests divided into verbal and performance sections. Within an individual subtest, the examiner begins with easy items and proceeds to a predetermined number of failures, then moves on to the next subtest. When completed, every Wechsler test yields a series of subtest scores normed to a mean of 10 and standard deviation of 3, and Verbal, Performance, and Full Scale IQs, each with the familiar mean of 100 and standard deviation of 15. These features have remained constant over several editions of his three instruments—a shrewd marketing decision which helps explain their enormous popularity. The current versions are the Wechsler Preschool and Primary Scale of Intelligence—Revised (WPPSI-R); the Wechsler Intelligence Scale for Children—III (WISC-III); and the Wechsler Adult Intelligence Scale—R (WAIS-R), which was re-

Table 3.1 Summary of Individual Intelligence Tests in Current Use

WAIS-III	1997	Wechsler Adult Intelligence Scale—III; ages 16 through 89; a slight revision and extension of the highly popular WAIS-R (1981).
KAIT	1992	Kaufman Adolescent and Adult Intelligence Test; ages 11 and up; based on the Cattell-Horn model of fluid/crystallized intelligence.
WISC-III	1991	Wechsler Intelligence Scale for Children—III; ages 6 to 16½; co-normed with the WIAT (Wechsler Individual Achievement Test).
DTLA-3	1991	Detroit Tests of Learning Aptitude—3; ages 6 through 17; the number of composite scores (16) exceeds the number of subtests (11).
DAS	1990	Differential Ability Scales; ages 2½ to 18; the subtests on this measure possess an unusually high degree of specificity.
K-BIT	1990	Kaufman Brief Intelligence Test; ages 4 to 90, this brief screening test (15–30 minutes) has excellent reliability and validity.
WPPSI-R	1989	Wechsler Preschool and Primary Scale of Intelligence—Revised; ages 3 to 7 years and 3 months; an excellent long-term predictor of intelligence and school performance.
SB:FE	1986	Stanford-Binet: Fourth Edition; ages 2 through adulthood; an excellent measure of general intelligence, but the factorial structure is still debated.
K-ABC	1983	Kaufman Assessment Battery for Children; ages 2½ through 12½; an intriguing test based on the distinction between simultaneous and successive processing.
SIT	1983	Slosson Intelligence Test; ages 2 through adulthood; a brief screening test based on the Stanford-Binet and Gesell schedules.
WAIS-R	1981	Wechsler Adult Intelligence Scale—Revised; ages 16 through adulthood; an excellent test of adult intelligence that has been superceded by the WAIS-III (1997).
MSCA	1972	McCarthy Scales of Children's Abilities; ages 2½ to 8½; a good measure of general intelligence that badly needs revision and renorming.

leased as a new edition (WAIS-III) in late 1997. These tests were designed for preschool, school-aged, and adolescent/adult populations, respectively, with some overlap in age ranges between adjacent tests. We focus attention here on the WAIS-R and WAIS-III, and remind the reader that the WPPSI-R and WISC-III are similar in approach—with age-appropriate difficulty level and a few modifications in subtests.

The WAIS-R consists of 11 subtests, which alternate between six verbal subtests and five performance subtests (Table 3.2). The WAIS-III includes a few additional subtests developed to assess abilities on a hypothesized third factor (Attention/Working Memory) and a fourth factor (Speed of Information Processing). Both tests are designed for ages 16 years and up. In addition to scores on the 11 subtests, the WAIS-R yields three summary scores: Verbal IQ, Performance IQ, and Full Scale IQ. The WAIS-III allows for an alternative model in which four composite scores are also reported:

Verbal Comprehension, Perceptual Organization, Working Memory, and Processing Speed. The three traditional IQ scores (Verbal, Performance, Full Scale) demonstrate exceptionally strong reliability, with test–retest coefficients as high as 0.97 for Verbal IQ and Full Scale IQ. From a practical standpoint, this means that Verbal and Full Scale IQ scores can be considered accurate to within ± 5 points. The reliability of Performance IQ is somewhat lower, about .90, but still quite robust. In fact, by traditional psychometric criteria (test–retest, internal consistency), the reliability of WAIS-R and WAIS-III IQs is about as good as could be expected for an instrument that takes less than 90 minutes to administer.

The validity of the WAIS-R/III is strongly supported by its substantial correlation with other intelligence tests (.8 to .9 in many studies) and its capacity to predict intelligence-related criteria such as high school rank and college grades. Test and subtest scores in various groups of persons are also con-

Table 3.2 Subtests and Typical Items on the WAIS-R and WAIS-III

SUBTEST	TYPICAL ITEMS
Vocabulary	Define: *summer, circumference, histrionic, synonymous, obstreperous.*
Information	What is the most common element in air? What is the population of the world? How does fruit juice get converted to wine? Who wrote *Madame Bovary*?
Comprehension	Why do people wear clothes? What does this saying mean: "A bird in the hand is worth two in the bush"? Why are Supreme Court judges appointed for life?
Arithmetic	If you have fifteen apples and give seven away, how many are left? John bought a stereo that was marked down 15 percent from the original sales price of $600. How much did John pay for the stereo?
Similarities	In what way are shirts and socks alike? In what way are a book and a newspaper alike? In what way are a box and a sack alike?
Digit Span	Repeat two- to nine-digit numbers forward; then the same in reverse order.
Block Design	Arrange 4 blocks to match 2 × 2 patterns; then 9 blocks for 3 × 3 patterns.
Object Assembly	Arrange cut-up pieces to resemble common objects, e.g., shoe, bicycle, cat, human face.
Picture Arrangement	Arrange four to six pictures so that they depict increasingly complex stories.
Picture Completion	Find the missing part in increasingly complex pictures.
Digit Symbol	Copy designs associated with digits 1 through 9 as quickly as possible.

Note: In addition to the core subtests listed above, the WAIS-III includes matrix reasoning and optional subtests designed to assess attention and processing speed.

sistent with prevailing theories of intelligence, which buttresses the construct validity of the instrument. For example, the WAIS-R subtests that rely on the retrieval of learned responses reveal far less decline in old age than do the subtests that require the solution of novel problems (Sattler, 1982). This finding has been widely substantiated in gerontological research and fits with the Cattell-Horn theory of intelligence (Horn, 1994).

The WAIS-R is surely an excellent test for the clinical assessment of adult intelligence, but it is not a perfect instrument. One of its notable weaknesses is a quirky anomaly in test scores for the teenagers in the standardization sample, which suggests that these individuals may not have been representative of the population at large. Standardization for the WAIS-III, the successor to the WAIS-R, was carefully planned to eliminate concerns about the representativeness of the standardization sample. This sample included 2,450 persons spanning ages 16 to 89. The sample was stratified on sex, educational level, ethnicity, and region of the country. For these variables, subjects in the standardization group closely mirrored census results for the U.S. population.

Stanford-Binet: Fourth Edition

Now in its fourth edition, the Stanford-Binet is the oldest individual intelligence test in existence. Based on a revision of the original Binet-Simon scales, the first edition of the test was produced by Lewis Terman at Stanford University in 1916. The current version is substantially more intricate—bordering on convoluted—than its predecessors. Whereas the first, second, and third editions (published in 1916, 1937, and 1960) featured only a global IQ score, the fourth edition consists of 15 subtests organized into four areas: verbal, abstract/visual, quantitative, and short-term memory (Table 3.3). The test is designed for ages 2½ and up. Not every subtest is suited to every age level. As a consequence, an examinee is administered only 8 to 10 subtests (depending on his or her age level). This makes the test more manageable but also introduces a problem—the lack of a comparable battery throughout the age levels covered by the test. Young examinees are not administered the same subtests as older examinees, which means that the test measures different aspects of intelligence at different ages.

The SB:FE produces up to 10 subtest scores, 4 area scores, and a composite score (no longer called an IQ) based on the entire test. The instrument possesses very strong psychometric qualities, at least insofar as the global score is concerned. The standardization sample is excellent, reliability of the composite score is substantial (test–retest coefficients in the .90s for most age groups), and the test is clearly valid as a measure of general intelligence. However, it is questionable whether intelligence can be accurately partitioned into the four areas claimed by the authors of the test. Most researchers prefer a two-factor model (verbal, nonverbal) for subjects up to 6 years of age and a three-factor model (verbal, nonverbal, and memory) for children 7 years of age and older (Laurent, Swerdlik, & Ryburn, 1992).

The SB:FE does possess several advantages over the more widely used Wechsler scales. For one thing, the test provides a good supply of very easy items on most subscales, which allows the examiner to obtain a more precise assessment of low-level functioning in children and young adults. Another advantage is that the test includes four subtests that tap different kinds of short-term memory.

Table 3.3 The Four Content Areas and Fifteen Subtests of the Stanford-Binet: Fourth Edition

VERBAL REASONING	QUANTITATIVE REASONING	ABSTRACT/VISUAL REASONING	SHORT-TERM MEMORY
Vocabulary	Quantitative	Pattern Analysis	Bead Memory
Comprehension	Number Series	Copying	Memory for Sentences
Absurdities	Equation Building	Matrices	Memory for Digits
Verbal Relations		Paper Folding/Cutting	Memory for Objects

therefore the instrument of choice
·rral issue provides a suspicion of
rment.

Other Intelligence Tests

Alan Kaufman has devised several innovative tests of intelligence which are gaining in popularity. The Kaufman Assessment Battery for Children (K-ABC) was the first intelligence test constructed within the framework of modern neuropsychology (Kaufman & Kaufman, 1983a, 1983b). Many of its subtests resemble neuropsychological tests. A subtest called Face Recognition, which assesses the ability to recognize a person from different photographs, is explicitly neuropsychological in nature. A highly similar test is found in a recent neuropsychological test battery (Benton, Hamsher, Varney, & Spreen, 1983). Another subtest is Hand Movements, in which the subject must imitate sequences of hand movements involving fist, palm, and side of the hand.

The K-ABC includes a Sequential Processing Scale (Hand Movements illustrates these subtests) and a Simultaneous Processing Scale (Face Recognition illustrates these subtests). All subtests are tied loosely to neuropsychological concepts of sequential or simultaneous processing and, as such, are thought to be more relevant to educational planning than the traditional verbal and performance subtests. In addition, the test includes an Achievement Scale with more traditional content such as Expressive Vocabulary, Arithmetic, and Reading subtests.

One intriguing feature of the K-ABC is that the disparity in global scores between white and minority children is minimal, on the order of 5 points (Kaufman, Kamphaus, & Kaufman, 1985). This is much smaller than for tests such as the WISC-III and Stanford-Binet: Fourth Edition, for which score differences on the order of 15 points, favoring whites, are common. Another noteworthy feature of the test is that children find it especially appealing because of its novel stimuli.

Kaufman has also devised a brief test of intelligence suitable for children and adults (Kaufman & Kaufman, 1990; Kaufman & Wang, 1992). As the name suggests, the Kaufman Brief Intelligence Test (K-BIT) is a short test of intelligence suitable as a screening measure. The test includes a Vocabulary section and a Matrices section. The Vocabulary test consists of two parts: Expressive Vocabulary (naming pictures) and Definitions (providing a word based on a brief phrase and a partial spelling). The Matrices test requires solving 2×2 and 3×3 analogies using abstract stimuli. The K-BIT is normed for subjects 4 to 90 years of age and can be administered in just 15 to 30 minutes. Internal consistency reliability is excellent (.94 for the overall composite), and concurrent validity with established instruments such as the WAIS-R and K-ABC is very strong.

NEUROPSYCHOLOGICAL TESTING

The distinguishing feature of neuropsychological tests is that performance on them is known to be sensitive to the effects of brain impairment. In fact, the original purpose of these instruments was to help diagnose neurological disorders. Experts, such as Ralph Reitan, could make highly accurate inferences as to the location, type, and cause of brain lesions. In the beginning, neuropsychological assessment provided valuable diagnostic information to neurologists and neurosurgeons.

With the advent of ultrasophisticated brain-imaging techniques such as magnetic resonance imaging (MRI) and computerized tomography (CT) scans, the role of neuropsychological testing has shifted from the medical perspective of diagnosis to the psychological perspective of assessment and treatment planning. It no longer makes any sense to ask the neuropsychologist to localize a tumor when an MRI can provide detailed, high-resolution, cross-sectional maps of the brain and reveal abnormalities smaller than the eraser on a pencil.

Neuropsychological test results now provide a basis for patient planning, rehabilitation, and treatment evaluation (Lezak, 1995). The most important function of neuropsychological test results is that they can identify and measure the behavioral consequences of brain damage. This information, in turn, provides a basis for planning interventions and, later, evaluating whether the interventions have had the desired effect.

Individual Neuropsychological Tests

One approach to neuropsychological assessment is to tailor a battery of tests to the specific needs of the individual client. For this approach, a practitioner might choose five to ten relevant instruments from hundreds of available tests such as those found in Lezak's (1995) encyclopedic review. In fact, the number and kinds of neuropsychological tests is so vast that we can only provide a few representative examples here.

Paced Auditory Serial Addition Task

The Paced Auditory Serial Addition Task (PASAT) was originally devised as a means of tracking the recovery of patients who had sustained a relatively minor form of head injury known as concussion. A concussion is a transitory alteration of consciousness from a blow to the head. The temporary consequences often include amnesia, dizziness, nausea, weak pulse, and slow respiration. Most persons make a full recovery from concussion, but the length of time needed to do so can vary from hours to months. The PASAT is helpful in determining whether a patient's capacities for attention and concentration have returned to normal.

The test consists of minimal equipment—audiotape, tape player, and answer sheet for the examiner. After the instructions are carefully explained, the examinee listens to a serious of digits presented on the audiotape and mentally adds together each successive pair of digits. For example, if the numbers presented are "...4...2...8...3 ...5..." the examinee should respond "...6...10... 11...8..."

After a practice set, the test begins with 61 digits, presented at one every 2.4 seconds. This is the first of four series, each consisting of 61 stimuli requiring 60 additions. The presentation speed increases with each series: 2.4, 2.0, 1.6, and 1.2 seconds between digits. The PASAT yields four scores: percentage correct at each of the four presentation speeds.

Although the test is conceptually simple, the information-processing requirements are complex. The examinee must hold two numbers in short-term auditory memory, add them together, verbalize the answer, retain the last of the two numbers, annex the ensuing digit to short-term memory, and then start the cycle over again. Some of these mental activities must be processed in parallel (simultaneously) rather than in simple sequence. Persons with impaired brain functions find the PASAT to be extremely difficult—often impossible.

Extensive age-graded norms are used to determine whether the performance is typical of normal functioning or indicative of continuing brain impairment. The PASAT is highly sensitive to the effects of concussion and identifies patients with ongoing impairment far better than other neuropsychological measures (Stuss, Stethem, Hugenholtz, & Richard, 1989). Because performance declines with age and improves as a function of practice, clinicians must use appropriate age norms and adjust the scores for practice when interpreting PASAT results.

Wechsler Memory Scale—Revised

Patients with brain impairment often complain of problems with memory, but so do depressed persons and others with no objective memory difficulties. A well-validated test of memory can help the clinician assess the reality of suspected brain impairment. The Wechsler Memory Scale—Revised (WMS-R, Wechsler, 1987) is among the best available tests for such purposes (Table 3.4) The WMS-R is an extensive measure of memory that taps auditory and visual modalities and examines both immediate and delayed memory. The 13 subtests yield scores for General Memory (which incorporates Verbal Memory and Visual Memory), Attention/Concentration, and delayed recall for General Memory, with scores on each based on the familiar mean of 100 and standard deviation of 15. The test functions well in the identification of memory deficits in alcoholism, head injury, and other conditions that produce memory impairment (Reid & Kelly, 1993).

Table 3.4 Component Subtests of the Wechsler Memory Scale—Revised

SUBTEST	CONTENT
Information and Orientation	Simple questions covering biographical data, orientation, and information
Logical Memory I	Recall for two brief stories read to examinee
Verbal Paired Associates I	Associative learning of word pairs
Figure Memory	Memory for abstract designs
Visual Paired Associates I	Learning colors associated with abstract line drawings
Visual Reproduction I	Drawing simple geometric designs from memory
Mental Control	Overlearned material such as the alphabet
Digit Span	Traditional digit-span test
Logical Memory II	Recall for Logical Memory I after 30-minute delay
Verbal Paired Associates II	Recall for Verbal Paired Associates I after 30-minute delay
Visual Paired Associates II	Recall for Visual Paired Associates I after 30-minute delay
Visual Reproduction II	Recall for Visual Reproduction I after 30-minute delay

The Halstead-Reitan and Other Fixed Batteries

Neuropsychological assessment can proceed upon one of two paths: a flexible, client-centered test battery tailored to specific referral issues, or a fixed test battery that evaluates the same broad range of capacities for every client. Each approach has strengths and weaknesses. The flexible battery appears more direct and relevant and avoids the use of unnecessary and inappropriate tests. But because this approach is not broad-range, areas of unsuspected weakness might be overlooked. One advantage of a fixed test battery is that the examiner can become an expert on these tests and does not need to keep abreast of the several dozen tests from which a flexible battery might be fashioned. Fixed batteries also tend to be broad-range, so the evaluation can be more thorough. A major disadvantage of the fixed approach, however, is that isolated areas of dysfunction not covered by the battery might be overlooked.

The Halstead-Reitan Neuropsychological Test Battery (Reitan & Wolfson, 1993) is probably the most widely used fixed battery. Certainly there is more validity evidence for this approach than for any other. Three versions are available: young children (5 to 8 years of age), older children (9 to 14 years of age), and adult (15 years and up), which we

discuss here. The core of the adult battery is five tests developed by Ward Halstead in the 1950s and then modified and extended by his protégé, Ralph Reitan, in the ensuing years. The entire battery consists of these five measures together with several ancillary tests and a few traditional measures such as the WAIS-R (Table 3.5). The full battery takes about 6 hours to administer. One disadvantage is that key aspects of the battery are not portable. In particular, the Category Test consists of a large, bulky plywood box with a carousel projector attached to the back.

The Halstead-Reitan provides a wealth of data, which are summarized in 42 variables scored from 0 (perfectly normal) to 3 (severely impaired). The sum of these scores (the General Neuropsychological Deficit Scale) is about 90% accurate in classifying examinees as normal versus brain-impaired. In the hands of a well-trained neuropsychologist, the test battery also provides enough information for reasoned inferences about the nature of any neurological problems. For example, here is Reitan's commentary on one battery of test results:

> For many psychologists, the confusing issue in interpreting W. L.'s results would be in effecting a meaningful integration of the poor and good scores. W. L. obviously did very well on many of the tests, including some most sensitive to cerebral

Table 3.5 Tests and Procedures of the Halstead-Reitan Neuropsychological Test Battery

[a]Category Test	A measure of abstract reasoning and concept formation that requires the examinee to find the rule for categorizing pictures of geometric shapes.
[a]Tactual Performance Test	A measure of kinesthetic and sensorimotor ability; the blindfolded examinee places blocks in appropriate cutouts on an upright board with dominant hand, then nondominant hand, then both hands; also tests for incidental memory of blocks.
[a]Speech Sounds Perception Test	Measures attention and auditory-visual synthesis; requires examinee to pick from four choices the written version of taped nonsense words.
[a]Seashore Rhythm Test	Measures attention and auditory perception; examinee listens to a tape of paired musical rhythms and responds "same" or "different."
[a]Finger Tapping Test	A measure of motor speed that requires examinee to tap a telegraph key–like lever as quickly as possible for 10 seconds.
Grip Strength	Measures grip strength with a dynamometer; the examinee squeezes the grip as hard as possible; separate trials with each hand.
Trail Making, parts A, B	easures scanning ability, mental flexibility, and speed; under pressure of time, the examinee must connect numbers (part A) or numbers and letters in alternating order (part B) with a pencil line.
Tactile Form Recognition	A measure of sensory-perceptual ability that requires the examinee to recognize simple shapes (e.g., triangle) placed in the palm of the hand.
Sensory Perceptual Exam	A measure of sensory-perceptual ability; requires examinee to respond to simple bilateral sensory tasks, e.g., detecting which finger has been touched, which ear has received a brief sound; assesses the visual fields.
Aphasia Screening Test	A measure of expressive and receptive language abilities; tasks include naming a pictured item (e.g., fork), repeating short phrases; copying tasks (not a measure of aphasia) included here for historical reasons.
Supplementary	WAIS-R, WRAT-R, MMPI-2, memory tests such as the Wechsler Memory Scale or Rey Auditory Verbal Learning Test.

[a]Core measures of the Halstead-Reitan Neuropsychological Test Battery

damage and disease. On other tests, though, his performances were definitely abnormal, and were characteristic of the responses seen only in persons with cerebral dysfunction. In this case, those performances related principally to the right cerebral hemisphere, but the pattern of test results would not suggest the presence of a specific, focal right cerebral lesion. The overall pattern of results is characteristic and typical for a particular condition, multiple sclerosis. (Reitan & Wolfson, 1993)

Another widely used fixed battery is the Luria-Nebraska Neuropsychological Battery (LNNB), which has the advantage of taking only two to three hours for administration (Golden, 1989). Separate forms of the LNNB are available for children and adults. The adult version comes in a single briefcase and consists of 269 discrete items, scored 0, 1, or 2. Though shorter than the Halstead-Reitan and also more portable, the LNNB is not as good at identify-

ing the type, location, and consequences of brain damage.

PERSONALITY TESTS

The purpose of personality tests is to measure the consistency and the distinctiveness of the traits and action patterns that characterize each individual. This information is useful for a variety of purposes, ranging from the prediction of job performance to the understanding of emotional problems. Psychologists have been unusually fruitful in devising ways to measure personality, so it is not possible to survey the entire range of approaches. Instead, we focus on major instruments that characterize each of the three major approaches to personality assessment: self-report, projective techniques, and behavioral methods.

Self-Report Inventories

In a self-report inventory, the examinee responds to relatively objective statements by making a choice (true–false), a rating (never, occasionally, often), or other structured answer. These are typically paper-and-pencil tests, which are usually computer-scored and frequently interpreted by computer as well. Self-report inventories may provide an omnibus overview of many personality dimensions or focus on one aspect of personality, such as anxiety, self-esteem, or depression.

MMPI-2

The Minnesota Multiphasic Personality Inventory—2 (MMPI-2) is a 1989 revision and restandardization of the MMPI, first released in 1943 (Butcher & Williams, 1992; Graham, 1993). The latest edition is a 567-item true–false inventory designed to assess clinical dimensions of personality such as health concerns, depression, antisocial behavior, schizophrenia, social discomfort, alcohol/ drug abuse, and many other areas discussed below. Though designed primarily as a measure of abnormal personality, the test provides information about normal, healthy functioning as well. Results are interpreted in relation to the latest normative sample of 2,600 adults loosely representative of the general population on major demographic variables (geographic location, race, age, occupational level, and income). Although persons with higher levels of education are slightly overrepresented, these are precisely the individuals most likely to take the MMPI-2. The MMPI-2 is intended for persons ages 18 years and up. An adolescent version, the MMPI-A, should be used for subjects younger than 18 years of age.

The MMPI-2 can be scored for 4 validity scales, 10 standard clinical scales, and an ever-expanding list of supplementary scales. The most important information is provided by the validity scales and the standard clinical scales, although more specific concerns (e.g., about drug abuse) can be reviewed with one or more of the supplementary scales. Most of the clinical scales were devised by means of the empirical-criterion approach, in which test responses of homogeneous clinical groups were contrasted with normal subjects to identify relevant scale items. For example, the item composition of the original 60-item Depression scale was determined by comparing endorsement frequencies (for each item) of 50 cases of relatively pure depression with endorsement frequencies of 724 normal subjects. With the revision and restandardization of the MMPI-2, three of these items were deleted and two were changed, resulting in a shorter scale (57 items) but a more sensitive index of depression.

Table 3.6 describes the traditional scales and provides items similar to those found on the MMPI-2. Raw scores on each scale are converted to T-scores with a mean of 50 and a standard deviation of 10. Scores that exceed T of 65 are considered clinically interesting because they often signify the presence of psychiatric symptomatology.

An MMPI-2 profile is reproduced in Figure 3.1. This patient was a 37-year-old single woman with a history of mental illness, including three hospitalizations for depression (Butcher, 1990). The patient exhibited a serious degree of depression coupled with confusion and disorganization. She was experiencing auditory hallucinations and showed some suicidal preoccupation. All of these problems are evident in her profile, which features prominent elevations on scale 2 (indicating serious depression) and scale 8 (signaling confusion and disorganization). The profile also reveals secondary elevations on scale 6 (suggesting the likelihood of paranoid features including auditory hallucinations) and scale 0 (indicating a dysfunctional degree of social introversion).

Increasingly, the MMPI-2 and other self-report inventories are interpreted by means of computer. Although it is always possible for the clinician to write an individualized report, computerized narrative reports have become so sophisticated that many clinicians are satisfied to let the computer do the work and then check for the possibility of an erroneous interpretation. This is a controversial practice, which we will discuss.

NEO-PI-R

The MMPI-2 excels in the identification of pathological characteristics but is less useful in por-

Table 3.6 MMPI-2 Validity and Clinical Scales and Simulated Items

Validity Scales	
? (Cannot Say)	Number of items left unanswered.
L (Lie)	15 items indicating unlikely virtues such as "I am never irritable with others." (true)
F (Frequency)	60 items endorsed less than 10% of the time by normal subjects, such as "I hear voices that tell me what to do." (true)
K (Correction)	30 items reflecting subtle defensiveness and a reluctance to admit problems, such as "Occasionally I feel like smashing things." (false)
Clinical Scales	
Hs or **1** (Hypochondriasis)	32 items indicating abnormal concern with health and bodily functions, such as "I rarely worry about my health." (false)
D or **2** (Depression)	57 items reflecting pessimism, dysphoria, and feelings of hopelessness, such as "I feel sad and blue much of the time." (true)
Hy or **3** (Hysteria)	60 items that suggest repression, denial, and the use of symptoms as a way of avoiding interpersonal conflicts or personal responsibilities, such as "I try to be friendly with those who have wronged me." (true)
Pd or **4** (Psychopathic Deviate)	50 items that indicate family conflicts, emotional shallowness, a disregard for social customs, and scrapes with the law, such as "I rarely have conflicts with those in authority." (false)
Mf or **5** (Masculinity-Femininity)	56 items that differentiate men and women, such as "I like to repair things." (true, for masculinity)
Pa or **6** (Paranoia)	40 items that reflect excessive sensitivity, suspiciousness, or paranoid delusions, such as "I believe that people are following me." (true)
Pt or **7** (Psychasthenia)	48 items showing unusual fears, rumination, guilt, and indecisiveness, such as "I rarely find myself worrying about things." (false)
Sc or **8** (Schizophrenia)	78 items indicating delusions, hallucinations, alienation, and unusual thoughts or behavior, such as "I feel alone almost all the time." (true)
Ma or **9** (Hypomania)	46 items that indicate overactivity, emotional excitement, and flight of ideas, such as "My speech is faster than it used to be." (true)
Si or **0** (Social Introversion)	69 items that portray shyness and introversion, such as "I like to go to parties." (false)

traying variations in normal personality. For this purpose the NEO Personality Inventory—Revised (NEO PI-R) would be a better choice. This test embodies decades of factor-analytic research with both normal and clinical adult populations. The NEO PI-R is based on a five-factor model of personality that has emerged from several lines of research (Costa & McCrae, 1992). It is available in two parallel forms of 240 items each. Unlike most self-report inventories, which use a true–false format, the NEO PI-R employs a five-point rating scale for items: strongly disagree, disagree, neutral, agree, strongly agree. The items assess emotional, interpersonal, experiential, attitudinal, and motivational variables.

Each of the five scales of the NEO PI-R is based on six trait subscales (Table 3.7). This test exhibits superb psychometric properties, with internal consistency reliabilities of .86 to .95 for the scales and test–retest stability coefficients of .51 to .83 in three- to seven-year longitudinal studies. The validity of the NEO PI-R is also very strong, based on correlations with other measures, correspondence of ratings between self and spouse, and concurrence of the five-factor model with other lines of research (Costa & McCrae, 1992; Piedmont & Weinstein, 1993). One of its most desirable features is that the trait subscales capture aspects of personality that are easily understood by psychologist and layperson alike.

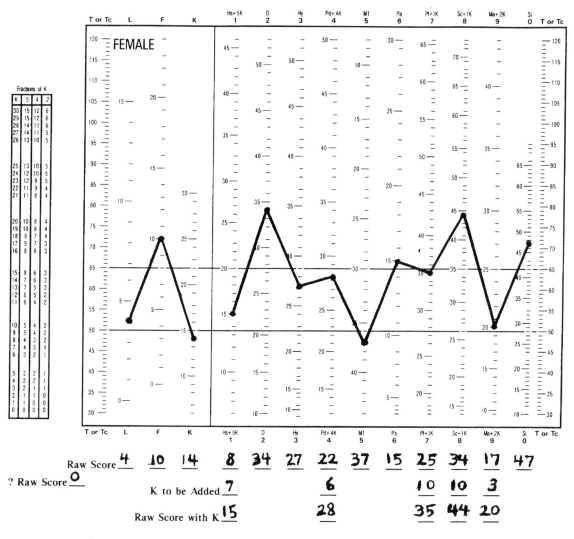

Figure 3.1. MMPI-2 clinical profile of a 37-year-old female with a history of mental illness.

Source: Reprinted with permission from Butcher, J. N. (1990). *The MMPI-2 in psychological treatment.* New York: Oxford University Press. (Minnesota Multiphasic Personality Inventory-2, Copyright © 1989 the Regents of the University of Minnesota. All rights reserved. "MMPI-2" and "Minnesota Multiphasic Personality Inventory-2" are trademarks owned by the University of Minnesota.)

Other Self-Report Inventories

Millon has developed the Millon Clinical Multiaxial Inventory, now in its third edition (MCMI-III) to aid in the classification of personality disorders such as schizoid personality disorder, borderline personality disorder, narcissistic personality disorder, and the like (Millon, 1994). The personality disorders are not explicitly assessed by major inventories such as the MMPI-2, and it was this omission that Millon sought to address with his 175-item true–false inventory. Many clinicians regard the MCMI-III as a useful supplement to the MMPI-2 because of its capacity to assess the lifelong influences that shape personality disorders.

Another widely used test is the Sixteen Personality Factor Questionnaire (16PF), a true–false inven-

Table 3.7 Scales and Trait Subscales of the NEO PI-R

SCALES	TRAIT SUBSCALES	
Neuroticism	Anxiety Angry Hostility Depression	Self-Consciousness Impulsiveness Vulnerability
Extraversion	Warmth Gregariousness Assertiveness	Activity Excitement Seeking Positive Emotions
Openness to Experience	Fantasy Aesthetics Feelings	Actions Ideas Values
Agreeableness	Trust Straightforwardness Altruism	Compliance Modesty Tender-Mindedness
Conscientiousness	Competence Order Dutifulness	Achievement Striving Self-Discipline Deliberation

tory predicated on a factor-analytic conception of personality (Cattell, Eber, & Tatsuoka, 1970). This test uses an unusual forced-choice item format of the following type:

I make decisions based on
  a. feelings
  b. feelings and reason equally
  c. reason

In a series of studies, Cattell determined that 16 dimensions of personality are needed to explain the structure of test responses, hence the name for this test. In addition to 16 bipolar scales that measure such attributes as warmth, dominance, impulsivity, sensitivity, and insecurity, the test also provides four summative indices of extraversion, anxiety, tough poise, and independence. An important use of the 16PF is for occupational testing and career guidance.

Projective Tests and Techniques

The term **projective method** was invented by Frank (1939) to describe a category of tests for studying personality with purposefully unstructured stimuli. The central assumption of this approach is that examinees will unknowingly reveal important aspects of personality (needs, motives, and conflicts) when asked to respond to vague, ambiguous stimuli. Proponents of the projective method typically believe that responses to such stimuli represent projections from the innermost unconscious mental and emotional processes of the examinee.

Rorschach

The most widely used projective test—indeed, one of the most widely used tests of any kind—is the Rorschach inkblot technique devised early in the twentieth century by Hermann Rorschach (1921). This test consists of 10 inkblots devised by dribbling ink on a sheet of paper and folding the paper in half to produce roughly symmetrical designs. Five of the inkblots are black or shades of gray, and five contain color. The Rorschach can be administered to children as young as age 5 but is more commonly used with adults. An inkblot similar to those found on the Rorschach is shown in Figure 3.2.

Administration of the Rorschach consists of two phases. In the free-association phase, the examiner presents the blots one at a time and asks "What might this be?" More than one response can be given. This is followed by an inquiry phase in which the examiner determines the location of the individ-

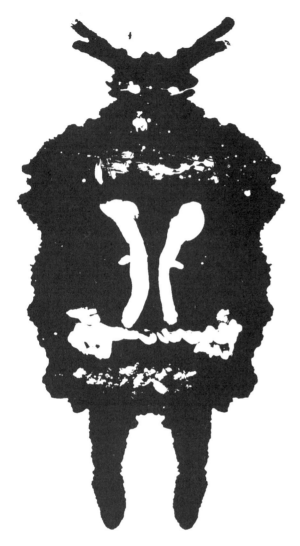

Figure 3.2. An inkblot similar to those on the Rorschach.

ual percepts and seeks to identify those aspects of the blot (such as form, color, and shading) that played a part in the creation of the response.

Although interpretation of the Rorschach can proceed on clinical lines ("Based upon my understanding of unconscious processes, the response of 'cat baring his fangs' to card I would appear to indicate..."), the preferable approach is to use a formal scoring and interpretive system like that provided by John Exner (1991, 1993). In Exner's Comprehensive Scoring System, each individual response is scored for location, determinants, con-

tent, originality, and other variables (Table 3.8). The individual scores are then collated to form various summary indices such as F+ percentage, which is the proportion of the total responses that use pure form as a determinant. These indices are then used to form reasonable, empirically based hypotheses about personality functioning. For example, when the F+ percent falls below 70%, the examiner should consider the possibility of severe psychopathology, brain damage, or intellectual deficit in the examinee (Exner, 1993).

Thematic Apperception Test

The Thematic Apperception Test (TAT) consists of 30 pictures illustrating a variety of themes and topics in black and white drawings and photographs; one card is blank. Most of the pictures depict one or more persons engaged in ambiguous ac-

Table 3.8 Summary of Major Rorschach Scoring Criteria

I. Location: Where on the blot was the percept located?		
W	Whole	Entire inkblot used
D	Common detail	Well-defined part used
Dd	Unusual detail	Unusual part used
S	Space	Percept defined by white space
II. Determinant: What feature of the blot determined the response?		
F	Form	Shape or outline used
F+	Form+	Excellent match of percept and inkblot
F–	Form–	Very poor match of percept and inkblot
M	Movement	Movement seen or implied in percept
C	Color	Color helped determine the response
T	Texture	Shading involved in the response
III. Content: What was the percept?		
H	Human	Percept of a whole human form
Hd	Human detail	Human form incomplete in any way
Ex	Explosion	An actual explosion perceived
Xy	X-ray	X-ray of any human part; involves shading
IV. Popular vs. Original		
P	Popular	Response given by 33% or more of normals
O	Original	Rare and creative response

Note: This table represents a consensus of several major scoring systems. The list is incomplete and is illustrative only.

tivities. Some cards are appropriate only for adult males (M), adult females (F), boys (B), or girls (G), such that exactly 20 cards are targeted for every subject. A picture similar to those on the TAT is shown in Figure 3.3. For each card, the examiner instructs the subject to make up a dramatic story, telling what led up to the current scene, what is happening at the moment, what are the characters thinking and feeling, and how will the story turn out. The responses are recorded verbatim for later scoring and analysis.

Even though many scoring systems have been proposed for the TAT, the most common method of interpretation is clinical-qualitative, in which the examiner infers the motivations, needs, and strivings of the subject on the basis of the content of the stories. A central postulate of this approach is the "hero" assumption, in which the subject is thought to project his or her own needs, strivings, and feelings onto the central character in each card. Wade and Baker (1977) reported that 82% of test-users employ this kind of "personalized" procedure for TAT interpretation. Unfortunately, there is no way to evaluate the validity of this approach because it is idiosyncratic to each examiner and not open to empirical research. Although new TAT scoring methods show much promise, this instrument is sorely in need of restandardization in both administration and scoring approaches. Another concern about the TAT is that many of the pictures depict dark, gloomy themes, so that the test tends to "pull" for unhappy stories. Perhaps it is time for someone to propose a completely new version of the TAT.

Other Projective Approaches

Sentence completion tests are popular because they often provide useful information with a minimal investment of testing time. In a sentence completion test, the examinee is provided with several sentence stems consisting of the first few words and asked to provide an ending. Examples include "My mother _____ " and "I only wish _____ ." The fundamental assumption of this technique is that the examinee will reveal underlying motivations, attitudes, conflicts, and fears in his or her responses. Interpretation can proceed along subjective-intuitive lines or the examiner can assign scores to each completed sentence according to a test manual. The Rotter Incomplete Sentences Blank (RISB), a popular and widely used sentence completion technique, provides an objective scoring system by which each completed sentence receives an adjustment score from zero (good adjustment) to 6 (very poor adjustment). The sum of all the scores for the 40 sentences yields an index of maladjustment (Lah, 1989; Rotter & Rafferty, 1950). This scoring system is highly reliable, but its validity as an index of maladjustment is more questionable as a result of high rates of misclassification. For example, the maladjustment index correctly classified delinquent youths only 60% of the time while identifying nondelinquent youths correctly 73% of the time (Fuller, Parmelee, & Carroll, 1982). These rates are much too low for individual decision making or effective screening.

Expressive techniques such as human figure drawing constitute another family of widely used projective tests. In the most common of these techniques, the examinee is given a blank piece of paper and asked to "draw a person." The pioneer in this

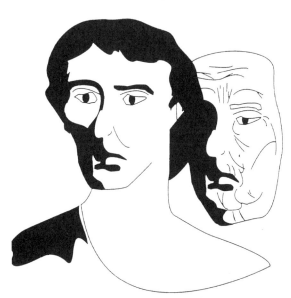

Figure 3.3. A picture similar to those on the thematic apperception test.

Source: Reprinted with permission from Gregory, R. J. (1996). *Psychological testing: History, principles, and applications* (2nd ed.). Boston: Allyn and Bacon.

approach was Karen Machover; her test, the Draw-A-Person Test (DAP), is still popular. Interpretation is entirely clinical-intuitive, with relevant sources providing numerous psychodynamically based hypotheses (Machover, 1949). For example, the omission of facial features is thought to indicate evasiveness about highly conflictual interpersonal relationships; a graphic emphasis of the neck suggests anxiety about the lack of control over impulses; the mouth drawn with a heavy line slash indicates a verbally aggressive and overly critical person.

An enduring problem with expressive drawing techniques such as the DAP is that empirical support for the colorful and plausible interpretations is virtually nonexistent. Every psychologist can cite anecdotal support for specific hypotheses, but these may be nothing more than illusory validation. **Illusory validation** is the empirically demonstrated phenomenon in which confirming instances are noticed but more numerous findings that contradict expectations are ignored (Chapman & Chapman, 1967). Even so, it is possible for the draw-a-person technique to possess an empirical foundation, as demonstrated by the successful application of this approach to the screening of children for behavior disorder and emotional disturbance (Naglieri & Pfeiffer, 1992). As with all projective techniques, the key to justifiable use resides in the development and validation of an objective scoring method.

Behavioral Approaches

Behavioral tests include a variety of straightforward approaches to personality evaluation. Unlike self-report and projective techniques, which focus on underlying traits, hypothetical causes, and presumed dimensions of personality, behavioral tests concentrate directly on behavior itself. A good review of behavioral techniques can be found in the *Dictionary of Behavioral Assessment Techniques* (Hersen & Bellak, 1988). We will illustrate this family of approaches by describing the behavioral avoidance test (BAT), an approach that is highly useful in gauging a patient's progress in overcoming fears such as the disabling fear of open spaces known as agoraphobia.

Hoffart, Friis, Strand, and Olsen (1994) devised a standardized BAT for patients with agoraphobia that is elegant in its simplicity:

> The patients were asked to walk alone as far as they could from the hospital along a mildly trafficated road that was 2 km long. The route was divided into eight intervals of equal length, and the patients rated their anxiety level on a 0–10 scale at the end of each interval. Uncompleted intervals were given a score of 10. An avoidance–anxiety score was computed by summing the anxiety scores for all intervals.

The reader will notice the direct relationship between a major goal of therapy (increasing the patient's capacity to venture alone into open spaces) and performance on the test. It is characteristic of behavioral tests that they capture—very directly—the desired features of a successful therapeutic outcome.

TESTING SPECIAL POPULATIONS

Testing Persons with Disabilities

Persons with disabilities present a special challenge in psychological testing because impairments in hearing, vision, speech, or motor control can invalidate traditional test results. A number of specialized tests have been developed for individuals with these disabilities, and we will discuss a few of them here. A first point, however, is that the examiner must recognize that a prospective subject has a disability—not always a straightforward matter. Particularly when testing children, referral for vision or hearing examination may be needed to identify a mild disability such as a fluctuating hearing loss due to periodic accumulation of fluid in the middle ear during episodes of illness. In other cases, considerable detective work may be needed to confirm that an adolescent has a mild case of cerebral palsy—which would invalidate performance-based test results requiring dexterity and motor speed. Several tests are available when an examinee's disability would invalidate traditional measures. We cannot review all of the relevant instruments, but a few examples will illustrate their variety.

For hearing-impaired children ages 3 to 17 years, the Hiskey-Nebraska Test of Learning Aptitude (H-NTLA) serves as a useful nonlanguage measure of ability. This test is unique in that it can be administered entirely through pantomime and requires no verbal response from the examinee. The H-NTLA consists of 12 subtests:

Bead Patterns	Block Patterns
Memory for Color	Completion of Drawings
Picture Identification	Memory for Digits
Picture Association	Puzzle Blocks
Paper Folding	Picture Analogies
Visual Attention Span	Spatial Reasoning

Correlation of global scores with WISC-R Performance IQ is substantial ($r = .85$), indicating that the H-NTLA is an excellent measure of performance-based intelligence (Hiskey, 1966; Phelps & Ensor, 1986).

A test that is both nonreading and motor-reduced is the Peabody Picture Vocabulary Test—Revised (PPVT-R; Dunn & Dunn, 1981). The PPVT-R can be used to obtain a rapid measure of vocabulary with speech-impaired persons, deaf individuals, and persons with problems of motor control (e.g., cerebral palsy) ages 2 ½ to 18. The test consists of a series of 175 plates, each with four line drawings of objects or everyday scenes. The examiner displays a plate, states a stimulus word orally, and asks the examinee to point to the picture that best portrays the stated word. The global score is normed to a mean of 100 and standard deviation of 15. Care must be taken with ethnic minorities (especially Native Americans) and persons with mental retardation, for whom PPVT-R scores can be much lower than IQ scores on standard instruments such as the Wechsler scales. Though not a substitute for a general intelligence test, the PPVT-R is a useful measure of hearing vocabulary.

Testing in Mental Retardation

Mental retardation refers to substantial limitations in present functioning as a consequence of significantly subaverage intellectual functioning (IQ of 70 to 75 or below) and related limitations in two or more adaptive skill areas. Onset must be before age 18 (American Association on Mental Retardation, 1992). With respect to psychological testing, the most important point to emphasize is that low IQ is an insufficient basis for the diagnosis of mental retardation. In addition, the examinee must manifest limitations in two or more of these ten adaptive skills areas:

- Communication
- Self-care
- Home living
- Social skills
- Community use
- Self-direction
- Health and safety
- Functional academics
- Leisure
- Work

Limitations in adaptive skill are more difficult to assess than a low IQ, but several instruments can aid in this process. The Vineland Adaptive Behavior Scales (Sparrow, Balla, & Cicchetti, 1984) is a revision and extension of the Vineland Social Maturity Scale (Doll, 1935, 1936), the first standardized instrument for assessing adaptive behavior. Another useful test is the Scales of Independent Behavior (SIB; Bruininks, Woodcock, Weatherman, & Hill, 1984), which we highlight here.

The SIB consists of a series of 14 subscales that are completed with the help of a parent, caregiver, or teacher. For each subscale, the examiner reads a series of items and enlists the aid of the parent, caregiver, or teacher in assigning a score from 0 (never or rarely does task) to 3 (does task very well). The 14 subscales are arranged into four clusters, as outlined in Table 3.9. A Broad Independence score with the usual mean of 100 (the adaptive functioning equivalent of an IQ score) is obtained from the average of the four cluster scores. SIB scores correlate very strongly with IQ scores ($r = .81$ to $.88$) and provide an essential confirmation that the examinee has limitations in adaptive functioning and not just a low IQ score.

Table 3.9 The 14 Subscales and 4 Clusters
of the Scales of Independent Behavior

---

1. Motor Skills
     Gross Motor
     Fine Motor

2. Social and Communication Skills
     Social Interaction
     Language Comprehension
     Language Expression

3. Personal-Living Skills
     Eating and Meal Preparation
     Dressing
     Personal Self-Care
     Domestic Skills

4. Community-Living Skills
     Time and Punctuality
     Money and Value
     Work Skills
     Home–Community Orientation

COMPUTER-BASED TEST INTERPRETATION

Computers are now widely used in psychological testing. The most straightforward and accepted uses include the presentation of test stimuli (such as the individual items on a self-report personality test), the recording of responses (including latency of response if needed), the scoring of test results, and the printing of summary data and test profiles. Of course, it is necessary to demonstrate that the computerized version of a test possesses the same psychometric properties as the original paper-and-pencil version—such equivalence should not be taken for granted. Fortunately, most tests prove to measure the same properties whether administered by printed questionnaire or computer screen, so the computer as handservant to the tester is rarely a matter of controversy.

Controversy does arise when the computer is used to *interpret* test results. With many tests, it is not unusual for a lengthy narrative report to emerge from the printer with no intervening input from the psychologist. This is a particularly commonplace practice in personality testing. The publishers of every major instrument now offer computerized narrative reports as part of their service. The psychologist is not obliged to use these reports, but many practitioners do. It is reasonable to ask whether computer-based test interpretations are a desirable

development in the practice of psychological testing.

A key question in resolving this issue is whether the interpretive statements in a computerized narrative report are based on quantitative research (more desirable) or the clinical opinion of experts (less desirable). Years ago, Meehl (1954) demonstrated that *actuarial* judgment (in which research-based formulas are used to diagnose, classify, or predict behavior) is almost always superior to *clinical* judgment (in which psychologists use experience and intuition to diagnose, classify, or predict behavior). This humbling truth has been demonstrated repeatedly in the ensuing years (Dawes, Faust, & Meehl, 1989; Kleinmuntz, 1990; Meehl, 1965, 1986).

Unfortunately, many computer-based test interpretations are based on clinical judgment and thus their validity is largely unproved. Lanyon (1984) points out that consumer professionals are predisposed to believe whatever is printed and unable to discriminate between more satisfactory (i.e., actuarially based) and less satisfactory (i.e., clinically based) computerized test interpretation systems:

> Particularly distressing is that the lack of demonstrated program validity has now become the norm, and there appear to be no checks against the further development of this untenable situation. Perhaps the time has now come when federal regulations for this industry are necessary for consumer protection.

Matarazzo (1986) has sounded a similar alarm. In addition, he has argued that the use of computerized narrative reports should not be confused with a comprehensive assessment. In a comprehensive assessment, the practitioner goes beyond test interpretations to *integrate* the findings as a cohesive response to referral issues surrounding the examinee. The danger in computer-based test interpretation is that simple testing will replace comprehensive assessment.

CURRENT STATUS AND ISSUES IN PSYCHOLOGICAL TESTING

The Enduring Question of Test Bias

An enduring question in modern psychology is whether psychological tests are biased. Much of the lay public and even many psychologists are quick to assert that individual tests (particularly ability-related tests) contain culture or gender bias and therefore discriminate unfairly against racial and ethnic minorities, women, or the poor. Are these criticisms warranted? To answer this question, we will need to objectify what is meant by *test bias*, since agreement on this concept is far from complete. An important starting point is to emphasize that appearances can be deceiving. The fact that certain test items "look" preferential to one race, sex, or social class does not prove test bias. Test bias must be defined in objective, empirically testable terms and not relegated to a matter of personal opinion.

The most widely accepted notion of test bias is that of differential validity. According to this approach, a test is biased if the same test score means something different for any definable, relevant subgroup of test-takers: "Bias is present when a test score has meanings or implications for a relevant, definable subgroup of test takers that are different from the meanings or implications for the remainder of the test takers" (Cole & Moss, 1989). Perhaps a simple example will clarify this definition. Consider an ability-related test that is used to predict the academic performance of school-aged children. This test would be considered biased if a low score accurately predicted poor school performance for one ethnic subgroup but the same low score showed no relationship with school performance for another subgroup.

From a technical standpoint, several methods are available for investigating test bias. One approach is to conduct factor analyses of test scores within definable subgroups. An unbiased test will show a similar factorial structure across subgroups. Regression equations also constitute a good basis for evaluating test bias. When test scores are used to predict relevant criteria (e.g., scores on a high school aptitude test are used to predict college grades) an unbiased test will reveal similar prediction equations and equal predictive power for different subgroups. Another approach involves the rank ordering of item difficulties within a test. For an unbiased test, the relative difficulty level of individual test items (i.e., their rank orderings) will be the same across definable subgroups. By these and other bias detection statistical methods, prominent psychological tests fare quite well. In fact, the consensus of all the major reviews is that the available research has failed to support the test bias hypothesis (Gregory, 1996; Reynolds, 1994).

These comments notwithstanding, the test bias controversy is unlikely to go away soon. The reason for this is that *tests in use* can produce social outcomes that are perceived as unfair and prejudicial. A case in point is the use of psychological tests to place disproportionate numbers of minority children in special education programs, ostensibly for their own good but in reality to their detriment. The problem here is not so much with tests and their bias (or lack thereof) as with well-meaning social policies that have unintended consequences. In truth, many compensatory education programs are stigmatizing and inferior—otherwise there would be no anguish in classifying children of any race, sex, or class as needing such placement. Perhaps we should speak of this larger social issue as *test fairness*, so as to distinguish it from the narrower technical issue of test bias. Unbiased tests still might be deemed unfair because of the prejudicial consequences of how they are used.

Abuses of Testing

Almost anything that is useful also has the potential for harmful social consequences, and this is certainly true of psychological testing. The demonstrated ill effects of testing tend to fall into one of two categories. The first type of negative impact stems from making important decisions on the basis of limited test data. A well-publicized case in this regard is that of Daniel Hoffman, who was placed in a class for mentally retarded persons when he was 5 years old because his Stanford-Binet IQ was only 74 (Sattler, 1988). Unknown to the examiner, Daniel's only real handicap was a speech impediment. However, the initial assessment was completed in a hurried manner, so the examiner never learned of this disability. Compounding the harm, Daniel was not retested for 11 years, at which time he received a normal-range WISC IQ of 94. Ironically, this test result was then used to deny him access to a special workshop program that he enjoyed!

At least three errors were made in the case of Daniel Hoffman (Gregory, 1987). First, important decisions should never be made on the basis of limited test information. As noted previously, when testing for mental retardation, it is always wise to obtain information about adaptive functioning in addition to IQ test scores. A second error was the failure to retest Daniel in a year or two, since the instability of IQ results is well known—at least to any well-trained psychologist. Finally, test cutoff scores should never be used in a rigid manner to include or exclude someone from special programs.

A second abuse of testing that has been highlighted more recently is the use of inappropriate tests for decision making. This is most likely to occur in preemployment screening than elsewhere, because employers need an efficient way to identify good prospects and weed out undesirable applicants. Unfortunately, in the quest to perform such functions expediently, it is easy to trample on the rights of job applicants. A case in point is the use of a 704-item true–false personality inventory by a major discount chain store as a screening test for security guards (Gregory, 1996). The problem with the use of this instrument was that its value in predicting job performance was not demonstrated prior to its use as a screening tool. From the standpoint of prospective employees, the test seemed arbitrary, irrelevant, and even bizarre. They sued the chain, citing a lack of evidence that the test helped identify good versus poor risks for employment. The case was settled out of court, and corporate officers agreed not to use the screening device for at least five years—time enough to discover whether the test was valid for this purpose.

The Future of Testing

Predicting the future of testing is difficult because the use of psychological tests is substantially affected by public opinion as translated into legal mandates—factors that are notoriously fickle and unstable. For example, at one point in the 1980s it was *illegal* in the state of California to use traditional intelligence tests for purposes of program placement—except under special and restrictive conditions. Another example is that many states now specify *exactly* which test(s) must be used to determine eligibility for programs such as SSI (Supplemental Security Income) rather than leaving it to a licensed psychologist to select the most appropriate instruments. Still another example is federal legislation outlawing the use of polygraph tests for most types of employment (probably a good idea). Increasingly, the practice of psychological testing is governed by legal and social influences, which makes predicting the future of testing a risky business.

If current trends continue, however, a few broad predictions would appear to be safe. The first has to do with the increasing computerization of psychological testing. Not only will existing tests be increasingly adapted to the computer, but new tests never before possible will emerge as a consequence of dramatic improvements in information technology. Consider the multimedia test being developed at IBM to assess job applicants for manufacturing positions. Whereas previous paper-and-pencil tests might have described work situations and then asked the examinee how he or she would respond, with computers it is now possible to display actual work scenes, including those that involve interactions between workers. As the applicant observes brief work vignettes, the screen freezes at crucial junctions and the computer then asks what the candidate would do in that situation. The work scenes have a highly realistic appearance that enhances the face validity of the test. Because of the realism inherent in the video display, computerized tests may provide a more valid assessment than paper-and-pencil tests of how an applicant would actually perform on the job (Gregory, 1996).

Another likely trend is that fewer and fewer wide-spectrum instruments—omnibus personality inventories and tests of general ability—will be released by test publishers. Instead, publishers will focus on tests designed to assess circumscribed areas of functioning for highly specific target populations. The reason for these complementary trends has to do with simple economics. Test publishing is big business, a respectable way for large corporations to earn a profit. Publishers will be reluctant to make the major investment needed to develop new instruments that have the grandiose ambition of assessing many aspects of personality or intellect for a wide range of subjects. The cost is too high and—in light of the existing competition—the risk is too great.

Instead, test designers and publishers alike will focus on less expensive and less risky forms of test development. These would be instruments that embody construct specificity (measuring highly specific aspects of functioning such as faulty cognitions in depressed persons or risky behaviors in adolescents or mental decline in the aged) and target specificity (designing tests for well-demarcated groups of patients such as maritally distressed couples or patients with pain or persons who appear suicidal). In short, we foresee a stagnation in the release of wide-spectrum tests of intelligence, personality, interests, and the like (with established instruments being revised and recycled periodically) amid an explosion of minor tests of highly focused constructs for use with well-defined subgroups of examinees.

REFERENCES

American Association on Mental Retardation. (1992). *Mental retardation: Definition, classification, and systems of supports*. Washington, DC: Author.

Anastasi, A. (1986). Emerging concepts of test validation. *Annual Review of Psychology, 37*, 1–15.

Benton, A. L., Hamsher, K., Varney, N. R., & Spreen, O. (1983). *Contributions to neuropsychological assessment*. New York: Oxford University Press.

Binet, A., & Simon, T. (1905). Méthodes nouvelles pour le diagnostic du niveau intellectuel des anormaux. *Année Psychologique, II*, 211–244.

Bruininks, R. H., Woodcock, R. W., Weatherman, R. F., & Hill, B. K. (1984). *Scales of Independent Behavior, Interviewer's Manual*. Allen, TX: DLM Teaching Resources.

Butcher, J. N. (1990). *The MMPI-2 in psychological treatment*. New York: Oxford University Press.

Butcher, J. N., & Williams, C. L. (1992). *Essentials of MMPI-2 and MMPI-A interpretation*. Minneapolis: University of Minnesota Press.

Campbell, D. P., Hyne, S., & Nilsen, D. (1992). *Manual for the Campbell Interest and Skill Survey*. Minneapolis, MN: National Computer Systems.

Cattell, J. McK. (1890). Mental tests and measurements. *Mind, 15*, 373–380.

Cattell, R. B., Eber, H. W., & Tatsuoka, M. M. (1970). *Handbook for the Sixteen Personality Factor Questionnaire*. Champaign, IL: Institute for Personality and Ability Testing.

Chapman, L. J., & Chapman, J. P. (1967). Genesis of popular but erroneous psychodiagnostic observations. *Journal of Abnormal Psychology, 74*, 271–280.

Cole, N. S., & Moss, P. A. (1989). Bias in test use. In R. L. Linn (Ed.), *Educational measurement* (3rd ed., pp. 201–220). New York: ACE/Macmillan.

Conoley, J. C., & Impara, J. C. (Eds.). (1995). *The twelfth mental measurements yearbook*. Lincoln: University of Nebraska Press.

Costa, P. T., Jr., & McCrae, R. (1992). *NEO PI-R test manual*. Port Huron, MI: Sigma Assessment Systems.

Dawes, R. M., Faust, D., & Meehl, P. E. (1989). Clinical versus actuarial judgment. *Science, 243*, 1668–1674.

Doll, E. A. (1935). The Vineland Social Maturity Scale. *Training School Bulletin, 32*, 1–7, 25–32, 48–55, 68–74.

Doll, E. A. (1936). Preliminary standardization of the Vineland Social Maturity Scale. *American Journal of Orthopsychiatry, 6*, 283–293.

Dunn, L. M., & Dunn, L. M. (1981). *Peabody Picture Vocabulary Test—Revised*. Circle Pines, MN: American Guidance Service.

Exner, J. E., Jr. (1991). *The Rorschach: A comprehensive system: Vol. 2. Current research and advanced interpretation* (2nd ed.). New York: Wiley.

Exner, J. E., Jr. (1993). *The Rorschach: A comprehensive system: Vol. 1. Basic foundations* (3rd ed.). New York: Wiley.

Frank, L. K. (1939). Projective methods for the study of personality. *Journal of Psychology, 8*, 389–413.

Fuller, G. B., Parmelee, W. M., & Carroll, J. L. (1982). Performance of delinquent and nondelinquent high school boys on the Rotter Incomplete Sentences Blank. *Journal of Personality Assessment, 46*, 506–510.

Gelb, S. (1986). Henry H. Goddard and the immigrants, 1910–1917: The studies and their social context. *Journal of the History of the Behavioral Sciences, 22*, 324–332.

Golden, C. J. (1989). The Luria-Nebraska Neuropsychological Battery. In C. S. Newmark (Ed.), *Major psychological assessment instruments* (Vol. II, pp. 165–198). Boston: Allyn and Bacon.

Gough, H. G., & Bradley, P. (1992). Comparing two strategies for developing personality scales. In M. Zeidner & R. Most (Eds.), *Psychological testing: An inside view* (pp. 215–248). Palo Alto, CA: Consulting Psychologists Press.

Graham, J. R. (1993). *MMPI-2: Assessing personality and psychopathology.* New York: Oxford.

Gregory, R. J. (1987). *Adult intellectual assessment.* Boston: Allyn and Bacon.

Gregory, R. J. (1996). *Psychological testing: History, principles, and applications* (2nd ed.). Boston: Allyn and Bacon.

Guilford, J. P., & Fruchter, B. (1978). *Fundamental statistics in psychology and education* (6th ed.). New York: McGraw-Hill.

Hersen, M., & Bellack, A. S. (Eds.) (1988). *Dictionary of behavioral assessment techniques.* New York: Pergamon Press.

Hiskey, M. S. (1966). *Manual for the Hiskey-Nebraska Test of Learning Aptitude.* Lincoln, NE: Union College Press.

Hoffart, A., Friis, S., Strand, J., & Olsen, B. (1994). Symptoms and cognitions during situational and hyperventilatory exposure in agoraphobic patients with and without panic. *Journal of Psychopathology and Behavioral Assessment, 16,* 15–32.

Horn, J. L. (1994). Theory of fluid and crystallized intelligence. In R. J. Sternberg (Ed.), *Encyclopedia of human intelligence* (Vol. 1, pp. 443–451). New York: Macmillan.

Kaufman, A. S., Kamphaus, R. W., & Kaufman, N. L. (1985). The Kaufman Assessment Battery for Children (K-ABC). In C. S. Newmark (Ed.). *Major psychological assessment instruments* (pp. 249–276). Boston: Allyn and Bacon.

Kaufman, A. S., & Kaufman, N. L. (1983a). *K-ABC administration and scoring manual.* Circle Pines, MN: American Guidance Service.

Kaufman, A. S., & Kaufman, N. L. (1983b). *K-ABC interpretive manual.* Circle Pines, MN: American Guidance Service.

Kaufman, A. S., & Kaufman, N. L. (1990). *Kaufman Brief Intelligence Test manual.* Circle Pines, MN: American Guidance Service.

Kaufman, A. S., & Wang, J. (1992). Gender, race, and education differences on the K-BIT at ages 4 to 90. *Journal of Psychoeducational Assessment, 10,* 219–229.

Kleinmuntz, B. (1990). Why we still use our heads instead of formulas: Toward an integrative approach. *Psychological Bulletin, 107,* 296–310.

Lah, M. I. (1989). New validity, normative, and scoring data for the Rotter Incomplete Sentences Blank. *Journal of Personality Assessment, 53,* 607–620.

Lanyon, R. I. (1984). Personality assessment. *Annual Review of Psychology, 35,* 667–701.

Laurent, J., Swerdlik, M., & Ryburn, M. (1992). Review of validity research on the Stanford-Binet Intelligence Scale: Fourth Edition. *Psychological Assessment, 4,* 102–112.

Lezak, M. (1995). *Neuropsychological assessment* (3rd ed.). New York: Oxford University Press.

Machover, K. (1949). *Personality projection in the drawing of the human figure.* Springfield, IL: Charles C Thomas.

Matarazzo, J. D. (1986). Computerized clinical psychological test interpretations: Unvalidated plus all mean and no sigma. *American Psychologist, 41,* 14–24.

Meehl, P. E. (1954). *Clinical versus statistical prediction.* Minneapolis: University of Minnesota Press.

Meehl, P. E. (1965). Seer over sign: The first good example. *Journal of Experimental Research in Personality, 1,* 29–32.

Meehl, P. E. (1986). Causes and effects of my disturbing little book. *Journal of Personality Assessment, 50,* 370–375.

Messick, S. (1989). Validity. In R. L. Linn (Ed.), *Educational measurement* (3rd ed., pp. 13–104). New York: American Council on Education/Macmillan.

Millon, T. (1994). *Manual for the Millon Clinical Multiaxial Inventory-III.* Minneapolis, MN: National Computer Systems.

Naglieri, J., & Pfeiffer, S. (1992). Performance of disruptive behavior disordered and normal samples on the Draw A Person: Screening Procedure for Emotional Disturbance. *Psychological Assessment, 4,* 156–159.

Phelps, L., & Ensor, A. (1986). Concurrent validity of the WISC-R using deaf norms and the Hiskey-Nebraska. *Psychology in the Schools, 23,* 138–141.

Piedmont, R. L., & Weinstein, H. P. (1993). A psychometric evaluation of the new NEO-PIR Facet Scales for Agreeableness and Conscientiousness. *Journal of Personality Assessment, 60,* 302–318.

Reid, D. B., & Kelly, M. P. (1993). Wechsler Memory Scale—Revised in closed head injury. *Journal of Clinical Psychology, 49,* 245–254.

Reitan, R. M., & Wolfson, D. (1993). *The Halstead-Reitan Neuropsychological Test Battery: Theory and clinical interpretation* (2nd ed.). Tucson, AZ: Neuropsychology Press.

Reynolds, C. R. (1994). Bias in testing. In R. J. Sternberg (Ed.), *Encyclopedia of human intelligence* (pp. 175–178). New York: Macmillan.

Rorschach, H. (1921). *Psychodiagnostik.* Berne: Birchen.

Rotter, J. B., & Rafferty, J. E. (1950). *Manual for the Rotter Incomplete Sentences Blank: College Form*. New York: The Psychological Corporation.

Sattler, J. M. (1982). Age effects on Wechsler Adult Intelligence Scale—Revised tests. *Journal of Consulting and Clinical Psychology, 50*, 785–786.

Sattler, J. M. (1988). *Assessment of children* (3rd ed.). San Diego, CA: Jerome M. Sattler, Publisher.

Sparrow, S. S., Balla, D. A., & Cicchetti, D. V. (1984). *Vineland Adaptive Behavior Scales*. Circle Pines, MN: American Guidance Service.

Stern, W. L. (1914). The psychological methods of testing intelligence (Über die psychologischen Methoden der Intelligenzprufung). (G. M. Whipple, Trans.). *Educational Psychology Monographs*, No. 13. Baltimore: Warwick & York. (Original work published 1912)

Stuss, D. T., Stethem, L. L., Hugenholtz, H., & Richard, M. T. (1989). Traumatic brain injury: A comparison of three clinical tests, and analysis of recovery. *The Clinical Neuropsychologist, 3,* 145–156.

Terman, L. M. (1916). *The measurement of intelligence*. Boston: Houghton Mifflin.

Thorndike, R. L., Hagen, E. P., & Sattler, J. M. (1986). *The Stanford-Binet Intelligence Scale: Fourth Edition, Guide for administering and scoring*. Chicago: Riverside Publishing Company.

Wade, T. C., & Baker, T. B. (1977). Opinions and use of psychological tests. *American Psychologist, 32*, 874–882.

Wechsler, D. (1987). *Wechsler Memory Scale—Revised manual*. New York: Psychological Corporation.

Wissler, C. (1901). The correlation of mental and physical tests. *The Psychological Review*, Monograph Supplement, *3*(6).

Yerkes, R. M. (1919). Report of the Psychology Committee of the National Research Council. *Psychological Review, 26*, 83–149.

FOR FURTHER READING

Anastasi, A., & Urbina, S. (1997). *Psychological testing* (7th ed.). New York: Macmillan. *This book is regarded as one of the best and most scholarly reviews of psychological testing.*

Eyde, L., Robertson, G., Krug, S., et al. (1993). *Responsible test use: Case studies for assessing human behavior*. Washington, DC: American Psychological Association. *A valuable and fascinating compendium of guidelines for responsible testing. The book also includes dozens of case studies that violate these guidelines.*

Goldstein, G., & Hersen, M. (Eds.). (1990). *Handbook of psychological assessment* (2nd ed.). New York: Pergamon Press. *A relatively high level textbook that summarizes the state of the art of psychological assessment.*

Gregory, R. J. (1996). *Psychological testing: History, principles, and applications* (2nd ed.). Boston: Allyn and Bacon. *A useful introduction to testing that includes extensive coverage of the history of testing.*

Zeidner, M., & Most, R. (Eds.). (1992). *Psychological testing: An inside view*. Palo Alto, CA: Consulting Psychologists Press. *The 12 chapters in this book include several topics not found elsewhere, such as the use of feedback from examinees in the revision of existing test procedures.*

CHAPTER 4

ETHICS AND ETHICAL REASONING

Mitchell M. Handelsman

Case #4-1

Dr. Newman is just getting started as a psychotherapist. He has just come from his new house (with a big mortgage) in his new car (with big payments) to his new office (with big rent due every month). One of his first appointments is with an attractive woman, Ms. Eldridge, who is deciding whether to come for therapy. She reports that she has been experiencing panic attacks ever since she inherited a large amount of money from a rich relative.

Dr. Newman has little experience with panic disorders and knows a colleague who could treat this client much better than he could. As he looks out the window at his big car from his expensive office, however, Dr. Newman decides not only to treat Ms. Eldridge, but to charge her twice his normal fee. Moreover, he assures the client that she needs two sessions a week. Ms. Eldridge does not know what psychologists usually charge, but she has heard that some clients need more than one session a week. She decides to enter treatment with Dr. Newman. After several weeks in therapy the client's condition worsens to the point that she requires hospitalization.

Dr. Newman engaged in unethical behavior. What do we mean by unethical behavior? What happens when psychologists behave unethically? And how can psychologists think about their professional behavior to prevent acting unethically? This chapter explores these questions and then applies ethical reasoning and principles to several major topics.

WHAT IS ETHICS?

If Dr. Newman had been selling shoes and overcharged a customer, we might not judge his behavior to be unethical. In most everyday business transactions the traditional principle is *caveat emptor*—"let the buyer beware." When customers buy psychological services such as psychotherapy, however, they may not have all the information they need to determine whether the service is appropriate, whether the psychologist is well qualified, or whether the service is for the benefit of the client—as it should be—or solely for the benefit of the psychologist. Thus, *professional ethics* can be defined as standards of correct professional behavior; these standards exist so that clients, students, research participants, and others are well served (see Table 4.1 for other key terms). Ethical standards are necessary in clinical psychology because professional relationships in psychology are based on trust. Psychologists have much more technical knowledge with which to make judgments; therefore, clients must trust psychologists to judge well.

Table 4.1 Some Key Terms in Ethics (with Short Definitions)

Ethical Principles

Autonomy: Respect people's rights to make their own decisions.
Beneficence: Do good, avoid harm, remove harm.
Justice: Treat people fairly.
Nonmaleficence: Do not cause harm.

Ethical Rules

Confidentiality: Keep what clients say private.
Fidelity: Keep promises.
Veracity: Tell the truth.

Other Terms

Fiduciary relationship: A relationship based on trust in a professional.
Informed consent: Clients have the option to accept or refuse services, and have the right to make that decision based on adequate information.
Paternalism: Overriding a person's autonomy for beneficent reasons.

A professional relationship that is built on trust because of the professional's greater knowledge is called a *fiduciary relationship*. Virtually all professional relationships can be characterized as fiduciary, including physician–patient, lawyer–client, and psychologist–client. Clinical psychologists play a variety of roles, including therapist, consultant, teacher, researcher, evaluator, and administrator, all of which involve elements of trust. In these roles, psychologists are bound by more than the principle of caveat emptor because the responsibility for making decisions is shared by psychologists and consumers.

A particular issue has an ethical component when something important is involved and when other people's welfare is at stake. Thus, ethical concerns can be differentiated from questions of etiquette. It is polite, for example, to wish a client Merry Christmas or a happy birthday, but not to do so is neither ethical nor unethical. One hallmark of ethical issues is that they involve the potential for significant impact on other people, rather than simple manners or personal preferences (Carroll, Schneider, & Wesley, 1985).

Ethics has become an increasingly important part of the training of psychologists because of the inherent dangers—to clients, students, research participants—of unethical behavior. Such dangers include harm, exploitation, and disrespect. In many cases these three dangers are interrelated. For ex-

ample, although disrespect can occur without exploitation or harm, exploitation of clients is almost always considered disrespectful and may also be harmful.

The first danger, *harm*, may occur because consumers cannot definitively evaluate the nature and effectiveness of the service provided. For example, Ms. Eldridge has not taken a graduate-level course on anxiety disorders, so she had no way of knowing that Dr. Newman did not do an adequate assessment of her condition and was not expert in treating it. Thus, she suffered more than she would have had Dr. Newman referred her to a more appropriate therapist.

The second danger of unethical behavior is *exploitation*. The fact that clients must trust psychologists, coupled with the fact that psychologists deserve compensation for their activities, produces an inevitable tension between the "professional" and "business" aspects of psychology. Exploitation may take the form of using clients to fulfill financial, emotional, sexual, neurotic, professional, or other needs. In Case #4-1, Dr. Newman clearly let his self-interest outweigh his professional judgment and exploited Ms. Eldridge.

The third danger of unethical behavior is *disrespect*—devaluing the client as an individual. Ms. Eldridge was devalued because of the harm done. But even if her condition had not worsened, she suffered a loss of dignity because Dr. Newman led her to believe that he would be the best therapist for her.

What Happens When Psychologists Behave Unethically?

Ethics Committees and Ethics Codes

The APA and most state psychological associations have ethics committees that will adjudicate complaints brought against psychologists. The APA committee receives written complaints against psychologists from clients, other psychologists, or anyone with knowledge of possible unethical behavior. The committee also can initiate an investigation itself if it learns of such behavior from newspapers or other public records.

The profession of psychology, like medicine, nursing, engineering, and other professions (Appelbaum & Lawton, 1990), has a written code of ethics that outlines basic ethical requirements. The original code for psychologists was published in 1953 by the American Psychological Association (APA, 1953) and has been revised several times. The current APA *Ethical Principles of Psychologists and Code of Conduct* (1992) comprises two major sections, "a set of principles that are aspirational, representing the professional ideals, and a set of enforceable standards that are intended to be specific enough to use as compelling rules resulting in sanctions should they be broken" (Keith-Spiegel, 1994, p. 315). There are six aspirational principles and 101 specific standards.

After Ms. Eldridge talks with her new therapist about her experiences with Dr. Newman, she decides that she should formally complain about Dr. Newman's behavior, both to punish him for his misdeeds and to prevent other clients from being harmed in the future. Ms. Eldridge has three options open to her: She can complain to state and national ethics committees, she can grieve against Dr. Newman's license, and she can file a malpractice suit. We shall explore each of these options.

If Ms. Eldridge decides to complain to the APA Ethics Committee, the committee would give Dr. Newman a chance to respond in writing, and gather whatever other evidence it could. The committee members would then determine if Dr. Newman's behavior violated one or more ethical standard. In this case, Dr. Newman seems to have violated Standard 1.04 regarding competent practice (see the section on Competence for a full discussion of this issue) and Standard 1.25, which states that "psychologists do not exploit recipients of services . . . with respect to fees" (APA, 1992, p. 1602).

In response to Dr. Newman's unethical behavior, the APA Committee can take a number of steps, depending on the amount of harm that was or could have been done, on Dr. Newman's prior record of ethics violations, and "on the basis of circumstances that aggravate or mitigate the culpability of the member" (APA Ethics Committee, 1996, p. 537). The mildest penalties would be letters of reprimand or censure. The most severe penalty available to the ethics committee is expulsion from APA

(APA Ethics Committee, 1996). A simple letter seems too mild for Dr. Newman, but expulsion may be too harsh. The most likely sanction might be a letter of reprimand, along with a requirement that Dr. Newman take steps to prevent future problems. Thus, Dr. Newman might need to obtain supervision for several years, obtain education about ethical issues, and/or enter personal therapy.

Legal Requirements

Because psychologists provide valuable but potentially harmful services to the public, all states require psychologists to acquire and maintain a license to practice. This license provides psychologists with recognized standing among consumers, but it also entails legal requirements embodied in state laws and regulations. Many of these laws are restatements of APA ethical standards, along with rules about such issues as privileged communication and sexual contact with clients.

If Ms. Eldridge decides to grieve against Dr. Newman's license, she would send her grievance to the state disciplinary board, which would investigate the complaint. The state board has the power—similar to that of ethics committees—to reprimand Dr. Newman and to require remediation in such forms as supervision, practice monitoring, and personal therapy. Unlike ethics committees, the board can also revoke Dr. Newman's license and prohibit him from practicing.

The APA (1992) code states that psychologists must obey the law. But just behaving legally is not always the same as behaving ethically. As Keith-Spiegel and Koocher pointed out, "ethical professional standards also expect behavior that is more correct or more stringent than is required by law" (1985, p. 7). They list many examples of behavior that would be judged unethical but that may not be illegal, including "administering psychological assessment techniques without adequate training, failing to give adequate or timely feedback to supervisees, or diagnosing people who call into a radio talk show" (p. 7). Most people in our society would probably agree that being a moral person is more than not breaking any laws.

Malpractice

The third option Ms. Eldridge has is to file a malpractice suit against Dr. Newman. To prove her case and collect monetary damages, she would have to prove four things: (1) that she was in a professional relationship with Dr. Newman, (2) that Dr. Newman acted negligently, (3) that she was harmed, and (4) that the harm was caused by Dr. Newman's negligence. Because of these legal criteria, even if Dr. Newman is guilty of unethical behavior, he may not be guilty of malpractice.

How Do Psychologists Make Good Ethical Decisions?: Ethical Reasoning

Dr. Newman's offense was a clear violation of the APA code of ethics; he should have known better. But sometimes knowing all the codes, laws, and guidelines is not enough to make good decisions. Ethical codes and guidelines have several shortcomings: First, they are not designed to provide answers to all ethical concerns in all circumstances. No code can encompass all the difficult decisions that clinical psychologists are called on to make; at best, the code may provide some specific rules, but more often it will provide more general directions that still leave room for judgment (Welfel & Lipsitz, 1984). Provisions of ethics codes need to be specific enough to be enforceable, but broad enough to apply to a range of situations. For this reason, they are sometimes vague and therefore not very useful (Keith-Spiegel, 1994).

A second problem with ethics codes is that psychologists often find themselves in situations where they have two conflicting obligations, each of which can be ethically justified. For example, decisions to hospitalize patients involuntarily nearly always involve a conflict between the requirement to respect the dignity and worth of individuals and the requirement to contribute to the welfare of individuals (Carroll et al., 1985). In these cases the issue is not simply right versus wrong, but a choice among options that appear equally right but are mutually exclusive. This choice is called an *ethical dilemma*.

Third, even if professional codes served all our current needs, new ethical dilemmas and decisions will arise. The profession gets more complex all the time: The roles of clinical psychologists have been expanding from researcher (Rosenthal, 1994; see Chapter 5), to psychotherapist, to psychoeducational assessor (Lakin, 1991; see Chapters 2 and 3), to family therapist (Vesper & Brock, 1991), to consultant, to expert witness (Golding, 1990), to police psychologist (Monahan, 1980), to custody evaluator (APA, 1994), to group leader (Gumaer & Scott, 1985; see Chapter 7). Further, the increasing cultural diversity of psychologists and their clients presents new ethical challenges (Aponte & Crouch, 1995; Sue, 1983). The financial climate in which clinical psychologists work is also becoming more complex as health care reforms are implemented (Dougherty, 1992; Haas & Cummings, 1991). Finally, new technologies present issues that need to be addressed. For example, psychologists are currently debating the ethics of various kinds of psychotherapy conducted over the phone ("APA's Ethics Committee," 1995; Haas, Benedict, & Kobos, 1996), by fax, by e-mail, through newsgroups, and on the World Wide Web. These questions could not have been anticipated only a few short years ago.

These drawbacks make it difficult to rely exclusively on ethics codes and laws to provide guidance in all cases. Many authors have developed ethical decision-making strategies to help psychologists explore both the obvious and subtle ethical pitfalls in their professional activities (Carroll et al., 1985; Handelsman, 1991; Kitchener, 1984; Tymchuk, 1981). One example is shown in Table 4.2.

Consider the following case:

Case #4-2
Dr. Anderson teaches in a clinical psychology graduate program. For his course in "Methods of Stress Management," Dr. Anderson wants to try something innovative to get students to feel what it is like to be acutely stressed. He plans to enter class one day and announce that half the class has failed the latest test so badly that they will be asked to leave the program at the end of the semester. After a short time, Dr. Anderson would ask students to reflect on their reaction to this news, which he would tell them was not true. Dr. Anderson anticipates a lively discussion about the physical, emotional, and cognitive reactions that each student had.

Table 4.2
An Ethical Decision-Making Procedure

I. Tentatively state the problem or the policy to be developed.

II. What are the relevant facts of the case?
   A. What empirical questions are involved?
   B. What facts might *not* be relevant?

III. To whom are we obligated (including the general public, institutions, the profession)? Who is our client?

IV. What sources of guidance are available?
   A. Professional codes of ethics
   B. Laws and regulations

V. How are general ethical principles relevant?
   A. Nonmaleficence, beneficence, autonomy, justice
   B. Confidentiality, fidelity, veracity
   C. What are the rights of the parties involved?

VI. Restate the problem in terms of the ethical issues involved.

VII. What are the alternative courses of action, or alternative policies?

VIII. What are the consequences of each of these?
   A. Long- and short-term consequences. Benefits and risks.
   B. What are the probabilities of these consequences?

IX. Is each of these possible actions morally consistent?
   A. Would we choose this option if positions were reversed?
   B. What would the decision be if there were no laws?
   C. What if all actions led to equally good outcomes?

X. What facts would have to change for our decision to change?

XI. How might our values be influencing our deliberations?
   A. Can the consequences be valued differently?
   B. Which facts of the case may be disguised values?
   C. What are my personal motivations?
   D. How might I benefit, personally or professionally, from the alternative courses of action?

Source: Based on Handelsman (1991).

Dr. Anderson checks the APA ethics code and finds nothing specifically prohibiting this activity, but he does feel some discomfort with it. He decides to consult with several colleagues on the faculty. He shares his idea before asking them, "Is my plan ethical?" How would you advise Dr. Anderson?

Steps in Ethical Reasoning

Although different authors have emphasized different aspects of ethical reasoning, they agree that psychologists must follow certain steps to think through their decisions. Initially, psychologists must determine the facts of the case. Disagreements about ethical courses of action often appear to be based on arguments about the merits of ethical principles when, in fact, they stem from incomplete knowledge of all the relevant facts. Once they have outlined the facts as clearly as possible, psychologists must clarify their own values and potential conflicts of interest, consider a range of alternative decisions, weigh the nature and likelihood of the consequences of the alternatives, and apply the relevant laws, ethical codes, and principles to each alternative. Also, a good strategy may be to consult with senior colleagues or ethics committees (Corey, Corey, & Callanan, 1993), as Dr. Anderson did. These steps help psychologists clarify the nature and extent of their obligations to their clients, their profession, the public, and themselves.

Dr. Anderson intuitively felt that his plan for class would be quite effective but might have some ethical problems. However, Kitchener (1984) argued that psychologists cannot rely on their intuition to make ethical decisions. She suggested that a comprehensive ethical reasoning process makes use of general principles that are typically employed in philosophy and medicine (Beauchamp & Childress, 1994). These principles include nonmaleficence, beneficence, autonomy, and justice; each of these principles is discussed in the next section.

The Incorporation of General Ethical Principles and Rules

Nonmaleficence

Physicians, psychologists, and other professionals learn early in their training, "Above all, do no harm." This states the ethical principle of *nonmaleficence*. The recent debates about physician-assisted suicide center on this principle when opponents argue that physicians should not kill people, as that is harm. Proponents do not argue that doctors *should* harm patients but, rather, that there are harms worse than death. The principle of nonmaleficence prohibits psychologists from such behaviors as acting incompetently and taking financial advantage of their clients, as we saw in Case #4-1.

Beneficence

Whereas nonmaleficence helps us decide what behaviors to avoid, the principle of *beneficence* obligates psychologists to perform behaviors that (1) prevent harm, (2) remove harm, and (3) provide benefit. Most clinical psychologists enter this field out of beneficent motivations—they very much want to ease suffering, to help people cope with life, and to contribute to the world's well-being by creating and imparting knowledge. Thus, beneficence is often the first principle used to justify their actions. They do therapy because it makes people feel better. They teach so students can have better lives. They report their suspicions of abuse to prevent harm to children. The principle of beneficence justifies virtually every professional activity.

Taken together, the principles of nonmaleficence and beneficence can be used to perform a "cost–benefit analysis" of a proposed behavior or policy. Few benefits come without some risk: Therapy clients may become depressed; students need to take tests and receive grades. Dr. Anderson wants his students to benefit from his course and also wants to avoid harm. He must ask himself, "What risk of harm exists in my teaching plan? And do the benefits to the students outweigh the risks?" Some of Dr. Anderson's colleagues tell him that students will get over his proposed "announcement" without lasting harm, and that what they learn will be worth the discomfort. Other colleagues tell Dr. Anderson that even if one student suffers for more than a few minutes, the benefit is not worth it.

Respect for Autonomy

Nonmaleficence and beneficence are always important, but psychologists must consider other principles before they make final judgments. Judgments about risks and benefits do not occur in a vacuum; psychologists are always acting on behalf of their consumers: students, clients, patients. Because these consumers are active participants in the professional relationship, one can argue that the entire profession of psychology stems from the inherent dignity and worth of individuals whom psychologists are helping.

The assumption that people are inherently worthy of respect leads to the ethical principle of *autonomy*. Beauchamp and Childress defined autonomy as "personal rule of the self that is free from both

controlling interferences by others and from personal limitations that prevent meaningful choice, such as inadequate understanding" (1994, p. 121). Because people deserve respect and because they have reasons for their actions, psychologists are obligated to consider them as free agents, whose choices and actions should not be interfered with except under unusual circumstances. Entering a professional relationship does not strip people of their dignity or their autonomy.

The principle of autonomy protects the right of people to make choices that others consider foolish. For example, one may believe that downhill skiing is unwise and self-destructive: The chances of injury are very high. People's judgments about the risks involved, however, do not justify their setting up roadblocks outside of Vail or Stowe to prevent skiers from entering. People who ski do so for their own reasons, and those reasons and actions need to be respected.

When people are not competent to make their own decisions, professionals need to step in for the clients' own good. When involuntary commitments are arranged, the principle of autonomy, because of limited competence, is overridden by the principle of beneficence. Psychologists sometimes override people's autonomy, for beneficent reasons, even when those people are competent. For example, a psychologist may suggest to a client that he must leave his marriage because doing so would be "mentally healthy." In fact, either choice—to stay or to leave—has both potential benefits and risks, and the client should be the one to decide, with the therapist helping to explore the options. Unfortunately, for various reasons, therapists may try to make a choice for clients. Perhaps the therapist is dealing with his own marriage vicariously through the client's; he may believe the benefits of leaving outweigh the costs and wants to hurry the client up. Or perhaps a therapist has political ideas about marriage that she wants to implement with the client. None of these reasons are ethically justifiable.

The relative weight given to the principles of beneficence and autonomy accounts for many of the toughest decisions in professional ethical reasoning. The conflict between autonomy and beneficence leads to concerns of *paternalism*, which can be defined as a judgment that beneficence overrides autonomy. Paternalistic actions can be justified or unjustified, depending on such factors as the degree of information available to clients, their level of competence to understand and use that information to make decisions, and the possible personal interests of the psychologist. In Case #4-2, for instance, Dr. Anderson would be making a paternalistic judgment that the learning of students is worth misleading them temporarily.

One way for psychologists to conceive of respecting autonomy is to facilitate and not inhibit clients' abilities and opportunities to make the best decisions they can. Psychologists must recognize that they may not always agree with those decisions. Clients' decisions are autonomous when they are unfettered by inappropriate restrictions placed on them by psychologists. In Case #4-1, Dr. Newman violated Ms. Eldridge's autonomy by providing incomplete and misleading information about his abilities, thereby restricting her choice.

The obligation to respect autonomy leads to three specific ethical rules (Beauchamp & Childress, 1994). (Of course, these rules also serve to promote good and prevent harm; thus, beneficence and non-maleficence can also justify them.) One rule is that of *fidelity*, or promise-keeping. If clients make decisions based on promises of psychologists, the decisions will be good only if the promises are kept. For example, if students enroll in a course that promises to be about statistics, they need to be taught about statistics and not about psychopathology, art history, or the professor's latest hobby.

A second ethical rule stemming directly from the principle of autonomy is *veracity*, or truth-telling: The information on which clients base their decisions needs to be accurate. Dr. Anderson's plan to mislead students raises important questions in this regard. A final rule is that of *confidentiality* (to be discussed), which refers to the obligation of psychologists to keep clients' disclosures private.

Justice

The fourth general ethical principle is *justice*. Although there are several meanings of justice, the most important for clinical psychologists is fairness—the obligation to treat equals equally and unequals, unequally (Beauchamp & Childress, 1994). Differential treatment should be based on ethically relevant dimensions; otherwise, the result is unethical behavior that can be called unfair, unjust, or discriminatory. Professors who base course grades on test performance, gains in knowledge and intellectual skill, and other indicators of learning are behaving justly. Professors who base grades on gender, ethnic background, or attractiveness are not behaving justly because they are using irrelevant dimensions. Therapists like Dr. Newman who base frequency of sessions on the clients' wealth, rather than on the need for treatment, are violating the principle of justice.

Ethical Reasoning in Practice

Ethical reasoning involves applying the foregoing general principles and rules as well as knowing the relevant professional codes and legal requirements. Even with full command of these principles, however, reasonable psychologists can find themselves disagreeing with each other about which principle or principles are primary. They also may hold differing values, which may affect their decisions. For example, many psychologists value the results of psychological research highly enough to justify deceiving research volunteers. Others believe that the results of research are not that important (Baumrind, 1985). Likewise, clients and therapists from different cultural groups may hold differing values that lead to different psychotherapeutic goals and strategies. For example, therapists and clients may disagree on whether a 20-year-old who is still living with his parents is showing a sign of an emancipation difficulty or simply of healthy family togetherness (McGoldrick, Pearce, & Giordano, 1982).

Throughout the remainder of this chapter, we will explore several important ethical issues by considering several additional cases. The cases focus primarily on psychotherapy, but the reasoning process applies as well to diagnosis, assessment, research, consultation, teaching, and the other professional roles of psychologists. Two points need to be stressed: First, the reader may become frustrated because many cases have no clear answers; the reader may think that psychologists can justify just about anything depending on the situation. In a given situation, it is sometimes true that all the alternatives are ethically acceptable and none is ethically pure. Even in the gray areas, however, ethical reasoning can help psychologists steer clear of unethical behavior and choose well among several ethical alternatives.

Second, the term *unethical psychologist* does not appear in this chapter; a phrase such as "psychologists engaging in unethical behavior" is more appropriate. Relatively few psychologists are "career wrongdoers." Many psychologists who violate ethical standards are well-meaning, generally good clinicians who may be lacking in some area of their training, who are going through a particularly rough personal or professional crisis at the moment, or who have made a mistake that has particularly serious consequences (Keith-Spiegel & Koocher, 1985). Being compassionate, having good intentions, and being dedicated to helping people does not make psychologists immune from unethical behavior.

COMPETENCE

As we saw in Case #4-1, psychologists must have the training, experience, knowledge, and skills to work with the clients they see. Here is another case that revolves around issues of competence:

Case #4-3
Dr. Davis, a clinical psychologist in private psychotherapy practice, has been working with Mrs. Edison for almost a year in individual therapy. They have worked on several issues, and now Mrs. Edison is introducing some marital problems. Dr. Davis has read a few articles on confrontive techniques in marital therapy, so she decides to have Edison bring in her husband for a therapy session in which she encourages both spouses to "let it all hang out" and share all their complaints about each other. Dr. Davis feels that the session went pretty well, but several months later Mr. Edison leaves his wife and complains to a local ethics committee that Dr. Davis has "ruined our marriage with her half-baked therapy."

The ethics committee will need to deal with several issues in this case, but the first one is professional competence. The APA code states: "Psychologists provide services ... only within the boundaries of their competence, based on their education, training, supervised experience, or appropriate professional experience" (APA, 1992, p. 1600, Standard 1.04). Did Dr. Davis act competently?

Dr. Davis may argue that she is a competent practitioner and may offer evidence by listing several of the general ways psychology has of assuring competence. She graduated from a regionally accredited institution. She went to a clinical psychology training program and completed an internship that were both accredited by APA, which sets standards for clinical (as well as counseling and school) psychology programs and internships (Sheridan, Matarazzo, & Nelson, 1995). She obtained a license to practice psychology in her state, based on her training, on receiving supervised post-doctoral experience, and on passing both oral and written examinations. On the basis of more supervised experience and another examination, she became a diplomate of the American Board of Professional Psychology, which signifies her professional excellence since becoming licensed. Although these methods of assuring competence have been criticized (see, for example, Greenberg, 1978; Hogan, 1979), they are generally recognized as a necessary, if not sufficient, indication of competence to the public and to agencies that hire psychologists.

The ethics committee will duly note Dr. Davis's background but will also recognize, as Corey, Corey, and Callanan note, that "most licenses and credentials are generic; that is, they usually don't specify the clients or problems that practitioners are competent to work with, nor ... the techniques that they are competent to use" (Corey et al., 1993, p. 182). No amount of training and experience, regardless of how flawless and extensive, can prepare psychologists for all possible problems, modalities of therapy, cultures, and so on. All psychologists have limits of competence. And even though psychologists are very bright people who enjoy challenges, they need to prepare adequately—via training and supervised experience—to meet those challenges.

For the ethics committee, the question remains: "In this case, did Dr. Davis—as good as she is in general—go beyond the limits of her competence?" Because marital therapy issues are not merely commonsense extensions of individual therapy issues, the committee will want to know if she had courses in marital therapy and if she had any supervised training dealing with issues in marital therapy, including ethical issues (Margolin, 1982; Vesper & Brock, 1991). The committee will want to know if she sought out consultation when she decided that marital therapy might benefit Mrs. Edison.

Three possibilities exist for how to characterize Dr. Davis's behavior. First, it could have been unethical because she was not competent. Let us assume, however, that Dr. Davis indeed sought consultation from another psychologist with expertise in marital therapy, a psychologist who was informed about the case and who concurred with Dr. Davis's treatment plan. Dr. Davis's consultant judged that the plan would work; unfortunately, in this case it didn't. Second, the possibility exists that the behavior was evidence of poor judgment on the part of Dr. Davis and her consultant. Poor judgment, however, does not necessarily mean that professionals were acting unethically. Third, Dr. Davis could have used good judgment that did not happen to have the predicted result. Therapy, after all, does not work all the time. Like any profession, psychology is not an exact science, and thus positive outcomes are not inevitable. Clients may not improve, students may not pass a course, research may not show the anticipated results.

To make their decision, the committee will look at the facts of the case, including the harm that was or might have been done to the Edison couple. It will attempt to determine whether harm should have been anticipated and whether Dr. Davis acted to avoid harm. It may also try to judge why Dr. Davis might have behaved incompetently: Was it laziness, arrogance, carelessness, ignorance, greed?

If we assume that Dr. Davis was not competent to practice marital therapy, the committee would judge her actions as unethical and would take some punitive actions. They would also educate her about how psychologists avoid acting incompetently. All psychologists are sometimes asked to do things that are beyond their ability; and they need to recognize their areas of incompetence. They should avoid engaging in these behaviors (nonmaleficence) and take alternative steps to help their client (beneficence). In this case, Dr. Davis could have referred Mrs. Edison to a well-trained person for marital therapy. Or, despite her level of academic training, Dr. Davis might have sought supervision for her work with the couple.

Psychologists need to recognize that their clinical and ethical reasoning skills may become temporarily diminished because of their own personal problems (see APA Ethical Standard 1.13). Dr. Davis, for example, may have experienced a recent divorce, which clouded her judgment enough to make her inappropriately confrontive of Mr. Edison. Psychologists, especially those in private practice, often avoid such lapses in judgment by staying professionally active; participating in workshops, conferences, and other continuing education; holding regular peer consultation sessions; and taking time away from the office to relax and satisfy their own personal needs.

Clearly, psychologists need to make sure they are acting according to generally accepted standards. Sometimes, however, there are no standards; in this case, the APA (1992) code requires psychologists to "take reasonable steps to ensure the competence of their work and to protect patients, clients, students, research participants, and others from harm" (p. 1600, Standard 1.04). Psychologists must act with caution; their compassion for clients and their desire to try anything that may work should be tempered with the recognition of the harm that may be done. In these situations, nonmaleficence clearly outweighs beneficence.

INFORMED CONSENT

All psychological services contain some element of risk; sometimes the service may not even be effective. When clients enter into a relationship with a psychologist as therapy clients, assessment clients, students, or research participants, they may not know enough about the nature of the relationship, the possible outcomes, the risks involved, or the alternatives available to them. At the same time, clients have the right either to refuse participation or to consent to it. Clients' right to consent to or refuse treatment as autonomous agents, and their right to make decisions based on adequate information provided by the professional, is called the doctrine of *informed consent* (Appelbaum, Lidz, & Meisel, 1987). On the basis of this doctrine, psychologists have two related obligations: (1) to provide information with which clients can make good choices, and (2) to secure clients' authorization, or consent, for participation in such activities as therapy, assessment, and research. The concept of informed consent has ethical, legal, and clinical components. We shall consider each as we follow Dr. Baker's process of ethical reasoning.

Case #4-4
Dr. Baker is a young psychologist just entering private practice. One of her first clients is Ms. Young, who seems very hesitant to enter therapy with Dr. Baker. "I was expecting a much older person," Ms. Young says. "Are you sure you can help me?" Dr. Baker merely answers, "You sound very upset," and avoids talking much about what therapy is or what it can and cannot accomplish. She knows she is ethically bound to provide certain information to the client about the nature of therapy, but she fears that if she tells Ms. Young about some of the risks of therapy, Ms. Young may not continue with the treatment. "Do I keep some of this information from her," Dr. Baker thinks to herself, "so she can benefit from therapy, or do I tell Ms. Young what she can expect in therapy and run the substantial risk that she will not get therapy at all?"

Laws and Codes

Dr. Baker's first question might be, "Does the ethical doctrine of informed consent apply to clinical psychologists?" Indeed, this doctrine did not start in psychology but in medicine; physicians are legally and ethically prohibited from touching patients or performing medical procedures without the patients' consent (Beauchamp & Childress, 1994; Lidz et al., 1984). Lidz et al. stated the legal requirement: "Unless a doctor discloses to a patient certain types of information before undertaking a diagnostic, therapeutic, or research procedure, the patient may collect damages from the doctor if he or she is injured by the procedure, even though the procedure itself was properly performed" (1984, p. 4). Physicians are legally and ethically obligated to provide patients with information about the nature and purpose of a procedure, the risks and benefits of the procedure, alternative procedures, their risks and benefits, and the risks and benefits of doing nothing.

The informed consent doctrine has become part of psychological practice as well (Haas, 1991). The APA code states, "Psychologists obtain appropriate informed consent to therapy or related procedures, using language that is reasonably understandable to participants. . . . When persons are legally incapable of giving informed consent, psychologists obtain informed permission from a legally authorized person, if such substitute consent is permitted by law" (APA, 1992, p. 1605, Standard 4.02).

The primary justification for informed consent, as noted, is autonomy. Consent is also justified by the principles of nonmaleficence and beneficence. An effective consent process guards against exploitation of clients (Hare-Mustin, Maracek, Kaplan, & Liss-Levinson, 1979) and provides potential positive effects such as facilitating the therapeutic relationship, allowing clients to make more rational and thus better decisions, and increasing the care that therapists take in thinking about the treatment (Appelbaum et al., 1987).

Once Dr. Baker understands the law, the APA Standard on informed consent, and their theoretical justifications, she must formulate her own informed consent policy for her practice. To apply the doctrine adequately, she will consider the two major parts of the doctrine: information and consent.

Information

Dr. Baker need not give her client a graduate course in therapy, but she must provide certain information in order to fulfill her obligation. Some guidance comes from the courts: Two major legal standards have been used to determine if professionals have provided adequate information to clients. The first is the *professional practice standard*, which states that "adequate disclosure is determined by a professional community's customary practices" (Beauchamp & Childress, 1994, p. 147). Using this standard, Dr. Baker needs to know what psychologists in similar situations usually disclose. Here, the empirical data are discouraging; psychologists appear not to be complete in their disclosure of information (Handelsman, Kemper, Kesson-Craig, McLain, & Johnsrud, 1986; Somberg, Stone, & Claiborn, 1993). Thus, the professional practice standard does not do enough to uphold the principles of autonomy and beneficence.

The second and more common legal standard is the *reasonable person standard*, articulated in *Canterbury v. Spence* (1972). This standard requires physicians "to disclose all information about a proposed treatment that a reasonable person in the patient's situation would consider material to a decision either to undergo or to forego treatment" (Lidz et al., 1984, p. 14).

Consistent with the reasonable person standard, the information provided to clients needs to be relevant and adequate (Beauchamp & Childress, 1994). *Relevance* refers to the likelihood that the information would possibly have an impact on one's decision to enter or refuse a particular service. *Adequacy* means that the psychologist must provide enough information to be useful. Dr. Baker cannot choose to omit certain information because it may make Ms. Young decide against therapy. This kind of information is exactly what Ms. Young needs to make an informed choice.

Very little research exists on what reasonable people want to know about therapy (Braaten, Otto, & Handelsman, 1993). However, authors have suggested that psychologists provide information about various aspects of therapy—in addition to the nature, risk, and benefits of the therapy and alternatives—including information about length of therapy, fees, record keeping, scheduling, insurance coverage, confidentiality and its limits (see below), credentials of the therapist, and grievance procedures (Handelsman & Galvin, 1988; Kovacs, 1984). Assessment clients also have the right to know the purposes and results of the assessment.

A few states, including Washington and Colorado, have recently passed legislation that requires psychologists to provide certain specific information to psychotherapy clients. For example, Colorado law (C.R.S. 12-43-214) requires psychologists to state, in writing, the credentials of the therapist, the address and phone number of the state grievance board, and the client's right to a second opinion. In addition, the "mandatory disclosure" form must state that "sexual intimacy is never appropriate" and that clients have the right to receive information about the methods and duration of therapy, fees, and confidentiality.

Understanding

The Colorado law requires therapists to disclose information, but the law says nothing about having clients understand what they read on the form. In order for information to achieve the goal of better client decisions, clients need to understand it.

Many authors have suggested that important information about therapy be presented in written format, for reasons such as increasing the understanding of the information (Handelsman et al., 1986; Miller & Willner, 1974; Morrow, Gootnick, & Schmale, 1978), increasing the autonomy of clients (Hare-Mustin et al., 1979), and even decreasing malpractice lawsuits against psychologists (Austin, Moline, & Williams, 1990; Kovacs, 1984). Unfortunately, research has found that most written information given to clients is very difficult to understand; many forms are written at the difficulty level of an academic journal (Handelsman et al., 1986, 1995). Having written forms that cannot be read by people below a certain educational level discriminates against them and therefore is unjust.

Dr. Baker should inform her clients in language that is clear. For example, instead of saying, "Communications about injurious behavior to minors warrants breeches of confidentiality," she could say, "If you tell me you've abused your child, I must report you to the Social Services Department." She should avoid using jargon and should give clients the opportunity to ask questions about the information she provides. Her answers should be intended to inform clients, not to persuade them to enter treatment. If a client is not a native English speaker, she needs to be especially careful about using slang expression or figures of speech, which are particularly difficult for people from other cultures to understand (Sue & Sue, 1990). If Dr. Baker decides to present information to clients in writing, she should make the information readable (Sullivan, Martin, & Handelsman, 1993), but she should not substitute the written form for a complete informed consent process, which includes talking with clients about therapy and about any questions they have (Vaccarino, 1978). Depending on the language ability of her clients, she may need to translate any written information into the clients' primary language (APA, 1991).

Consent

Voluntariness

Consent to therapy or other psychological services must be voluntary; a coerced client or subject cannot give valid consent. "To coerce a person is to put him or her in a position where there is no meaningful alternative, a position in which the person can do nothing about the options and is forced to make a strongly biased choice" (Carroll et al., 1985, p. 30). For example, making a course grade dependent on participation in research, without allowing students to fulfill the research requirement in an alternative way, is unethical. Also coercive is the case in which the alternative to research participation is so odious that no reasonable student would choose it. Sometimes the line between persuasion and coercion is difficult to draw. In many forensic situations, such as court-ordered assessment and treatment within prisons, voluntary consent becomes more complicated, and psychologists must take care to respect the rights of clients (Clingempeel, Mulvey, & Reppucci, 1980).

If Dr. Baker leaves out important information about risks or about alternative sources of help, she runs the risk of coercing Ms. Young into treatment. However, if Dr. Baker really thinks that her therapy will do Ms. Young some good, she can give her professional recommendation; she must consider and reject the possibility (perhaps with help from a consultant) that she is acting solely out of self-interest. She also needs to frame her recommendation in a way that is not intimidating, that is respectful of Ms. Young's autonomy and right to refuse. "Recommending a course of action can be seen as promoting the client's welfare. However, when a course of action is insisted upon by the therapist, the client's right to free choice is diminished" (Hare-Mustin et al., 1979, p. 7).

Competence to Consent

For a consent to be valid, the client should be competent to make a rational choice. "The basic question is, Can the person engage in rational thought to a sufficient degree to make competent decisions about his or her life? Competence is assumed unless a person has been legally declared to be 'mentally incompetent'" (Everstine et al., 1980, p. 831). There are no perfect tests of competence. However, psychologists should be careful about judging a person incompetent merely on the basis of the fact that they disagree with the person's choice. One way to judge competence is to see if clients can give reasons for their decisions, keeping in mind that reasoned choices need not be perfect ones.

Even though the specific age of consent varies among the states, minors, by definition, are incompetent to consent to treatment. Developmental disabilities and other significant cognitive impairments may also lead to a judgment of incompetence. However, competence is not always an all-or-none judgment; even people with severe mental disorders can make some decisions at some times.

In cases of incompetence to consent, a proxy—usually a family member or court-appointed guardian—needs to give informed consent. But proxy consent does not reduce the psychologists' obligation to provide information to both the proxy and the incompetent person. According to the APA code, "Psychologists (1) inform those persons who are legally incapable of giving informed consent . . . in a manner commensurate with the persons' psychological capacities, (2) seek their assent to those interventions, and (3) consider such persons' preferences and best interests" (APA, 1992, p. 1605, Standard 4.02). People "assent" rather than "consent" when they understand that they will be involved in a relationship with a psychologist, even though they have no opportunity to refuse.

Exceptions to Informed Consent

The doctrine of informed consent includes four exceptions: incompetence, emergency, waiver, and therapeutic privilege.

1. *Incompetence*: When incompetence is used to denote an exception to informed consent, it refers to the inability of clients to make a reasoned decision as a result of age, crisis, mental illness, or other factors. However, psychologists must not assume that all clients coming for treatment are in a crisis severe enough to warrant an exception. If Dr. Baker felt that Ms. Young was in crisis and would not understand the information well enough to make a good decision, or needed help before she could explain all the ins and outs of therapy, Dr. Baker might *not* have to provide information and get consent.

2. *Emergency:* The second exception is emergency situations. In medicine, unconscious patients brought in by ambulance might die before they are physically able to give consent. In this case, providing treatment until the patient is able to give consent is not only justifiable but ethically obligatory. In psychotherapy, few clients are unconscious, yet emergency situations do occur. Psychologists may treat clients in emergencies without obtaining consent.

3. *Waiver:* The third exception to informed consent is waiver. Clients have the right to refuse information (*Cobbs v. Grant*, 1972), and some research in medicine has shown that some patients will exercise that right. For example, Alfidi (1975) told hospital patients that their upcoming medical procedures had some risks. When he asked patients if they wanted to be told what the specific risks were, over 60% of them said no. Thus, they waived their rights to information about risks. To be valid, waivers must be informed and voluntary; clients must know that they have a right to information.

4. *Therapeutic privilege:* The fourth and most controversial exception to informed consent is

called therapeutic privilege. In medicine, "a physician may legitimately withhold information, based on a sound medical judgment that to divulge the information would be potentially harmful to a depressed, emotionally drained, or unstable patient" (Beauchamp & Childress, 1994, p. 150). This exception is controversial because of the potential for abuse; for example, Dr. Baker can claim that all her clients come into her office highly distressed and thus that any information would be harmful. Ethics committees would be highly suspicious of such arguments and might encourage Dr. Baker to consider that she is using this exception as a cover for less noble motives such as self-interest or discomfort in providing information. The decisions clients need to make are important ones, and the process of informed consent need not be free of pain in order to be effective.

CONFIDENTIALITY

As Bersoff noted, "Except for the ultimate precept—above all, do no harm—there is probably no ethical value in psychology that is more inculcated than confidentiality" (1995, p. 143). The first theoretical justification for confidentiality is beneficence; it is widely believed that clients will be more favorably disposed toward therapy, and toward the self-disclosure involved, if they know that the information they provide will be kept private (Siegel, 1979).

The second major justification for confidentiality is respect for autonomy, and is rooted in the general notion in our society of a right to privacy. The information disclosed by clients still belongs to them, and not to the therapists. Therefore, therapists are not at liberty to decide what to do with that information. This basic right to privacy is established in common and constitutional law.

With these two justifications for confidentiality in mind, consider the following case:

Case #4-5
Dr. Braff is seeing a client, Joe, who is working on his ability to deal with stress in the workplace. Joe is a very cooperative client and is making some progress in the early stages of therapy. But Dr. Braff knows that even with the best clients, unanticipated issues about confidentiality may arise.

He has also read Standard 5.02, which says, in part, "Psychologists have a primary obligation and take reasonable precautions to respect the confidentiality rights of those with whom they work . . ." (APA, 1992, p. 1606). Dr. Braff considers the following possible scenarios so he can be prepared:

1. A concerned coworker of Joe's calls and asks how Joe is doing.
2. Joe tells Dr. Braff that he is going straight home after the session to kill his mother with the knife he has with him.
3. Joe tells Dr. Braff that he killed his mother last night, and nobody suspects.
4. Joe tells Dr. Braff that he plans to embezzle money from his company.
5. Joe tells Dr. Braff that he was just tested and is HIV-positive, and plans to have unprotected sex with his sexual partner or partners.

Dr. Braff wonders, "Assuming that Joe does not give me permission to speak to anybody in these situations, under which of these circumstances can I or should I violate Joe's confidentiality?"

This case highlights some major decisions to be made relevant to confidentiality, as well as some important elements of ethical reasoning. One should always anticipate the unanticipated to be prepared for a range of outcomes. One way to be prepared, and to understand one's ethical position, is to consider alternative scenarios that vary, starting with situations in which the ethical obligations are clear on each side. For example, Dr. Braff would certainly not break confidentiality in situation #1. According to the principles of beneficence and autonomy, Dr. Braff has no good reason to report Joe's progress in situation #1. Dr. Braff cannot even divulge whether or not Joe is a client. However, Dr. Braff has a clear duty to break confidentiality to protect the victim in situation #2. Once the "easy" scenarios are established, one can progress toward the gray areas (see below) in which judgments are more difficult. Situation #5 is such a gray area. This procedure helps define the ethical issues more precisely, defines the gray areas, and allows for full empirical and ethical consideration.

Confidentiality and Privilege

Whereas confidentiality is an ethical and legal obligation to keep disclosures private, privilege is a more limited legal right of clients not to have their disclosures revealed in legal proceedings. States grant privileged status to communications in several professional relationships, including attorney–client, doctor–patient, and psychologist–client. In some states the privilege is extended to family and group therapy in which more than one client is present. In other states, there is no privileged communication under these circumstances.

The privilege belongs to clients, and only they have the option of waiving the privilege. If clients waive the privilege, psychologists could testify in court even if their professional judgment is that such testimony will hurt the client. Once again, the choice of clients overrides the possible good that therapists believe they can do.

Limits of Confidentiality

Exceptions to confidentiality only occur when clients give permission or when other ethical obligations take precedence. Psychologists must never breach confidentiality simply to benefit the client, even when the benefit would be significant. For example, if Dr. Braff told a co-worker about Joe's progress, Joe might be eligible for a raise. Without Joe's consent, however, such behavior would still be unethical because it violates the rule of confidentiality and the principle of respect for autonomy. Confidentiality is a stringent requirement. Beneficence toward the client does not outweigh autonomy; paternalism is not justified in this case.

The APA code tells psychologists to inform clients of the limits of confidentiality. "Psychologists discuss with persons and organizations with whom they establish a scientific or professional relationship . . . (1) the relevant limitations on confidentiality . . . , and (2) the foreseeable uses of the information generated through their services" (APA, 1992, Standard 5.01, p. 1606).

Waiver

Clients may waive their right to confidentiality. Indeed, this is a relatively common event, as clients will want their therapists to convey information to other professionals (physicians, other therapists, etc.), to insurance companies in order to receive third-party payment, and to the psychologists' supervisors or consultants. If clients raise their psychotherapy or their mental status as an issue in court proceedings such as divorce and custody battles, job-related actions, and criminal proceedings, they automatically waive their right to confidentiality.

Child Abuse

Other situations involve breaking confidentiality without clients' permission. In these cases psychologists are obliged to violate confidentiality due to a legal obligation that society—via courts and legislatures—has deemed weightier than the clients' rights to privacy. One such situation is suspected abuse: All states have laws that obligate psychologists to report suspected child abuse or neglect (Kalichman, 1993). Some states also require the reporting of suspected elder abuse. The theory behind these laws is that the welfare of the child (or elder) outweighs considerations of confidentiality, and that the benefits accruing to the child compensate for the potential harm done to the therapeutic relationship. Whether the benefits outweigh the harms is still an open empirical question (Melton et al., 1995), one that is difficult to answer.

Dangerousness to Self or Others: The Duty to Protect

Psychologists must also take steps to prevent clients from committing suicide. If clients appear to be in imminent danger of doing so, psychologists must arrange for the safety of the clients, which means anything from contracting with clients to involuntary hospitalization (Bongar, 1991, 1992).

Many states have laws that obligate psychologists and others to break confidentiality when clients have made a threat of imminent physical harm to a reasonably identifiable victim or victims, and to take reasonable steps to prevent harm to the intended victims. These laws were enacted after the California Supreme Court, in *Tarasoff v. Board of Regents of California* (1976), found a therapist at fault for not taking appropriate steps to prevent a murder after a client had threatened the action.

The prevailing view in *Tarasoff* is that an immediate threat of imminent physical danger is enough

to override confidentiality. Because this exception to confidentiality occurs rarely and in specifically defined circumstances, the overall level of trust in therapy is not significantly diminished.

The opposing side in the *Tarasoff* case argued that confidentiality was a necessary part of psychotherapy; society benefits more in the long run when clients are not afraid to enter therapy. Clients will be more likely to feel free to disclose personal information in therapy when they can trust their therapists to maintain privacy. The empirical assumption is that getting therapy prevents people from committing serious crimes and that making it easier and safer for more people to get help reduces the number of crimes.

Notice that the principle of beneficence is invoked on both sides. This is an example in which the implementation of a principle, rather than which principle is at stake, defines the core ethical issue. The resolution of these issues rests on empirical questions, some of which cannot be answered easily, or at all.

Because the major purpose of breaking confidentiality is to protect clients or third parties, there is no obligation to report past crimes that clients have committed, or current or future crimes that do not involve significant physical harm. The only past harm that should be reported is child abuse or elder abuse if state law requires. Thus, Dr. Braff must not violate confidentiality to report a past murder (#3) or embezzlement (#4).

Circumstance (#5), in which Joe is HIV-positive, represents a current gray area in psychology. Dr. Braff's first obligation is to attend to the clinical needs of his client. Clinical sensitivity and the trust that has developed between therapist and client may prevent an ethical dilemma if Dr. Braff can convince Joe to inform his partner(s) about his status and practice safer sex.

If there were clear legal precedents, therapists' decisions would be easier. In the absence of such legal guidance, however, therapists must still consider their ethical obligations (Knapp & VandeCreek, 1990). One way some writers have attempted to do this is to judge the extent to which an AIDS-related situation is similar to a *Tarasoff* situation (Gray & Harding, 1988; Melton, 1988;

Schlossberger & Hecker, 1996). Thus, therapists must explore the following questions: Is unprotected sex "imminent danger"? What is the risk of HIV infection in each case of unprotected sex? Is HIV infection "significant physical harm"? Finally, how identifiable is the victim? The harm, in the form of AIDS, takes time to develop but is obviously significant. If Joe is married and threatens to have unsafe sex with his wife, Dr. Braff may have a clearer obligation to break confidentiality than if Joe is not sexually active and is talking about possible future events. In the absence of clear guidance, therapists are urged to act with clinical sensitivity and openness, be knowledgeable about state laws, and consult with senior colleagues and/or lawyers (McGuire, Nieri, Abbott, Sheridan, & Fisher, 1995).

Confidentiality in Other Contexts

This discussion of confidentiality has focused primarily on therapy situations, but confidentiality also governs psychologists' work in assessment, supervision, consultation, and other contexts. However, considerations of confidentiality may become less clear under various circumstances and need to be discussed in advance with the parties involved. For example, confidentiality may not exist between psychologists and those whom they are assessing if the assessment is done at the request of a third party such as a court or business. As mentioned before, clients in group and family therapy may not be protected to the same extent as individual clients (Arthur & Swanson, 1993). When minors are seen for therapy or assessment, parents may have access to the information disclosed (Gustafson & Mc-Namara, 1987).

Several issues related to confidentiality concern psychologists as teachers (Keith-Spiegel, Wittig, Perkins, Balogh, & Whitley, 1993). When psychologists use actual case examples from their own practice to illustrate points in the classroom or during workshops, they are ethically bound either to get permission from those clients or to disguise the identity of the clients. Questions of confidentiality also arise when final course grades are posted on the department wall. For example, are grades the prop-

erty of students and therefore private? Is posting grades by the last digits of students' social security numbers enough of a guarantee of anonymity?

The following case illustrates a few of the difficult choices teachers face about the information they receive from students in classroom discussions, papers, and office meetings:

Case #4-6
Dr. Gillespie, a college professor, is sitting down for what she hopes will be a quiet evening of grading papers for her "Abnormal Psychology" class. In the first paper, her student mentions that he has done drugs. In the second paper, the student seems to be admitting to having plagiarized her paper for another class. The third paper is by a seriously depressed student.

Students do not enjoy privileged communication or legal confidentiality with their instructors. Therefore, keeping written material confidential is a matter of ethics rather than law. In all three cases, Dr. Gillespie's first option may be to meet with the students who wrote the papers. Because there is no immediate threat of harm, Dr. Gillespie's initial impulse to turn in the first two students and to alert the counseling center about the third needs to be weighed against students' rights to privacy in addition to issues of respect. Dr. Gillespie may be justified in telling another professor because her loyalty to the college or to the welfare of the students may be stronger than her obligations of confidentiality.

Dr. Gillespie's dilemma could have been avoided had she reasoned through these scenarios in advance and developed a policy that she could communicate to students in class or on the syllabus. Of course, she needs to consult with officials and attorneys at the college to see if there are policies that relate to these cases.

PROFESSIONAL BOUNDARIES AND DUAL RELATIONSHIPS

Most people have heard or read stories about therapists who have sex with their clients, and most people accept that such behavior is unethical. Psychologists should know that sexual relationships with their clients, students, research participants, and others are forbidden. But there are many other behaviors that may or may not have a place in a professional relationship, and psychologists often have difficulty judging when they might be crossing the line between acceptable and unacceptable professional conduct. The following case introduces specific boundary questions psychologists confront in their professional work.

Case #4-7

Dr. Rodney is a psychologist in private practice. He calls his local ethics committee with a series of questions. He has been receiving, or anticipates receiving, many kinds of invitations from clients. He would like to know if he should or can accept any of these invitations, and what the ethical issues are. Some of the invitations Dr. Rodney receives are one-time events; others invite Dr. Rodney to become part of a different kind of relationship. These invitations all begin with "I would like you to . . .

. . . come to my wedding."
. . . attend my family reunion; they've all heard about you."
. . . accompany me to the movies Friday night."
. . . join me for a dinner party—just us two."
. . . come to a meeting with my lawyer to discuss our case."
. . . visit me in the hospital after my transplant."
. . . come to a barbecue for the other members of my cancer support group and their therapists."
. . . use my tickets to tonight's baseball game; I can't go."
. . . have this Christmas card."
. . . have this Picasso for your office as a token of my thanks."
. . . loan me $1,000."
. . . talk some about *your* problems for a change."
. . . hug me."
. . . do a custody evaluation on my son; my husband and I are divorcing."
. . . become a partner in my new couch business."

Ethics committees are happy to respond to psychologists who are looking to prevent ethical problems. Some prior consultation with psychologists might save the committee the painful task of investigating unethical behavior later. Unfortunately, the committee will not always be able to provide definitive answers because the decisions sometimes hinge on the specific facts of a given case, such as the type of therapy, the issues dealt with in therapy, the meaning to the client of a particular behavior, the cultural issues involved, and the personal situation of the therapist. But the committee can provide help to psychologists as they think through cases by highlighting the relevant ethical issues, including the concepts of boundaries and dual relationships.

Boundaries

The term *boundaries* refers to the parameters of professional relationships. Some behaviors are clearly standard procedures in various types of professional relationships. For example, interpreting a transference, doing hypnosis, charging a fee, and suggesting termination when therapy is not working are all behaviors that are appropriate for psychotherapists. Holding office hours, giving exams, and attending graduation ceremonies are appropriate behaviors for professors. On the other hand, some behaviors clearly are not part of such relationships. For example, going to the movies with psychotherapy clients or sending them sentimental birthday cards is not an appropriate behavior. Other behaviors, such as visiting clients in the hospital, may or may not be appropriate.

Gutheil and Gabbard (1993) differentiated between boundary *crossings*—which merely refer to behaviors that are not typically associated with the relationship—and boundary *violations*, which are crossings that are harmful. Boundary violations violate the principle of nonmaleficence and constitute conflicts of interest. We have seen such a conflict before, when Dr. Baker (Case #4-4) considered withholding information to increase the likelihood that a client will stay in therapy. Whenever the needs of clients, research participants, students, and other consumers become subordinate to the personal interests of psychologists, a conflict of interest occurs. Also, satisfying the psychologists' needs instead of the clients' is a violation of fidelity. Because boundary violations compromise the ability of psychologists to provide effective service, they violate the principle of beneficence. Whether actual or perceived, these conflicts can diminish the trustworthiness of psychologists in the eyes of clients, peers, and the public.

Gutheil and Gabbard (1993) provided a long list of boundary violations and crossings that may occur in psychoanalytically oriented psychotherapy. Many of the boundaries concern structural aspects of the relationship: time, space, and money. Starting or ending sessions early or late, taking phone calls at odd hours, meeting with clients during lunch or in cars, and letting a client's debt accumulate too much are all structural boundary crossings.

Another boundary crossing is giving or accepting gifts; the meaning and value of the gifts may determine whether they constitute a violation. A small token of thanks may be acceptable, whereas a priceless painting is not. Giving gifts as part of a professional relationship is also more characteristic of some cultural groups than others. Dr. Rodney would have to examine each of these factors to determine his policy about accepting gifts.

Another controversial issue is self-disclosure by psychotherapists. Disclosing their professional credentials, of course, is an essential part of the relationship. Some disclosures about the therapist's life may have a positive impact in therapy (Hendrick, 1988). However, therapists must carefully examine their own motivations to avoid crossing or violating a boundary. Therapists who talk about their own lives may indicate that they are seeking "personal gratification that is beyond the professional satisfaction derived from being a part of the therapeutic process" (Smith & Fitzpatrick, 1995, p. 500). In addition, self-disclosure is often a precursor to sexual involvement (Simon, 1991).

Nonerotic touch is another very controversial boundary issue (Kertay & Reviere, 1993). Handshakes are generally considered an acceptable part of a professional relationship (Pope, Tabachnick, & Keith-Spiegel, 1987), but pats on the shoulder, hugs, and other forms of touching can be easily misinterpreted by clients as having some sexual connotation. Again, however, theoretical orientation may be an important factor: Touching clients in certain ways may be acceptable in some humanistic therapies under certain conditions (Holub & Lee, 1990), but anything more than a handshake may be out of bounds in psychoanalytic psychotherapy (Gutheil & Gabbard, 1993).

The same behavior may be a crossing or a violation depending on what the therapist does clinically. "The difference between a harmful and a harmless boundary crossing may lie in whether it is discussed or discussable; clinical exploration of a violation often defuses its potential for harm" (Gutheil & Gabbard, 1993, p. 190). For example, going to a family reunion may be acceptable if the purposes, nature, and meanings of the event were discussed in therapy. But the fact that clinical sensitivity may decrease the risk of boundary crossings does not absolve psychologists of the responsibility for avoiding boundary violations.

Dual Relationships

Dual relationships are magnified boundary violations that add an entirely new relationship to an established one. The additional relationship violates the principles of nonmaleficence and autonomy. Sonne (1994, p. 336) defined dual relationships as

> those situations in which the psychologist functions in more than one professional relationship, as well as those in which the psychologist functions in a professional role and another definitive and intended role (as opposed to a limited and inconsequential role growing out of and limited to a chance encounter).

The APA (1992) ethics code obligates psychologists to avoid potentially harmful dual relationships, although the code recognizes that these are sometimes difficult to avoid. In small towns, for example, a client may have few options for psychological services; the only psychologist in town may be a customer at the client's store. These situations demand extra caution and clarity when psychologists negotiate these relationships. Indeed, all the issues of informed consent become even more important (Sleek, 1994).

The major rationale behind the prohibition of dual relationships, like other boundary violations, is nonmaleficence. The objectivity necessary for good decision making in a professional relationship is lost when it is contaminated by the demands of a second relationship. For example, clients may not feel comfortable telling a friend who is also their therapist that they are not benefiting from therapy and want to stop. In the same light, therapists may find it hard to confront clients about inappropriate behaviors in therapy when they enjoy or benefit from those very behaviors as friends or when such confrontations may jeopardize the friendship. Even objectivity in other professional relationships might be jeopardized: Therapists may not provide the best custody evaluation when their clients are involved.

Dual relationships also violate the principle of autonomy. When a dual relationship occurs, clients no longer know whether the therapists' actions are based on sound professional judgment or concerns about sex, friendship, money, and the like. Further, the ethical obligations of autonomy and fidelity are compromised when dual relationships become exploitive. For example, a therapist who loans a client money may be tempted to keep the client in therapy until the loan is paid off.

Dual relationships can exist either simultaneously or sequentially. For example, the actual or perceived conflicts of interest are equally great whether Dr. Rodney did a custody evaluation for the son of a current or a former client. In other words, the perceptions, expectations, obligations, and power involved in professional relationships do not necessarily end when the relationship ends.

Kitchener (1988) explored the factors that make dual relationships so potentially harmful. She isolated three specific aspects of relationships—expectations, obligations, and power—and hypothesized that the greater the difference in these three variables between each of the relationships, the more potential for harm. For example, the differences in expectations between the role of therapist and the role of friend are usually much greater than the differences in expectations between the roles of employer and research supervisor. Thus, the former dual relationship may be more dangerous than the latter.

Sexual Relationships

The APA (1992) code specifically prohibits sexual intimacies with psychotherapy clients (Standard 4.05), recognizing that sexual relationships in therapy are a very severe form of dual relationship. Several states have also made therapist–client sex illegal (Strasburger, Jorgenson, & Randles, 1991). Research has shown that psychotherapy clients involved in sexual relationships with their therapists can suffer very severe negative effects, from loss of trust to suicide (Pope, 1988; Pope & Bouhoutsos, 1986).

The issue of sexual relationships with former clients was not addressed by the APA ethics codes until the current version was published in 1992. The current code prohibits sexual relationships with former clients for two years after termination of the professional relationship. Even after two years, the burden is on the psychologist to prove that the relationship is not harmful or exploitive. The code states, "because such intimacies undermine public confidence in the psychology profession and thereby deter the public's use of needed services, psychologists do not engage in sexual intimacies with former therapy patients . . . even after a two-year interval except in the most unusual circumstances" (APA, 1992, p. 1605, Standard 4.07). This provision of the code is very controversial; some have argued that all posttermination sexual relationships should be prohibited (Gabbard, 1994).

Psychotherapy is not the only professional relationship that is incompatible with sexual intimacies. The APA code explicitly bans sexual relationships with students: "Psychologists do not engage in sexual relationships with students or supervisees in training over whom the psychologist has evaluative or direct authority, because such relationships are so likely to impair judgment or be exploitive" (APA, 1992, p. 1602; Standard 1.19b). Although the APA code is silent about relationships with former students, professors may still be considered to be in a relationship with students even after the end of particular courses or graduate programs; for example, they may be asked by students to write letters of recommendation or to provide references for jobs.

Other Dual Relationships

Although sexual dual relationships have received the most attention (Smith & Fitzpatrick, 1995) and are the only ones mentioned specifically in the APA code, other dual relationships, including friendships and business relationships, can also be harmful. Some authors consider bartering, in which clients pay for therapy with goods or services, to be a dual relationship. Even accepting expensive gifts may change the relationship so much that it can be judged a dual relationship (Keith-Spiegel & Koocher, 1985).

Sometimes one relationship naturally evolves into others. For example, when students graduate from a clinical psychology graduate program, they often interact with their former professors as colleagues at professional meetings, as research collaborators, and sometimes as faculty members at the same institution. However, some progressions of one professional relationship to another are not as natural, and should be avoided. For example, clinical supervisors should not become therapists to those they formerly supervised.

Handling Potential Boundary Violations and Dual Relationships

Concerns about dual relationships and other boundary issues are very common among psychologists (Pope & Vetter, 1992). Smith and Fitzpatrick (1995) urge a conservative stance: "In the face of uncertainty, therapists are advised to err on the side of caution and abstain from crossing a boundary when there is a potential that their behavior, however well-intentioned, could be construed as misconduct by clients or peers" (p. 504). For example, Gutheil and Gabbard (1993) noted that ethics committees and other disciplinary bodies may be more likely to conclude that sexual behavior occurred in a therapeutic relationship if a psychologist routinely scheduled the client for the last time slot of the day. Small boundary crossings often lead to harmful dual relationships. Accepting invitations even for a cup of coffee may be misinterpreted by both client and psychologist as a sign that therapy may or should turn into a friendship or romantic relationship. Even such a subtle behavior as writing a letter on a client's behalf or wearing particular clothing (e.g., seductive or too casual) may be considered a possible crossing, especially when several small behaviors are combined (Gutheil & Gabbard, 1993).

One way Dr. Rodney can determine whether a particular behavior constitutes a boundary violation is to ask the following question: Is this behavior part of recognized professional practice in this context (Gutheil & Gabbard, 1993)? For example, romantic and sexual behaviors are not part of psychotherapy. Performing psychotherapy is not part of a custody evaluation. Business partnerships are not part of the therapeutic relationship.

Another question that Dr. Rodney can ask is, "Is this behavior an exception to my policies, my usual way of doing things?" Such exceptions are always cause for concern because they may be based on bias rather than on sound judgment. For example, if a psychoanalytic therapist has a policy against self-disclosure and then "begins to indulge in even mild forms of self-disclosure, it is an indication for careful self-scrutiny regarding the motivations for departure from the usual therapeutic stance" (Gutheil & Gabbard, 1993, p. 194).

Evidence of biased judgments may show itself in exceptions or in behavior based on professionally irrelevant factors. If Dr. Rodney were to argue that some clients need hugs for therapeutic reasons, he needs to question his judgment if on reflection he finds, for example, that only attractive female clients seem to need his hugs (Holroyd & Brodsky, 1980).

When psychologists attempt to determine and label dual relationships, they will always encounter gray areas. For example, professors and students are often engaged in several types of interactions with each other. A professor may be a classroom instructor, an academic advisor, an internship supervisor, and a research collaborator to the same student. At times it may be unclear whether these are multiple roles or merely multiple aspects of the same role. In any case, professors must be careful not to exploit their relationships with students by violating the boundaries of the professor–student relationship, however broadly conceived. Regardless of the label attached to a "dual relationship" or a "multifaceted professional relationship," the potential for harm exists, and Kitchener's (1988) approach of looking at disparities in expectations, obligations, and power will still be useful.

In Dr. Rodney's case, all the invitations and behaviors he is exploring are boundary crossings; they go beyond the therapeutic contract. Although Dr. Rodney did not initiate any of the invitations in this case, as the psychologist he is always responsible for avoiding boundary violations (Smith & Fitzpatrick, 1995). When considering whether he should go to a client's wedding, reunion, apartment, or lawyer's office, his thinking might include the following: A visit with a lawyer may be related to the therapy; the other visits are not. The wedding is a public event and a recognized ritual that may be acceptable depending on how it was handled in the therapy. The reunion and dinner for two are personal and private events that would be harder to justify.

Gottlieb (1993) formulated a decision-making strategy to help psychologists judge whether adding a new relationship to an existing relationship will be problematic. He suggested using three dimensions of the relationship: power, duration, and termination. The first step in Gottlieb's process is to consider the existing relationship; if the power is high, the duration long, and the termination indefinite, no other relationship should be considered. Thus, if Dr. Rodney is doing long-term therapy, he should be especially careful not to accept personal invitations, gifts, or business opportunities. If Dr. Rodney had taught a one-session class on smoking cessation to a class of 75 people, the low power, short duration, and definite termination may mean that he could consider forming another relationship. If, however, Dr. Rodney did a custody evaluation, the duration is relatively short and the termination is definite, but the power is very high. Thus, by looking at all possible boundary violations in terms of Gottlieb's dimensions, as well as the potential for exploitation, harm, and compromise of trust, psychologists will prevent many unfortunate outcomes.

A final relevant issue arises when a psychologist learns of a colleague who has engaged in dual relationships. Consider the following case:

Case #4-8
A client comes into see Dr. Terry and tells Dr. Terry that she had sex with her previous therapist.

Dr. Terry immediately tells the client that this incident needs to be reported to the state ethics committee and licensure board. The client says, "I'd prefer not to," and refuses to sign a release of information form or to initiate a complaint against her previous therapist. What should Dr. Terry do?

The options for Dr. Terry include: (1) making the report herself, stating the client's name; (2) going to see the previous therapist and confronting him with her client's charges; (3) making an anonymous report; (4) letting the client know about her options and working within clinical boundaries to encourage reporting; and (5) ignoring the entire incident.

Dr. Terry should first look for guidance in the APA code. In most cases, psychologists handle ethical violations informally by "bringing it to the attention of that individual" (APA, 1992, p. 1611, Standard 8.04). However, with serious violations like sexual misconduct, the code requires reporting the violation to ethics committees and/or state licensing boards. These guidelines would seem to leave out option #2 and require either option #1 or #3. However, the APA code also states that informal resolution or reporting can be done "unless such action conflicts with confidentiality rights in ways that cannot be resolved" (APA, 1992, p. 1611, Standard 8.05). The client's right to confidentiality, which she does not want to waive, outweighs the psychologist's obligation to report. Remember that past harm is not a valid exception to confidentiality.

Though frustrating to Dr. Terry because of the probability that the other therapist is exploiting other clients, her best course of action is to let her client know of the options. Perhaps the client will feel stronger and more comfortable after she works in therapy and develops trust in Dr. Terry, and will make a report at a future time.

ISSUES OF CULTURAL DIVERSITY

We have noted throughout this chapter that cultural variables affect the decisions we make about ethical issues. Lack of sensitivity to the diversity of the people psychologists interact with can lead to serious ethical problems. Consider the following case:

Case #4-9

Ms. Cheatham, a graduate student therapist under the supervision of Dr. Armstrong, is currently seeing two families in treatment. By coincidence, both families have sons who recently graduated from distant colleges and moved into houses next door to their parents. However, the two families have very different reactions. Family A, who have lived in this town for generations, come to the next therapy session in great distress over their son moving back so close to them, and Ms. Cheatham enthusiastically begins work on getting the son to feel independent enough to move further from home. When Family B, who immigrated to this country several years ago, comes to the next session, Ms. Cheatham is surprised to learn that they are terminating treatment; they see their son's move back close to them as the best possible solution to their problems.

During her next supervision, Ms. Cheatham tells Dr. Armstrong about her impulse to talk Family B out of leaving therapy and to convince them that having an adult son living next door is a sign of family pathology. They discuss the fact that Ms. Cheatham shares the Western cultural background of Family A and must become aware of the values and attitudes of Family B. Dr. Armstrong congratulates Ms. Cheatham for being open to her own reactions and values, and for her decision to talk to her supervisor before inappropriately imposing those values on her clients.

The potential for imposing psychologists' own values on clients to the detriment of those clients exists in all professional relationships (Corey et al., 1993). The possibility of harm being done by imposing values is increased when many of the basic, often unverbalized, assumptions psychologists make differ from those of their clients. Differences in values may be much more likely when psychologists deal with clients from cultural groups different from their own.

Awareness of Self

The groups of people who are considered under the term *cultural diversity* are different for different psychologists, depending on their own backgrounds, values, and tolerance. Such variables as nationality, ethnic background, religion, gender, sexual preference, age, geographic location, social class, and even professional affiliation can all be dimensions along which people can be classified as different. For example, Ms. Cheatham may have felt differently about the "pathology," and less likely to object, if the child renting a house next to the parents was a woman versus a man, a homosexual versus a heterosexual, or a member of a rich, politically well-connected family versus a poor, working-class family.

Psychologists may find it difficult to admit negative attitudes—such as dislike or fear—toward members of other groups. The behaviors that demonstrate these attitudes are often very subtle. For example, psychologists might quickly judge that a particular client will not score well on an intelligence test and therefore might not wait as long for the client to answer the questions before counting answers wrong.

Even well-meaning, compassionate psychologists may have difficulty admitting their lack of competence to treat or assess all clients. Psychologists are not able to work with all clients because of their lack of knowledge and skill in dealing with various groups and/or their own attitudes. Working with members of different cultural groups is more than a simple extension of our unconditional positive regard and lack of prejudice (Dana, 1993; Sue, 1990). Ramirez, Wassef, Paniagua, and Linskey (1996) found that psychologists knew that it was quite important to recognize cultural variables when assessing clients, but they also did not feel competent actually dealing with such issues. They recommended more education about multicultural issues, and found that when psychologists learned more about different cultural groups, they reported more enjoyment working with members of those groups.

Awareness of Clients in Context

Sue and Sue (1990) discussed three types of barriers to effective cross-cultural counseling, but these barriers also exist in assessment, teaching, research, and other professional endeavors. The first type of barrier they discussed concerns language and communication. For example, eye contact can mean engagement, interest, and comfort in a Western culture, but may signify disrespect in another culture. If eye contact is inappropriately used in a mental status exam, members of certain cultural groups could be systematically mislabeled.

The second type of barrier Sue and Sue (1990) discussed concerned class variables. Once again, traits such as apathy, indifference, or dependence could be inappropriately attributed to people on the basis of behaviors that are due to poverty and unemployment rather than to psychopathology.

The third type of barrier consists of cultural variables. Psychotherapy and assessment place a high value on self-disclosure, opening up to strangers about personal problems, straightforward answers to questions, and rational analytic processes. These values are not shared by all cultures. Western values that underlie psychotherapy include individual uniqueness, free choice, and self-assertion. Eastern values, by contrast, include interdependence, the collective, and acceptance of one's environment (Saeki & Borow, 1985).

Also, the goals of therapy may vary greatly depending on one's cultural values. Traditional therapy focuses on developing independence, autonomy, and rational thought. These goals do not fit with cultures that place more value on collective life, spirituality, and relationship to the world.

Sue and Sue (1990) encouraged psychologists to be aware that people can have widely disparate world views based on their cultural experiences and background. In Western-majority cultures, many people believe that their own hard work will yield rewards, and if not, they must be at fault. But people who have experienced oppression as a group have not seen their efforts pay off, and they may believe that their lack of rewards is due to influences of society rather than to laziness, poor work habits, or mental illness.

Not all members of each cultural group have the same world view. Members of particular groups differ among themselves on the basis of such variables as subcultural patterns, age, social class, geography, and level of acculturation (Aponte & Barnes, 1995). Assuming that differences exist between cultural groups is just as dangerous as assuming that all people are the same. For example, members of a minority group who have a high level of acculturation—have adopted the values and mo-

res of the majority culture—may be more different from recent immigrants from their own group than they are from members of the majority group.

Differences in world view reflect actual differences in the experiences of various groups in our society and lead psychologists to rethink the role of society in the generation of psychopathology. The internal world view of Western psychology and psychotherapy creates the assumption that many symptoms are the result of individual dynamics and bad choices; thus, changes in the person's own thoughts and emotions will lead to improvement. However, feminist therapists and others have explored the role society plays in the development of behavioral and emotional problems (Lerman & Porter, 1990). They believe that many symptoms are generated not by imperfect individual processes but by the experience of socialization, which includes oppressive aspects. Reactions to oppression would then be more common among women and minorities, and these may be diagnosed as mental illness by members of the majority culture.

Part of being culturally aware is recognizing the meaning of diagnosis, assessment, and treatment for the individuals involved. But cultural awareness also means acknowledging the meaning of these professional functions in the larger societal context. (See Chapter 15 for a full discussion of cultural issues.)

Ethical Issues and Cultural Variables

To the extent that lack of sensitivity and consequent lack of clinical skill compromises the effectiveness of assessment, therapy, and other clinical work, psychologists violate the principles of nonmaleficence and beneficence. To the extent that they treat members of all groups the same, to the detriment of some individuals, they are behaving unjustly. To the extent that clients cannot make good decisions, psychologists compromise the principle of autonomy.

Psychologists need to be aware of those aspects of their practice that bear directly on ethical issues. As mentioned before, cultural background will influence perceptions of informed consent, boundaries, and other issues. For example, in cultures that hold strong paternalistic views about who runs the family, asking for consent to family treatment from both a son and his elderly mother may be meaningless to clients. In discussing confidentiality, Arthur and Swanson encouraged therapists to "acknowledge and remain sensitive to how cultural differences about privacy and disclosure may affect client expectations, interpretations, and understandings regarding confidentiality" (1993, p. 41).

The potential for exploitation is heightened when dealing with diverse groups because of the nature of the power relationship. Pope and Vasquez (1991) noted that "the differential power between therapist and client . . . may lose its enabling, healing, or therapeutic force and become instead a reflection of the power differential that is frequently perceived between the rich and the poor, between the racial majority and minorities, and between other social, economic, or political groupings" (p. 131). Psychologists may unwittingly maintain a status quo that includes elements of discrimination, bias, and prejudice. Therapists need to balance the tendency to accept clients' stereotypic views without question and the tendency to transform clients' world views into their own (Margolin, 1982).

Finally, given that maladaptive behavior may be influenced by societal factors in addition to individual factors, psychotherapy may not be the best way to help individuals who are experiencing difficulties in their lives. Rather, social and political action may be more effective at helping people. Psychologists may have some ethical responsibility to engage in such social action—for example, lobbying or community organizing—to fulfill their professional mission to improve the condition of people's lives.

On a broader level, psychologists must understand that some of their fundamental notions about principle-based ethics exist in a limited cultural context. Alternatives to principle-based ethical reasoning are discussed next.

EMERGING TRENDS AND ISSUES

Clinical psychology changes rapidly; new issues, techniques, and findings make it difficult to predict what will happen even a few years from now. The ethical reasoning that psychologists have been developing will need to be applied to emerging areas of involvement, such as prescribing medication (Buelow & Chafetz, 1996) and working with recovered memories (Handelsman, Bershenyi, Whetsel, Maestas, & Boynton, 1996; Polusny & Follette, 1996). In this section, however, we highlight several trends that represent more significant changes in the way psychologists might need to think about the ethics of their work: managed care, the enforcement of ethics codes, and alternatives to principle-based ethical reasoning.

Ethical Practice and Managed Care

The therapeutic context in which clinical psychologists work is changing drastically. Traditionally, psychologists could "hang out their shingle" and have clients consult them in confidence for help in solving personal problems. The clients or their insurance companies would pay the psychologists' "reasonable and customary" fees. Those days are over.

In the last twenty years, the health care industry, including mental health, has developed new models of service delivery in an attempt to curb escalating costs (Broskowski, 1991). *Managed care* refers to a variety of agencies and techniques designed to contain the costs of treatment (Winegar, 1992). Managed care agencies, such as health maintenance organizations and preferred provider organizations, have instituted new types of cost containment mechanisms that create ethical problems for psychologists.

Perhaps the most fundamental change in the managed care approach is "utilization review," which refers to "techniques . . . used to . . . evaluate the necessity or appropriateness of care for the purposes of insurance coverage or provider reimbursement" (Winegar, 1992, p. 331). Traditionally, clients and psychologists decided between themselves what kinds and amounts of services were needed. Insurance companies typically paid for the services that psychologists judged appropriate. Now, however, managed care agencies typically employ case managers to decide, either before or during treatment, whether a particular psychological service is "medically necessary." Thus, case managers become an active third party in the provision of mental health care (Haas & Cummings, 1991).

Utilization review by case managers presents several potential ethical problems. The first problem concerns autonomy: Most managed care agencies offer clients a limited choice of providers and less variety in the kinds of treatment available. A second problem concerns confidentiality: Information traditionally shared only between psychologist and client must now be reviewed by third parties.

The third and most fundamental ethical problem with utilization review concerns the definition of the helping relationship and the potential loyalties of psychologists. Who are the clients in the typical managed care scenario—the people seeking therapy, or the managed care agencies who actually contract with and pay the psychologists? The goal of saving money often conflicts with the goal of helping clients.

Although most psychologists are involved in potential conflicts because they make money, managed care brings the conflict into sharper focus. "Managed care entities often give their participating providers financial incentives . . . to hold down the actual cost of care" (Newman & Bricklin, 1991, p. 26). Thus, psychologists may feel more temptation to end therapy prematurely, thereby causing harm to clients. Another managed care strategy is to put caps or limits on the number of psychotherapy sessions they will pay for. Psychologists then need to deal with clients who can no longer afford treatment as they had under existing insurance systems (Haas & Cummings, 1991). Their options are to refer the client to another therapist or to see the client for a reduced fee. In fact, the APA (1992) code prohibits psychologists from abandoning their clients and encourages them to provide some of their service for little or no financial gain.

Haas and Cummings (1991) correctly pointed out that the short-term treatments favored by managed care agencies are not necessarily bad and often provide effective and efficient help. However, limited treatment will not meet all clients' needs. Thus, psychologists in managed care risk violating beneficence for two reasons. First, risks increase when

psychologists who sign up to work for managed care agencies are not competent to provide shorter term treatment. The changing paradigm of care delivery presents ethical challenges for those who train clinical psychologists. For example, training psychologists to do only long-term psychotherapy without an awareness of the current demands for shorter term treatment leads to graduates who may be considered incompetent to practice.

The second threat to beneficence is that psychologists often are not the ones making decisions about the length of treatment. Case managers place limits on care for reasons other than clinical effectiveness. Psychologists who judge that their clients need more than the allotted number of sessions must petition the managed care agency for more time (Appelbaum, 1993) and appeal decisions that certain treatments are not medically necessary (*Wickline v. State of California*, 1987). This role of advocate for a client's reimbursement is a new one with many gray areas (Appelbaum, 1993). The behaviors of "advocate" in addition to behaviors of "psychotherapist" may constitute a boundary violation or a dual relationship, depending on the nature of the treatment, the intensity of the advocacy, and other aspects of the situation.

Also, issues of informed consent arise when psychologists are encouraged or required by some agencies not to tell clients about financial and other arrangements (Haas & Cummings, 1991). Psychologists need to inform clients about situations that rarely occurred under the old paradigms: Clients may run out of benefits before therapy is over, they may be referred to other therapists after a limited number of sessions, and they may be denied "medically unnecessary" treatment even before their benefits run out (Appelbaum, 1993).

A managed care paradigm may increase the importance of ethical reasoning as a way to ensure that concerns about cost do not hinder the mission of the profession to render service to clients.

Enforcing Ethics Codes

Just as shrinking health care resources and other societal pressures make attention to ethics as important as ever (Wolf, 1994), several trends have converged to make enforcing ethics codes more difficult for state psychological associations. Society has become more litigious; consumers are more likely to sue psychologists for malpractice, and psychologists are more likely to sue ethics committees and licensing boards when an unfavorable decision is rendered. Indeed, one North Carolina court found that a previous version of the APA ethics code was unconstitutionally vague and could not be used as grounds for revoking a psychologist's license (*White v. North Carolina State Board of Examiners of Practicing Psychologists*, 1990). As the legal and ethics realms have fused more and more, psychologists find themselves confronting difficult choices when they simultaneously face ethics complaints and malpractice suits. They would like to cooperate with their local ethics committees, but such cooperation may increase their liability in court.

Several state associations have recently decided no longer to investigate complaints of ethical violations. Seaman (1996) noted that many ethics committees began their investigative activities before there were state licensing boards. Licensing boards can take more effective actions, and state associations often do not have the financial and legal resources to support their volunteer committee members (Nagy, 1996). These factors, combined with an increased risk of lawsuits against ethics committees, have led some association ethics committees to choose to concentrate exclusively on their education and consultation functions.

Alternatives to Principle-Based Ethical Reasoning

Virtue Ethics

Applying ethical principles to a series of cases and dilemmas is a standard way of approaching ethical reasoning; indeed, this chapter has followed such an approach. However, Jordan and Meara (1990) argued that "principle ethics" is incomplete and flawed. The application of ethical principles runs the risk of becoming too intellectual and too disconnected from the actors, the psychologists making the decisions.

Meara and her colleagues (Jordan & Meara, 1990; Meara, Schmidt, & Day, 1996) have advocated the introduction of *virtue ethics* as a supplement to the use of ethical principles in psychology. "Virtue ethics focuses on the ideal rather than the obligatory and on the character of the agent or professional rather than on the solving of specific ethical dilemmas" (Meara et al., 1996, p. 47). In principle ethics, the major question for defining ethical behavior is "What should I do?" Advocates of virtue ethics consider that question incomplete and argue that a more comprehensive approach adds the question "Who shall I be?" Jordan and Meara postulated that "achieving professional maturity and internalizing professional virtue are prerequisite to competent application of ethical principles" (1990, p. 109).

Virtues refer to elements of one's character. There is no definitive set of virtues, but Meara et al. (1996) proposed a list of four basic virtues for consideration. The first is *prudence*, which includes being cautious, planful, and "knowing when one does not know" (p. 39). The second virtue is *integrity*, which refers to having a stable and coherent value system over time and acting in accordance with it (Beauchamp & Childress, 1994). The third virtue is *respectfulness* of individuals and communities "in the terms they themselves (not the professionals) define" (Meara et al., 1996, p. 44). The fourth virtue is *benevolence*, the desire to do good. To the extent that these and other virtues are present, professional decisions and behaviors will be grounded in a sound ethical context.

Meara et al. (1996) recognized that virtue ethics is not a substitute for but, rather, a supplement to, principle ethics. Whereas principle ethics alone provides a basis for a series of rules to be adhered to, virtue ethics challenges psychologists to explore an ethical idea to which they can aspire. An emphasis on virtues and ideals may also lead to better ethical behavior in a multicultural environment by placing more emphasis on self-awareness and awareness of the customs, values, and traditions of the communities that help define desired virtues. For example, Meara et al. (1996) stated that "a prudent individual is aware that another's definition of the situation is not necessarily one's own" (p. 40).

The concept of virtue ethics applied to psychology is still in its infancy, and many questions remain to be answered (Kitchener, 1996; Vasquez, 1996). The approach has been criticized for being too idealistic and incomplete (Bersoff, 1995). However, virtue ethics may help psychologists expand their ability to counteract some of the problems that accompany an exclusive reliance on principles. Discussion of the virtues necessary in good psychologists may help the profession articulate and actualize its core values.

Ethics of Care

The *ethics of care* grew out of research by Gilligan (1982) and others who studied how women develop and articulate their ethical stance. In general, women, unlike many men, are not driven by dispassionate analysis of rights and obligations, which Gilligan calls the *justice* orientation. Rather, women tend to conceive of ethics in terms of the relationships in which they find themselves; this conception is called the *care* orientation. Ethics flows from the internal, emotionally charged characteristics of the relationship, which carry more weight than the imposition of external, intellectual, theoretical principles. Both men and women can approach ethical issues using either approach, but men are more likely to take the justice orientation and women tend toward the care orientation (Gilligan, Ward, & Taylor, 1988).

There are some fundamental differences between the care and justice orientations (Carse, 1991). For example, the principle or justice orientation appears to treat professional relationships as if they were always among equals, free agents, who choose their relationships. As any student in a required course will attest, many helping relationships are involuntary and based on vulnerability rather than equality. Therefore, "as a framework for moral decision, care is grounded in the assumption that the other and self are *interdependent*" (Gilligan, 1982, p. 24, emphasis added). This interdependence creates a need for psychologists to appreciate the specifics of each particular relationship and their responsibilities to particular individuals, in addition to the abstract and universal qualities of rights and obligations (Carse, 1991).

Like virtue ethics, the ethics of care discusses desirable aspects of professionals, but focuses on traits or characteristics that occur primarily in relation to others, traits such as sympathy, compassion, and love. The ethics of care also emphasizes the role of emotions; being a responsible professional has as much to do with the emotional experience of relationship as the cognitions of impartial ethical analysis. For example, in Case #4-4, in which Dr. Baker struggled with what to tell Ms. Young about the risks of therapy, Dr. Baker's feelings—including sympathy, concern, and frustration with Ms. Young—would be an integral part of ethical decision making rather than obstacles to be overcome by the use of principles. "Our moral experience suggests that our responses rely on our emotions, our capacity for sympathy, our sense of friendship, and our knowledge of how caring people behave" (Beauchamp & Childress, 1994, p. 88).

The ethics of care and principle ethics are not mutually exclusive. As Carse (1991) noted, for example, "We still need to articulate a clear set of standards by which we can distinguish morally good from morally problematic (or even morally debased) forms of 'care'" (p. 24). However, the relative weight given to care versus principles is still controversial. The next ten years should see increased debate about the role of the care orientation in psychology, the practical applications of that orientation, and the integration of care and justice orientations.

Neither the ethics of care nor virtue ethics by themselves give psychologists concrete guidelines for how to act in particular situations. However, these two approaches can be part of a complete decision-making process that is relevant when psychologists need to make real-world decisions. They compel psychologists to reflect from new perspectives and to question the assumptions that are so easy to take for granted. An openness to the wisdom of different approaches to complex issues may help guard against professional shortsightedness and arrogance.

CONCLUSION

Like any profession, psychology is constantly evolving. As psychologists continue to face the challenges of new technologies, new paradigms, and new perspectives, they will certainly continue to reap wonderful rewards from a profession designed to allow people growth and fulfillment. In a pluralistic and ever-changing social climate, psychologists are also certain to continue facing regulations, along with practical, legal, and ethical constraints. The key to professional fulfillment is to see these rules only as part of a larger process by which psychologists strive to perfect their art and science. As Smith and Fitzpatrick noted, "in the final analysis, ethical practice is governed less by proscriptions than by sound clinical judgment bearing on the . . . interventions that will advance the client's welfare" (Smith & Fitzpatrick, 1995, p. 505). Ethical decisions demand more than merely good intentions and technical competence. The abilities to think, feel, reason, reflect, and explore will always be critical to the practice of clinical psychology.

REFERENCES

Alfidi, R. J. (1975). Controversy, alternatives, and decisions in complying with the legal doctrine of informed consent. *Radiology, 114,* 231–234.

American Psychological Association. (1953). *Ethical standards of psychologists.* Washington, DC: Author.

American Psychological Association. (1987). *Casebook on ethical principles of psychologists.* Washington, DC: Author.

American Psychological Association. (1991). *Guidelines for providers of psychological services to ethnic, linguistic, and culturally diverse populations.* Washington, DC: Author.

American Psychological Association. (1992). Ethical principles of psychologists and code of conduct. *American Psychologist, 47,* 1597–1611.

American Psychological Association. (1994). Guidelines for child custody evaluations in divorce proceedings. *American Psychologist, 49,* 677–680.

American Psychological Association Ethics Committee. (1996). Rules and procedures: June 1, 1996. *American Psychologist, 51,* 529–548.

APA's ethics committee adopts statement on telephone therapy. (1995, October). *APA Monitor,* p. 15.

Aponte, J. F., & Barnes, J. M. (1995). Impact of acculturation and moderator variables on the intervention and treatment of ethnic groups. In J. F. Aponte, R. Y. Rivers, & J. Wohl (Eds.), *Psychological interventions and cultural diversity* (pp. 19–39). Boston: Allyn and Bacon.

Aponte, J. F., & Crouch, R. T. (1995). The changing ethnic profile of the United States. In J. F. Aponte, R. Y. Rivers, & J. Wohl (Eds.), *Psychological interventions and cultural diversity* (pp. 1–18). Boston: Allyn and Bacon.

Appelbaum, D., & Lawton, S. V. (1990). *Ethics and the professions.* Englewood Cliffs, NJ: Prentice-Hall.

Appelbaum, P. S. (1993). Legal liability and managed care. *American Psychologist, 48,* 251–257.

Appelbaum, P. S., Lidz, C. W., & Meisel, A. (1987). *Informed consent: Legal theory and clinical practice.* New York: Oxford University Press.

Arthur, G. L., Jr., & Swanson, C. D. (1993). *Confidentiality and privileged communication.* Alexandria, VA: American Counseling Association.

Austin, K. M., Moline, M. E., & Williams, G. T. (1990). *Confronting malpractice: Legal and ethical dilemmas in psychotherapy.* Thousand Oaks, CA: Sage Publications.

Baumrind, D. (1985). Research using intentional deception: Ethical issues revisited. *American Psychologist, 40,* 165–174.

Beauchamp, T. L., & Childress, J. F. (1994). *Principles of biomedical ethics* (4th ed.). New York: Oxford University Press.

Bersoff, D. N. (1995). *Ethical conflicts in psychology.* Washington, DC: American Psychological Association.

Bongar, B. (1991). *The suicidal patient: Clinical and legal standards of care.* Washington, DC: American Psychological Association.

Bongar, B. (1992). The ethical issue of competence in working with the suicidal patient. *Ethics and Behavior, 2,* 75–89.

Braaten, E. B., Otto, S., & Handelsman, M. M. (1993). What do people want to know about psychotherapy? *Psychotherapy, 30,* 565–570.

Broskowski, A. (1991). Current mental health care environments: Why managed care is necessary. *Professional Psychology: Research and Practice, 22,* 6–14.

Buelow, G. D., & Chafetz, M. D. (1996). Proposed ethical practice guidelines for clinical pharmacopsychology: Sharpening a new focus in psychology. *Professional Psychology: Research and Practice, 27,* 53–58.

Canterbury v. Spence, 464 F.2d 772 (D.C. Cir. 1972).

Carroll, M. A., Schneider, H. G., & Wesley, G. R. (1985). *Ethics in the practice of psychology.* Englewood Cliffs, NJ: Prentice-Hall.

Carse, A. L. (1991). The "voice of care": Implications for bioethical education. *Journal of Medicine and Philosophy, 16,* 5–28.

Clingempeel, W. G., Mulvey, E., & Reppucci, N. D. (1980). A national study of ethical dilemmas of psychologists in the criminal justice system. In J. Monahan (Ed.), *Who is the client? The ethics of psychological intervention in the criminal justice system* (pp. 126–153). Washington, DC: American Psychological Association.

Cobbs v. Grant, 502 P. 2d 1 (Cal. 1972).

Corey, G., Corey, M. S., & Callanan, P. (1993). *Issues and ethics in the helping professions* (4th ed.). Pacific Grove, CA: Brooks/Cole.

Dana, R. H. (1993). *Multicultural assessment perspectives for professional psychology.* Boston: Allyn and Bacon.

Dougherty, C. J. (1992). Ethical values at stake in health care reform. *Journal of the American Medical Association, 268,* 2409–2412.

Everstine, L., Everstine, D. S., Heymann, G. M., True, R. H., Frey, D. H., Johnson, H. G., & Seiden, R. H. (1980). Privacy and confidentiality in psychotherapy. *American Psychologist, 35,* 828–840.

Gabbard, G. O. (1994). Reconsidering the American Psychological Association's policy on sex with former patients: Is it justifiable? *Professional Psychology: Research and Practice, 25,* 329–335.

Gilligan, C. (1982). *In a different voice: Psychological theory and women's development.* Cambridge, MA: Harvard University Press.

Gilligan, C., Ward, J., & Taylor, J. (Eds). (1988). *Mapping the moral domain.* Cambridge, MA: Harvard University Press.

Golding, S. L. (1990). Mental health professionals and the courts: The ethics of expertise. *International Journal of Law and Psychiatry, 13,* 281–307.

Gottlieb, M. C. (1993). Avoiding exploitive dual relationships: A decision-making model. *Psychotherapy, 30,* 41–48.

Gray, L., & Harding, A. (1988). Confidentiality limits with clients who have the AIDS virus. *Journal of Counseling and Development, 71,* 297–305.

Greenberg, M. D. (1978). The examination of professional practice in psychology (EPPP). *American Psychologist, 33,* 88–89.

Gumaer, J., & Scott, L. (1985). Training group leaders in ethical decision making. *Journal for Specialists in Group Work, 10,* 198–204.

Gustafson, K. E., & McNamara, J. R. (1987). Confidentiality with minor clients: Issues and guidelines for therapists. *Professional Psychology: Research and Practice, 18,* 503–508.

Gutheil, T. G., & Gabbard, G. O. (1993). The concept of boundaries in clinical practice: Theoretical and risk-management dimensions. *American Journal of Psychiatry, 150,* 188–196.

Haas, L. J. (1991). Hide and seek or show and tell? Emerging issues of informed consent. *Ethics and Behavior, 1,* 175–189.

Haas, L. J., Benedict, J. G., & Kobos, J. S. (1996). Psychotherapy by telephone: Risks and benefits for psychologists and consumers. *Professional Psychology: Research and Practice, 27,* 154–160.

Haas, L. J., & Cummings, N. A. (1991). Managed outpatient mental health plans: Clinical, ethical, and practical guidelines for participation. *Professional Psychology: Research and Practice, 22,* 45–51.

Handelsman, M. M. (1991, August). An ounce of prevention: Proactive ethical reasoning. In D. J. Lutz (Chair), *Full-time academics in part-time practice: Ethical and legal concerns.* Symposium conducted at the meeting of the American Psychological Association, San Francisco.

Handelsman, M. M., Bershenyi, K., Whetsel, D., Maestas, D., Jr., & Boynton, K. (1996, April). *Thanks for the memory?: Ethical judgments of memory recovery strategies.* Paper presented at the meeting of the Rocky Mountain Psychological Association, Park City, Utah.

Handelsman, M. M., & Galvin, M. D. (1988). Facilitating informed consent for outpatient psychotherapy: A suggested written format. *Professional Psychology: Research and Practice, 19,* 223–225.

Handelsman, M. M., Kemper, M. B., Kesson-Craig, P., McLain, J., & Johnsrud, C. (1986). Use, content, and readability of written informed consent forms for treatment. *Professional Psychology: Research and Practice, 17,* 514–518.

Handelsman, M. M., Martinez, A., Geisendorfer, S., Jordan, L., Wagner, L., Daniel, P., & Davis, S. (1995). Does legally mandated consent to psychotherapy ensure its ethical appropriateness? The Colorado experience. *Ethics and Behavior, 5,* 119–129.

Hare-Mustin, R. T., Marecek, J., Kaplan, A. G., & Liss-Levinson, N. (1979). Rights of clients, responsibilities of therapists. *American Psychologist, 34,* 3–16.

Hendrick, S. S. (1988). Counselor self-disclosure. *Journal of Counseling and Development, 66,* 419–424.

Hogan, D. B. (1979). *The regulation of psychotherapists* (Vols. 1–4). Cambridge, MA: Ballinger.

Holroyd, J. C., & Brodsky, A. (1980). Does touching patients lead to sexual intercourse? *Professional Psychology, 11,* 807–811.

Holub, E. A., & Lee, S. S. (1990). Therapists' use of nonerotic physical contact: Ethical concerns. *Professional Psychology: Research and Practice, 21,* 115–117.

Jordan, A. E., & Meara, N. M. (1990). Ethics and professional practice of psychologists: The role of virtues and principles. *Professional Psychology: Research and Practice, 21,* 107–114.

Kalichman, S. C. (1993). *Mandated reporting of suspected child abuse: Ethics, law, and policy.* Washington, DC: American Psychological Association.

Keith-Spiegel, P. (Ed.). (1994). The 1992 ethics code: Boon or bane? [Special section]. *Professional Psychology: Research and Practice, 25,* 315–387.

Keith-Spiegel, P., & Koocher, G. P. (1985). *Ethics in psychology: Professional standards and cases.* New York: Random House.

Keith-Spiegel, P., Wittig, A. F., Perkins, D. V., Balogh, D. W., & Whitley, B. E., Jr. (1993). *The ethics of teaching: A casebook.* Muncie, IN: Ball State University.

Kertay, L., & Reviere, S. L. (1993). The use of touch in psychotherapy: Theoretical and ethical considerations. *Psychotherapy, 30,* 32–40.

Kitchener, K. S. (1984). Intuition, critical evaluation and ethical principles: The foundations for ethical decisions in counseling psychology. *The Counseling Psychologist, 12*(3), 43–55.

Kitchener, K. S. (1988). Dual role relationships: What makes them so problematic? *Journal of Counseling and Development, 67,* 217–221.

Kitchener, K. S. (1996). There is more to ethics than principles. *The Counseling Psychologist, 24,* 92–97.

Knapp, S., & VandeCreek, L. (1990). *What every therapist should know about AIDS.* Sarasota, FL: Professional Resource Exchange.

Kovacs, A. L. (1984). The increasing malpractice exposure of psychologists. *The Independent Practitioner, 4*(2), 12–14.

Lakin, M. (1991). *Coping with ethical dilemmas in psychotherapy.* New York: Pergamon Press.

Lerman, H., & Porter, N. (Eds.). (1990). *Feminist ethics in psychotherapy.* New York: Springer.

Lidz, C. W., Meisel, A., Zerubavel, E., Carter, M., Sestak, R. M., & Roth, L. H. (1984). *Informed consent: A study of decisionmaking in psychiatry.* New York: Guilford Press.

Margolin, G. (1982). Ethical and legal considerations in marital and family therapy. *American Psychologist, 37,* 788–801.

McGoldrick, M., Pearce, J., & Giordano, J. (Eds.). (1982). *Ethnicity and family therapy.* New York: Guilford Press.

McGuire, J., Nieri, D., Abbott, D., Sheridan, K., &

Fisher, R. (1995). Do *Tarasoff* principles apply in AIDS-related psychotherapy? Ethical decision making and the role of therapist homophobia and perceived client dangerousness. *Professional Psychology: Research and Practice, 26,* 608–611.

Meara, N. M., Schmidt, L. D., & Day, J. D. (1996). Principles and virtues: A foundation for ethical decisions, policies, and character. *The Counseling Psychologist, 24*(1), 4–77.

Melton, G. B. (1988). Ethical and legal issues in AIDS-related practice. *American Psychologist, 43,* 941–947.

Melton, G. B., Goodman, G. S., Kalichman, S. C., Levine, M., Saywitz, K. J., & Koocher, G. P. (1995). Empirical research on child maltreatment and the law. *Journal of Clinical Child Psychology, 24*(Suppl.), 47–77.

Miller, R., & Willner, H. S. (1974). The two-part consent form. A suggestion for promoting free and informed consent. *New England Journal of Medicine, 290,* 964–966.

Monahan, J. (1980). *Who is the client? The ethics of psychological intervention in the criminal justice system.* Washington, DC: American Psychological Association.

Morrow, G. R., Gootnick, J., & Schmale, A. (1978). A simple technique for increasing cancer patients' informed consent to treatment. *Cancer, 42,* 793–799.

Nagy, T. F. (1996, January/February). Ethics committees: Investigate or educate? *The National Psychologist,* pp. 15–16.

Newman, R., & Bricklin, P. M. (1991). Parameters of managed mental health care: Legal, ethical, and professional guidelines. *Professional Psychology: Research and Practice, 22,* 26–35.

Payton, C. R. (1994). Implications of the 1992 ethics code for diverse groups. *Professional Psychology: Research and Practice, 25,* 317–320.

Polusny, M. A., & Follette, V. M. (1996). Remembering childhood sexual abuse: A national survey of psychologists' clinical practices, beliefs, and personal experience. *Professional Psychology: Research and Practice, 27,* 41–52.

Pope, K. S. (1988). How clients are harmed by sexual contact with mental health professionals: The syndrome and its prevalence. *Journal of Counseling and Development, 67,* 222–226.

Pope, K. S., & Bouhoutsos, J. (1986). *Sexual intimacy between therapists and patients.* New York: Praeger.

Pope, K. S., Tabachnick, B. G., & Keith-Spiegel, P. (1987). Ethics of practice: The beliefs and behaviors of psychologists as therapists. *American Psychologist, 42,* 993–1006.

Pope, K. S., & Vasquez, M. J. T. (1991). *Ethics in psychotherapy and counseling.* San Francisco: Jossey-Bass.

Pope, K. S., & Vetter, V. (1992). Ethical dilemmas encountered by members of the American Psychological Association. *American Psychologist, 47,* 397–411.

Ramirez, S. Z., Wassef, A., Paniagua, F. A., & Linskey, A. O. (1996). Mental health providers' perceptions of cultural variables in evaluating ethnically diverse clients. *Professional Psychology: Research and Practice, 27,* 284–288.

Rosenthal, R. (1994). Science and ethics in conducting, analyzing, and reporting psychological research. *Psychological Science, 5,* 127–133.

Saeki, C., & Borow, H. (1985). Counseling and psychotherapy: East and West. In P. Pedersen (Ed.), *Handbook of cross-cultural counseling and therapy* (pp. 223–229). Westport, CT: Greenwood Press.

Schlossberger, E., & Hecker, L. (1996). HIV and family therapists' duty to warn: A legal and ethical analysis. *Journal of Marital and Family Therapy, 22,* 27–40.

Seaman, H. (1996, January–February). Future of ethics complaint investigations by state associations is questioned. *The National Psychologist,* pp. 8–9.

Sheridan, E. P., Matarazzo, J. D., & Nelson, P. D. (1995). Accreditation of psychology's graduate professional education and training programs: An historical perspective. *Professional Psychology: Research and Practice, 26,* 386–392.

Siegel, M. (1979). Privacy, ethics, and confidentiality. *Professional Psychology, 10,* 249–258.

Simon, R. I. (1991). Psychological injury caused by boundary violation precursors to therapist–patient sex. *Psychiatric Annals, 21,* 614–619.

Sleek, S. (1994, December). Ethical dilemmas plague rural practice. *APA Monitor,* p. 26.

Smith, D., & Fitzpatrick, M. (1995). Patient–therapist boundary issues: An integrative review of theory and research. *Professional Psychology: Research and Practice, 26,* 499–506.

Somberg, D. R., Stone, G. L., & Claiborn, D. C. (1993). Informed consent: Therapists' beliefs and practices. *Professional Psychology: Research and Practice, 24,* 153–159.

Sonne, J. L. (1994). Multiple relationships: Does the new ethics code answer the right questions? *Professional Psychology: Research and Practice, 25,* 336–343.

Strasburger, L. H., Jorgenson, L., & Randles, R. (1991). Criminalization of psychotherapist–patient sex. *American Journal of Psychiatry, 148,* 859–863.

Sue, D. W. (1990). Culture-specific strategies in counseling: A conceptual framework. *Professional Psychology: Research and Practice, 21,* 424–433.

Sue, D. W., & Sue, D. (1990). *Counseling the culturally different: Theory and practice* (2nd ed.). New York: Wiley.

Sue, S. (1983). Ethnic minority issues in psychology: A reexamination. *American Psychologist, 38,* 583–592.

Sullivan, T., Martin, W. L., Jr., & Handelsman, M. M. (1993). Practical benefits of an informed consent procedure: An empirical investigation. *Professional Psychology: Research and Practice, 24,* 160–163.

Tarasoff v. Board of Regents of California, Cal. Rptr. 14, No. S.F. 23042 (Cal. Sup. Ct., July 1, 1976) 131.

Tymchuk, A. J. (1981). Ethical decision-making and psychological treatment. *Journal of Psychiatric Treatment and Evaluation, 3,* 507–513.

Tymchuk, A. J. (1982). Strategies for resolving value dilemmas. *American Behavioral Scientist, 26,* 159–175.

Vaccarino, J. M. (1978). Consent, informed consent, and the consent form. *New England Journal of Medicine, 298,* 455.

Vasquez, M. J. T. (1996). Will virtue ethics improve ethical conduct in multicultural settings and interactions? *The Counseling Psychologist, 24,* 98–104.

Vesper, J. H., & Brock, G. W. (1991). *Ethics, legalities, and professional practice issues in marriage and family therapy.* Boston: Allyn and Bacon.

Welfel, E. R., & Lipsitz, N. E. (1984). The ethical behavior of professional psychologists: A critical analysis of the research. *The Counseling Psychologist, 12*(3), 31–42.

White v. North Carolina State Board of Examiners of Practicing Psychologists, 97 N.C. App. 144, 388 S.E.2d 148 (1990), *review denied,* 326 N.C. 601, 393 S.E.2d 891 (1990).

Wickline v. State of California, 239 Cal. Rptr. 805, 741 P.2nd 613 (1987).

Winegar, N. (1992). *The clinician's guide to managed mental health care.* New York: Haworth.

Wolf, S. M. (1994). Health care reform and the future of physician ethics. *Hastings Center Report, 24*(2), 28–41.

FOR FURTHER READING

For students who are interested in delving deeper into ethics, Bersoff's (1995) collection of readings presents a comprehensive treatment of ethics in psychology. Corey et al. (1993) look at ethics more generally from the perspective of helping professionals, and present excellent cases, questions, and self-assessment instruments for discussion. APA (1987) published a book of ethics cases that is useful despite being based on a previous version of the ethics code.

Several good books deal specifically with psychotherapy, including Lakin (1991) and Pope and Vasquez (1991). Austin et al. (1990) present issues from a legal perspective, and Lerman and Porter (1990) present feminist perspectives. Vesper and Brock (1991) specialize in ethical and legal issues pertaining to marital and family therapy.

The best book about the ethics of teaching is Keith-Spiegel et al. (1993).

To put psychological ethics in perspective, students can read Beauchamp and Childress's (1994) classic text on biomedical ethics. Appelbaum and Lawton (1990) look at ethics in a variety of professions, including health care, business, and criminal justice.

CHAPTER 5

EVALUATING WHAT WE DO

David L. Streiner

WHY WE SHOULD EVALUATE

As the chapters of this book illustrate, clinical psychology encompasses a wide range of activities: conducting individual and group therapy with people who suffer from a variety of psychological problems; designing rehabilitation programs for people who have experienced some injury to their brains through accident or stroke; implementing interventions to help people change maladaptive behaviors, such as smoking or abusing drugs; evaluating individuals for vocational purposes; assessing parents and children to help decide issues of custody and access; and using a host of other techniques for a variety of different purposes.

As the range of activities in which clinical psychologists engage has increased, so has the number of therapeutic and assessment techniques that are available. Until the early 1960s, for example, if a patient came to a psychologist complaining of anxiety, he or she would be treated with some form of psychotherapy, most likely based on psychoanalytic or ego-analytic theory. Although practitioners argued mightily among themselves about the details of the theories, an outside observer would have had great difficulty distinguishing one form of

therapy from another. Today, on the other hand, it appears as if there are as many types of therapies for anxiety as there are therapists. For example, flooding, implosion, desensitization, cognitive, cognitive-behavioral, object relations, eye movement desensitization, and psychodynamic therapies have all been used, to say nothing about the wide variety of drugs being offered by psychiatrists and family physicians.

If we ask, "Has this growth in the number of techniques been good or bad?," we would have to answer, "Yes." On the one hand, many of these newer procedures have been more effective than the older ones in terms of the number of people who can be helped and the speed with which they can be treated. On the other hand (and there is always an "other hand"), some of the new methods are less than helpful, and some may actually do more harm than good. The plethora of available therapies places an additional burden on practitioners: How do they select which among the techniques they should use, and which they should avoid? At another level, how do they know that this particular form of therapy, which may have been shown to work in studies using large numbers of patients, is actually working when applied by them to the individual patients sitting in their offices? The more research-oriented clinical psychologist often asks the first type of question and designs studies involving large groups of patients, randomly assigned to receive one type of therapy or another, and using sophisticated statistics to analyze the results. The more clinically oriented psychologist (who could be the same person, wearing a different hat) is more interested in the second type of problem: evaluating whether the particular therapy is working at an individual patient level. Needless to say, although this example has focused on therapeutic techniques, the same considerations apply to assessment procedures, community-based interventions, or anything else we do that is designed to make a difference in the lives of the people we see.

In addition to this altruistic reason for evaluating what we do, to ensure that we are really helping the people who are requesting (and paying for) our services, there is another important reason to evaluate. Crass as it may sound, we are in an era in which health services are seen as a commodity, and in which access to these services is coming under the scrutiny and control of accountants and "cost containment managers." Insurance companies and other third-party payers will not approve payment for services unless it can be proved that the interventions really work and make a difference in the lives of the people who are our clients. It is no longer sufficient to say, "Trust me, I'm a doctor"; now we have to earn that trust with hard data. Within the last few years, medical interventions such as chelation therapy for calcium overload, and surgical procedures like extracranial/intracranial bypass surgery have been removed from insurance company reimbursement schedules (and thus effectively eliminated from practice) because their effectiveness could not be demonstrated. Many third-party payers also have procedures in place by which external appraisers review psychotherapy records if they feel that too many sessions have taken place without enough progress to show for them. In order to continue what we are doing (and, we hope, to keep improving what we do), we must be in a position to show that our techniques work in general and that they are being applied effectively with our particular cases.

In this chapter, we will cover some of the research strategies that can be used by the researcher and the practitioner: how to critically evaluate studies of therapeutic and diagnostic effectiveness; and the ethical issues that arise when we are conducting any form of evaluation. Entire textbooks have been written about each of these topics, so all we can do is skim the surface and highlight the important points. For those who hunger for greater knowledge, though, there is a section at the end of this chapter, called "For Further Reading," which lists some books that cover these topics in greater depth.

HOW TO EVALUATE OUR INTERVENTIONS

Ideally, before any technique is adopted into practice, it has been shown to be effective. This may seem so self-evident that it hardly needs to be said. However, the history of psychology is replete with examples of procedures employed because it seemed "logical" that they should work, or because some respected person in the field reported his or her impression that they do work, but with no evidence to back up those claims. In this section, we will consider some of the research strategies that can be used to evaluate the effectiveness of therapeutic and diagnostic interventions, and the strengths and weaknesses of those procedures.

Designs Appropriate for Larger Studies

Strengths and Weaknesses of Various Study Designs

There are many ways to determine whether a therapeutic intervention is effective, and each of these procedures has its own strengths and limitations. Perhaps the easiest type of study to do is one using *historical controls*, in which the outcomes of patients who have had some form of therapy is compared to some earlier time when that therapy was not yet available. On the basis of this type of design, for example, it was concluded that since the number of chronic patients in large state and provincial hospitals dropped dramatically just about the time that psychoactive drugs like chlorpromazine (CPZ) were introduced in the mid-1950s, it must have been these drugs that were responsible for the dramatic decrease in the number of patients. The major drawback of this design is the assumption that nothing else changed during this time that could have affected the observed phenomenon. In fact, some researchers have postulated that the hospitals were starting to empty out *before* CPZ was introduced into the medical community, as a result of changes in administrative policies and a trend toward more open hospitals (Kiesler & Sibulkin, 1987; Mechanic, 1980; Warner, 1994). The reality is that it is not only extremely difficult to ensure that nothing else has changed, but also quite unreasonable to do so. We would require a thorough knowledge of what all the other factors are that may influence the results, and what happened to those factors over the decade or so separating the treated from the untreated cases. For the most part, studies using historical control groups may be useful for hypothesis generation, but rarely can prove that the change in the outcome was due to the particular intervention.

Closely related to the historical control design is the *before–after* trial, also referred to as a *one-group prestest/posttest* study. In the before–after design, however, each person is compared to the way he or she was before therapy, as shown in Figure 5.1. For example, it has been hypothesized that phobic patients are selectively attentive to cues in their environment that may signal a threat. Lavy, van den Hout, and Arntz (1993) tested phobic patients before and after behavior therapy to determine if there were any changes in their attentional bias for threat-relevant information (there were). There are a number of advantages of this design over historical controls; the major one is the shortened time span, so that there is less opportunity for other factors to have been operating. In addition, the same person is compared at both times, eliminating the possibility that the attributes of the patients themselves may have changed over the time period in question (e.g., because of the wider availability

of insurance, less disturbed people may be seen now than previously). The question, however, is very similar to the one found with historical controls: Could the people have improved without the therapy, simply because of other changes in their lives or the nature of the condition itself? We know that many disorders, such as the milder forms of depression, are time-limited (Hankin & Locke, 1982; Mann, Jenkins, & Belsey, 1981). If these patients seek help when they are most distressed, then the natural history of the disorder dictates that they will improve over time *whether or not the therapy works*, and we may be deluding ourselves (and the public) in attributing their progress to our intervention. This before–after design can work, however, if we know from other studies that the natural history of the disorder is that it will remain the same or get worse without treatment. This seems to be the case, for example, in some forms of anxiety disorders (Turner & Beidel, 1989; Wittchen & Essau, 1993), so that it is relatively safe to conclude that without therapy, the patients would not have improved.

A somewhat more sophisticated design involves a *nonequivalent control group*. This is referred to as a "quasi-experimental design" and includes studies "that have treatments, outcome measures, and experimental units, but do not use random assignment to create the comparisons from which treatment-caused change is inferred" (Cook & Campbell, 1979, p. 6). In a nonequivalent control group study, shown schematically in Figure 5.2, people who have had the therapy are compared with another group that, for one reason or another, has not had therapy. In epidemiological research, this is referred to as a *cohort study* (Streiner & Norman, 1996). In one of the earliest examples of this design in therapy research, Eysenck (1952) compared the outcome of neurotic patients (who today would be diagnosed as suffering from an anxiety-related disorder) who underwent psychotherapy with a group of people who filed disability claims for psycho-

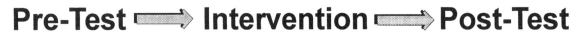

Figure 5.1. Design of a before–after trial.

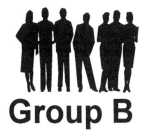
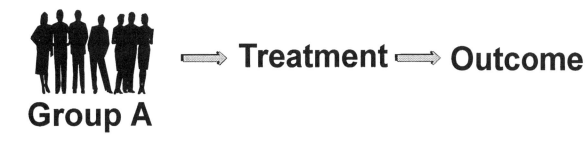
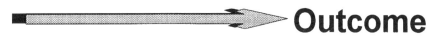

Figure 5.2. Design of a nonequivalent group trial.

neuroses with insurance companies and who were treated "by their own physicians with sedatives, tonics, suggestion, and reassurance" (p. 320). Eysenck found that about two-thirds of each group showed substantial improvement after two years, and concluded that psychotherapy was ineffective.

The major problem of the nonequivalent control group design is ensuring that the two groups of people are similar in all other regards that may affect the results—that is, that the factors that influence which people do and do not seek therapy have no impact on their eventual outcome. We have known for quite a while, however, that patients who seek therapy differ from those who do not on a number of variables, many of which, like helplessness, social isolation, demoralization, and a sense of failure and worthlessness, are related to treatment outcome (e.g., Galassi & Galassi, 1973; Garfield, 1986; Kellner & Sheffield, 1973; Vaillant, 1972). It is possible, then, that the patients who had therapy may have been worse off initially than those who did not seek help. In this case, the groups looked similar at the end of two years *because* therapy ef-

fectively brought them up to the level of those who did not need therapy. Thus, while Eysenck's conclusion is tantalizing, it cannot be considered to be conclusive.

The most powerful research design to evaluate the effectiveness of an intervention is called a *true experiment* or, in epidemiology, a *randomized controlled trial* (RCT; Streiner & Norman, 1996). In this type of study, schematized in Figure 5.3, people are assigned *at random* and *by the experimenter* to the different conditions. For example, to determine whether the therapy works at all, people would be allocated either to the therapy group or to a control group. The control group often consists of people receiving a placebo treatment, one that should not affect their condition. For example, Kemp, Hayward, Applewhaite, Everitt, and David (1996) wanted to determine whether compliance with medication could be increased among psychotic patients. They randomly assigned 47 patients to either a "compliance therapy" group or a placebo condition consisting of nonspecific counseling. Both groups needed less medication after the inter-

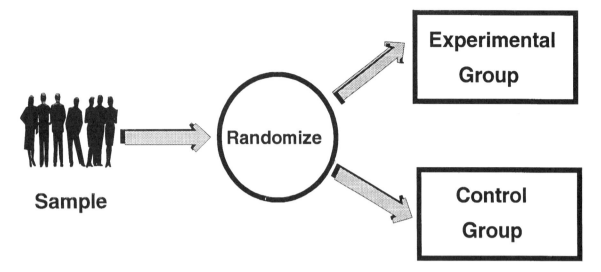

Figure 5.3. Design of a randomized controlled trial.

vention, but the experimental group took their drugs more regularly, showed more improvement in their symptoms, and had fewer subsequent hospitalizations.

When the aim of the study is to determine which of two forms of therapy is better, the people would be randomly assigned to receive either one treatment or the other. One major study, for instance, compared two forms of brief psychotherapy (interpersonal and cognitive-behavioral) both with each other and against clinical management with and without the use of antidepressant medication (Elkin, Parloff, Hadley, & Autry, 1985; Elkin et al., 1989). A total of 250 patients were randomly assigned to one of these four treatments. All patients improved; those in the drug-plus-management condition did best, whereas those receiving only clinical management improved least. The other two therapies showed intermediate levels of improvement.

The reason that this design is preferred over all others is that it *minimizes bias* between the groups. Bias in this context means any factor, other than the intervention itself, that may affect the results. These factors may include the severity of the disorder, age, verbal ability, or motivation. Because group membership is randomly determined and under the con-

trol of the researcher, these other factors should, in the long run, be equally distributed between or among the groups. Furthermore, most of our statistical tests are based on the assumption of randomization. For example, despite all of our care in randomly assigning people to groups, we still find that they differ at baseline on some crucial variables. If random allocation had been used, then techniques such as analysis of covariance can be used to take these differences into account; if assignment were not random, then there is very little we can do after the fact to adjust for them.

Internal and External Validity of the Study

Differences between internal and external validity. Proper design is a necessary ingredient for a study to assess therapeutic effectiveness, but it is not sufficient. A strong design allows us to have more confidence in the *internal validity* of the study (Cook & Campbell, 1979)—that is, to have greater assurance that the results are due to the intervention and not to other factors such as bias in the assignment of subjects to the different treatment conditions, or changes in the patient due to factors other than the intervention. Of equal, if not greater, concern is the *external validity* of the study—to what degree can we generalize from the somewhat artificial conditions of an experimental study to what goes on in real life? There is very often a trade-off between these two types of validity. To minimize potential sources of error, we have to sacrifice verisimilitude. Conversely, the more we try to mirror the reality of the therapeutic encounter, the greater the chances are that factors outside of our control (and perhaps of our knowledge) may be responsible for the results. The difference between "real life" and the laboratory was nicely documented by Weisz, Donenberg, Han, and Weiss (1995). Combining the results of many well-controlled studies of child psychotherapy, they found that children in the treatment condition scored about 0.75 standard deviations higher on various outcome measures than those in the control group; a very respectable improvement. However, looking at studies that were conducted in traditional clinics (and which therefore presumably mirrored more closely what therapists actually do, and with whom), the difference between the two groups virtually disappeared. Thus, careful experimental control over what occurs in therapy and to whom increases the internal validity of the study (as evidenced by the large difference) but jeopardizes external validity (seen in the difference between lab- and clinic-based studies)—what has been called the lack of "transportability" of findings from research to service (Kendall & Southam-Gerow, 1995). We will now take a closer look at some of the factors that may affect the internal and external validity of studies of therapy.

Control over the procedures. Increasingly over the years, studies of therapy have become "manualized," whereby the therapists must follow a structured guide governing what they can and cannot say or do during the sessions (Clarke, 1995; Luborsky & DeRubeis, 1984). As a check on compliance, the sessions are often tape recorded so that an external evaluator can determine if the therapist deviated from the script. For example, in a study comparing cognitive-behavioral with supportive-expressive therapy for eating disorders (Garner et al., 1993), each therapist had a manual for the type of therapy he or she was doing. As a further check on the therapists' compliance, the patients were given questionnaires at the end of therapy to tap their perceptions of what the therapists did. Some of the items asked about things a therapist using that form of therapy should have done, and other items tapped things the therapist should not have done. The purpose of this standardization is twofold. First, if differences between the treatments are found, then it is easier to determine which aspects of the therapy may have been responsible. Second, if therapists in one condition use techniques from the other type of therapy, this would tend to dilute the specific effects of each intervention. The ultimate effect of this would be to make the two groups similar to each other, thereby lessening the chances that any differences would be found. The drawback is that, in reality, therapists are rarely this rigid; they may combine techniques, sacrificing theoretical purity for therapeutic improvement, and basing their judgment of what to do on everything from empirical studies to hunches (Clarke, 1995; Persons, 1991).

The number of sessions. A related problem concerns the number of sessions: whether there is a fixed number of sessions for all patients, or if patients are seen as many times as necessary. The argument in favor of a fixed number of sessions is that we are studying a known intervention—a specific form of therapy for a given number of sessions. The disadvantage, again, is that this is rarely how therapy is done. Some people progress in therapy faster than others, either because their problems are not as severe, or because they make changes faster, or for some other reason. Even if the therapist and the patient agree beforehand regarding how long treatment should last, other issues may arise that require additional sessions. Sticking to a fixed number of sessions means that some patients must remain in therapy after they have derived all the benefit they can, while others may be terminated before all of their issues are dealt with. On the other hand, a variable number of sessions not only makes what is being studied a moving target, but also makes it more difficult for patients in the comparison group to receive the same amount of attention. As with many decisions that have to be made in therapy research, there are no right or wrong answers, only trade-offs between advantages and disadvantages.

Selection of subjects. Another issue that affects the internal and external validity of a study is the set of criteria used for selecting the people who will be the subjects in the study. In an attempt to gain a better understanding of the procedure being studied, and to reduce the within-group variability, researchers try to form homogeneous groups and may exclude, for example, people who have two or more diagnoses, who were in therapy previously, or who have used any psychoactive medication during the past six months. These exclusion criteria are sensible ways of improving the internal validity of the study and increasing the chances of finding a significant difference if one exists. At the same time, however, they also limit the generalizability of the results. Therapists rarely have the freedom to turn patients away for these reasons, so the question remains the degree to which the conclusions of the research can be applied in the clinical situation. The comparability of patients becomes even more acute when the subjects are not even patients. It is very common in studies of psychological tests to use college students (e.g., Frost, Steketee, Krause, & Trepanier, 1995; Roper, Ben-Porath, & Butcher, 1995), and though less common, this also exists in therapy research (Heller, 1971). However, the generalizability of results from this mainly middle-class, young, well-educated, and nonclinical group to a clinical population may be tenuous at best.

The choice of a control group. As was mentioned earlier, the hallmark of the randomized controlled trial (RCT) is random assignment to treatment or control conditions. The problem, however, is: What do we mean by control? If we are comparing two or more forms of therapy, then the issue is simple: "Control" is simply another, usually the older, more traditional, form of therapy. We saw this design previously in the study of various treatments for depression (Elkin et al., 1985, 1989). In some situations, however, the objective is to determine whether the therapy has any effect at all. In this situation, the appropriate control group would be one that receives either no therapy (e.g., half of the subjects are placed on a waiting list for the duration of the study), or a sham, placebo treatment. These people are given some form of structured activity that is

felt to be therapeutically ineffective for the presenting problem. The purpose of this is to control for any nonspecific effects of therapy, such as attention, or what has been called the Hawthorne effect (which likely never existed but still remains as a very handy rubric; Bramel & Friend, 1981; Jones, 1992). However, there are a number of problems with this type of control group. People seek therapy because they need (or at least want) help. They are often unwilling to wait 6 to 12 months if alternatives are available, so that those who remain on the waiting list are likely less disturbed than the group as a whole. Even if they remain on the list, the people may seek out other, less formal, helpers such as clergy, friends, bartenders, or hairdressers. Finally, we are not really sure what a "placebo" is in therapy. Simply seeing an individual whom the patient perceives as a therapist, or meeting with other people in a group, may provide elements that are therapeutic, such as a feeling of being understood or social contact (Clarke, 1995; Strupp, 1977). The result of people deriving nonspecific benefits from placebo conditions is to lessen any differences between the experimental and control groups and to increase the probability of a Type II error (erroneously concluding that there is no difference). Thus, if differences *are* found, we can be even more confident that they are real. But if no difference is found, we cannot know if it is because the therapy was ineffective or because there was some form of co-intervention with the control group. On the other hand, more healthy people dropping off a wait list would result in the control group being more disturbed than the treatment group, possibly leading to a significant, but spurious, difference. So dropouts may (1) make the control group more like the treatment group; (2) make it less like the treatment group, or (3) have no effect. There is no easy solution, except to minimize dropping out and co-intervention as much as possible. Methods for evaluating the effects of attrition will be discussed later in this chapter.

The Choice of Outcomes

In many situations, the outcome of a study is dictated by the nature of the problem being treated. If the therapy is designed to help bulimics, then the outcome measures would focus on the number of episodes of binging and purging; a therapy for ago-raphobia would focus on the person's ability to venture outside of the house; and interventions to help children with Attention-Deficit/Hyperactivity Disorder might consider school performance. However, there are many situations in which behavioral outcomes are not available or are not sufficient. Programs designed to improve self-esteem, for example, must rely to a great extent on the clients' reported feelings of worthiness. Some of the criteria used in evaluating the psychometric properties of scales have been discussed in Chapter 3; here the focus will be on three other issues: the *comprehensiveness* of the outcomes, what has been called the *substitution game*, and whether the outcome should be *continuous or discrete*.

Comprehensiveness. Even when therapy is directed toward specific target behaviors, such as weight gain for anorectics or fear reduction with phobic patients, for a number of reasons, change is rarely limited to just these areas. First, with the exception of hermits and social isolates (who rarely seek therapy in any case), people are embedded within a social matrix—their friends, family, work mates, and others. The patients' symptoms affect not only themselves but also those around them. If an agoraphobic woman cannot leave the house on her own, then other members of the family must change their habits to accommodate this. They must do the shopping or accompany her when she goes, visits to family and neighbors become problematic, and vacations may be curtailed or eliminated completely. By the same token, the husband may be secretly reassured that his wife will never divorce him, since she would find it nearly impossible to live on her own. Second, disorders often arise in reaction to real or perceived areas of conflict. Some people have hypothesized, for example, that anorexia results from fears about adult sexuality (Crisp, 1980). By starving herself, the woman remains prepubescent, with arrested development of her secondary sexual characteristics, and amenorrheic. Consequently, any change in weight may also affect the patient's perception of herself and how she sees people, especially males, who interact with her. Third, the treatment itself involves costs. Even

if the sessions are covered by an insurance plan (and these rarely cover all the charges), the person incurs indirect costs such as lost time from work, babysitting charges, transportation fees, and the like.

The implication of this is that it is rarely sufficient for the outcome measures to focus solely on the target behaviors. Changes occur in many aspects of the lives of the patients and their families. Some of these other changes may be positive and will further strengthen the effectiveness of the therapy. Others, however, may be negative and may detract from the overall picture. For example, a reduction in phobic anxiety may have the added benefit of increasing the woman's self-esteem, so that she is better able to assert herself. At the same time, this may lead to greater marital disharmony, because the equilibrium of the family has been disrupted. Ideally, studies of therapy effectiveness should include assessment of as many of the eight *D*s as possible:

- Dysfunction (difficulties in psychosocial functioning)
- Disability (the inability to carry out daily activities)
- Distress (symptoms)
- Disease (morbidity and side effects from treatment)
- Disharmony (problems with marital functioning)
- Debt (direct and indirect costs to the patient and society)
- Dissatisfaction (unhappiness with the therapy itself)
- Death (in studies, for example, of the treatment of depression or of suicide prevention programs)

Naturally, no one study can examine all potential outcomes, but they should be as comprehensive as possible and should take potential negative effects into account.

Substitution. Another aspect of the measurement of outcomes is *what* is measured. People do not enter therapy because their score on a Depression scale is too high or their reaction time on a choice discrimination task is too slow. Rather, they seek help because of the disruption in their lives caused by the depression, or because they have received some injury to their brain, or some other factor that has affected their daily lives. Many of the measures used to evaluate therapy are surrogates for the underlying problems, which are used because they have the advantage of being available, handy, less time-consuming, or standardized. However, these advantages should not blind us to the fact that a substitution has occurred: replacing what we would *like* to measure with what we *can* measure. For example, Brubaker and Wickersham (1990) reported on the "success" of a program to improve testicular self-examination in order to detect early cancer. However, their outcome measure was a scale tapping the men's *intention* to do the procedure; whether or not they actually followed through and *performed* the examination was not assessed. Although intention is a necessary component in changing behavior, it is only a first step and should not be used as a substitute for the desired outcome. In a different realm, Rudd et al. (1996) evaluated a program targeted at suicidal young adults. Their outcome measures consisted of scales of suicidal ideation, hopelessness, depression, substance abuse, and other indices of affect and cognitions—but not, unfortunately, actual suicidal behavior.

It is easy to see why these substitutions took place. It is difficult to measure compliance with self-examination except by self-report, which itself is susceptible to social desirability bias (Edwards, 1957). Suicidal behavior, fortunately, is relatively rare, even in high-risk groups, so a long follow-up would be needed, with a very large sample of patients, in order to determine if the program were effective. Surrogate end points cannot be considered adequate substitutes for what we want to measure unless the association between them is very strong and has been demonstrated in previous studies.

Continuous versus discrete. In some situations there can be a choice of outcomes, some of which are continuous and others that are discrete. For example, if we were evaluating a relapse prevention program for alcoholics, we could assess whether or not the person resumed drinking (discrete), if the person were subsequently arrested on alcohol-related charges (discrete), the length of time until the person resumed drinking (continuous), the number of ounces of alcohol consumed per week one year after discharge (continuous), or a host of other outcomes. One advantage of discrete outcomes is that there is rarely any ambiguity about them—the person was either admitted or not, or resumed drinking or not. With continuous measures, on the other hand, the person may admit to having some drinks but may minimize the reporting of his or her intake, leading to some degree of error. Similarly, we may know that the person was convicted of impaired driving, but not know exactly when. A second advantage of discrete measures is that each person has a definite outcome: yes or no, present or absent. But if the outcome is time to relapse, we may be in a position of having to terminate follow-up because the study has ended, but may know only that the person had not relapsed up to that time. The person may remain sober for the rest of his or her life, or may resume drinking the next day. Hence, any number we record for length of sobriety (e.g., the interval between discharge and the end of the study) is arbitrary and represents only a lower bound.

Counterbalancing these advantages of discrete outcomes is one major drawback: They are much less powerful than continuous measures. By this we mean that in order to show statistical significance, we would need many more subjects with discrete outcomes than with continuous ones. For example, a dichotomous outcome is, at best, only 67% as efficient as a continuous one (Suissa, 1991); if we need 100 subjects per group to show significance with a continuous measure, we would need at least 150 if the results were measured as a dichotomy. Further, the more the two outcomes differ from a 50:50 split in subjects, the more power is lost (Hunter & Schmidt, 1990). Low power jeopardizes the internal validity of the study because it increases the likelihood of a Type II error. The bottom line, then, is to use continuous measures whenever possible.

Handling Attrition and Losses to Follow-Up

Another issue in therapy research is how to handle the data for patients who drop out of therapy prematurely or who are lost to follow-up. Although sophisticated techniques have recently been developed to handle the statistical problems (which are many and knotty), they all assume to one degree or another that patients are lost randomly—that is, that the reasons they discontinued therapy are unrelated to the treatment they received (or did not receive, if they were in a wait-list control group), or to any other factor that may affect the outcome. We know that this is unrealistic; people rarely drop out for trivial reasons. For instance, Hansen, Hoogduin, Schaap, and de Haan (1992) found that in comparison to people who completed behavioral treatment for obsessive-compulsive disorders, dropouts said more often that therapy did not meet their expectations, that the therapists showed little or no understanding of them, and that they were less pressured by family to get help. Similarly, Emmelkamp and van den Hout (1983) found that agoraphobics who discontinued therapy were less able to remain in phobic situations until the anxiety decreased than were patients who completed treatment.

The problem of dropouts and patients lost to follow-up is even more acute when the reason for attrition may be related to a failure of the treatment program. "Especially in dealing with life-threatening disorders, it cannot be assumed that inability to find a person means that he or she has simply moved; it may be related to the failure of the program, culminating in the patient's suicide" (Streiner & Adam, 1987, pp. 98–99).

Higginbotham, West, and Forsyth (1988) outline a three-step procedure that researchers can follow to detect possible biases introduced by differential attrition from the various groups. First, the dropout rate is compared across groups. If there is a significant difference, then attrition is likely due to the effects of therapy or being in a control group. Unfortunately, any other findings may be due to unequal attrition. The second step is to compare the study participants in terms of baseline characteristics, using analyses where group membership is one factor, and dropping out versus remaining in the study is the other factor. Last, if the data are available, the reasons for dropping out should be compared for those in the active treatment condition versus those in the control group. The difficulty with all of these strategies, however, is that there may not be enough people in the groups to detect significant differences (i.e., the problem of a Type II error).

The problem for the consumers of research is to determine how much the dropouts may have biased the findings, since they do not have the raw data to do the analyses suggested by Higginbotham et al. (1988). A good rule of thumb is to assume that all of the dropouts are treatment failures. If we ascribe no improvement to them, and the results still look good, then the results can be believed; otherwise, we would have to conclude that the study did not show that the treatment was effective.

Statistical Significance and Clinical Importance

The bottom line in all studies of effectiveness is the p level: Were the differences among the groups statistically significant or not? If the study found that p was less than .05, then the conclusion is that, under the assumption of the null hypothesis that there are no group differences, it is highly unlikely—less than one chance in 20—that these results could have been due to chance. But there are three factors which affect the p level: (1) the choice of the Type I error level (i.e., the probability of finding a significant difference when there is none); (2) the ratio of the difference between the means relative to the variability within the groups (what is called the effect size, or ES); and (3) the sample size. This means that if we set the Type I error level at the customary 5%, then there is a reciprocal relationship between the ES and the sample size. If the sample size is small, then we will find statistical significance only if the ES is large; we would have to find a big difference between the means relative to how much the people in each of the groups differ among themselves. Conversely, if we have a very large number of people in the study, then very small ESs will be statistically significant.

The implication of this inverse relationship is that it is possible to have statistical significance, but that the magnitude of the effect of the intervention is very small. The question that then arises is whether that size difference is *clinically important*. What do we mean by clinically important? Basically, is it

worth changing what we do, and implementing the
new procedure, in order to achieve those results?
For example, Thompson, Nanni, and Schwankovsky (1990) designed a program to encourage patients to ask questions of their obstetricians/gyne-
cologists regarding their medical conditions. At the
end, the women in the experimental groups asked
an average of 5.2 questions; those in the control
condition had a mean of 4.9 questions asked. Although this difference was statistically significant,
the issue remains that, on average, for every 10
women, three asked one additional question of the
doctors.

The converse of statistical significance with very
small ESs is what is called the *power problem*. Studies that have small sample sizes need very large ESs
to yield statistical significance, so that a small study
may end up with an effect of treatment that looks
clinically important, but has insufficient power to
reject the null hypothesis. Cohen (1962), who developed the technique of determining sample size a
priori in order to achieve a given power in an experiment, did so because his review of the literature indicated that the mean power to detect a medium ES
was only .48—that is, "the chance of obtaining a
significant result was about that of tossing a head
with a fair coin" (Cohen, 1992, p. 155). This was
true among *published* studies; it is impossible to determine how many studies never saw the light of
day because low power led to nonsignificant results, and there is a bias against publishing null results (Dickersin, 1990; Greenwald, 1975). A study
24 years later found that the situation had not
changed at all (Sedlmeier & Gigerenzer, 1989).

What can we conclude from studies that yield
clinically important but statistically nonsignificant
results? Strictly speaking, not much. Using the
logic of significance testing, we cannot conclude
that the difference between the groups is anything
other than zero. In fact, it is just as likely from a statistical perspective that the groups could differ by
this amount in the opposite direction. But, as we
shall see in a later section on meta-analysis, ever-
resourceful statisticians have found ways of turning
sows' ears into silk purses—methods to combine
the results of many nonsignificant studies to deter-

mine whether, overall, the intervention does have
any effect.

Designs Appropriate for
Clinical Practice

As Weisz et al. (1995) pointed out, the ESs of
studies done under highly controlled conditions are
considerably higher than those of studies carried
out under more natural conditions. The lessons
from that review are sobering: There may be a
marked difference between what an intervention
can do in ideal circumstances (what is called *efficacy*) and what it *does* do when applied in the real
world to the range of patients who walk through the
door (referred to as *effectiveness*). Even if you dili-
gently search the literature to find the most efficacious treatment for a given disorder, there is no
guarantee that it will work when it is implemented
by you with the specific patient whom you are seeing. You might not have had the same training in the
technique as did the therapists in the studies, or the
patient may be different in some way from those
who served as subjects, or a host of other reasons
may result in a poorer (or better) outcome in the individual case. The implication of this is that it is necessary to evaluate your effectiveness, ideally with
each person you see, or at the very least, each time
you modify your practice. The techniques that are
appropriate for doing large studies (e.g., RCTs, cohort designs) clearly cannot be used when you are
seeing only a few people at any given time.

Perhaps the simplest, and most widely used, way
of assessing change in an individual patient is a *before–after* design: The patient is assessed at the start
of therapy and then at the conclusion. For reasons
that will be discussed in Chapter 6, the evaluations
should be done using a validated instrument rather
than simply accepting the patient's statement that
he or she feels better. Two issues immediately arise:
(1) how best to measure the change, and (2) how
much change is clinically important? Simply sub-
tracting one test score from the other is not sufficient, because all scores have some error of measurement associated with them (Streiner &
Norman, 1995). To determine if the change is

greater than what would be expected on the basis of measurement error, we can use the formula suggested by Christensen and Mendoza (1986) to assess significant change (SC):

$$SC = \frac{X_2 - X_1}{SE_D} \qquad (5.1)$$

where X_1 is the pretest score, X_2 the posttest score, and SE_D is the standard error of the difference between the two scores, defined as:

$$SE_D = \sqrt{2\,(SEM)^2} \qquad (5.2)$$

where SEM is the standard error of measurement of the test. Unlike other equations, this one does not assume that either the pretest or the posttest score is measured without error. If SC exceeds ±1.96, then the change in scores is more than what would be expected simply on the basis of measurement error. But is this enough? Here, unfortunately, statistics cannot help us. One recommendation (Jacobson, Follette, & Revenstorf, 1984) is to say that clinical change has occurred if (1) the pretest score is in the dysfunctional range; (2) the posttest score is similar to those of the functional population; and (3) the index of change is statistically significant. This assumes, though, that norms exist for well-functioning people, which is not always the case. In these situations, Jacobson et al. recommend that the second criterion be replaced by using a score that is at least two standard deviations above the mean for patients.

However, the major threat to the validity of large before–after trials also applies when we look at individuals in therapy: We cannot rule out that change may have occurred because of factors other than treatment, such as the natural history of the disorder or other events in the person's life. A number of other methods have been proposed to minimize this bias (Barlow & Herson, 1984; Cook & Campbell, 1979), but here we will focus on just three: the *reversal* design, *interrupted time series*, and the *multiple-baselines* design.

Reversal studies. Reversal studies, also called A-B-A or A-B-A-B designs, were first used in a sys-

tematic way in evaluating the ability of behavior modification programs to eliminate maladaptive behaviors (e.g., head banging in children) or to establish positive ones (e.g., the token economies used on the wards of psychiatric hospitals, which were aimed at improving social interactions). The basic design involves first determining the baseline level of the behavior prior to therapy (A), then instituting the program to elicit or suppress the target behavior (B), and finally removing the intervention (A). If the change were due to the therapy, then the behavior should return to baseline during the third phase. Of course, this can be repeated any number of times, leading to the A-B-A-B design, and any number of other variants, such as A-B-A-C-A, where C is a different intervention. An example of an A-B-A-B design used to evaluate a behavioral program is the study by Dugan et al. (1995), who looked at the ability of cooperative learning groups (CLG) to integrate autistic children into regular classes, focusing on the amount of learning that took place and the time spent in peer interaction. Their results for the two children in the program are shown in Figure 5.4. It is obvious that interaction time increased during CLG and returned to baseline when the children were removed from the groups. Also typical of this type of study is the lack of any formal statistical analysis. Rather, the focus is on reading the graph; the desired behavior increased during the intervention, and reached a level deemed to be clinically important. One difficulty, however, is that what may be clinically meaningful for one person may seem trivial to another; the lack of statistics results in some degree of subjectivity. Consequently, we would recommend that statistical procedures—in particular, randomization tests (Edgington, 1996; May & Hunter, 1993)—be used in this and other single-subject trials.

The major assumption of the reversal design is that the behavior change is not permanent but will return to its pretherapy level when the reinforcement is withdrawn. Consequently, it cannot be used, for example, to evaluate the effectiveness of desensitization for agoraphobia. If avoidance behavior returns when the therapy is stopped, then the patient could justifiably request a refund. The re-

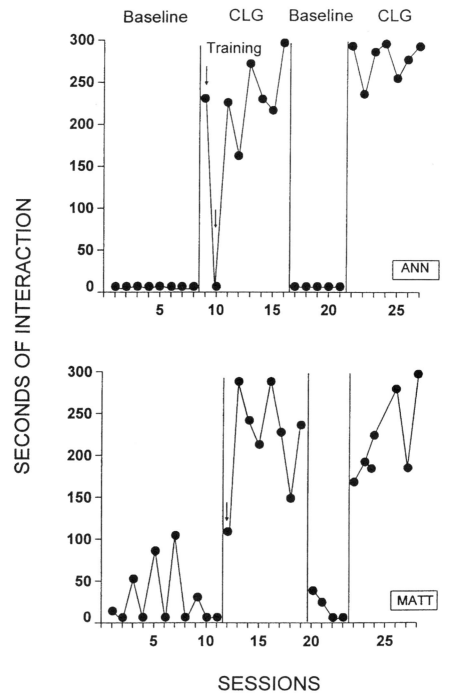

Figure 5.4. Example of results from an A-B-A-B design.

Source: From Dugan, E., et al. (1995). Effects of cooperative learning groups during social studies for students with autism and fourth-grade peers. *Journal of Applied Behavior Analysis, 28,* 175–188.

versal design is also difficult to use to assess therapy involving antidepressant and antipsychotic drugs, which have relatively long half-lives, and stay in the bloodstream for days or weeks after the last pill is taken (Hardman & Limbird, 1996), although some studies in this area have been done (e.g., Cook, Guyatt, Davis, Willan, & McIlroy, 1993). From an ethical perspective, it may also be problematic to withdraw reinforcement if that results in an increase in self-destructive behavior (Barlow & Hersen, 1984). Finally, the clinician can never be sure that simply because the behavior changed after the intervention, that the change was because of the intervention. Some other event may have happened concurrently that led to the modification, as we discussed earlier within the context of historical control groups and before–after designs. Each time that a reversal occurs followed by a change in the target behavior, however, the less likely it is that something else is affecting the outcome. In situations where the assumptions can be met and the ethical problems can be avoided, the reversal design can be a powerful method, and the more reversals that occur, the more powerful it is.

Interrupted time series. When the intervention results in a nonreversible outcome, so that a reversal design is not feasible, it is sometimes possible to use an *interrupted time series.* An example of one is shown in Figure 5.5, where the intervention was the 1974 law setting the speed limits on federal highways to 55 miles per hour (mph), and the dependent variable (DV) is the proportion of cars exceeding 65 mph. As can be seen, there is a series of preintervention data points, the intervention itself, and another series of points after the intervention. In this case, there is a clear change in the slope of the line, from slowly increasing to about 50% prior to 1974, dropping to 10% immediately after the law was passed, and remaining at that level. Figure 5.6, however, shows a somewhat different picture. The fatality rate was dropping even prior to 1974, and there is no indication that it began to fall more quickly afterwards; if anything, the decrease in fatalities appears to slow down after 1974, but we cannot infer causality on the basis of this correlation. We would con-

clude from these results that the law was effective in modifying driving behavior but that it would be difficult to attribute any decrease in deaths to its passage.

The requirements for this design are an outcome measure that can be taken repeatedly and enough data points before and after to minimize variations and obtain a stable estimate of the slopes. To analyze the data statistically, we generally want at least 30 observations before and 30 after the change (Norman & Streiner, 1997). But, as is the case with A-B-A designs, clinicians often rely on "eyeball" tests of significance. Possible measures, therefore, could include daily weights for the treatment of anorexia or obesity, the number of blocks ventured from the home on each day if the problem was agoraphobia, or daily severity ratings of headaches before and after frontalis muscle biofeedback. It would not be possible to use interrupted time series to look at the effects of early childhood education on intelligence, because it would be impractical to administer IQ tests often enough to get stable estimates of slope. A before–after design would be required in this case.

Multiple baselines. Another solution to the problem of separating the effects of treatment from natural history is to use *multiple baselines.* As the name implies, this design involves getting measures of two or more behaviors but intervening to change only one of them at a time. The rationale is that if the person is improving for reasons other than the therapy, he or she should show gains in all areas. On the other hand, if the therapy is targeted at one specific behavior, then only that one should change, and other, independent behaviors should remain constant. So, for example, if therapy were aimed at helping a person overcome extreme shyness, one measure (the target) could count the number of times the person initiated conversations with other people. A second symptom, such as driving anxiety, would also be assessed, because it is expected that this phobia would be unrelated (or only weakly related) to the shyness, and therefore should show little change. It would not make sense, however, to select a problem such as self-esteem to be the sec-

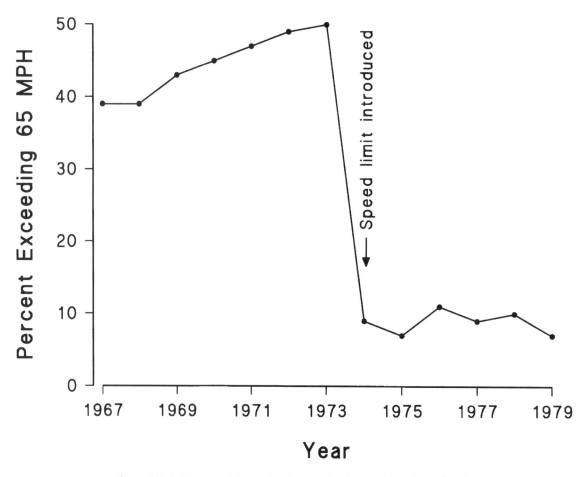

Figure 5.5. An interrupted time-series showing that the speed limit law reduced the proportion of people driving faster than 65 mph.

ond symptom, since we would assume that it would improve as the shyness were overcome. As Figure 5.7 shows, we can start therapy for the second problem at a later date. Now we have data showing that (1) treatment targeted at the first symptom was followed by improvement in it, (2) the therapy did not affect the second symptom, and (3) therapy aimed at the second symptom led to its amelioration. This does not guarantee that the therapy was the important change factor, but it is relatively convincing.

Barlow and Hersen (1984) state that the multiple-baseline technique is much weaker than the A-B-A design because the effects of treatment are inferred from the untreated behaviors and are not directly

demonstrated. That is, the assumption is made that if the target behavior changed and the others did not, that natural history or maturation could not have played a role. But if the behaviors are independent of each other, it is quite possible that these factors could have influenced the target behavior and not the others. The absence of change in these other areas does not preclude maturation from having affected just the target behavior. When the reversal design is not feasible, however, multiple baselines provide more solid evidence of effectiveness than measuring only the target behavior. As with the reversal design, the more the better. In this case, the more areas which are measured and subsequently

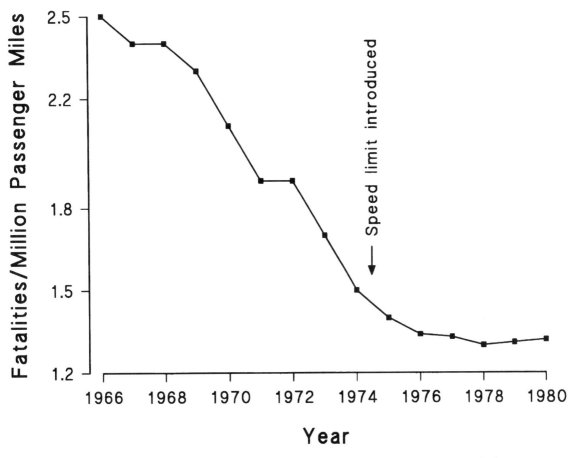

Figure 5.6. An interrupted time-series showing that the speed limit law did not affect motor vehicle fatality rates.

treated (up to four or so, that is the limit of feasibility), the more confident we are that the changes were due to the treatments.

Evaluating Meta-analyses

If any aspect of psychology can be said to be a growth industry, then that part must be meta-analysis. Meta-analyses are studies of studies—that is, comprehensive and systematic syntheses of previous research. One of the leading journals in psychology, *Psychological Bulletin*, has virtually become a compendium of these analyses. The reasons for this relatively recent spurt of interest are many and compelling. First, if we are to base any change in what we do on empirical studies (as we

should), then if one study provides good evidence, the weight of many studies with similar findings would give us much firmer ground on which to base our decision. Second, the traditional way of summarizing the literature, by having a reviewer rely solely on his or her expert opinion of which articles to include in a survey and what they conclude, can introduce bias. For example, Munsinger (1975) and Kamin (1978) reviewed the same set of articles addressing the issue of the effects of the environment on children's intelligence, and came to diametrically opposing conclusions. Not surprisingly, what they found was consistent with their beliefs about this issue, which they had expressed before their reviews. Third, simply counting the number of articles that report results in one direction or the other,

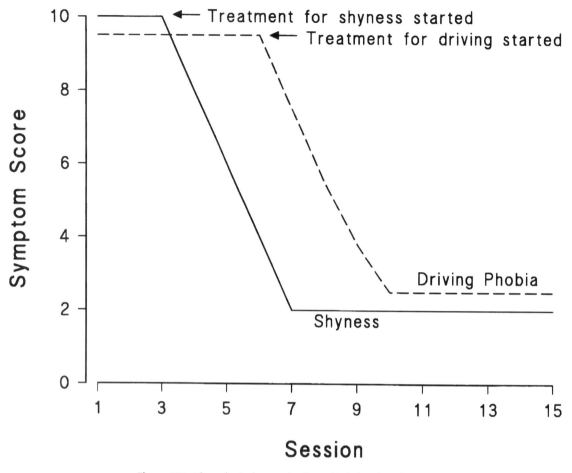

Figure 5.7. A hypothetical example of a multiple-baseline design.

though an improvement over nonquantitative methods, still leads to difficulties. Sobal and Stunkard (1989) found 27 articles reporting an association between obesity and socioeconomic status in men. Of these, 12 reported a positive correlation, 12 a negative one, and the remaining 3 found no association. Furthermore, this vote-counting method does not take into account the magnitude of the findings. It is possible, for instance, that all of the studies reporting results in one direction had very small ESs, whereas those showing findings in the opposite direction had much larger ESs; but all studies would be given equal weight if they were simply counted.

Meta-analysis tries to avoid these problems in a number of ways. First, the search for the articles should be thorough and systematic. The usual starting points are computerized databases: *PsychInfo*, which covers most of the psychological literature, *Medline*, which does the same for the medical and much of the clinical psychological literature, CINAHL (*Cumulative Index of Nursing and Allied Health Literature*), and a few others. Although these have made searching for articles much easier than going through each volume of *Psychological Abstracts* and *Index Medicus* by hand, it is not sufficient to stop here. Because the indexing of the articles into the databases by key words is done by people who may have only limited expertise in the subject matter, retrieval is somewhat of a hit-or-miss proposition. Some studies have found that only 20% of relevant articles are found in this way, even by people who are expert in database searching (McKibbon et al., 1990). Inexperienced users, not surprisingly, do much worse. To increase the coverage, the reference lists of the retrieved articles are searched for studies that may have been missed by the computerized searches. If the field is relatively small, with only a limited number of people actively working in it, some meta-analysts write to these people to determine if they know of other studies in the area, or if they have any unpublished manuscripts lying around in file drawers. Later, we'll see why this may be important.

At the same time that the articles are being retrieved from the library, the analysts should be drawing up a list of criteria to use for including or excluding articles. Depending on the type of meta-analysis being done, these may include the type of study (e.g., for therapy trials, looking only at those that used random assignment of subjects, or that compared treatment to a placebo condition, or compared two treatments), what to do with studies that had multiple outcomes (e.g., select only one or use an average of all the outcomes), sample size (e.g., only using studies that had a minimum number of subjects), and the subjects themselves (e.g., real patients versus analog studies, patients' diagnoses established through structured interviews). Using these criteria, at least two reviewers should evaluate a sufficient number of articles independently, in order to determine the interrater reliability of the decision to accept or reject the studies. This somewhat elaborate procedure helps ensure that articles are not excluded simply because their conclusions do not match the preconceived biases of the reviewers.

The next step is to calculate an ES for each study. If group means and standard deviations (SDs) are given, then this is relatively simple, since the ES is:

$$ES = \frac{\overline{X}_{Group_1} - \overline{X}_{Group_2}}{SD_{Pooled}} \qquad (5.3)$$

and the pooled SD is:

$$SD_{Pooled} = \sqrt{\frac{(n_1 - 1)\, s_1^2 + (n_2 - 1)\, s_2^2}{n_1 + n_2 - 2}} \qquad (5.4)$$

There are ways to estimate the ES on the basis of other data such as proportions, correlations, the value of a t-test, or even just the p level (Glass, McGaw, & Smith, 1981; Hedges, 1985). The last step in summarizing each study is to weight each ES by the sample size of the study (Rosenthal & Rubin, 1982), so that larger studies contribute more to the overall conclusions than do smaller ones.

These weighted ESs can now be combined to determine if the combined evidence indicates that there is or is not an effect. Because it is in SD units, the mean ES also reflects the size of that effect. A mean ES of 0.5, for instance, shows that there is one-half a standard deviation difference between the groups or conditions being compared. A table of the normal curve tells us that the area up to 0.5 SDs is 0.69, so we can conclude that half of the people in one group have scores higher than 69% of the other. The ESs from the individual studies can also be used as dependent variables, in order to tease apart why some studies found large differences and others found small ones or none at all. For example, Joffe, Sokolov, and Streiner (1996) reported that in studies of antidepressant medication, those that used structured interviews to determine diagnosis had significantly larger ESs than studies that relied on the psychiatrists' judgment.

Previously, we mentioned the "file drawer" problem—that there may be studies tucked away in researchers' filing cabinets, unloved and unpublished. Because the bias is against publishing studies that do not show significant findings (Greenwald, 1975), these would tend to lessen the magnitude of the final ES or even make it disappear completely. It may be impractical to write to all researchers in the area to ask them to retrieve these manuscripts, and many people may never even have published in the area because their initial studies were so disappointing. Rosenthal (1979), however, has worked out a way around this problem. He derived an equation to determine how many unpublished studies must exist with ESs of zero in order to make the results of the meta-analysis nonsignificant. If the number is large, then the reviewer can be assured that it would be highly unlikely that this many studies actually exist; but if the number is small, the reviewer should be a bit worried. Unfortunately, no one really knows what this magic number "large" really is.

If you're looking for a fast way to review the literature regarding the effectiveness of some intervention, a well-conducted meta-analysis can save you considerable time. But bear in mind that this approach is not infallible. Because various reviewers may search different data bases, use different criteria in selecting articles, or combine ES differently, they do not always agree. Abrami, Cohen, and d'Apollonia (1988) reviewed six meta-analyses of the validity of students' evaluations of teaching effectiveness, and found major differences in their conclusions; as did Chalmers et al. (1987), who looked at a variety of meta-analyses in medicine.

ETHICAL ISSUES IN CLINICAL RESEARCH

Until the early 1970s, conducting research in clinical psychology was relatively simple: The investigator would formulate an idea, perhaps discuss it with a few colleagues to iron out any wrinkles in the design, and then start the study. If the research could be conducted using college students, so much the better, since they were a captive audience, and many introductory psychology classes mandated that students participate in a minimum number of experiments as part of the course requirements (in fact, in 1946, McNemar called psychology "the science of the behavior of sophomores"). Even research that focused on patients in psychotherapy was done with minimal external oversight and without any need for the people involved even to be told that they were subjects in a study (e.g., Goldstein et al., 1967). The situation today is very different. Researchers are responsible to external boards, and there are strict rules regarding what can and cannot be done to study participants. In this section, we will

explore some of the history of this transformation, and what the obligations of the investigator are.

The major impetus for the change in the relationship between the researcher and the study subjects was World War II and the subsequent revelations about the horrific "medical experiments" carried out on concentration camp victims. In response to this, the international medical community drafted the Nuremberg Code, followed shortly after by the World Health Organization's Declaration of Helsinki (Levine, 1986). Despite later revisions and modifications, the essence of these documents remains unchanged, and serves as the cornerstone of all ethical codes: the *autonomy of the individual*. This seemingly simple phrase, which means that people should be free to decide what happens to them, has major implications for the conduct of all research. It has been operationalized to mean that all potential study participants (with a few exceptions, which will be mentioned later) must give their *free and informed consent* in order to participate in studies. Let us consider what is meant in the research context by the terms *free* and *informed* (these were discussed in more detail in Chapter 4 as they pertain to clinical practice).

Free consent means that the person can refuse to participate or can withdraw from a study without fear of any negative consequences. Although this may appear to be so self-evident that it hardly needs mentioning, it has been ignored by psychologists in a number of situations in the past (and we hope *only* in the past). The most widespread violation of this precept was the requirement that introductory psychology students had to serve as subjects for a certain number of hours or in a minimum number of studies. Although the vast majority of studies are relatively innocuous, some may ask questions about sexual practices (e.g., St. Lawrence et al., 1994), involve the use of deception (e.g., Scher & Cooper, 1989) or of an electric shock as an unconditional stimulus (e.g., Cacioppo, Marshall-Goodell, Tassinary, & Petty, 1992), or use other procedures that some people may find objectionable to such a degree that they would not participate if they had a choice. The most recent code of ethics of the American Psychological Association (APA, 1992) now stipulates that students must be offered some alternative to serving as a research participant, such as writing a paper.

A more subtle form of coercion exists when professors ask their graduate students or research assistants to be subjects. Because there will be a time when the supervisor has to give a grade or write a letter of reference, the subordinates may find it extremely difficult to say no, even if they have misgivings about participating. The easiest solution is to avoid this situation completely. Any time there is even the perception of a power imbalance, those in a superior position should never ask people under them to be subjects in studies. [This recommendation is actually stronger than the APA's (1992), which states only that when students or subordinates are approached, "psychologists take special care to protect the prospective participants from adverse consequences of declining or withdrawing from participation" (p. 1608).]

Another situation in which freedom of withdrawal may be jeopardized occurs when participants are paid. This is especially true if they are paid only if they complete the study. Although this is a less common practice in psychological than in biomedical research, it does exist and is likely necessary when subjects have to be drawn from the community at large. Few people work for free, and we cannot expect people to participate in studies simply out of a sense of altruism, obligation, or curiosity. At the very least, they should be reimbursed for any out-of-pocket expenses such as parking or travel, and most people expect some remuneration for their time as well. The important issue is how much to pay the study participants. It must be enough so that they will sign up, but not so much that it coerces them to take risks or endure pain (either physical or psychological) they ordinarily would not. Especially if the research involves discomfort or inconvenience, it may also be ethically questionable to pay people only if they remain until the study is completed. It is understandable why the researcher would want participants to complete the study: When subjects quit an experiment early, the result is lost data and time and possible bias of the results, since dropouts very often differ from those

who continue. A more satisfactory solution would be to pay people in proportion to their participation time, and perhaps with a "bonus" for completing the study. Again, the trade-off is between treating people fairly on the one hand versus coercing them on the other.

Being free to participate in or withdraw from a study does not mean much, however, if the people do not know what it is they are consenting to. Consequently, *free* consent also implies *informed* consent. Potential subjects should be told what the study is about, what will happen to them, how long it will take, and anything else that could affect their decision to participate or not. As is the case with freedom of consent, though, what appears simple in principle becomes problematic in practice. There are at least three situations where informed consent is not possible: (1) when the study involves naturalistic observations of a large number of people; (2) when telling subjects the purpose of the study would affect the results; and (3) with subjects who have a limited capacity to understand.

The first situation is relatively straightforward. The Office for Protection from Research Risks (OPRR; 1995), part of the National Institutes of Health, as well as the APA (1992), have stated that informed consent need not be obtained in surveys or observational studies if the individual subjects cannot be identified. Similarly, studies that use hospital or clinic records do not need the informed consent of every patient or client, if they will not be identified on the data collection forms.

The second situation, in which the participant either is not informed about the purpose of the study or is deliberately deceived, is much more difficult to justify. Some studies, especially those looking at processes of decision making, opinion formation, or attitudes, would be impossible to do if the participants were aware of the purpose of the research. For example, Luchins and Luchins (1961) told subjects that their visual acuity was being assessed as part of a new intelligence test, and they had to indicate which of two lines was shorter. In fact, three confederates of the experimenters could be overheard giving the wrong answer, and the actual purpose of the study was to determine whether the research subjects would conform to the majority (but wrong) opinion. In another classic study, Milgram (1963) studied obedience by telling subjects that they were taking part in a study of the effects of punishment on memory. The participant's job was to increase the level of shock given to another person (the "learner") each time the learner in the next room made a mistake. Despite strong protests and cries of pain from the learner (who was, in fact, a confederate of the experimenter and did not receive the shocks), the subjects followed orders to increase the shock, even up to levels marked in red on the machine and designated "Extreme Shock" and "Danger: Severe Shock."

It is obvious that had the subjects not been deliberately deceived, and if they had been told the true purpose of the study, the results would not show how people actually behave when their opinion runs counter to the majority (Luchins & Luchins, 1961) or when they are ordered to carry out distasteful acts by an authority figure (Milgram, 1963). Is either one of these studies ethical; and when, if ever, is it ethical to do a study that involves deception?

According to the APA's Ethical Principles (1992), deception is permitted as long as all of the following conditions are met:

- The study has prospective scientific or educational value;
- No feasible alternative methods exist;
- The subjects are not deceived about any aspect of the study that could affect their willingness to participate (e.g., pain, humiliation, discomfort);
- The subjects are debriefed about the deception as early as is feasible.

Following these guidelines, the Luchins and Luchins (1961) study would be considered ethical (although it is not clear whether the subjects were debriefed). It is doubtful, however, whether the Milgram (1963) study would be deemed ethical, since the nature of the deception most likely affected their willingness to participate.

The third area in which gaining informed consent may be problematic occurs where the potential participants' ability to understand is compromised. Such groups would include (1) children; (2) those

whose cognitive abilities are limited because of mental retardation, psychosis, brain trauma, or dementia; and (3) people from different linguistic or cultural backgrounds. One solution would be to say that these people should never serve in experiments because it is impossible to get truly informed consent from them. However, the ones who would be most harmed by this fairly Draconian measure would be the very groups we are trying to protect, since it would be impossible to study, for example, methods to detect Alzheimer's disease early in its course, or the problems that immigrants may have in adapting to a new culture, or the effects of radiation therapy on the cognitive development of children with leukemia. The issue is more one of being able to enroll these subjects in a way that best protects their welfare.

The usual procedure with children and with adults with limited cognitive ability is to seek consent from a surrogate—a person who would act in the best interests of the potential participant and would be in the best position to know whether the subject would want to participate. The surrogate is most usually one of the parents in the case of children, and a spouse, child, or sibling when the subject is an adult. This does not mean that the subjects should not be asked. Even if they cannot legally give consent, the study should be explained to adults and older children (an age defined more in terms of cognitive ability than in years) in terms they can understand. If both the potential participant and the surrogate agree, then the person can be enrolled in the study. But, if the potential participant says "No," then this would override the surrogate's "Yes." There are still some people who would not be covered by these procedures, such as older people who have been in a hospital for many years and who do not have any family members willing to act as surrogates. Here, the solution may vary from one state or province to another. Many jurisdictions have patient advocates or government-appointed surrogate decision makers who can be called in. However, this is still an evolving area with regulations changing very rapidly.

Working with people from different cultures presents other issues. The most obvious one, language, is perhaps the easiest to manage. Especially in larger cities and university settings, it is possible to find people who can translate informed consent forms or serve as interviewers. The more difficult problems are the cultural differences in the *process* of gaining consent. For example, in some cultures a woman would not give consent without her husband's approval, or people would look to a religious or secular leader of the group for direction (e.g., Barry, 1988). We may not necessarily approve of these situations, but it would be presumptuous of us to ignore these cultural norms and impose our values on the potential participants; this has been termed "ethical imperialism" (Angell, 1988). What is needed is a balance, so that the cultural values of both groups—theirs and ours—are preserved. For example, if the group's mores dictate that the husband give consent for the wife, then his approval must be gained. At the same time, though, because of our ethical system, we must also get approval from the wife, even if this is not required by the group's norms.

Earlier, we mentioned some situations in which informed consent is not required, such as surveys or observational studies where individuals cannot be identified, and reviews of records (again, where the people remain anonymous). There are some other types of studies for which either the APA (1992) or the OPRR (1995) state that consent can be waived. One is the completion of questionnaires. Because people who do not want to fill them out can leave them blank or sabotage the results in other ways (e.g., by answering randomly), it is assumed that completing the forms constitutes a form of implicit consent. Last, educational research is exempted from the requirements of consent, either because it is felt that nothing in education can do any harm (or any good), or perhaps because students are the last indentured servants in the developed world!

A very different issue from informed consent is whether there is some research that should not be done at all, even if it can be done well. For example, Rushton (1992; Rushton & Ankney, 1996) has proposed that there are genetically determined differences among Caucasians, African Americans, and Japanese, affecting attributes ranging from intelligence to sexuality. Though not as extreme in its conclusions, the book called *The Bell Curve*

(Herrnstein & Murray, 1994) has also proposed that genetics plays a major role in intelligence. These authors have been criticised as much for *what* they are studying as for the methodology employed (e.g., Ramos, 1995). In a similar vein, a proposed conference on genetics and violence had to be cancelled following objections by some groups that the conference would conclude that African Americans were genetically more predisposed to antisocial behavior than other groups. These critics contend that science is not ethically neutral. Study results have implications that may affect people and, as in the two cases cited here, may adversely affect groups that are already disadvantaged in other ways.

The difficulty is that *not* conducting research in certain areas has ethical implications as well. This dilemma was highlighted very well by Rosenthal and Rosnow (1984). They were addressing the issue of not doing research because of invasion of privacy, but the same points are true whether the problem is privacy, deception, or taboo topics:

> The psychologist whose study might reduce violence or prejudice or mental illness, but who refuses to do the study because it involves an invasion of privacy, is making a decision that is to be evaluated on ethical grounds as surely as the decision of a researcher to investigate psychological problems with a procedure that carries a certain cost. The psychologist has not solved an ethical problem but only traded one problem for another. (p. 562)

As with most ethical problems, there are no easy answers, just competing sets of demands and principles.

The final issue we will deal with concerns the very definition of *research*, because this influences when consent need or need not be sought. At first glance, the situation seems simple: Research is what is done when we want to understand or discover some phenomenon. However, the problem is quite a bit more complicated (Woodward & Streiner, 1995). Either as clinicians in private practice, or as researchers in health care, we should be evaluating what we do. If we decide to pull the charts of the last 50 patients seen by us or in our service, and rate whether termination was successful or not, do we have to get the patients' consent? The answer is "No" for three reasons: (1) Chart review is exempted from the requirements for informed consent; (2) the patients are not being asked to do anything different because of the review; and (3) assessing what we do—quality assurance (QA)—is also seen as an activity that should be ongoing and exempted from review. The rationale of QA is that it exists to inform clinical practice, not to produce new knowledge.

Let us take this a few steps further, though. If we now ask the patients to complete some questionnaires for the purposes of QA, then we *are* changing what the patient has to do—complete forms for our benefit, not theirs. Further, let us assume that the results are so interesting that we submit them for publication; that is, the outcome of the QA (intended or not) is the production of new knowledge. Is this research, which would require informed consent and review by an ethics committee, or is it QA, which requires neither? The answer is very definite: We don't know. Research and QA are not two completely different activities but, rather, ends of a spectrum, with no clear demarcation point between them. Where a particular project falls on this continuum depends both on the procedures (Did the patients have to do anything different?) and on the intention (Was the work carried out primarily to improve clinical service at one setting, or to increase knowledge in general?). Both may change over the course of the project, as information starts accumulating. In such circumstances, it is best to be somewhat cautious and to discuss the project with the head of the ethics review board or a senior colleague.

In most aspects of research, such as experimental design or data analysis, change occurs slowly and by the accumulation of new knowledge. Ethics, however, is somewhat different. What is considered ethical at one time (e.g., the requirement of research participation for introductory psychology students) may not be a short time later, in response to changes in society at large. Within two years of the latest revision of the APA's ethical code, there were calls for even further modifications. Researchers therefore must constantly keep abreast of not only the profession's standards, but also legisla-tion affecting who can participate in studies, and under what circumstances.

REFERENCES

Abrami, P. C., Cohen, P. A., & d'Apollonia, S. (1988). Implementation problems in meta-analysis. *Review of Educational Research, 58*, 151–179.

American Psychological Association. (1992). Ethical principles of psychologists and code of conduct. *American Psychologist, 47*, 1597–1611.

Angell, M. (1988). Ethics in international collaborative clinical research. *New England Journal of Medicine, 319*, 1081–1083.

Barlow, D. H., & Hersen, M. (1984). *Single case experimental designs: Strategies for studying behavior change* (2nd ed.). New York: Pergamon Press.

Barry, M. (1988). Ethical considerations of human investigation in developing countries. *New England Journal of Medicine, 319*, 1083–1086.

Bramel, D., & Friend, R. (1981). Hawthorne, the myth of the docile worker, and class bias in psychology. *American Psychologist, 36*, 867–878.

Brubaker, R. G., & Wickersham, D. (1990). Encouraging the practice of testicular self-examination: A field application of the theory of reasoned action. *Health Psychology, 9*, 154–163.

Cacioppo, J. T., Marshall-Goodell, B. S., Tassinary, L. G., & Petty, R. E. (1992). Rudimentary determinants of attitudes: Classical conditioning is more effective when prior knowledge about the attitude stimulus is low than high. *Journal of Experimental Social Psychology, 28*, 207–233.

Chalmers, T. C., Berrier, J., Sacks, H. S., Levin, H., Reitman, D., & Nagalingam, R. (1987). Meta-analysis of clinical trials as a scientific discipline: II. Replicate variability and comparison of studies that agree and disagree. *Statistics in Medicine, 6*, 733–744.

Christensen, L., & Mendoza, J. L. (1986). A method of assessing change in a single subject: An alteration of the RC index. *Behavior Therapy, 17*, 305–308.

Clarke, G. N. (1995). Improving the transition from basic efficacy research to effectiveness studies: Methodological issues and procedures. *Journal of Consulting and Clinical Psychology, 63*, 718–725.

Cohen, J. (1962). The statistical power of abnormal-social psychological research: A review. *Journal of Abnormal and Social Psychology, 65*, 145–153.

Cohen, J. (1992). A power primer. *Psychological Bulletin, 112*, 155–159.

Cook, D. J., Guyatt, G. H., Davis, C., Willan, A., & McIlroy, W. (1993). A diagnostic and therapeutic N of 1 randomized trial. *Canadian Journal of Psychiatry, 38*, 251–254.

Cook, T. D., & Campbell, D. T. (1979). *Quasi-experimentation: Design and analysis issues for field settings.* Boston: Houghton Mifflin.

Crisp, A. H. (1980). *Anorexia nervosa: Let me be.* London: Academic Press.

Dickersin, K. (1990). The existence of publication bias and risk factors for its occurrence. *Journal of the American Medical Association, 263*, 1385–1389.

Dugan, E., Kamps, D., Leonard, B., Watkins, N., Rheinberger, A., & Stackhaus, J. (1995). Effects of cooperative learning groups during social studies for students with autism and fourth-grade peers. *Journal of Applied Behavior Analysis, 28*, 175–188.

Edgington, E. S. (1996). Randomized single-subject experimental designs. *Behaviour Research and Therapy, 34*, 567–574.

Edwards, A. L. (1957). *The social desirability variable in personality assessments and research.* New York: Dryden.

Elkin, I., Parloff, M. B., Hadley, S. W., & Autry, J. H. (1985). NIMH treatment of depression collaborative research program: Background and research plan. *Archives of General Psychiatry, 42*, 305–316.

Elkin, I., Shea, T., Watkins, J. T., Imber, S. D., Sotsky, S. M., Collins, J. F., Glass, D. R., Pilkonis, P. A., Leber, W. R., Docherty, J. P., Fiester, S. J., & Parloff, M. B. (1989). National Institute of Mental Health treatment of depression collaborative research program: General effectiveness of treatments. *Archives of General Psychiatry, 46*, 971–982.

Emmelkamp, P. M. G., & van den Hout, A. (1983). Failure in treating agoraphobia. In E. B. Foa & P. M. G. Emmelkamp (Eds.), *Failures in behavior therapy* (pp. 58–81). New York: Wiley.

Eysenck, H. J. (1952). The effects of psychotherapy: An evaluation. *Journal of Consulting Psychology, 16*, 319–324.

Frost, R. O., Steketee, G., Krause, M. S., & Trepanier, K. L. (1995). The relationship of the Yale-Brown Obsessive Compulsive Scale (YBOCS) to other measures of obsessive-compulsive symptoms in a non-clinical population. *Journal of Personality Assessment, 65*, 158–168.

Galassi, J. P., & Galassi, M. D. (1973). Alienation of college students: A comparison of counselling seekers and nonseekers. *Journal of Counselling Psychology, 20*, 44–49.

Garfield, S. L. (1986). Research on client variables in psychotherapy. In A. E. Bergin & S. L. Garfield (Eds.), *Handbook of psychotherapy and behavior change: An empirical analysis* (3rd ed., pp. 213–256). New York: Wiley.

Garner, D. M., Rockert, W., Davis, R., Garner, M. V., Olmstead, M. P., & Eagle, M. (1993). Comparison of cognitive-behavioral and supportive-expressive therapy for bulimia nervosa. *American Journal of Psychiatry, 150*, 37–46.

Glass, G. V., McGaw, B., & Smith, M. L. (1981). *Meta-analysis in social research.* Bevrley Hills, CA: Sage Publications.

Goldstein, A. P., Gassner, S., Greenberg, R. P., Gustin, A. W., Land, J., Liberman, B., & Streiner, D. L. (1967). The use of planted patients in group psychotherapy. *American Journal of Psychotherapy, 21*, 767–773.

Greenwald, A. G. (1975). Consequences of prejudice against the null hypothesis. *Psychological Bulletin, 82*, 1–20.

Hankin, J. R., & Locke, B. Z. (1982). The persistence of depressive symptomatology among prepaid group practice enrollees: An exploratory study. *American Journal of Public Health, 72*, 1000–1007.

Hansen, A. M. D., Hoogduin, C. A. L., Schaap, C., & de Haan, E. (1992). Do dropouts differ from successfully treated obsessive-compulsives? *Behaviour Research and Therapy, 30*, 547–550.

Hardman, J. G., & Limbird, L. E. (Eds.). (1996). *Goodman and Gilman's the pharmacological basis of therapeutics* (9th ed.). New York: McGraw-Hill.

Hedges, L. V. (1985). *Statistical methods for meta-analysis.* Orlando, FL: Academic Press.

Heller, K. (1971). Laboratory interview research as an analogue to treatment. In A. E. Bergin & S. L. Garfield (Eds.), *Handbook of psychotherapy and behavior change: An empirical analysis* (pp. 126–153). New York: Wiley.

Herrnstein, R. J., & Murray, C. A. (1994). *The bell curve: Intelligence and class structure in American life.* New York: Free Press.

Higginbotham, H. N., West, S. G., & Forsyth, D. R. (1988). *Psychotherapy and behavior change: Social, cultural, and methodological perspectives.* New York: Pergamon Press.

Hunter, J. E., & Schmidt, F. L. (1990). Dichotomization of continuous variables: The implications for meta-analysis. *Journal of Applied Psychology, 75*, 334–349.

Jacobson, N. S., Follette, W. C., & Revenstorf, D. (1984). Psychotherapy outcome research: Methods for reporting variability and evaluating clinical significance. *Behavior Therapy, 15*, 336–352.

Joffe, R., Sokolov, S., & Streiner, D. L. (1996). Antidepressant treatment of depression: A meta-analysis. *Canadian Journal of Psychiatry, 41*, 613–616.

Jones, S. R. G. (1992). Was there a Hawthorne effect? *American Journal of Sociology, 98*, 451–468.

Kamin, L. J. (1978). Comment on Munsinger's review of adoption studies. *Psychological Bulletin, 85*, 194–201.

Kellner, R., & Sheffield, B. F. (1973). The one-week prevalence of symptoms in neurotic patients and normals. *American Journal of Psychiatry, 130*, 102–105.

Kemp, R., Hayward, P., Applewhaite, G., Everitt, B., & David, A. (1996). Compliance therapy in psychotic patients: Randomized controlled trial. *British Medical Journal, 312*, 345–349.

Kendall, P. C., & Southam-Gerow, M. A. (1995). Issues in the transportability of treatment: The case of anxiety disorders in youths. *Journal of Consulting and Clinical Psychology, 63*, 702–708.

Kiesler, C. A., & Sibulkin, A. E. (1987). *Mental hospitalization: Myths and facts about a national crisis.* Newbury Park, CA: Sage Publications.

Lavy, E., van den Hout, M., & Arntz, A. (1993). Attentional bias and spider phobia: Conceptual and clinical issues. *Behaviour Research and Therapy, 31*, 17–24.

Levine, R. (1986). *Ethics and regulations of clinical research* (2nd ed.). Baltimore: Urban and Schwarzenber.

Luborsky, L., & DeRubeis, R. (1984). The use of psychotherapy treatment manuals: A small revolution in psychotherapy research style. *Clinical Psychology Review, 4*, 5–14.

Luchins, A. S., & Luchins, E. H. (1961). On conformity with judgments of a majority or an authority. *Journal of Social Psychology, 53*, 303–316.

Mann, A. H., Jenkins, R., & Belsey, E. (1981). The twelve-month outcome of patients with neurotic illness in general practice. *Psychological Medicine, 11*, 535–550.

May, R. B., & Hunter, M. A. (1993). Some advantages of permutation tests. *Canadian Psychology, 34*, 401–406.

McKibbon, K. A., Haynes, R. B., Walker Dilks, C. J., Ramsden, M. F., Ryan, N. C., Baker, L., Flemming, T., & Fitzgerald, D. (1990). How good are clinical MEDLINE searches? A comparative study of clinical end-user and librarian searches. *Computers and Biomedical Research, 23*, 583–593.

McNemar, Q. (1946). Opinion–attitude methodology. *Psychological Bulletin, 43*, 289–374.

Mechanic, D. (1980). *Mental health and social policy.* Englewood Cliffs, NJ: Prentice-Hall.

Milgram, S. (1963). Behavioral study of obedience. *Journal of Abnormal and Social Psychology, 67*, 371–378.

Munsinger, H. (1975). The adopted child's IQ: A critical review. *Psychological Bulletin, 82*, 623–659.

Norman, G. R., & Streiner, D. L. (1997). *PDQ Statistics* (2nd ed.). St. Louis: Mosby.

Office for Protection from Research Risks. (1995). *Exempt research and research that may undergo expedited review.* OPRR Reports, No. 95–02. Rockville, MD: National Institutes of Health.

Persons, J. B. (1991). Psychotherapy outcome studies do not accurately represent current models of psychotherapy: A proposed remedy. *American Psychologist, 46*, 99–106.

Ramos, D. (1995). Paradise miscalculated. In S. Fraser (Ed.), *The bell curve wars: Race, intelligence, and the future of America* (pp. 62–69). New York: Basic Books.

Roper, B. L., Ben-Porath, Y. S., & Butcher, J. N. (1995). Comparability and validity of computerized adaptive testing with the MMPI-2. *Journal of Personality Assessment, 65*, 358–371.

Rosenthal, R. (1979). The "file drawer problem" and tolerance for null results. *Psychological Bulletin, 86*, 638–641.

Rosenthal, R., & Rosnow, R. L. (1984). Applying Hamlet's question to the ethical conduct of research: A conceptual addendum. *American Psychologist, 39*, 561–563.

Rosenthal, R., & Rubin, D. B. (1982). Comparing effect sizes of independent studies. *Psychological Bulletin, 92*, 500–504.

Rudd, M. D., Rajab, M. H., Orman, D. T., Stulman, D. A., Joiner, T., & Dixon, W. (1996). Effectiveness of an outpatient intervention targeting suicidal young adults: Preliminary results. *Journal of Consulting and Clinical Psychology, 64*, 179–190.

Rushton, J. P. (1992). Cranial capacity related to sex, rank and race in a stratified random sample of 6,325 U.S. military personnel. *Intelligence, 16*, 401–413.

Rushton, J. P., & Ankney, C. D. (1996). Brain size and cognitive ability: Correlations with age, sex, social class and race. *Psychonomic Bulletin and Review, 3*, 21–36.

Scher, S. J., & Cooper, J. (1989). Motivational basis of dissonance: The singular role of behavioral consequences. *Journal of Personality and Social Psychology, 56*, 899–906.

Sedlmeier, P., & Gigerenzer, G. (1989). Do studies of statistical power have an effect on the power of studies? *Psychological Bulletin, 105*, 309–316.

Sobal, J., & Stunkard, A. J. (1989). Socioeconomic status and obesity: A review of the literature. *Psychological Bulletin, 105*, 260–275.

St. Lawrence, J. S., Reitman, D., Jefferson, K. W., Alleyne, E., Brasfield, T. L., & Shirley, A. (1994). Factor structure and validation of an adolescent version of the Condom Attitude Scale: An instrument for measuring adolescents' attitudes toward condoms. *Psychological Assessment, 6*, 352–359.

Streiner, D. L., & Adam, K. S. (1987). Evaluation of the effectiveness of suicide prevention programs: A methodological perspective. *Suicide and Life-Threatening Behavior, 17*, 93–106.

Streiner, D. L., & Norman, G. R. (1995). *Health measurement scales: A practical guide to their development and use* (2nd ed.). London: Oxford University Press.

Streiner, D. L., & Norman, G. R. (1996). *PDQ Epidemiology* (2nd ed.). St. Louis: Mosby.

Strupp, H. (1977). A reformulation of the dynamics of the therapist's contribution. In A. S. Gurman & A. M. Razin (Eds.), *Effective psychotherapy: A handbook of research* (pp. 3–22). New York: Pergamon Press.

Suissa, S. (1991). Binary methods for continuous outcomes: A parametric alternative. *Journal of Clinical Epidemiology, 44*, 241–248.

Thompson, S. C., Nanni, C., & Schwankovsky, L. (1990). Patient-oriented interventions to improve communication in a medical office visit. *Health Psychology, 9*, 390–404.

Turner, S. M., & Beidel, D. C. (1989). Social phobia: Clinical syndrome, diagnosis, and comorbidity. *Clinical Psychology Review, 9*, 3–18.

Vaillant, G. E. (1972). Why men seek psychotherapy: I. Results of a survey of college graduates. *American Journal of Psychiatry, 129*, 645–651.

Warner, R. (1994). *Recovery from schizophrenia: Psychiatry and political economy* (2nd ed.). London: Routledge.

Weisz, J. R., Donenberg, G. R., Han, S. S., & Weiss, B. (1995). Bridging the gap between laboratory and clinic in child and adolescent psychotherapy. *Journal of Consulting and Clinical Psychology, 63*, 688–701.

Wittchen, H-U., & Essau, C. A. (1993). Epidemiology of panic disorder: Progress and unresolved issues. *Journal of Psychiatric Research, 27* (Suppl. 1), 47–68.

Woodward, C. A., & Streiner, D. L. (1995). Editorial. *International Journal for Quality in Health Care, 7*, 323–324.

FOR FURTHER READING

How to Evaluate Our Interventions

Designs Appropriate for Larger Studies

Cook, T. D., & Campbell, D. T. (1979). *Quasi-experimentation: Design and analysis issues for field settings*. Boston: Houghton Mifflin.

Higginbotham, H. N., West, S. G., & Forsyth, D. R. (1988). *Psychotherapy and behavior change: Social, cultural and methodological perspectives*. New York: Pergamon Press.

Streiner, D. L., & Norman, G. R. (1996). *PDQ epidemiology* (2nd ed.). St. Louis: Mosby.

Designs Appropriate for Clinical Practice

Barlow, D. H., & Hersen, M. (1984). *Single case experimental designs: Strategies for studying behavior change* (2nd ed.). New York: Pergamon Press.

Kazdin, A. E. (1982). *Single case research designs: Methods for clinical and applied settings*. New York: Oxford University Press.

Kratochwill, T. R., & Levin, J. R. (1992). *Single-case research design and analysis: New directions for psychology and education*. Hillsdale, NJ: Erlbaum.

Long, C. G., & Hollin, C. R. (1995). Single case design: A critique of methodology and analysis of recent trends. *Clinical Psychology and Psychotherapy, 2*, 177–191.

Evaluating Meta-analyses

Glass, G. V., McGaw, B., & Smith, M. L. (1981). *Meta-analysis in social research*. Beverly Hills, CA: Sage Publications.

Light, R. J., & Pillemer, D. B. (1984). *Summing up: The science of reviewing research*. Cambridge, MA: Harvard University Press.

Ethical Issues

American Psychological Association. (1992). Ethical principles of psychologists and code of conduct. *American Psychologist, 47*, 1597–1611.

Levine, R. (1986). *Ethics and regulations of clinical research* (2nd ed.). Baltimore: Urban and Schwarzenber.

CHAPTER 6

TREATING THE INDIVIDUAL

Jerold R. Gold
George Stricker

WHAT IS PSYCHOTHERAPY?

"Psychotherapy is an undefined technique applied to unspecified problems with unpredictable outcome. For this technique we recommend rigorous training" (Raimy, 1950, p. 93).

In all seriousness, the best answer to this question might be, "It depends whom you ask." Another answer, one that resembles a dreaded stereotype of the psychotherapist's response to a patient's question, is, "What would you like it to be?"

These answers reflect an interesting, troubling, and perhaps extraordinary state of affairs within the scholarly discipline and professional practice of psychotherapy: We do it, we know that it exists, we believe in its effectiveness, we recommend it to people and defend it from attacks from politicians, newspapers, colleagues, and patients—but we cannot describe or define psychotherapy in a precise way.

Yet, is this dilemma, in fact, so extraordinary? Many of the experiences or ideas that push human beings along—that cause wars, start families, build hospitals, change things in momentous ways—cannot be described fully in words. Just think of love, honor, gratitude, among many other concepts, and try to offer precise definitions that will enjoy universal consensus.

Psychotherapy cannot be defined precisely because there is no single enterprise, discipline, or activity to which the term is attached. At the date of this writing, over four hundred forms or schools of psychotherapy can be identified (Gold, 1996), each of which defines itself somewhat differently from the other types of therapy. A recent conference that was organized to define psychotherapy offered its participants the chance to select from 81 different contributions, none of which was identical to any other (Zeig & Munion, 1990). These students of psychotherapy at least were able to group the hundreds of types of psychotherapy into a much smaller number of categories, and then to extract some skeletal consensus with regard to a beginning definition of the term. Nine broad types of psychotherapy were noted: (1) psychodynamic, (2) humanistic/experiential, (3) behavioral, (4) cognitive, (5) philosophical, (6) family/systemic, (7) group, (8) hypnotherapy, and (9) eclectic/integrative.

The generic definition offered is a good one and is consistent with other attempts to capture the elusive essence of all these psychotherapies in a few words. *Psychotherapy* has been defined as an interpersonal relationship that contains within it an implied or overt theory of psychological distress and of the conditions that are necessary for psychological change to occur. The relationship and the interpersonal interactions that mark that relationship are structured in such a way that the conditions for psychological change are optimized. One party in the relationship (the therapist) has as her or his task the provision of experiences that promote change. The other party (the patient) participates to her or his best ability in order to improve.

This definition does not do justice to any particular form of psychotherapy. Psychotherapy is a complex, frustrating, puzzling, and at times exhilarating experience that may often defy words. Each system of psychotherapy is built on an expanded definition that includes a theory of psychopathology, a theory of psychological change, a theory of technique and interpersonal influence, and a conception of the interpersonal relationship that best promotes change. In the pages that follow we will review the major systems of psychotherapy and will attempt to convey to the reader a more vivid description of just what the varied psychotherapies are.

THE HISTORY OF PSYCHOTHERAPY

Psychotherapists and psychotherapeutic activities have existed in some form at every point in history, but only in the last hundred years or so have these persons and experiences been identified with the term *psychotherapy.* Consistent with our generic definition of psychotherapy, each historical precursor of modern psychotherapy was built on some theoretical explanation of psychological suffering and the necessary conditions for correcting this pain, and singled out a specific interpersonal arena for alleviating the person's suffering as central to the process.

Ancient and Medieval Precursors of Psychotherapy

In the classical past of Rome and Greece, psychological distress was attributed to supernatural forces: to the malevolence of the gods, to magical spells cast by sorcerers, to the hatred of the gods, or

to one's enemies. The folk versions of psychotherapy that were prescribed for these ills included sacrifices meant to appease an offended deity; the intercession of a shaman, priest, or other healing or religious official who would perform an expiatory ritual; or the use of counterspells or overt aggression against the person who cast or commissioned the black magic. Sometimes, as in certain South American tribal societies, hallucinogenic drugs or primitive psychosurgical methods also were employed. With the transition to Christianity as the dominant religion in Western society, explanations of psychopathology found a basis both in the supernatural and in failures of faith and morality. As an early, influential example, St. Augustine describes, in his Confessions, a prolonged period of uncertainty and anxiety that today might be diagnosed as an identity crisis of late adolescence. He found solace in the teachings of the Church and in a strict adherence to its moral tenets. From Augustine's time until the early modern period, the role of folk psychotherapist usually was assigned to the religious leaders of each community, who treated the psychologically distressed of their flock through confession, assignment of penance, counseling based on the Bible and its teachings, and occasionally, exorcism and other supernatural means as well.

The Early Modern Era (Eighteenth and Nineteenth Centuries)

The emergence of modern psychotherapy has its roots in the European Enlightenment and in the development of modern science and medicine in the eighteenth and nineteenth centuries. The empirical study of the human body and of the natural world included the application of scientific methods and ideas to the human mind and its abnormalities. Modern psychiatry began to coalesce in the nineteenth century, as the authority to confine and to treat madness moved away from lay persons and religious orders into the hands of the medical profession. The middle of the nineteenth century found the new field of psychiatry dominated by biological theories about the causation of mental illness, and by the work of such psychiatrists as Emil Kraepelin, who established the first broadly accepted classification system of psychiatric disorders. The mad were confined to asylums, while more moderately troubled persons found themselves under the care of a physician for some "nervous disorder," usually attributed to a congenital weakness or abnormality of the nervous system. Psychotherapy involved following the physician's prescriptions of rest, warm baths, mild electrical stimulation of afflicted areas of the body, "taking the cure" at a sauna or warm springs, and other supportive measures.

The Emergence of Psychoanalysis (Late Nineteenth Century–World War 1)

Sigmund Freud and psychoanalysis moved psychotherapy onto the world stage and laid the foundation for its current status. Freud's work grew out of experimentation with hypnosis as a treatment for hysteria, pioneered by such figures as Jean Charcot and Hippolyte Bernheim. He was also influenced by other psychotherapeutic explorers of the time, including particularly Pierre Janet. Freud's original ideas, however, including his theories of the unconscious, of infantile sexuality, and of transference, coupled with his innovative methods of free association and interpretation, made Freudian psychoanalysis the dominant psychotherapeutic system during the early part of the twentieth century.

Deviations and schisms within European psychoanalysis led, by 1930, to the establishment of alternative systems and methods, including most prominently Jung's analytical psychology, Adler's individual psychology, existential psychotherapy, and many others. In the United States, during the 1920s and 1930s, Freudian psychoanalysis and its offshoots had a great impact on a segment of the psychotherapeutic community that became more dogmatic and rigid in its approach to psychoanalysis than its founder had ever intended. Other American psychotherapists found inspiration in Freud's ideas but combined them with homegrown insights and an appreciation for environmental variables and the impact of culture, politics, and economics. This was particularly important in a nation that was struggling through a massive economic depression and was heading toward war. The chief contributors

to these advances included Karen Horney, Erich Fromm, and Harry Stack Sullivan.

As Europe moved toward war during the mid- and late 1930s, many European analysts fled the Nazi regime and moved to England, North America, and South America, bringing with them an orthodox version of psychoanalysis that was to dominate psychoanalysis for at least the next thirty years.

American Psychotherapies During the 1940s

During the years surrounding World War II, other nonpsychoanalytic psychotherapies were developed in the United States. Carl Rogers offered the public his client-centered therapy, based on an experiential theory that placed psychological growth and actualization of human potential at its center. Learning theorists and behavioral psychologists, drawing on the writings of Pavlov, Watson, Hull, Spence, and other laboratory-based psychologists, began to explain psychopathology within a stimulus–response framework, and to see the cure for emotional suffering as residing in new learning and in the correction of faulty habits and behavior patterns. The foundations of modern cognitive psychotherapy were laid in the research and applied work of such early clinical psychologists as George Kelly and Julian Rotter, who attempted to apply the rigor of behaviorism to covert thought processes. These pioneering efforts were to take center stage during the postwar decades as the foundations of modern behavior therapy.

Postwar Psychotherapy (1945–1980)

The early postwar period saw a huge increase in public interest in, and consumption of, psychotherapy, as a more educated, psychologically sophisticated, and economically advantaged population sought to soothe itself in a threatening and alienated era. The period immediately following the war also saw psychotherapy emerge as a professional activity shared, though not always congenially, by several disciplines: psychiatry, clinical and counseling psychology, social work, nursing, and pastoral counseling. The field was split by heated debates between client-centered therapists, psychoanalysts, the newly important and influential group of behavior therapists, and several other new therapeutic systems and practitioners: rational-emotive therapy, Gestalt therapy, personal-construct therapy, experiential therapy, and many others.

During this period, the research literature suggested that behavior therapy would emerge as the treatment of choice for most psychological disorders. The impact of this perspective was felt in a number of ways. Many training programs in clinical psychology abandoned or decreased their training experiences in psychoanalytic and humanistic approaches (Rogerian and related therapies) and moved heavily toward behavioral models. Psychiatry, becoming disillusioned with psychoanalytic models, moved more heavily into psychopharmacological approaches and away from a general reliance on psychological methods.

The Current Era (1980–Present)

In the midst of this competition and animosity were a group of research-oriented psychotherapists who were finding that no single psychotherapy could substantially outperform its rivals, and practitioners who began to look across the boundaries of traditional psychotherapies. The ultimate failure of behavior therapy to demonstrate its superior effectiveness, together with all of the external challenges to psychotherapy that have emerged in our society (the health care crisis, the prospect of limited insurance funding, the emphasis on the use of drugs to treat mental illness) have actually been helpful to the field in many ways, forcing many therapists to stop squabbling and to consider other ideas more seriously.

The last 25 years have been marked by the emergence of cognitive psychotherapy as an influential theory and method, the integration of cognitive theories and methods with mainstream behavioral approaches, the revitalization of psychoanalytic and humanistic psychotherapies through an expansion of their theories and methods, and a general interest in combining or integrating the best of the various therapies into more powerful and effective treatments.

THE CULTURAL CONTEXT OF PSYCHOTHERAPY

As Jerome Frank (1961) pointed out in his classic work, *Persuasion and Healing,* psychological suffering is not limited to "modern" Western societies. Psychotherapeutic experiences and authorities are present in traditional cultures, although those events and persons are described in other terms, within the language of healing that is associated with each group of people.

Frank's (1961) study indicated that certain psychological phenomena seem to cause or contribute to emotional distress in all cultures. These variables include the loss of purpose and direction in one's life, the loss of hope, and the erosion of realistic optimism. The disturbed person is demoralized, pessimistic, discouraged, and defeated. In all cultures, Western or Eastern, technical and modern or traditional and "undeveloped," a variety of interpersonal relationships exist whose purpose is to remoralize and to instill hope in those who suffer psychologically. In the middle-class, psychologically oriented segments of our society, psychotherapists have to some extent replaced parents, grandparents, clergy, teachers, and other traditional caretakers in this role. In other segments of our culture and in other societies, the witch doctor, shaman, fortune teller, bartender, rabbi, parish priest, imam, or community organizer may serve people in the same ways. Each is capable of offering an interpersonal relationship in which there exists a theory that explains the person's suffering, and out of which can be prescribed experiences that can lead to change. It was Frank's (1961) tremendous insight that any and all of these relationships can offer the sufferer new hope, optimism, and direction, thus making these relationships the functional equivalents of psychotherapy. In fact, many students of psychotherapy have suggested that people turn to formal psychotherapy only after these folk psychotherapies have failed or have been found to be unavailable.

This last point may speak to the tremendous expansion of the profession of psychotherapy during the last 50 years, and to the uneasy status that psychotherapists have attained during this period. Those who have detailed the development of the profession in a historical and cultural context have suggested that the alienation inherent in an industrial, materialistic society has led inevitably to a loss of community ties and of the natural healing relationships that formerly existed within the extended family and rural society (Cushman, 1995; Fromm, 1955). As people live more isolated and autonomous lives, it becomes all too easy to experience despair, discouragement, and demoralization. At the same time, the isolation that spawns these conditions also prevents people from having as resources those relationships that in the past were "naturally" psychotherapeutic. Hence the need for psychotherapy, a specific profession to satisfy the need for such healing interpersonal experiences.

AN OVERVIEW OF THE MAJOR SYSTEMS OF PSYCHOTHERAPY

This review of the major systems of psychotherapy is organized according to the general definition of psychotherapy that we developed earlier. We will include the ways in which each system understands the etiology and maintenance of psychopathology, the conditions and experiences through which psychological change occurs, and the perspective of each school of psychotherapy with regard to the nature of the optimal psychotherapeutic relationship.

Psychodynamic Approaches to Psychotherapy

The term *psychodynamic* refers to any form of psychotherapy that uses the concept of unconscious motivation as introduced by Freud (1900) and that sees psychopathology as caused by intrapsychic factors. There are many approaches to psychodynamic psychotherapy. The oldest, classical psychoanalysis, is the variant of psychodynamic psychotherapy that remains closest to the ideas and practice introduced by Freud (1900, 1912) and his contemporaries. It involves multiple sessions per week, can last for many years, and is based on current versions of Freud's biological approach to psychopathology.

Relational psychoanalysis developed more recently and resembles classical psychoanalysis in its length and frequency of sessions, but is based on a modified theory of psychodynamics that includes acknowledgment of environmental factors in emotional suffering. Psychodynamic psychotherapy, as opposed to psychoanalysis, refers to any therapy that relies on psychodynamic concepts and methods while operating within more limited parameters of time and frequency. Despite many announcements of the death of psychoanalysis (Klein, 1971), a psychodynamic orientation still remains prominent among clinical psychologists and psychotherapists.

Psychodynamic Theories of Psychopathology

Psychoanalysis and its offshoots offer a long and rich tradition of conceptualizing human behavior in terms of motivation, conflict, and defense. All versions of psychodynamic theory stress the unconscious determination of conscious cognition, affect, and behavior. They differ predominantly in terms of the particular motives, conflicts, and developmental issues that are viewed as most influential. Classical psychoanalysis posits that personality develops along a path of universal, biologically determined stages of psychosexual wishes. Psychopathology reflects a fixation at, and regression to, unknown and unresolved conflicts stemming from one or more of these fixation points. Symptoms and problematic behaviors are understood to be reflective of several simultaneous covert conflicts, and to be the manifestation of a compromise between the wish to express the unconscious desire and the defensive processes that alter that wish into an unrecognizable form. These psychological processes that the person uses (also without awareness) to remain unaware of these strivings are known as the defense mechanisms of the ego (A. Freud, 1936). Contemporary psychoanalytic theories have retained the emphasis on unconscious motivational factors but have moved toward etiological models that are more interpersonally and socially conditioned. This conceptual shift within psychoanalysis has been influenced by clinical studies and by the emergence of psychodynamically informed studies of child development (cf. Mahler, Pine, & Bergman, 1975; Stern, 1985). Collectively, these theories have been described as making up the "relational structure model" (Greenberg & Mitchell, 1983), which emphasizes the interaction between the growing child and the significant persons in his or her life. (These variants of psychoanalysis represent the "nurture" side of the so-called nature–nurture debate that runs through most areas of psychology, whereas classical psychoanalysis falls heavily in the "nature" camp.)

The early parent–child interactions are considered to be crucial in the formation of psychological structures, motivational conflicts, and representations of the self and of others. Relational-structure theorists are most concerned with the processes through which the child internalizes, identifies with, and represents productive and maladaptive patterns of relatedness, and the ways in which these largely unconscious structures skew and distort present-day perception, thinking, affective functioning, and interpersonal engagement.

The relational structure perspective within psychodynamic thinking refers to any number of separate schools and leading theorists, including self psychology (Kohut, 1977), interpersonal psychoanalysis (Sullivan, 1953; Fromm, 1955), object relations theory (Greenberg & Mitchell, 1983), and Bowlby's (1980) representational model of attachment.

Theories of Change and of Therapeutic Technique

Two broadly defined conceptualizations of change processes exist within current psychodynamic thinking. The more traditional view, which emphases insight into unconscious processes, is derived directly from Freud's (1912) earliest work in psychoanalysis. The second view of change is considered more radical within the psychoanalytic world and is a result of the work of such revisionists as Alexander and French (1946), who emphasized the centrality of new experience (the "corrective emotional experience") within therapy as leading to changes in behavior, symptoms, character, and in-

trapsychic processes and structures. This latter theory of change is typical of relational forms of psychoanalysis.

Insight involves the patient learning something about his or her unconscious psychological activity. This learning is of a specific sort: The patient becomes aware of some forbidden, frightening, and painfully evocative wish, emotion, motive, fantasy, or memory that has been influencing his or her mental life in unknown but powerful ways. Complete insight also contains the entrance into awareness of the ways in which the patient kept himself or herself unknowing (defense mechanisms, inhibitions, and character traits). The final component of insight involves learning about the anxieties, painful affects, self-images, and anticipated interpersonal consequences that led to the original warding off or disavowal of the particular issue. The emotional process of experiencing and integrating previously warded-off conflicts is known as *abreaction* and always is cited as crucial to therapeutic change. Intellectual awareness of one's conflicts never leads to change in isolation from such abreaction.

Insight and abreaction sometimes occur spontaneously as the patient associates freely in the presence of the therapist. Most often, these experiences follow some interpretation offered by the psychoanalyst, in which the patient is told about the contents of the unconscious conflict, its historical roots, and its present-day manifestations. An accurate interpretation seems to lead to the recovery of memories, to affective arousal, and to greater awareness of previously hidden feelings, desires, self-images, and object representations. As these mental contents become conscious, a decrease occurs in the consequent anxiety, guilt, shame, or other affective correlates of those inner states. As insight and abreaction occur with some regularity over the course of therapy, the patient is freed of the burdensome psychic task of drastically limiting his or her intrapsychic life through defenses, symptoms, and distortions of behavior. Relational psychoanalysis relies on insight into problematic self-images and images of others that are regressive and evocative of anxiety. This allows the patient to revise those representations and to form a more benign and productive representational system.

Insight essentially is an intrapsychic event that theoretically requires little interpersonal interchange (Greenberg & Mitchell, 1983). Since at least the 1930s, however, analysts have been aware that the therapeutic interaction is at least as important as insight in promoting change (cf. Strachey, 1934). This thesis was formulated most clearly by Alexander and French (1946), who argued that a "corrective emotional experience" in psychoanalysis caused the patient to change. In their view, insight followed intrapsychic and interpersonal change as frequently as it preceded change, or more so.

The "corrective emotional experience" proposed by Alexander and French (1946) is the forerunner of relational psychoanalytic concepts that describe the ways in which new, ameliorative experiences are provided for the patient by the therapist (see the work of Kohut, 1977; Levenson, 1983; and Winnicott, 1971, for some examples of these approaches). Essentially, the analyst interacts with the patient in ways that differ considerably from past interactions in which the patient was slighted, hurt, abused, neglected, or made unable to act as a unique individual. The therapist becomes the prototype for new representations of others that correct and replace fearsome, hateful, or ineffective parental images, while the emotional sense of being responded to thoughtfully, sensitively, and compassionately becomes the core of a new, stable sense of self and process of thinking about, and relating to, the self.

The Therapeutic Relationship in Psychodynamic Psychotherapy

Psychoanalytic therapies divide the interaction between patient and therapist into three overlapping components: (1) the "real" relationship, (2) the therapeutic alliance, and (3) the transference–countertransference relationship. The *"real" relationship* consists of the social aspects of the interaction between the two therapeutic participants. This part of the interaction is thought to be an inevitable by-product of the frequent, regular contact between patient and therapist. The *therapeutic alliance* is the working, task-oriented bond that develops between the rational, investigative, and psychologically observant aspects of the personalities of the patient and the therapist. Out of the alliance comes the analytic process, which includes the patient's freedom to communicate fully about inner experience and to remain open to the interpretations offered by the therapist. *Transference* and *countertransference* refer to the historically determined, irrational, idiosyncratic perceptions, affects, and portrayals of the therapist by the patient (transference) and of the patient by the therapist (countertransference). Transference is the unconscious process through which the patient mistakes or actively transforms the therapist into someone from the patient's past or current life outside of the therapeutic realtionship. Countertransference involves a similar, unwitting misperception of the patient by the therapist. Transference and countertransference influence the immediate interaction in a repetitive and initially unacknowledged way, and are among the most frequent causes of resistance and blockages in the flow of the communication between patient and therapist.

At the heart of this form of psychotherapy is the analysis of the transference: the unconscious transformation of the patient's relationship to the psychoanalyst into a reproduction of his or her childhood relationships with parents and other significant people. The patient unknowingly transfers or displaces the pathogenic wishes and defense mechanisms from the past into her or his perceptions of, and reactions toward, the analyst. These wishes then are analyzed in the here and now as they come to dominate the therapeutic interaction. Most classical analysts believe that the analysis of the transference allows the most important opportunity for gaining insight and for cathartic release from the past.

Relational analysts share the view of the importance of the transference relationship but differ in their understanding of just what is transferred. This group suggests that patients unconsciously reproduce the interactions in which they were traumatized, neglected, abandoned, or made to feel ashamed, anxious, and guilty. As these old images of, and ways of relating to, significant persons from the past become conscious, the patient is able to revise her or his ways of looking at ongoing relationships. The ability of the therapist to understand these hurts, to communicate about them effectively, and to provide the curative experiences that the patient has always needed lead to new intrapsychic structures.

Humanistic/Experiential Psychotherapies

This school of psychotherapy includes the client-centered approach, Gestalt therapy, and existential psychotherapy.

Client-Centered Therapy

Client-centered psychotherapy was developed by Carl Rogers (1951), who was concerned with the ways that psychological growth, authenticity, and integration are achieved or thwarted. Realization of the person's abilities, values, and goals; emotional and cognitive flexibility and openness; a capacity for genuine self-acceptance; and warm, empathic regard for others are some of the signs of self-actualization or psychological health that are mentioned in the literature (cf. Maslow, 1954; Rogers, 1961).

Psychopathology. Rogers (1951) was among the first of the therapists to adopt a phenomenological orientation to the study of other persons. This refers to the study and clinical use of the person's immediate experiences and to the ways in which each person makes sense out of the vast flow of images, sensations, ideas, and feelings that pass through consciousness from moment to moment. Rogers's chief empirical and clinical concerns were the meanings that the person attaches to experience— meanings that reflect either moments of authentic living, or moments of unhealthy and avoidant functioning. Client- centered therapists (Raskin & Rogers, 1989) emphasize the ability to symbolize consciously what one is experiencing as a crucial factor in the process of self-actualization. Psychopathology is thought to result from chronic anxiety or other threats that become associated with particular experiences, emotions, or thoughts. Any event or inner state that is associated with some subjective danger to the person thus may lead to the closing down, interruption, or distortion of awareness. Client-centered therapists (Rice & Greenberg, 1992) see anxiety as resulting from a conflict between the

need to preserve a learned image of the self and any experience that is incompatible with that image. Learned self-images—the "ideal self" referred to by Rogers (1961)—result from repeated evaluations of the person by parents and other significant persons during childhood. To the degree that important constructive experiences are disapproved of by these authorities (e.g., the need to express disappointment in one's parents), then those tendencies will mean danger to that person in the future. At those moments, gaining the approval of others supersedes actualization of the potentials and abilities of the self as an aim. Furthermore, those experiences will be excluded from the ideal self-image that the person constructs, meaning that any awareness of such trends will lead to incongruity, anxiety, and limitations of awareness.

Theory of change and of technique. Client-centered therapy emphasizes the role of the person's present phenomenology and perceptions of the future in shaping the experience of the present. Therefore, Rogerian therapists tend to deemphasize developmental models and the role of past experiences in therapeutic discussions. Instead, the prime topics are the person's immediate, ongoing flow of thoughts, feelings, sensations, images, and fantasies. Rogers (1951) originally called his therapy "nondirective therapy." This was an accurate title for a model of psychotherapy in which assessment and diagnosis were shunned as irrelevant at best and damaging at worst, and in which the therapist's technical expertise was downplayed almost entirely. It is impossible to discuss Rogers's view of therapeutic change apart from his conceptualization of the therapeutic relationship. Therapy was no more and no less than the totality of the interaction between client and therapist. Client-centered therapy is built upon the premise that the therapeutic interaction provides the "necessary and sufficient" conditions for change and growth (Rogers, 1957). Those relationship conditions included the provision by the therapist of an utterly safe and accepting atmosphere, in which the client is responded to with unconditional positive regard or prizing, warmth, and accurate empathy. These conditions can be offered only if the therapist functions out of the experience of being as fully integrated or self-congruent as he or she can be. Any significant shift away from self-congruence by the therapist is likely to result in anxiety that will interfere with the therapist's ability to respond to the patient in a nonevaluative and open way.

The relationship conditions in this therapy allow the patient gradually to broaden and deepen his or her ability to live in feelings and experiences, and to symbolize consciously that experience to the fullest degree possible. This is because internalized "conditions of worth" (Rogers, 1957) that were instilled in early family life can be unlearned actively in the interaction with the therapist (Bohart, 1993). As the patient finds unconditional acceptance, regardless of the nature of his or her ongoing internal experiences, he or she learns to prize, accept, and symbolize those experiences as well. The final result of this process is self-congruence and a greatly expanded potential for phenomenological authenticity on the part of the patient.

The therapeutic relationship. Client-centered therapy is a process-oriented therapy in which the relationship and technique are considered to be fully identical and inseparable (Rice & Greenberg, 1992). The "real," forward-looking, and growth-oriented aspects of the relationship are considered indispensable, to the exclusion of any meaningful consideration of regressive or transferential components or distortions of the interaction. Shlein (1984) has argued that reliance on the concept of transference by a client-centered therapist may be a way of negating or avoiding a real but painful perception of, or appropriately negative response to, the therapist by the patient. Such defensive behavior contradicts the authentic, unconditionally accepting, and congruent attitudes that typify client-centered therapy.

Gestalt Therapy

Psychopathology. Gestalt therapy is most concerned with the person's openness to the processes of moment-to-moment bodily, cognitive, and emotional experience (Perls, Hefferline, & Goodman, 1951). Gestalt therapy suggests that the person lim-

its his or her awareness of wishes, needs, feelings, and bodily states because of anxiety. This anxiety occurs because the person has accepted interpersonal and societal sanctions on certain types of experience. For example, in certain segments of American culture it is unacceptable for boys or men to cry when they are hurt or sad. Having noticed signs of ridicule and disapproval from parents, teachers, and peers for crying, in later life many males will unwittingly restrict their experience of sadness and vulnerability, replacing these experiences with anger, bodily tension, or other symptoms.

Gestalt therapists suggest that the ability to recognize and contact a pressing internal need or interpersonal encounter, and to attend fully to shifts in the interactional field and in the body, are the characteristics of the individual who has reached a state of holistic organization (Perls et al.,1951). Gestalt therapists also point out that the disturbed person suffers from a habitual restriction of consciousness and behavior due to socialized anxiety. Direct contact with the phenomenology of the environment and the body is replaced by mechanistic functioning aimed at repeating learned patterns of interaction that are protective and avoidant. The patient remains unaware of what he or she feels, thinks, senses, and does. Even basic bodily functions of breathing, posture, movement, vocal quality and tone, and muscular tension are affected and lose their freedom and spontaneity.

Theory of change and therapeutic technique. The expansion of awareness, particularly of bodily and emotional needs and states, is the goal of Gestalt therapy and, as Perls (1973) demonstrates, is accomplished through a series of active exercises and confrontations. The mechanisms that produce change involve focusing of awareness on the ways that the person distorts, avoids, or transforms emotions, fantasies, desires, and bodily states. Attentional focusing, experiential exercises, and the resultant heightened awareness eventuate in a conscious sense of the levels of faulty, self-estranged, and falsified modes of living that produce psychopathology. Authentic experience and an expansion of awareness emerge as the person becomes able to acknowledge his or her own role in limiting conscious experience, and becomes aware of the pain and anxiety that set such processes in motion. The patient thus is able gradually to accept spontaneous emotions, needs, and wishes.

The therapist suggests and designs exercises meant to increase the patient's awareness of the bodily distortions, interpersonal habits, and internalized figures and prohibitions that limit the scope of awareness. These exercises, tailored to the immediacy of the clinical situation, may be as simple as asking a patient to focus on the level of tension in a limb as she moves, or to listen carefully to the timbre and tone of her voice as she speaks. Technique in Gestalt therapy asks the patient to reflect on the here and now, often simply through questions such as "What are you doing at this moment?" The most well known Gestalt exercises involve enactment of an interaction with an internalized other or with a part of the self. These techniques, known as the *empty-chair* or *two-chair* technique, involve a discussion in the here and now with the imagined partner. The goal of all Gestalt techniques is contact with the authentic need, feeling, or perception that is repressed or disavowed through the restriction of awareness (Rice & Greenberg, 1992).

The therapeutic relationship. Gestalt therapy relies on an affectively charged encounter between patient and therapist. The therapist confronts the patient's habitual patterns of behavior and defense, and refuses to engage the patient in these repetitive interactions. Gestalt therapists do not stress the efficacy of the therapeutic interaction to the extent that client-centered therapists do, but they agree that an authentic encounter is necessary for significant change to occur (Rice & Greenberg, 1992). Contemporary Gestalt therapy stresses the need for an honest, open, and emotionally charged exchange between patient and therapist, in which the patient is confronted immediately with his or her ways of avoiding contact with the self and with the therapist. This respectful but potent "I-Thou" experience is considered to be as important as the technical experiments and exercises that mark the formal Gestalt approach (Yontef, 1981).

Existential Psychotherapy

Existential psychotherapies share with client-centered therapy and Gestalt therapy an emphasis on unimpeded awareness, but they are more concerned with the individual's capacity to stay with and to experience fully life's painful existential realities. Most writers in this tradition have attempted explicitly to focus on issues of individual free will and choice in behavior and adaptation (Bugental & Kleiner, 1993). These therapists focus on the active role each of us takes in making choices and in determining the nature and directions of our relationships and lives.

Psychopathology. Existential therapists (May, 1977; Yalom, 1981) suggest that anxiety is an inevitable consequence of human existence. The "thrown," helpless nature of the person in the face of life's inevitable limits (including death, freedom, meaninglessness, finitude, isolation, and separation) yields a sense of uncertainty and insecurity that is part of the experience of each of us. To the degree that the person is unable or unwilling to acknowledge these issues and anxieties, his or her experience and way of life will be guided by the goal of avoidance and escape. When such goals predominate, psychic disturbance results.

Theory of change and therapeutic technique. Existential therapy does not have a well-delineated theory of technique. In general, it is characterized by active questioning by the therapist about the subjectivity of the patient, within a charged and mutually open relationship that is meant to heighten the urgency of the process. Bugental and Kleiner (1993) liken the stance of an existential therapist to that of a consultant who assists patients in mastering the process of inner exploration that the therapist calls "searching." Existential therapists compare searching to free association and other means of turning inward, and suggest that it brings into immediate focus both previously unacknowledged aspects of experience and the resistances to that expansion of consciousness. Confrontation of resistances to self-exploration is a major task of the therapist, and after many repetitions this may yield understanding by the patient of the sources of such actions. This insight may allow the resistances to be abandoned, and a major gain in authentic living is then achieved.

Existential therapists attend to and communicate with their patients about the ways in which neurotic anxiety causes patients to distort their experience of themselves and the world, and to enter into a mode of inauthentic and mechanical experience. Existential writers appear to be in great agreement with their client-centered and Gestalt colleagues in emphasizing the curative role of immediate, spontaneous therapeutic experience (cf. Bugental & Kleiner, 1993; Yalom, 1981). Existential therapy depends on active confrontation of the way in which the person retreats into inauthentic modes of experience in order to avoid responsibility and the existential givens that he or she fears. The interaction with the therapist is crucial in this regard. The therapist's confrontation of these inauthentic patterns and processes, and his or her refusal to accept and participate in them, makes such activity more and more untenable. As a result, the person may come to an active decision to face his or her anxieties. Complete change occurs as these anxieties are faced and accepted, with the result that important spheres of experience can be integrated.

The therapeutic relationship. The relationship with the therapist is a crucial factor in this process of attaining authenticity. Sharing one's distress in the presence of another who does not impose solutions or flee from the pain allows the therapist to be internalized as a schematic support with which the realities of life can be faced more openly. As the patient admits both anxieties and potentials into experience, a more genuine state of existence emerges, with a corresponding reduction in pathology.

Existential therapists do not perceive technique and relationship to be equivalent. The relationship is considered to be the sphere in which active change processes and experiential learning are encouraged and provoked (Bugental, 1965). Existential writers often incorporate notions of the real relationship, the therapeutic alliance, and distortion and transference into the consideration of the therapeutic relationship (Bugental & Kleiner, 1993; May & Yalom, 1989). However, they differ from psychoanalysts in emphasizing the current motives for inauthentic and defensive behavior, which center around the patient's existential anxieties, with the therapist. The therapist responds to the patient's defensive and transferential attitudes and behaviors by remaining as real and authentic as possible, leading to a powerful and unsettling clash or encounter that shakes and disables the patient's ways of avoiding choices and responsibility. The "presence" of the therapist (May & Yalom, 1989) is a crucial variable in this process. It is defined as the therapist being with the patient in his or her most fully human, authentic, unique, and open way possible. Support, acceptance, exploration, advice, and confrontation all are part of this relationship. Existential therapists (Bugental & Kleiner, 1993; May & Yalom, 1989) often rely on notions of transference and countertransference that are very similar to psychoanalytic ideas. However, this group of therapists see the source of these phenomena as existential anxiety and the retreat from the pain of an authentic existence. The patient reacts to the therapist as he or she does and did with others when threatened. Gradually, these transference reactions are confronted and interpreted, and a more authentic expression of self in the therapeutic exchange may emerge.

Behavior Therapy

Psychopathology. The earliest versions of behavior therapy were based on mainstream versions of learning theory that emphasized the ways in which maladaptive habits, behavior patterns, and symptoms were acquired through the processes of classical and operant conditioning (cf., Salter, 1949; Wolpe, 1958). Contemporary versions of behavior theory include a reliance on social learning processes as well as on Pavlovian and Skinnerian models (Goldfried & Davison, 1994). Modern behavior therapists place the acquisition of behavior solidly in the context of social interactions (Bandura & Walters, 1963; Mischel, 1973). Social learning theorists accept the power of learning through classical and operant conditioning, but also stress the importance of observational learning, modeling of social behavior, and identification with peers and with authorities. These authors also report on the impressive role of the person's subjective organization of, and expectancies about, the social context in the determination of behavior.

Psychopathology, therefore, always is the result of faulty learning. Faulty learning includes the association of excessive levels of responding to a particular stimulus, as in phobias, where a dog, an airplane, or open spaces elicit paralyzing levels of anxiety. Faulty learning also can refer to the relative absence of response in situations where more behavior would be better. Examples would be a person's inability to answer a question in class or to behave assertively in a social situation. These kinds of behavioral deficits typically are mediated by fear. A third class of behavioral disturbance is that of a deviant response to a stimulus or social situation—for example, sadness that occurs when the person has achieved a success.

Many contemporary behavior therapists are guided by an integrative theory that combines explanatory concepts from cognitive therapy with social learning principles. This hybrid theory, and the cognitive-behavior therapy associated with it, is perhaps the leading example of the integrative psychotherapies that will be discussed later in this chapter.

Theory of change and therapeutic technique. Behavior therapy is built upon the notion that the patient must actively learn to function differently and must go through corrective experiences as a necessary precondition for change. These therapies stress the correction of deviant behavioral and cognitive processes and the gradual acquisition of productive, adaptive skills. Concepts drawn from social learning theory, cognitive psychology, and classical and operant conditioning form the theoretical framework for understanding how a person changes and improves through psychotherapy

Behavioral therapies strongly place action, repetition, and practice at the center of therapeutic gain. New experience becomes the basic stuff of restructured patterns of interpersonal relatedness, and of revised and more open cognitive structures. Many of the standard techniques of traditional behavior therapy, such as systematic desensitization, assertiveness training, or flooding, rely on processes of

exposure and extinction to lessen anxious, phobic, or other fearful responses (Goldfried & Davison, 1994; Wolpe, 1958). Assisting a patient in the task of gradually abandoning a pattern of avoidance that is motivated by fear, and facing the internal or external stimuli that provoke that fear, may be the change principle most frequently relied upon in this group of interventions. This is accomplished in desensitization procedures by constructing with the patient a series of scenes in which he or she can face, gradually and comfortably, the situation or stimulus that provokes anxiety. For example, for a patient who is afraid of heights, 20 or so scenes might be employed, starting with some that elicit little or no anxiety (standing outside a tall building, being in a room on the third floor) through moderate levels of fear (taking an elevator to the sixth floor) to high levels of distress (standing on the observation deck of a 100-story skyscraper). Desensitization usually is carried out in the therapist's office by having the patient imagine each scene, with each exposure limited in time and often accompanied by a relaxation procedure. When appropriate, desensitization may be employed in real life settings as well, and then is known as in-vivo desensitization. *Flooding* and *implosion* are highly charged variants of desensitization that also aim at exposing the patient to the object of his or her fears. These methods rely on immediate and prolonged exposure to the fear-producing situation or stimulus, without the gradual buildup provided in systematic or in vivo desensitization.

Operant principles of positive and negative reinforcement, habituation, and shaping also play a frequent and important role in promoting exposure, and in building up new, adaptive patterns of thinking and of action. Social learning, through observation of effective models, is an essential part of techniques such as behavior rehearsal, social skills training, communication training, and parent training, to name only a few. This type of learning effectively corrects deviant actions, allows the acquisition of new behaviors as replacements or to fill in deficits, and also is an aid in promoting exposure and reduction of anxiety. In each of these techniques, new behaviors are identified as desirable and then are acquired by the patient in a variety of ways. He or she might be exposed to a model (the therapist or colleague in a role-playing situation, film, tape, or real-life event), might practice the new behaviors in and out of sessions, and then would receive feedback from the therapist. This feedback then is incorporated into further practice and refinement of the new skills.

Therapeutic relationship. Behavioral therapies are built upon the explicit acknowledgment of the need for a comfortable, secure therapeutic relationship. Early writers on behavior therapy decried the positive effects of the therapeutic relationship and argued that behavior therapy's impact could be traced entirely to its techniques (e.g., Eysenck, 1960). However, most clinically sophisticated behaviorists abandoned this view long ago. As Goldfried and Davison (1994) pointed out, technical expertise without interpersonal skill will not result in continuance in, or cooperation with, the tasks and goals of cognitive-behavioral therapy. Fishman and Lubetkin (1983) observed that the technical aspects of behavior therapy often take up only a small percentage of the time spent in sessions, with more minutes devoted to the therapeutic provision of empathy, understanding, encouragement, support, and the generation of alternative behavioral solutions. O'Leary and Wilson (1987) suggested that issues within the therapeutic relationship in behavior therapy could not and should not be relegated to the junk pile of "nonspecific" factors. In their view, the patient's expectations, the intricacies of the therapist's response to the patient, and the repetition of deviant patterns in the therapeutic interaction all were as important in determining outcome as were experimentally derived techniques. Most recently, Goldfried (1995) has compared the role of the therapeutic relationship in cognitive-behavioral therapy to the role of anesthesia in surgery: it is absolutely necessary to enable the patient to accept and tolerate the pain that is caused by the procedure. Goldfried (1995) also sees the therapeutic relationship as an important source of real-life data, about which hypotheses concerning the patient's general interpersonal functioning can be generated. He includes his own reactions to the patient, and the

patient's appraisals of his feelings, as useful points for cognitive and behavioral intervention.

A formal theory of the specific components of the therapeutic relationship that are most important clinically has not yet been worked out by cognitive-behavioral therapists. A number of studies have indicated that cognitive-behavioral therapists are as adept as therapists of other orientations, or more so, at establishing a positively charged, warm, unconditionally accepting relationship (Gold, 1980; Sweet, 1984; Raue & Goldfried, 1994). Also, retrospective studies of patients' experiences in behavior therapy indicate repeatedly that those patients found the relationship at least as important in their progress as they did the technical aspects of the treatment (Gold, 1980; Raue & Goldfried, 1994). Most writers within this orientation also argue that a major source of resistance or noncompliance to cognitive and behavioral techniques derives from failures of interpersonal contact by the therapist (Gold, 1980; Goldfried & Davison, 1994; Lazarus, 1989).

Cognitive Psychotherapy

A close cousin of behavior therapy, cognitive therapy has its roots in the work of Piaget (1926) and such early clinical psychologists as George Kelly (1955), who were concerned with the ways in which the person's thought processes and ways of organizing experience were implicated in psychopathology. The two pioneers of modern cognitive therapy are Albert Ellis, who is the force behind rational-emotive therapy (RET), and Aaron Beck, the "father" of cognitive therapy.

Psychopathology. Both of these innovators have concluded that disturbances in emotion, behavior, and relatedness usually follow from disturbed or dysfunctional thoughts. Ellis (1984) has argued that humans have a biological predisposition toward irrational modes of construing experience. This tendency leads many people to think poorly of themselves and blame themselves for events that are uncontrollable, and also leads them to irrational emotions such as guilt, anxiety, depression, and shame. Ellis (1984) breaks down dysfunctional behavior into an *A-B-C* sequence. *A* refers to the antecedents, or the situation in which the person's emotional distress becomes apparent. The irrational belief that is elicited by that event is the *B* in the chain, whereas *C* represents the emotional and behavioral consequences of the belief. An example would be the young man who calls his girlfriend; finds that she is not home (*A*); begins to worry about the possibility that she is out with another man (*B*); and as a result becomes anxious, angry, and depressed (*C*).

Beck (1976) is more of an environmentalist, who suggests that many irrational or inaccurate beliefs are inferred or are taken directly from difficult or disappointing experiences in one's early life. But he, like Ellis, would focus, in the example just cited, on the unfounded and empirically unsupported thought as the critical factor in psychopathology.

Psychological change and therapeutic technique. Cognitive therapists are unanimous in the view that the task of therapy begins with the identification of the dysfunctional thoughts, images, opinions, and attitudes that precede troubling emotions and interactions in the patient's life. Often these pathogenic beliefs exist at the edge of the person's awareness, in the self-talk that we all engage in as we go about our business in life. Troubled individuals engage in self-talk that predicts danger where it is not present and that evaluates the person's relationships and situation, present and future, in pessimistic and dour ways. Improvement in one's psychological state occurs when these persons are able to identify the cognitive errors or misattributions that they have made, and then can substitute more rational and productive modes of thinking and of perception.

Cognitive therapy relies heavily on the Socratic method: The patient is questioned about, and encouraged to learn to question, the conclusions he or she has drawn from his experiences. To return to the previous example, the young man would be asked to provide support or empirical evidence for concluding that an unanswered phone meant what he thought it meant. Once able to see that he had leapt to very upsetting conclusions without any data to support them, he would be asked to think about

other, more likely ways of interpreting the absence of his friend. Beck (1976) has written that, in cognitive therapy, the patient comes to resemble a scientist who seeks data to confirm or disconfirm his or her hypotheses. The patient learns that her or his ideas and beliefs are not written in stone and often do not fit well with the data of experience. In making this discovery, the patient, like the researcher, has the opportunity to revise currently held but inaccurate thoughts and perceptions. A variety of forms, logs, and other recording devices are used to help the person to keep track of his or her self-talk and to build skills in asking such questions as, "What's the evidence for this thought?" or "What's another way of looking at it?" Rational emotive therapists also engage in active confrontation of irrational beliefs and disputation of those ideas (Ellis, 1984). Most cognitive therapy is heavily didactic and, like behavior therapy, involves a great deal of homework wherein new cognitive skills are tested and practiced in between therapy sessions.

Cognitive and RET therapists frequently use behavioral techniques in addition to cognitive interventions. The former are employed both to intervene in troubling symptoms and behavior problems, and also as indirect means to change dysfunctional thoughts. Sometimes the patient must achieve a new level of behavioral competence or social success in order to revise or to give up a negative outlook.

The psychotherapeutic relationship. The patient–therapist interaction in cognitive therapy most often is described as "collaborative empiricism" (Beck, Rush, Shaw, & Emory, 1979). This term refers to the joint venture in which therapist and patient are engaged, with the focus being correction or modification of the patient's symptoms and interpersonal problems. As in behavior therapy, the importance of a warm, supportive, and respectful relationship is acknowledged as the platform for therapeutic activity, but the relationship in itself is not considered to be the source of much therapeutic gain. Typically, the relationship becomes the explicit focus of therapeutic discussion only when things are not going well. In instances when the patient is not complying with the therapist's suggestions, fails to complete homework assignments, or misses several sessions, factors within the relationship may be explored in order to restore a workable collaboration.

RESEARCH IN PSYCHOTHERAPY

Psychotherapy Outcome Studies: "Has Everyone Won, So All Shall Have Prizes?"

Outcome research in psychotherapy has focused on two related questions:

1. Does psychotherapy work, and, if so, to what degree?
2. Does one type of psychotherapy work better than other types, and, if so, with whom and for what types of problems?

The answers to these questions, a bit facetiously, are yes for question 1 and no for question 2. To go on in more useful depth: The effectiveness of psychotherapy as compared to no treatment, to placebo effects, or to alternative forms of intervention (such as medication) has been studied in hundreds, if not thousands, of investigations. One powerful method that is a relatively recent addition to outcome studies is the technique of meta-analysis, in which effect sizes for an intervention are obtained by combining the data from a group of studies (see Chapter 5 for a more complete description of the technique of meta-analysis). These techniques suggest that the average effect size for psychotherapy is large; for example, it is powerful as or even more effective than psychiatric medication in a meta-analytic study of the treatment of depression (Lambert & Bergin, 1994). When psychotherapy is compared to no treatment and placebo conditions in meta-analytic studies, the findings are similar: an effect size that is twice as great as a placebo and triple that of no treatment (Lambert & Bergin, 1994). Although we may all catch our breath in relief with this support for the efficacy of psychotherapy, we may become a little shaky as we turn to our question about the relative effectiveness of the different forms of psychotherapy.

Despite early claims for the superiority of one form of psychotherapy over another, the data have been unsupportive of any brand or school of psychotherapy. As Luborsky (1995) pointed out, most comparative treatment studies find nonsignificant differences. He cites, as a typical example, a "box score" that summarized 16 studies in which dynamic psychotherapy was compared to other treatment modalities. Dynamic therapy was superior in one study, it was inferior in two, and there were nonsignificant differences in the other 13 reports. Important meta-analytic work in this area, such as the Smith, Glass, and Miller (1980) review of 475 outcome studies, also fails to find one type of therapy to be more effective than any other.

Common-Factors Research

One important response to the empirical "dodo bird verdict" (Luborsky, 1995), which suggests strongly that all psychotherapies are equally effective, is common-factors research. This field involves the search for the underlying curative factors that are included in all psychotherapies. It has its roots in Frank's (1961) studies of cross-cultural psychotherapy and in Rogers's (1957) effort to tease out the effective ingredients in client-centered therapy. At this point, a fair degree of consensus exists with regard to the common factors that allow all therapies to have some considerable impact.

Weinberger's (1995) review of the common-factors literature identified five commonly cited variables: (1) the therapeutic relationship, (2) expectations of therapeutic success, (3) confronting or facing the problem, (4) provision of an experience of mastery or cognitive control over the problematic issue, and (5) attributions for therapeutic success and failure. He notes that, although all five factors may in fact be operative in all therapies, the theories and methods of the specific therapies tend to emphasize or neglect certain factors differentially. For example, as we have seen earlier, the impact of the therapeutic relationship is stressed in client-centered and psychodynamic therapy, but downplayed in behavior therapy and cognitive therapy.

Patients' Perceptions of Psychotherapy Outcome: "Good News for Psychotherapy"

One important but often overlooked source of data about the effectiveness of psychotherapy is the perceptions and experiences of the consumers of psychotherapy. After all, people go to therapists to feel better; to improve their relationships; and to find more adaptive ways to work, to learn, and to enjoy themselves. Information about whether people achieve these goals can and does tell us a great deal about our practice and theories.

The few early studies of patients' perceptions of psychotherapy (Gold, 1980; Strupp, Wallach, & Wogan, 1964) found that two-thirds to three-quarters of subjects reported significant improvement in their problems, regardless of the type of therapy involved. However, these studies suffered from being based on relatively small samples. The field awaited a broader and more powerful investigation.

The data are in from such a study, and as one prominent psychologist has announced, the news for psychotherapy is good (Seligman, 1995). A major study of patients' satisfaction with psychotherapy was published in *Consumer Reports* magazine in 1995. Supplementary mental health questionnaires had been added to the annual products survey that was sent to over 180,000 subscribers to the magazine, and 7,000 of these mental health instruments were returned. This enormous database dwarfs the sample size of any preceding study of satisfaction with psychotherapy by an enormous factor.

The researchers found that, of these 7,000, about 2,900 had seen a mental health professional, 1,300 joined a support group, and 1,000 used the services of a family physician to treat an emotional problem. The remaining subjects tried to manage by talking to friends, relatives, or a member of the clergy.

The "good news" was that the vast majority of respondents felt that psychotherapy had been very useful. Subjects were asked to compare how they felt prior to treatment, and then following psychotherapy. Of those who were feeling very poorly before therapy, 87% reported that they were feeling between so-so and very, very good at the present time. Of those who rated themselves as starting out feeling fairly poor, 92% reported an improvement rate to so-so or very, very good. There was a robust dosage effect for psychotherapy: Long-term psychotherapy led to significantly greater perceptions of improvement than did short-term psychotherapy. The use of psychiatric medications in combination with psychotherapy did not add to the effectiveness of psychotherapy.

Those subjects who worked with mental health professionals (psychologists, psychiatrists, and social workers) reported greater improvement than those who saw marriage counselors. Treatment by family doctors and by mental health professionals yielded equivalent results in the short run, but improvement by the physician-treated group leveled off after six months, whereas subjects who saw psychologists, psychiatrists, and social workers continued to make gains beyond the six-month point. Finally, and consistent with the outcome literature discussed earlier, different modalities of psychotherapy yielded equivalent levels of change and patient satisfaction.

Seligman (1995) suggested that these data are highly consistent with the claims made by psychotherapists for the field: Long-term therapy with a trained therapist was found to be highly effective and to outperform other, less formal types of psychotherapeutic services. This study cannot be considered conclusive because of its methodological limitations. It is essentially an opinion survey and is not firmly grounded in experimental design. It lacked a control group, included potential sampling bias in that those who were dissatisfied with psychotherapy might have chosen to avoid responding, and is subject to the biases of memory and subjectivity on the part of the subjects. Its size and scope, however, make it a persuasive document for the effectiveness of psychotherapy. It is hoped that these encouraging results will be followed up by more empirically rigorous corroboration.

Process Research: Therapist and Patient Variables

Another burgeoning sphere of research activity is concerned with identifying the impact of characteristics of both therapist and patient on the process of psychotherapy and on its outcome. Among the patient variables that have been studied are socioeconomic status, race, age, gender, psychiatric diagnosis, personality characteristics as measured on psychological tests, and patient expectations. These factors have been evaluated with regard to their power in predicting continuation in psychotherapy and the outcome of psychotherapy. Unfortunately, as Garfield (1994) concluded in reviewing this literature, little can be said about the empirical utility of these variables.

Therapist characteristics that have been studied include age, sex, ethnicity, socioeconomic level, personality traits and coping styles, emotional well-being and level of disturbance, values, expectancies, and skill in engaging in productive interpersonal relationships. Beutler, Machado, and Neufeldt (1994) concluded, from a review of this research, that there were a number of therapist variables that were correlated with therapeutic effect size. The most powerful effects had to do with therapist choice of intervention and use of therapeutic manuals (to be discussed). That is, therapists who carefully followed an explicit manual for intervention tended to be more successful. Therapist directiveness was highly and negatively correlated with outcome. Therapist ability to provide a warm and accepting atmosphere was positively but moderately associated with effect size.

FUTURE TRENDS IN PSYCHOTHERAPY

To conclude this chapter, we will review some of the more exciting and important developments that perhaps predict what psychotherapy will look like into the next century.

Manualized Psychotherapy

These projects are concerned with the development of technical, prescriptive guides for practice and research in psychotherapy. They strive to produce replicable, reliable, and consensual methods through which a patient's psychological organization can be assessed and which, therefore, can form the focus of a testable set of interventions. In turn, both clinical investigation and empirical research

are aimed at understanding the relationships between these operationally defined psychological processes and more overt manifestations, including patient and therapist actions and characteristics, techniques and procedures, and outcome.

The model for manualized psychotherapy can be found in the pioneering work of behavioral and cognitive authors, who were the first to offer other psychotherapists these step-by-step guides to the conduct of psychotherapy. Beck and his colleagues at the Center for Cognitive Therapy at the University of Pennsylvania stand out as exemplars in these efforts. This group has systematically turned out manuals for cognitive therapy of depression (Beck et al., 1979), cognitive therapy of anxiety disorders and phobias (Beck & Emory, 1985), cognitive treatment of personality disorders (Beck, Freeman, & Associates, 1989), and cognitive therapy of substance abuse (Beck, Wright, Newman, and Liese, 1993). Other cognitive-behavioral therapists have produced manuals that are useful in the therapy of schizophrenic patients (Perris, 1989), panic disorders (Barlow & Cerny, 1988), and bipolar (manic-depressive) disorder (Basco & Rush, 1996).

These manuals provide therapists with clear cognitive-behavioral formulations of the disorders or problems, followed by step-by-step guides to the techniques that have been found through research to be effective in correcting the cognitive and behavioral underpinnings of the problems. For example, in their ground-breaking *Cognitive Therapy of Depression* (Beck et al., 1979), the authors organize the cognitive treatment of the disorder around the "cognitive triad" of dysfunctional beliefs that causes people to become depressed: negative conceptions of the self, of the environment, and of the future. Specific interventions are suggested for each part of this triad, as well as for alleviating the bodily, behavioral, and emotional symptoms of depression that are triggered by this way of thinking. Methods for establishing a viable therapeutic relationship within the context of the specific disorder with which the patient is suffering also are provided, as are techniques for assessing the therapy as it progresses.

Therapists who work within an interpersonal framework also have produced important psychotherapy manuals. Perhaps the most significant of these is the work of Klerman, Weissman, Rounsaville, and Chevron (1984). This group has produced a manual for a short-term therapy of depression that is based on interpersonal principles and processes. Their conceptualization of depression follows from the assessment of the problematic relationships in which the patient is currently engaged. Dysfunctional thinking, affect, mood, and behavior are assumed to be consequences of these interactional deficits or conflicts. Four problem areas are considered to be contributory to the onset and maintenance of depression to one degree or another: (1) grief and bereavement; (2) interpersonal conflict with significant others in the patient's immediate life; (3) role transitions and changes in areas such as employment, residence, economic status, marriage, and parenting; and (4) deficits or gaps in interpersonal skills that inhibit successful engagement with others and so lead to isolation and loneliness. As each person's depression is understood in terms of the unique and relative contribution of each of these four interpersonal components, an individualized treatment plan is devised. Interpersonal therapy has been evaluated in the treatment of acute depression, as a maintenance therapy for people who have recovered from depression, and as a treatment for serious and chronic depressions (Klerman et al., 1984; Kiesler, 1996). The therapy has been found to be superior to placebo treatment in a number of populations, and to produce roughly equivalent treatment gains when compared to cognitive therapy and to pharmacological intervention. Interestingly, the comparison with medication revealed different types of outcomes than are seen with antidepressants, even though the mean level of improvement seemed to be about the same. Interpersonal therapy resulted in rapid and stable improvement in mood, enhanced interest in and ability to perform at work, and decreases in suicidal ideation and guilt. Drug therapy was most efficacious in reducing vegetative symptoms of depression, including sleep disturbance, loss of appetite, and somatic distress.

Psychodynamic therapy also has been influenced by manualized approaches to therapy in the past two decades. Luborsky's (1984) supportive-expressive, psychodynamically oriented psychotherapy is guided by a general manual for assessment and practice that is applicable to both short- and long-term psychotherapy. Clinically, Luborsky (1984) notes that this therapy resembles traditional psychodynamic psychotherapy in most respects, with its emphasis on interpretation of unconscious conflict. It differs in its specificity of intervention. The manual instructs the therapist as to the type and timing of interventions, which are of two sorts: (1) supportive or relationship-building comments that are empathic and convey acceptance of the patient's pain and of his or her point of view, and (2) expressive or interpretive remarks that point out to the patient the ways in which his or her wishes and fears influence relationships with others and with the therapist. This manual is supplemented by specific manuals that have been created for use with several discrete populations, including heroin addicts, cocaine abusers, and persons with major depression. Research has demonstrated that supportive-expressive therapy is efficacious with all of the populations with which it has been tested (Luborsky, 1984).

Another important manualized psychodynamic psychotherapy was developed by Strupp and his colleagues (Strupp, 1995; Strupp & Binder, 1984) in the Vanderbilt Psychotherapy Project. This therapy, known as time-limited dynamic psychotherapy (TLDP), is a 25-session, interactional, psychoanalytically informed method that places distinct emphasis on the formulation of the cyclical maladaptive pattern (CMP), an unconsciously motivated and dysfunctional pattern of construing the self and others. The CMP is manifested in the ways in which the patient skews ongoing interpersonal behaviors and thus confirms the self and object images. The CMP is taken as the main therapeutic focus from its earliest manifestations in the therapeutic interaction and in the patient's descriptions of other relationships. Time-limited dynamic psychotherapy grew out of the collection of psychotherapy research studies known as Vanderbilt I (Strupp, 1995). This project investigated the technical and interactional variables that might be predictive of positive results in dynamic therapy. The most important results of Vanderbilt I were concerned with the ways in which both novice and experienced therapists failed to engage more difficult or unusual patients in flexible, open, humane relationships and, instead, reacted in stereotyped, theory-bound, and inflexible ways. These findings were the impetus to create a flexible, dynamically oriented, interpersonally focused therapy in which positive and necessary relationship factors could be operationalized and taught systematically.

The evaluation of TLDP was a central component of the Vanderbilt II psychotherapy project (Strupp, 1995). Significant validity and reliability for the formulation of CMPs according to manualized criteria were demonstrated, as was adherence to the protocol of therapy as described in the manual.

Short-Term Psychodynamic Psychotherapies

These therapies address the increasing demands of third parties (the government, insurance companies, health maintanance organizations [HMOs], and managed care) for therapies that are empirically proved to be effective within externally determined time and cost constraints (see Chapter 8 for a more complete discussion of brief therapy). These new short-term process therapies also demonstrate greater concern with precision and with demonstrable outcomes than has been the case in traditional psychoanalysis. They therefore suggest a movement toward the goals and ideologies of outcome-oriented therapies such as cognitive and behavioral therapy.

Short-term dynamic therapies rely on the rapid and reliable formulation of a central, organizing psychodynamic issue or conflict. This formulation is pursued and studied in the context of the patient's intrapsychic functioning, her or his current and past interpersonal relationships, and especially in the interaction with the therapist. High activity is prescribed for the therapist, and most of these models concur on the importance of early and accurate transference interpretation as a critical factor in producing a positive outcome. A number of the individual systems have been subjected to empirical validation of process and outcome factors, with

most studies yielding moderate to major therapeutic effects on target complaints, general ratings of symptoms via such instruments as the SCL-90, and patient and therapist objective and subjective ratings (Crits-Cristoph & Barber, 1991).

Advances in Cognitive-Behavioral Therapy

A process orientation and a concern with inferential and intrapsychic phenomena also have crept into cognitive and behavioral theories and therapies. Cognitive and behavioral therapists have begun to focus their attention on personality disorders (Beck, Freeman, & Associates, 1989), on developmental processes and the structure of personality, and on schemas and unconscious cognitive processing (Guidano, 1987). Other cognitive therapists have placed their clinical work squarely in an interactional context (Safran & Segal, 1990), with the result that their theories and methods overlap significantly with some of the dynamic and experiential positions that were described in this chapter. This move toward a process orientation probably reflects the same clinical and research pressures that have led to an interest in psychotherapy integration among many clinicians. That is to say, as students of therapy investigate more complicated pathology or look at clinical work in more depth-oriented ways, all perspectives seem to blend at some point.

Advances in Humanistic Psychotherapy

The experiential and humanistic therapies have continued to make steady progress. Work in this area has centered around ways in which to make therapy more tightly focused (a theme that arises again and again in this discussion) and more specifically tailored to the needs of individual patients and their unique problems. Experientially oriented therapists also have made important progress in integrating clinical theory and practice with emerging findings in information processing and emotion research (Guidano, 1987; Safran & Greenberg, 1991). Others (Rice & Greenberg,

1992) have explored ways in which the client-centered therapist may enhance active learning and internalization of new experiences within the context of positive regard and therapist congruence. Bohart (1993) has discussed the role of experiencing as a curative factor in psychotherapy and has provided clinical guidelines for assisting patients to grow in this area. Greenberg, Rice, and Elliot (1993) recently contributed a major study of the role of emotional experience as an organizing factor in psychotherapeutic change. These authors are able to demonstrate six methods of intervening in and producing emotional shifts on a moment-to-moment basis in therapy sessions. Their work is built on a substantial body of empirical research and brings together the process orientation with outcome data.

Psychotherapy Integration

Psychotherapy integration is both a set of theories and a group of technical procedures, innovations, and scholastic pursuits. In the last decade, integrative therapies have assumed a more legitimate and prominent place in psychotherapeutic practice and theory. Norcross and Newman (1992) identified eight variables that have encouraged this growth:

1. The expansion in the number of separate psychotherapies
2. The failure of any therapy to demonstrate superior efficacy
3. The lack of success of any theory in adequately explaining and predicting pathology, or personality and behavioral change
4. The growth in number and importance of shorter term, focused psychotherapies
5. Greater communication between clinicians and scholars that has resulted in increased willingness to, and opportunity for, experimentation
6. The intrusion into the consulting room of the realities of limited socioeconomic support by third parties for long-term psychotherapies
7. The identification of common factors in all psychotherapies that are related to outcome

8. The development of professional organizations, conferences, and journals that are dedicated to the discussion and study of psychotherapy integration.

The Modes of Psychotherapy Integration

The three most commonly discussed forms of integration are technical eclecticism, the common-factors approach, and theoretical integration. *Technical eclecticism* is the most clinical and technically oriented form of psychotherapy integration. Techniques and interventions drawn from two or more psychotherapeutic systems are applied systematically and sequentially. The series of linked interventions usually follows a comprehensive assessment of the patient. This assessment allows target problems to be identified and identifies the relationships between different problems, strengths, and the cognitive, affective, and interpersonal characteristics of the patient. Techniques are chosen on the basis of the best clinical match to the needs of the patient, as guided by clinical knowledge and by research findings.

The *common-factors approach* to integration stems from common-factors research described earlier. Common-factors integration starts from the identification of specific effective ingredients of any group of therapies, followed by exploration of the ways in which particular interventions and psychotherapeutic interactions promote and contain those ingredients. The integrative therapies that result from this process are structured around the goal of maximizing the patient's exposure to the unique combination of therapeutic factors that will best ameliorate his or her problems.

Theoretical integration is the synthesis of concepts of personality functioning, psychopathology, and psychological change from two or more traditional systems. Integrative theories of this kind explain psychological phenomena in interactional terms, by looking for the ways in which environmental, motivational, cognitive, and affective factors influence and are influenced by each other. Perhaps the best known version of theoretical integration was identified earlier: cognitive-behavioral therapy. This system is based on a theory of psychopathology and of personality change that is greater than the sum of its behavioral and cognitive parts. This theoretical synthesis then guides the therapist in the selection and use of interventions that are drawn from each school of therapy (Goldfried, 1995).

A particular subset of theoretical integration that has been written about with much recent interest is assimilative integration (Messer, 1992; Stricker & Gold, 1996). The term *assimilative* refers to the impact that new techniques have on the existing conceptual foundation of the therapy. As these interventions are used in a context other than that in which they originated, the meaning, impact, and utility of those techniques are changed in powerful ways. In his discussion of assimilative integration of psychotherapies, Messer (1992) points out that all actions are defined and contained by the interpersonal, historical, and physical context in which those acts occur. As any therapeutic intervention is an interpersonal action (and highly complex at that), those interventions are defined, and perhaps even re-created, by the larger context of the therapy. Thus a behavioral method such as systematic desensitization will mean something entirely different to a patient whose ongoing therapeutic experience has been largely defined by psychodynamically oriented exploration than that same intervention would mean to a patient in traditional behavioral therapy. We (Stricker & Gold, 1996) have found that our use of cognitive-behavioral, Gestalt, and systems approaches are assimilated into our psychodynamically framed therapy in just this way. The impact of such interventions often is uniquely experienced by both patient and therapist, and can lead to very novel results.

With assimilation, the process of accommodation is an inevitable partner. Psychodynamically oriented ideas, styles, and methods are recast and experienced differently in an integrative system as compared to traditional dynamic therapies. When we choose to intervene actively in a patient's cognitive activities—his or her behavior, affect, and interpersonal engagements—we change the meaning and felt impact of our exploratory work and our emphasis on insight as well.

The Major Systems of Psychotherapy Integration

Multimodal therapy. This psychotherapeutic system (Lazarus, 1989) is perhaps the best known, most widely cited, and most influential version of technical eclecticism in contemporary psychotherapy. Multimodal therapy is organized around an extensive assessment of the patient's strengths, excesses, liabilities, and deviant behavior that follows the acronym of the BASIC ID: Behavior, Affect, Sensation, Imagery, Cognition, Interpersonal relations, and Drugs (or biology). As the firing order or causal sequence of variables in the BASIC ID is known, interventions are selected and are implemented. More microscopic BASIC ID profiles of discrete or difficult problems and of components of a firing order can be attempted once the initial, global assessment and interventions are completed.

Lazarus (1989) states that he prefers to use methods that have been demonstrated through empirical tests to be effective with specific problems and skill, and his theory and technical strategies are more heavily aligned with social learning theory and with cognitive-behavioral therapy than with any other therapeutic school. In his broad-spectrum approach, however, he often includes imagery work, techniques drawn from couples and family therapy, Gestalt exercises, and some affective and insight-oriented interventions.

Systematic eclectic psychotherapy. This system of psychotherapy integration was developed by Beutler and his colleagues (Beutler, 1983; Beutler & Consoli, 1992; Beutler & Hodgson, 1993). It is a second-generation system of integration that attempts to incorporate some of the findings of common-factors theorists into an advanced eclectic approach. This is an empirically informed system in which a thorough assessment of the patient is followed by the prescription of techniques, if available, that have received the most research validation for efficacy with that specific clinical profile. When such research-based matching is not possible, techniques are selected according to accumulated clinical findings drawn from the literature and from the experience of the individual therapist. Beutler (Beutler & Hodgson, 1993) bases the selection of techniques on the interaction of three factors: (1) the stage of psychotherapeutic involvement that the patient has reached, (2) the necessary change experiences for which the patient is prepared, and (3) the dominant aspects of the patient's immediate clinical status. As necessary and appropriate, interventions can be matched to the ongoing assessment of the patient's needs at four levels: (1) overt dysfunctional behavior, (2) faulty thinking, (3) inhibitions of affective and sensory experience, and (4) repressed unconscious conflict. The choice of intervention also is influenced by each patient's coping style, ability to engage in a collaborative therapeutic relationship, and level of resistance to any type of therapeutic experience. Techniques that can be included in this model range from the interpretive, to exercises that enhance the patient's ability to integrate affect and sensation, to behavioral and cognitive interventions.

Transtheoretical psychotherapy. This common-factors system (Prochaska & DiClemente, 1992) prescribes interventions on the basis of three elements of assessment: (1) the required change mechanisms, (2) the stage of change at which the patient seeks help, and (3) the level of change that is required. Behavior therapy is indicated in this system for patients who require change at the level of overt symptoms and of maladaptive patterns of dealing with the environment. These interventions are best prescribed when the patient is at the stage of action, which means that the person has a sense of self-liberation and is able to perceive him- or herself as capable of self-control and independent change. The required change mechanisms are those that are intrinsic to behavioral interventions, including counterconditioning, stimulus control, and contingency management. When the patient requires the change mechanisms of self-reevaluation and self-liberation, suffers from maladaptive cognitions, and is at the stage of contemplation or preparation, then cognitive techniques are prescribed. The two stages of change mentioned refer to the readiness to examine one's psychological processes and experi-

ence, and to be willing to use self-knowledge as a stimulus to change.

Cyclical psychodynamics. Perhaps the single most influential system of psychotherapy integration, cyclical psychodynamics is a theory that represents the theoretical integration of concepts and methods drawn from interpersonal psychoanalysis, family systems theory, social learning theory, and behavior therapy (Gold & Wachtel, 1993; Wachtel, 1977; Wachtel & Wachtel, 1986). Cyclical psychodynamic theory is organized around a radically recast view of the causes, role, and meaning of unconscious motives, fantasies, and conflict. This revision suggests that an individual's ongoing social interactions cause and reinforce pathogenic unconscious processes and anxieties. As such, unconscious factors in psychopathology may be considered to be dependent variables that provide information about the patient's current adaptation, perceptions, and relationships. The effects of the past impinge on the present insofar as the patient's thinking, behavior, and ways of perceiving the self and others were skewed and deformed through anxious interactions with others. Cyclical psychodynamics assigns an ironic status to much of a patient's struggles, in that the patient is seen as unintentionally re-creating past internal conflicts and interpersonal binds. As he or she tries to have new experiences, the anxiety-driven warping of perception, thought, and relatedness causes the person to enlist others as "neurotic accomplices" (Wachtel & Wachtel, 1986). Integrative psychodynamic therapy (Gold & Wachtel, 1993) is based on this theoretical model and is an open-ended amalgam of methods. It is most influenced by psychodynamic, behavioral, and systemic techniques, but can include any intervention that can interrupt or correct the ongoing, ironic vicious circles in which the patient is caught.

Behavioral psychotherapy. As developed by Fensterheim (1993), this system is an example of theoretical integration that leads to integrated interventions. Fensterheim (1993) divides the psychological totality of the patient into three levels, with level 1 being the behavioral and level 3 being the psychodynamic. Level 2 refers to the level of obstacles, and is conceptualized from both the behavioral and the dynamic positions. Its explanatory value lies in formulating the patient's difficulties in working successfully at level 1. Dynamic conflict, transference and countertransference, and conditioning and reinforcement factors all may be considered here, either in isolation or in complex interrelationships. Fensterheim concentrates most of his assessment efforts at the first, behavioral level.

Because behavioral formulations and interventions are much simpler and easier to test than are psychodynamic ones, the behavioral level is preferred for both assessment and therapy. Work at the dynamic level proceeds when the patient is not able to make productive use of work at the behavioral level, thus necessitating assessment and therapy at levels 2 and 3. Behavior at level 1 is examined with regard to the identification of the interpersonal and intrapsychic factors that are fueling and maintaining symptoms. When resistances are noted and become too great an interference, other behavioral and dynamic factors are added to the formulation. Dynamic issues of greatest importance in Fensterheim's system are defenses. He notes that when pathological defenses are made inoperable or are given up, both behavioral change and insight will result. Therapy usually proceeds from level 1 to 2 and 3 only as necessary. Standard behavioral techniques often are sufficient for instilling changes in the organization of behavior that render the person's defenses obsolete and inoperable. In such cases, change at levels 2 and 3 occurs spontaneously, as resistances to insight are abandoned and conflicts are resolved. When straightforward behavioral work is not completely successful, the behavioral measures must be modified, and or complemented by interpretation, in order to deepen and expand the treatment

Assimilative psychodynamic psychotherapy. This integrative therapy, developed by the authors of this chapter, is a theoretical synthesis that in some ways is the mirror image of Fensterheim's model. We (Gold & Stricker, 1993; Stricker & Gold, 1996) have argued that the psychological functioning of

the person can be approached at three levels or tiers: Tier 1 refers to behavior, tier 2 to conscious cognitive and emotional experience, and tier 3 to unconscious motivation and conflict. Dynamic interrelationships between the three tiers can occur in any direction, but our theoretical and clinical emphasis (Stricker & Gold, 1996) is on the role of tier 3 (unconscious phenomena) in psychopathology and in change. We employ cognitive, behavioral, and experiential interventions when they might be clinically useful, but always within an assimilative context: We are as, or more, concerned with the unconscious impact and meaning of these techniques as we are with their immediate effect on behavior, thinking, or feelings.

A FINAL THOUGHT

So, our tour through this ill-defined but exciting and most important activity is now complete. Obviously, those of you who managed to get to this point in the chapter have had only a sketchy introduction to psychotherapy. Any of the individual systems of therapy, the research topics, or the new directions in the field can be learned about more thoroughly by obtaining the original citations that are mentioned. However, we hope that our firm conviction that this field is valuable; useful to those we serve; and deserving of future funding, study, and discussion has been made plain in the preceding pages. One part of the definition of psychotherapy that we did not include earlier is that it is an activity in which we are engaged as therapists for the large part of our working week, and a field of inquiry that dominates much of our more productive thinking. Perhaps some of the readers of this chapter might be encouraged by what has been discussed here to join us in this enterprise.

REFERENCES

Alexander, F., & French, T. (1946). *Psychoanalytic therapy.* New York: Ronald.

Bandura, A., & Walters, R. (1963). *Social learning and personality development.* New York: Holt, Rinehart, and Winston.

Barlow, D. H., & Cerny, J. A. (1988). *Psychological treatment of panic.* New York: Guilford Press.

Basco, M. R., & Rush, A. J. (1996). *Cognitive-behavioral therapy for bipolar disorder.* New York: Guilford Press.

Beck, A. T. (1976). *Cognitive therapy and the emotional disorders.* New York: New American Library.

Beck, A. T., & Emory, G. (1985). *Anxiety disorders and phobias.* New York: Guilford Press.

Beck, A. T., Freeman, A., & Associates (1989). *Cognitive therapy of personality disorders.* New York: Guilford Press.

Beck, A. T., Rush, A. J., Shaw, J., & Emory, G. (1979). *Cognitive therapy of depression.* New York: Guilford Press.

Beck, A. T., Wright, F. D., Newman, C. F., & Liese, B. S. (1993). *Cognitive therapy of substance abuse.* New York: Guilford Press.

Beutler, L. E. (1983). *Eclectic psychotherapy: A systematic approach.* New York: Pergamon Press.

Beutler, L. E., & Consoli, A. J. (1992). Systematic eclectic therapy. In J. C. Norcross & M. R. Goldfried (Eds.), *Handbook of psychotherapy integration* (pp. 264–299). New York: Basic Books.

Beutler, L. E., & Hodgson, A. B. (1993). Prescriptive psychotherapy. In G. Stricker & J. R. Gold (Eds.), *Comprehensive handbook of psychotherapy integration* (pp. 151–164). New York: Plenum Press.

Beutler, L. E., Machado, P. P., & Neufeldt, S. A. (1994). Therapist variables. In A. E. Bergin & S. L. Garfield (Eds.), *Handbook of psychotherapy and behavior change* (4th ed., pp. 229–269). New York: Wiley.

Bohart, A. C. (1993). Experiencing: The basis of psychotherapy. *Journal of Psychotherapy Integration, 3,* 51–68.

Bowlby, J. (1980). *Loss.* New York: Basic Books.

Bugental, J. F. T. (1965). *The search for authenticity.* New York: McGraw-Hill.

Bugental, J. F. T., & Kleiner, R. (1993). Existential psychotherapies. In G. Stricker & J. R. Gold (Eds.), *Comprehensive handbook of psychotherapy integration* (pp.101–112). New York: Plenum Press.

Crits-Cristoph, P., & Barber, J. (Eds.). (1991). *Handbook of short term dynamic psychotherapy.* New York: Basic Books.

Cushman, P. (1995). *Constructing the self, constructing America.* Boston: Addison-Wesley.

Ellis, A. (1984). Rational-emotive therapy. In R. J. Corsin (Ed.), *Current psychotherapies* (3rd ed., pp. 331–378.) Itaska, IL: Peacock.

Eysenck, H. J. (1960). *Behavior therapy and the neuroses.* New York: Pergamon Press.

Fensterheim, H. (1993). Behavioral psychotherapy. In G. Stricker & J. Gold (Eds.), *The comprehensive handbook of psychotherapy integration* (pp. 73–86). New York: Plenum Press.

Fishman, S. T., & Lubetkin, B. S. (1983). Office practice of behavior therapy. In M. Hersen (Ed.), *Outpatient behavior therapy* (pp. 21–41). New York: Grune & Stratton.

Frank, J. D. (1961). *Persuasion and healing.* Baltimore: Johns Hopkins University Press.

Freud, A. (1936). *The ego and the mechanisms of defense.* New York: International Universities Press.

Freud, S. (1900). The interpretation of dreams. In J. Strachey (Ed. & Trans.), *The standard edition of the complete psychological works of Sigmund Freud* (Vols. 4, 5.) London: Hogarth Press.

Freud, S. (1912). Dynamics of transference. In J. Strachey (Ed. & Trans.), *The standard edition of the complete psychological works of Sigmund Freud* (Vol. 12, pp. 97–108). London: Hogarth Press.

Fromm, E. (1955). *The sane society.* New York: Henry Holt.

Garfield, S. L. (1994). Research on client variables in psychotherapy. In A. E. Bergin & S. L. Garfield (Eds.), *Handbook of psychotherapy and behavior change* (4th ed., pp.190–228). New York: Wiley.

Gold, J. R. (1980). A *retrospective study of the behavior therapy experience.* Unpublished doctoral dissertation, Adelphi University.

Gold, J. (1996). *Key concepts in psychotherapy integration.* New York: Plenum Press.

Gold, J. R., & Stricker, G. (1993). Psychotherapy integration with personality disorders. In G. Stricker & J. R. Gold (Eds.), *Comprehensive handbook of psychotherapy integration* (pp. 323–336). New York: Plenum Press.

Gold, J., & Wachtel, P. L. (1993). Cyclical psychodynamics. In G. Stricker & J. R. Gold (Eds.), *Comprehensive handbook of psychotherapy integration* (pp. 59–72). New York: Plenum Press.

Goldfried, M. (1995). *From cognitive behavior therapy to psychotherapy integration.* New York: Springer.

Goldfried, M. R., & Davison, G. (1994). *Clinical behavior therapy* (Expanded ed.). New York: Holt.

Greenberg, J., & Mitchell, S. (1983). *Object relations in psychoanalytic theory.* Cambridge, MA: Harvard University Press.

Greenberg, L. S., Rice, L., & Elliot, R. (1993). *Process-experiential therapy: Facilitating emotional change.* New York: Guilford Press.

Guidano, V. F. (1987). *Complexity of the self.* New York: Guilford Press.

Kelly, G. (1955). *The psychology of personal constructs* (Vol. 1). New York: Norton.

Klein, G. S. (1971). *Psychoanalytic theory: An exploration of essentials.* New York: International Universities Press.

Kiesler, D. J. (1996). *Contemporary interpersonal therapy and research.* New York: Wiley.

Klerman, G. L., Weissman, M. M., Rounsaville, B. J., & Chevron, E. S. (1984). *Interpersonal psychotherapy of depression.* New York: Basic Books.

Kohut, H. (1977). *The restoration of the self.* New York: International Universities Press.

Lambert, M., & Bergin, A. E. (1994). The effectiveness of psychotherapy. In A. E. Bergin & S. L. Garfield (Eds.), Handbook of psychotherapy and behavior change (4th ed., pp. 143–189). New York: Wiley.

Lazarus, A. A. (1989). *The practice of multimodal therapy.* Baltimore: Johns Hopkins.

Levenson, E. R. (1983). *The ambiguity of change.* New York: Basic Books.

Luborsky, L. (1984). *Principles of psychoanalytic psychotherapy: A manual for supportive-expressive treatment.* New York: Basic Books.

Luborsky, L. (1995). Are common factors across different psychotherapies the main explanation for the dodo bird verdict that "Everyone has won so all shall have prizes?" *Clinical Psychology: Science and Practice, 2,* 106–109.

Mahler, M. S., Pine, F., & Bergman, A. (1975). *The psychological birth of the human infant.* New York: Basic Books.

Maslow, A. H. (1954). *Motivation and personality.* New York: Harper & Row.

May, R. (1977). *The meaning of anxiety.* New York: Norton.

May, R., & Yalom, I. (1989). Existential therapy. In R. J. Corsini & D. Weddings (Eds.), *Current psychotherapies* (pp. 363–402). Itaska, IL: Peacock.

Messer, S. (1992). A critical examination of belief structures in integrative and eclectic psychotherapy. In J. C. Norcross & M. R. Goldfried (Eds.), Handbook of psychotherapy integration (pp. 130–168). New York: Basic Books.

Mischel, W. (1973). Toward a cognitive social learning reconceptualization of personality. *Psychological Review, 80,* 252–283.

Norcross, J. C., & Newman, C. (1992). Psychotherapy integration: Setting the context. In J. C. Norcross & M.

R. Goldfried (Eds.), *Handbook of psychotherapy integration.* New York: Basic Books.

O'Leary, K. D., & Wilson, G. T. (1987). *Behavior therapy: Application and outcome.* Englewood Cliffs, NJ: Prentice-Hall.

Perls, F. (1973). *The Gestalt approach: An eyewitness to therapy.* New York: Science and Behavior Books.

Perls, F., Hefferline, R. F., & Goodman, P. (1951). *Gestalt therapy.* New York: Julian Press.

Perris, C. (1989). *Cognitive therapy with schizophrenic patients.* New York: Guilford Press.

Piaget, J. (1926). *The language and thought of the child* (Trans. M. Worden). New York: Harcourt, Brace.

Prochaska, J. O., & DiClemente, C. C. (1992). The transtheoretical approach. In J. C. Norcross & M. R. Goldfried (Eds.), *Handbook of psychotherapy integration* (pp. 300–334). New York: Basic Books.

Raimy, V. (1950). *Training in clinical psychology.* New York: Prentice-Hall.

Raskin, R., & Rogers, C. R. (1989). Person centered therapy. In R. J. Corsini & D. Weddings (Eds.), *Current psychotherapies* (pp. 155–196). Itaska, IL: Peacock.

Raue, P. J., & Goldfried, M. R. (1994). The therapeutic alliance in cognitive-behavior therapy. In A. O. Horvath & L. S. Greenberg (Eds.), *The working alliance: Theory, research and practice* (pp. 131–152). New York: Wiley

Rice, L. N., & Greenberg, L. S. (1992). Humanistic approaches to psychotherapy. In D. K. Freedheim (Ed.), *History of psychotherapy* (pp. 337–363). Washington, DC: American Psychological Association.

Rogers, C. R. (1951). *Client centered therapy.* Boston: Houghton Mifflin.

Rogers, C. R. (1957). The necessary and sufficient conditions of therapeutic personality change. *Journal of Consulting Psychology, 21,* 95–103.

Rogers, C. R. (1961). *On becoming a person.* Boston: Houghton Mifflin.

Safran, J. D., & Greenberg, L. S. (Eds.). (1991). *Emotion, psychotherapy, and change.* New York: Guilford Press.

Safran, J. D., & Segal, Z. D. (1990). *Interpersonal processes in cognitive therapy.* New York: Basic Books.

Salter, A. (1949). *Conditioned reflex therapy.* New York: Creative Age.

Seligman, M. E. P. (1995). The effectiveness of psychotherapy: The *Consumer Reports* study. *American Psychologist, 50,* 965–974.

Shlein, J. M. (1984). A countertheory of transference. In R. F. Levant & J. M. Shlein (Eds.), *Client-centered therapy and the person centered approach* (pp. 176–207). New York: Praeger.

Smith, M. L., Glass, G. V., & Miller, T. I. (1980). *The effectiveness of psychotherapy.* Baltimore: Johns Hopkins University Press.

Stern, D. (1985). *The interpersonal world of the infant.* New York: Basic Books.

Strachey, J. (1934). The therapeutic action of psychoanalysis. *International Journal of Psychoanalysis, 15,* 127–159.

Stricker , G., & Gold, J. (1996). An assimilative model for psychodynamically oriented integrative psychotherapy. *Clinical Psychology: Science and Practice, 3,* 47–58.

Strupp, H. H. (1995). The psychotherapist's skills revisited. *Clinical Psychology: Science and Practice, 2,* 70–75.

Strupp, H. H., & Binder, J. (1984). *Psychotherapy in a new key.* New York: Basic Books.

Strupp, H. H., Wallach, M. S., & Wogan, M. (1964). Psychotherapy experience in retrospect: A questionnaire study of former patients and therapists. *Psychological Monographs, 78.*

Sullivan, H. S. (1953). *The interpersonal theory of psychiatry.* New York: Norton.

Sweet, A. A. (1984). The therapeutic relationship in behavior therapy. *Clinical Psychology Review,* 8, 253–272.

Wachtel, E. F., & Wachtel, P. L. (1986). *Family dynamics in individual therapy.* New York: Guilford Press.

Wachtel, P. L. (1977). *Psychoanalysis and behavior therapy: Toward an integration.* New York: Basic Books.

Weinberger, J. (1995). Common factors aren't so common. *Clinical Psychology: Science and Practice, 2,* 45–69.

Winnicott, D. W. (1971). *The maturational processes and the facilitating environment.* New York: International Universities Press.

Wolpe, J. (1958). *Psychotherapy through reciprocal inhibition.* Stanford, CA: Stanford University Press.

Yalom, I. (1981). *Existential psychotherapy.* New York: Basic Books.

Yontef, G. (1981). The future of Gestalt therapy. *The Gestalt Journal, 4,* 69–83.

Zeig, J. K., & Munion, W. M. (Eds.). (1990). *What is psychotherapy?* San Francisco: Jossey-Bass.

FOR FURTHER READING

Cushman, P. (1995). *Constructing the self, constructing America.* Reading, MA: Addison-Wesley. *A historical and clinical exploration of the role of psychotherapy in determining the path of personality development in the United States.*

Gold, J. R. (1996). Key *concepts in psychotherapy integration.* New York: Plenum Press. *A review of the major systems of psychotherapy and of progress in psychotherapy integration.*

Greenberg, L. S., Rice, L. E., & Elliot, R. (1993). *Process-experiential psychotherapy: Facilitating emotional change.* New York: Guilford Press. *An updated version of client centered, experiential psychotherapy that incorporates techniques and concepts from Gestalt therapy and cognitive therapy.*

Wachtel, P. L. (1997). *Psychoanalysis, behavior therapy, and the representational world.* Washington, DC: American Psychological Association. *A revision and expansion of the classic text that made discussion of psychotherapy integration possible, it is an excellent introduction to current thinking and practice in psychodynamic, behavioral, and cognitive therapies.*

CHAPTER 7

PSYCHOTHERAPY IN GROUPS

Rae Dezettel Perls

GROUP PSYCHOTHERAPY

Historical Perspective

Psychotherapy in groups grew out of an evolving interest in placing the client in a therapeutic environment that more realistically reflected real-life social situations, that encouraged more equality both among members of the group and between the clients and the leader, and that offered psychotherapeutic opportunity at a lower cost than individual psychotherapy.

Particular theoreticians are associated with the group therapy movement. Alfred Adler, an early follower of Freud, was most interested in social and cultural issues. Adler, in 1922, founded an institute because he was so intrigued by the idea of therapy in groups with the focus away from the power and influence of the leader, to the power and influence of the therapy group members on one another. His focus on the support and encouragement of group members for one another has been an important basic element in the development of group theory.

In the early 1940s the social psychologist Kurt Lewin was particularly interested in group dynamics. Lewin pointed the way toward group-as-a-whole concepts and social systems theory. He sug-

gested that we look at the influence of the group as more than the sum of its parts. This concept was influenced by the early Gestalt psychologists who taught about *Gestalt* as a configuration representing the whole, as more than the sum of its parts. Lewin postulated that as each individual in the group influences each other member and alters behavior, so do the group values and group environment influence each individual member. This concept was called *field theory*. To view the group as an entity with its own qualities, values, and personality was a major contribution to group therapy process concepts.

In the late 1940s the National Training Laboratories developed the concept of "training groups," which became known as T-groups. These were intended to be educational learning groups rather than therapy groups. As T-groups became more widely available, large numbers of people joined sessions because of the opportunity to learn new ways to relate to others, cut through feelings of isolation, and become more effectively connected to others.

The 1960s' human potential movement spawned "growth groups" that "normal" people eagerly joined to gain self-understanding. Although the goals were therapeutic in nature, these were not proclaimed as psychotherapy groups. At this stage in the development of group psychotherapy the preponderance of therapy groups were either psychodynamic, with its emphasis on nondirective long-term group process and analytic interpretations, or activity groups for children based on the Slavson group play therapy model. Many "growth" movement facilitators used psychodrama techniques based on the work of Jacob Moreno, the Gestalt therapy experiments of Fritz Perls, and the creation of a warm supportive environment modeled by Carl Rogers. Sometimes Eastern philosophies and meditation were added to the mix to create workshop approaches to self-awareness that appealed to people's need to know more about themselves, while making more authentic contact with others.

The 1970s shifted philosophically away from psychotherapies that appeared more authoritarian, focused on past events, and/or called for extensive interpretation by the therapist, to psychotherapy theories that focused more on the here and now, cognitive understanding by the client, and practical problem solving. The therapist was framed more as an emotionally available consultant, and the stage was set for the increased demand for professionally trained group psychotherapists.

William Powles (1983, p. 71) summarizes these developments: " Group psychotherapy is a general mode of psychotherapy oriented to the social nature of man and characterized by the exploitation of group relationships and processes by a trained expert . . . little of certainty is known regarding what patient should be most cost effectively offered what type of group." Dr. Powles also points out the polarity between the various theoretical viewpoints about the way a group should be conducted. We continue to see the struggle within the profession between those espousing more nondirective or psychodynamically based group approaches, and the more problem-solving behaviorally focused therapist-directed approaches.

Therapeutic Considerations

Inpatient groups have characteristics particular to the restricted settings in which they are used. Most typically, hospital psychiatric units separate crisis patients from longer term care individuals.

Each defined patient group will have their own therapy groups. These groups will be organized around the needs and goals of each population. Some of the inpatients are mandated to be in the facility. Other patients agree that a hospital stay will best serve them.

Acute inpatients will meet in group daily to sort out the pressures and dilemmas that drove them to attempt suicide, or to sort out the stressors that triggered a severe clinical depression. The level of therapeutic work is likely to be intense. With the guidance of staff therapists, strategies for more effective living will be explored. Psychotropic medications will likely also be used during the hospital stay, and their effectiveness will be evaluated to some extent during these group sessions. The goal will be to establish enough emotional stability for the patient to leave the hospital setting and return to work, family life, and the community. Most often, new patients come into the group each day, so that the group population is ever-changing. Termination from group signals leaving the hospital, so good-byes can be a daily or weekly experience.

The more chronic inpatient adult will be in a long-term protected setting. The stay could be from several weeks on a periodic basis (if for example the person is struggling to stabilize a bipolar disorder), to many months (if suffering a debilitating psychotic condition such as schizophrenia). The group therapy will still be provided on a daily basis, but the level of functioning of the group members may be lower and the progress only modest over time. The goal is to rehabilitate the patient sufficiently to cope in a less restricted environment.

Most children and adolescents suffering from acute emotional and behavioral disorders will be treated in facilities separate from adults. They too will be in daily therapy groups with goals similar to those of the adult populations. More focus will likely be on peer relationships, school problems, and family issues. Many facilities for youth also incorporate family group therapy into their programs because of the significant continued involvement and impact the family will have on the young patient.

Outpatient groups come in a wide variety of settings and populations. Most often these are voluntary groups, with stable membership during agreed-on time parameters. Group members tend to be more alike than different in that they most often are of similar educational and socioeconomic background. These individuals are typically grouped together on the basis of similar needs and interests. They also will be functioning at similar levels in their daily lives outside the group setting.

Outpatient clients are most often seen in clinics and private practices. There are also topic-specific counseling groups attached to schools, community centers, and religious congregations. These groups may focus on grief, divorce adjustment, living with an elderly relative, parenting a disabled child, or any of many subgroups in the community. Typically the group meets weekly for a given number of weeks.

Sometimes the time-limited, topic-focused counseling group evolves into an ongoing long-term support group. Sometimes groups take on a life of their own and move from a therapy or counseling focus with a professional leader, to an ongoing support mode that is leaderless or led by an experienced member. Out of such a progression come self-help groups.

Psychotherapy groups are distinguished from support groups in the clear definition of the goals leading to new depths in self-understanding, healing, and behavior change. The group therapy facilitator is trained specifically in the concepts of group dynamics and the practice of group therapy as a change agent. Group therapists who are certified through a program sponsored by the American Group Psychotherapy Association must demonstrate their skills through completion of particular coursework and supervision of their work by senior group therapists.

Trained group therapists may be counselors, social workers, psychologists, or psychiatrists. They all share certain training experiences, have similar ethical understandings about confidentiality in groups, and share an understanding of the therapeutic factors crucial to successful therapeutic outcomes. These therapeutic factors, which are rather generally accepted, were formulated by Irvin Yalom (Vinogradov & Yalom, 1989) as follows:

1. Instillation of hope
2. Universality
3. Imparting of information
4. Altruism
5. Development of socializing techniques
6. Imitative behavior
7. Catharsis
8. Corrective recapitulation of the primary family group
9. Existential factors
10. Group cohesiveness
11. Interpersonal learning

Group Formation

The matter of participant selection for a given therapy group is a challenging clinical assessment issue for the group therapist. A starting point is to define and understand the type of group for which we are screening individuals.

An inpatient group that meets daily on a hospital unit will necessarily be based on the population on the unit each day. The staff may decide either that individuals recently admitted to the program will be in a special "observation" group that is part of the assessment process, or that these newer patients will enter the ongoing group once they are stable enough to sit, listen, and share. Attending staff will observe each day whether an individual is free from psychotic delusions and thus able to benefit from the group and avoid disrupting the group process unnecessarily. Attention to screening for group membership is usually an ongoing daily process on an inpatient unit.

Outpatient psychotherapy groups tend to fall into two major categories: long-term and short-term. Each type of group will have certain variations depending on the theoretical assumptions and the personal style of the therapist. The histories, presenting problems, educational levels, and relational styles of the members also contribute to the "personality" of a group. These groups typically meet weekly in the group room of the therapist. They use a space that often resembles a living room, with couches and/or chairs in a circle. Most typically there is a set time duration of either one hour, one and one-quarter hour, one and one-half hours, or two hours.

Long-term therapy groups are typically considered "open" groups, in that long-time members will leave when it is determined that their therapeutic work is complete, and new members will be added when the group has space. How the transitions of members in and out of group are handled is based on several factors related to the orientation of the facilitator. Because the therapist in a long-term group may be psychodynamic, cognitive-behavioral, or some combination of these and other approaches, the process for membership change will vary from one group to another.

It is most common for participants in long-term groups to appear fairly stable in their daily lives in the world outside of group. Inside group, they can share their fears, problems with relationships, neurotic impulses, and preoccupations, and seek help from both the therapist and peers as they experience being "stuck" in their lives. The group becomes a family that is safe and attentive to the needs of its membership. Over time, the participants explore, at ever deepening levels, the many complex aspects of their personalities. Individuals gradually allow themselves to open areas of their psyche for expression, exploration, consultation, and ultimately change.

In short-term psychotherapy groups there is usually a stated contract of 6 to 20 "closed" sessions with the same participants for the duration. Most often the members are selected for the similarity of their issues and the similarity of their status. Thus, they may all be recently divorced individuals, or children of parents going through divorce. They could be women who were raped or battered and requested the opportunity to do some therapeutic work around this particular traumatizing experience. These participants may attend to general issues of well-being, or focus on a particular type of problem that they have in common. Most often the group population is unchanged for the duration of the group. If members drop out, they are not usually replaced. The "contract" to meet may be renewed, and then new people will be added to those who choose to continue.

For any potential psychotherapy group member, it is expected that the therapist will have done at least one initial session individually. The group therapist or a referring colleague will most often have engaged the client in some individual psychotherapy sessions prior to the start of the group therapy experience. These individual sessions either would have been the earlier phase of psychotherapeutic work for the client, or would have been simply the screening for group psychotherapy.

Initial sessions with the group therapist are necessary for several reasons. Most important, each group member must have some understanding of the therapist's philosophical orientation and style. Then the prospective participant needs to understand the reasons for engaging in this form of therapy. Individual needs and goals for group participation should be explored before entering a group. Questions and concerns about joining the group can be addressed before starting the group. With careful preparation, the new group member will feel more ready and secure about the coming group psychotherapy experience.

Regardless of the kind of psychotherapy group, the group participant can expect to experience support, inclusion, attention, information, feedback, and encouragement to make constructive change. Judith Schoenholtz-Read (as cited in Barnard & MacKenzie, 1994) stated the most commonly held basic assumption about group psychotherapy: "The social environment created by the interpersonal interactions of the members of a group becomes the powerful vehicle for therapeutic change. Group psychotherapies use the group members' interactions as a main focus for the therapeutic work . . ." (p. 162).

Practice Models

Certain factors are common to all psychotherapy groups regardless of the theoretical orientation of the therapist. There will be a set time and place for the group to meet that is private. The importance of confidentiality will be discussed at every first session. In the early sessions, the task of building a sense of group cohesion will be in the forefront. Attention will be paid less to individual issues than to group themes that emerge from the group members. As the weeks go by and the members attend regularly, they come to be acquainted with and interested in one another. Their sense of trust, self-disclosure, and risk-taking abilities will increase.

As time and opportunity move along, the work of the group intensifies. The role of the therapist and the nature of the therapist's interventions will vary depending on the particular training of the therapist. Generally, however, it is agreed that among experienced group psychotherapists there is more in common than in dispute. Qualities of intelligence and kindliness, mixed with a nonhostile and nonjudgmental disposition, are common to the best group therapists regardless of theoretical orientation.

The theoretical differences between one therapist and another do influence the themes and activity of the group. It is to these differences that the following five summaries will be addressed.

Basic Elements of Psychodynamic Group Psychotherapy

The followers of Freud subscribe to the primary principles of psychoanalysis. Thus, the psychoanalytically trained group therapist will focus first on transference issues, where the client experiences the therapist and/or other members of the group as significant figures from the past. Thus, the therapist interprets client statements, reactions, and feelings within a context that is referential to the client's past important relationships.

The psychodynamic therapist looks for resistance in both the group members and the group as a whole. By sharing verbal interpretations, the therapist points out the ways that defenses are used to protect against anxiety and to protect the system from threatening feelings of change. The therapist may also speak about that of which the client (or group) is unaware, thereby making the unconscious thought or feeling, conscious.

When asked a direct question by a group member, the psychodynamic group therapist is less likely to answer directly or to put the question back to the group than to ask for the associations the question triggers for the questioner. The tendency is for the facilitator to be nondirective. When speaking, the therapist is most apt to be reflecting feelings, probing for deeper meaning, making an interpretation, or moving the group process forward with an open-ended question to the group.

The psychoanalytically trained group therapist will also be strict regarding the time when group begins and ends. The issue of keeping to therapist-prescribed boundaries will come up in different forms over time in the group. The therapist will insist that a certain structure be followed that likely will include the prohibition against any physical contact between group members, instructions not to eat or bring food items into group, and instructions to avoid social contacts outside of the group.

Noted contemporary psychodynamic group psychotherapist trainers include Anne Alonso, Howard Kibel, Scott Rutan, Sol Scheidlinger, and Walter Stone. All are either psychologists or psychiatrists who are past presidents of the American Group Psychotherapy Association and have written extensively in the field (Klein, 1992).

Cognitive and Behavioral Group Psychotherapy

Albert Ellis wrote and lectured widely about old and faulty thought processes as an interference with change. Dr. Ellis was the first of the cognitive therapists to clearly present the concept that maladaptive behaviors are learned and therefore can be unlearned. He called his approach *rational emotive therapy.* The psychotherapist was viewed as a teacher who challenges and trains others to think differently about experiences (Corey 1990).

Joseph Wolpe (1982) was another pioneer in behavior therapy who believed that bad habits are learned. He taught that behavior is learned through reinforcement, so destructive behavior can change when that reinforcement stops and the behavior becomes extinct in the face of new and better responses that are rewarded.

Cognitive and behavior therapies do not ask for deep understanding of the question "Why?" The cognitive-behavioral therapist comes to the group seeking a contract with each member, and with the group as a whole, to share concerns, think out loud, and problem-solve around the question: " How can I most effectively change particular aspects of my life so that I am more constructively functional?" Group members will be encouraged to challenge one another to think more objectively and clearly, and to practice different ways of communicating and behaving. The therapist and the group will offer positive ways of viewing oneself; they will urge and encourage group members to experiment by doing "homework" outside the group that will provide practice for new ways of thinking and new ways of responding to old messages.

In the group, members will share difficult experiences and will be "coached" about strategies to assist in viewing these negative experiences in ways that are more constructive. This *reframing* of events can loosen the emotional hold of old, self-destructive ways of thinking and functioning. Behavior "rehearsal" offers an opportunity to experiment with doing something in ways very different from present habits. Use of relaxation techniques is usually a part of this therapy process. Through learning to think differently, to relax, and to respond differently, more positive feelings can be developed.

The group therapist using cognitive-behavioral theories and methods will be an active participant, eager to facilitate group members' efforts to reach their stated goals for entering the therapy group. The therapist will reinforce positive group interaction and will encourage new and creative ideas that move members toward change. Members will enjoy congratulating and rewarding each other for therapeutic work well done.

In these groups, therapist and members may bring "treats" for celebration of successful events or accomplishments. For example, after practicing various approaches in group to prepare for seeking a raise from a supervisor who is seen as intimidating, a participant brought cookies to thank the group for their involvement in his practice session role playing. He was able to enjoy his success openly and to accept congratulations, while group members also were rewaded for constructive thinking and creative effort in their work with him. These group celebrations support and encourage the group therapy goals.

Members are not discouraged from having casual social contact outside of group, as long as the experience is shared with the group so that it can be processed and used as part of new social learning. Observations from a group member about appearance or behavior out in public can provide useful data within the group.

Any group member can offer ideas, share information, ask facilitating questions, and receive praise for taking that initiative. The group becomes a laboratory for trying out new ways of being with people. The therapist and the other group members become models for different ways of seeing an issue and for demonstrating positive behaviors. This system can be very empowering to clients as they experience themselves functioning with as much usefulness to others as the therapist.

The therapist challenges assumptions and insists that group members face important issues. Support and encouragement are offered when a client struggles to formulate a new way of thinking and doing. The cognitive-behavioral therapist looks for opportunities to analyze "scripts" or "schemas" to help in understanding the burdens of old negative thinking and reacting that are carried from youth to adulthood. Permission is explicitly given to discuss any topic or feelings.

A summary statement about this approach was written by Elaine Cooper-Lonergan (cited in Bernard & MacKenzie, 1994).

> . . . Cognitive therapists are interested in the spontaneous thought process of their patients. Behavior therapists try to change maladaptive behaviors. Both make the assumption that if certain negative thinking changes or if maladaptive behaviors change, the person will also change; that is, if you change one part of the system, the entire system will necessarily change. (p. 209)

Training in the area of cognitive and behavioral applications is available through the Institute for Rational-Emotive Therapy in New York City (Corey, 1990) or the works of Dr. Simon Budman, who writes and speaks widely on the topic of brief therapies using a mixture of cognitive and behavioral approaches in time-limited settings (1988).

Gestalt/Existential Therapy in Group

Fritz Perls, the creator and first teacher of Gestalt therapy in the early 1950s, challenged most of the basic assumptions of psychoanalytic psychotherapy. He preferred to begin psychotherapeutic work with the here and now. Perls conceptualized an existential therapy that focused first on awareness in the present moment. The group setting was viewed as the ideal place for learning. In the early demonstration groups, one individual would volunteer to take the "hot seat" and work with the therapist while the other members observed. Group members shared observations and engaged in interactions after the initial one-on-one was complete. This model is often misunderstood as the totality of Gestalt group work.

Polster and Polster (1973) presented some of the ways in which the second generation of Gestalt therapists expanded the use of the group modality. They described the "floating hot seat," which allows the focus of attention to shift around the group and encourages any of the members to participate spontaneously. Meaningful contact between participants is encouraged. Looking and listening with care is the responsibility of every member. Observations about one another become the basis of the therapeutic work in the group. Attention is paid to body language, breathing, posture, voice volume and tone, and hesitations—all contributing to heightened awareness in the moment.

The Polsters point out the value of this method for self-discovery. "... People learn to be tuned in to their inner process, to articulate it, and to behave in terms of it ... The opportunity to set up experiments joins contactfulness and awareness... Almost invariably there is support somewhere in a group for whatever behavior anyone may try. The group has a wisdom of its own that extends beyond the wisdom of the leader alone ... " (1973, p. 297).

The use of "experiments" in the group is a basic Gestalt method. A group member may be invited by either the therapist or a group member to practice a new behavior—for example, by role playing with another group member, or by having dialogue with parts of himself that are in conflict, or by expressing a feeling in an exaggerated way in order to experience the feeling more fully. The existential group method encourages the participants to use themselves creatively to confront themselves and others in a joint effort to change behavior.

The Gestalt group therapist is a fully present participant-facilitator. The therapist questions and reflects, as do therapists from other theoretical orientations. However, the Gestalt therapist also challenges the status quo and confronts reactions that appear overly guarded and/or ritualistic. The Gestalt therapist does not make interpretations but, rather, shares perceptions. Gossip and reporting are discouraged. Speaking in general terms like "one does" is also discouraged; participants are encouraged by the therapist to use "I" in order to take ownership of their feelings and ideas. The therapist will facilitate dream work and guided fantasies in the group when that appears useful. The therapist supports and encourages the group interaction and will ask group process questions. The questions are likely to be framed as "What is happening now?" rather than "Why did that happen?"

Small-group existential methods, combined with Gestalt experiments, led to the encounter group movement which in turn spawned the growth group movement. Lieberman, Yalom, and Miles (1973), writing about encounter groups, explain that "... the most common effect on participants is in the area of value shifts and, particularly, in increasing the valuation of personal growth and change" (p. 447).

Gestalt therapy institutes for training exist in most major cities, notably New York, Cleveland, and Los Angeles. Senior Gestalt therapists Miriam and Erving Polster continue to conduct professional training groups internationally and in La Jolla, California.

Eclectic, Integrative, and Other Group Therapy Approaches

Interest in "group-as-a-whole" approaches have continued to be a focus of attention that looks more at the group as metaphor for the therapeutic process, and less at the individual transactions. For example, the Tavistock method draws on object relations work combined with group dynamics theory. Interpretations by the leader are focused away from individual issues to group issues such as conflict and competition, or tasks and authority. Attention is directed to understanding the group behavior and the influences of the social structure on individuals. Personal change comes through exploration of these relationships.

Social systems theory places emphasis on the concept of *boundary*, which is that region of experience that separates the individual from the group or the group from the rest of the environment. Edward Klein (1992, p. 106) is definitive in his statement: "All systems theorists agree that every group has a boundary that distinguishes it from the environment. The leader's role involves boundary identification and regulation." As the group is ever evolving, a change in an individual stimulates a change in the group system, as a change in a group subsystem will effect change in the individuals. These are complex dynamics.

Helen Durkin (1964) was an early leader and writer about a group-focused therapy grounded in psychodynamic psychotherapeutic assumptions that became known as general systems theory (GST). The GST approach examines the structural systems while exploring the transferential and resistance issues. Attention is paid to what is expressed rather than what is concealed. This is also considered to be a growth-oriented approach that can be readily integrated with object relations and self psychology theories (Klein, Bernard, & Singer, 1992).

In the past ten years more attention has been paid to focal group psychotherapy. These groups are developed around homogeneous groups focused on a specific client population. The therapy subgroups are formed around a particular issue like spouse dependency, or an experience such as shyness. In a recent book about these groups (McKay & Paleg, 1992), the following description of qualities common to focal groups was provided:

- Have a high degree of structure.
- Have a specific and limited target issue.

- Be strongly goal-oriented.
- Place a high value on efficiency—homework and structured exercises designed to promote rapid change.
- Have a high educational function.
- Discourage attention to transference issues.

Most topic- or interest-focused groups are time-limited, with clear "contracts" stated at the start of each group regarding goals, membership, and date of completion. Some of these groups are facilitated by professionally trained group therapists, and many are not. Sometimes these groups are a part of a larger organization that sponsors series of support groups that can be easily confused with psychotherapy groups established to deal with similar issues.

A growing number of well-trained group psychotherapists call themselves *eclectic* or *integrative* therapists. Generally this refers to the thoughtful integration of a variety of theoretical positions, mixed with group techniques that experience dictates work most effectively in a given situation. Rather than adhering rigidly to any particular formulation or system, there is an orderly use of various approaches that make sense to the therapist.

So we find that experienced group therapists may work with similar populations of clients in a variety of ways.

A depressed young man may find himself weekly in a small group of eight other men and women of various ages with assorted presenting concerns for an undefined period of time. The mood of the group may be highly energized around a different issue each time they meet, or they may spend a significant amount of time each session rather slowly working to draw into the circle of intimacy one particularly fearful new member. If the same young man were in a different group, he might find himself asked questions about his activities of the week before, with an emphasis on encouragement for him to do something different in between sessions. Another group might combine both kinds of group involvement.

A recently divorced older woman might find herself referred to a group made up entirely of single women or of a group of men and women who are all recently divorced; or she might be in a group with the depressed young man mentioned earlier here.

She could find attention paid to her past losses that are triggered by the divorce and combine to leave her feeling sad and hopeless. Or she might be drawn into intense group process discussions that keep all of the feelings and awareness in the room.

No one group therapy method is best for any one person. Perhaps future research will better illuminate the choice process for the group therapy consumer.

Research Data and Future Trends

Although the status of current group psychotherapy outcome research is limited, it is informative to review briefly both the problems and the conclusions available.

Research findings indicate that group therapy is as effective as individual therapy, in most cases (Dies, 1992). Because it is less expensive, practitioners will be challenged to explain why group therapy is not more often the therapy of choice for most patients.

Empirical data concerning client selection criteria are too limited and currently unavailable to hold up. Many of the findings are based on such small populations that the patterns reported may be a product of chance. Few such studies have been replicated. One problem is that most intake or screening sessions for group therapy are "clinical" interviews, in which the therapist asks the potential group member questions and notes the responses. Thus, the therapist has selection criteria that are predominantly subjective and difficult to measure. Most therapists have clearer criteria for screening "out" members than for selecting "in" members. The typical reasons given for screening "out" potential group members are:

1. Client in acute crisis
2. Reported psychotic episodes
3. Inability to sit quietly and listen
4. Brain damage
5. Drug-dependent
6. Suicidal
7. Sociopathic personality disorder

An interesting but mostly untested approach is the screening group, a group specifically designed to provide a short-term group experience for a limited number of individuals. This provides an opportunity for the therapist both to orient the new referrals to group and to observe them. A screening group is not practical in a small outpatient practice, but it can be of value in either an institutional setting or a large group practice that offers a variety of therapy group settings. This is another area for future research attention.

Systematic preparation for group therapy participation has been described and advocated by Yalom (1985). Some practitioners suggest that clients who participate actively in the therapy group by giving and receiving feedback obtain the most benefits. Studies indicate that clients experience fewer bad outcomes when the style of the therapist is warm and accepting (Lieberman et al., 1973). There is no definitive research that instructs about the optimal size for a therapy group. The common collective wisdom shared by most group therapists is that five to eight participants is the best number. If there is an absence or two, there are still enough members to keep the process viable. The next most discussed number for a therapy group is ten.

The most often referenced studies about group therapy continue to be those that compare the effectiveness of group therapy with the effectiveness of individual therapy. In the preface to a textbook on group psychotherapy one of the editors, Harold Bernard, reports:

> Over the last decade and a half, there has been a concerted effort to demonstrate that psychotherapy is effective. Hundreds of controlled studies are now available that indicate an overall therapeutic effect of about 0.85; that is, about 85% of patients receiving psychotherapy do significantly better than control group patients. That the results are essentially the same whether the psychotherapy is delivered in an individual or group format is not well known. (Bernard & MacKenzie, 1994, p. viii)

With convincing evidence that group therapy is as effective for most people as individual therapy, and the clear cost-effectiveness of group when compared to individual therapy work, there will continue to be an increased interest in group psychotherapy. It will remain a challenge to future researchers to help us discriminate which kind of group therapy for which kind of personal problems will provide the best outcome.

FAMILY THERAPY

Introduction

The use of conjoint family therapy initially evolved out of concern for children being unfairly identified as "patient." It appeared to many clinicians that too often parents held the belief that if their "problem" child could be "cured," then their entire family atmosphere would be made "healthy." This viewpoint came out of a medical-model concept that a troubling child must be "mentally ill" and so could be made "well" with the proper study, diagnosis, and treatment.

In historical context, interest in the family as a unit also came out of the social sciences and the interest in communication theory. Family communication patterns could be observed, and the functioning of the family unit could be viewed in the context of its having a system. Within this framework, an individual can be seen as learning information, processing nonverbal signals, and being stimulated in certain ways that become internalized into life patterns.

As challenges to individual psychoanalytic psychotherapy emerged, it seems reasonable that different ways of understanding individual experience, pain, growth, and change would be developed.

For many practitioners of psychotherapy, there was too much emphasis on the individual as having a problem. In fact, it too often appeared that one member of a family "carried" the symptoms for the family. So the focus took a shift to the environment of the client. Many problems would now be conceptualized as not existing within the individual but, rather, reflecting systemic dysfunctioning in the patterns and experiences of the family unit.

Philip Barker, in his 1981 textbook, *Basic Family Therapy*, wrote:

> It will now be clear that it is possible to use systems theory as a model for understanding how families function, but nevertheless to use a wide variety of methods to change their functioning.... The literature suggests that any of the different theoret-

ical approaches can be the basis for successful therapy ... there are a variety of ways of bringing about change in any particular troubled family. (1981, pp. 7, 40)

Practice Models

Several psychotherapist–theoreticians significantly contributed to the early formulations about working with families in therapy. Although the current trend is integrative, it is still of value to have an overview of the progression in theory and practice that brought us to the present.

Nathan Ackerman is generally considered the grandfather of family therapy. He was a psychodynamic child analyst and part of the child guidance movement. In the 1930s he was looking at the family unit as having significant impact on the status of the child. By the 1940s he was observing the family unit together as part of the assessment study. He would see the family both in their home and in his office. The diagnostic process became a part of the treatment. As he explored issues and interacted with families, family members became more aware, sharing, and intimate (Ackerman, 1958, 1984).

In the 1950s Murray Bowen (Papero, 1991) began to involve family members of hospitalized schizophrenic patients in the treatment process. From that early work he created an evolving set of theories about the influences of the family on the defined patient. He assumed that the family "caused" the patient's problems. A basic position that resulted from his research is that family therapy should be used when the family appears to be the reason for the reported problems. He created the term *emotional system* to describe the complex of life forces, genetic and experiential, that establishes an individual behavior system. Bowen explained this phenomenon as a complex of influences involving both biology and feelings that govern "the dance of life."

By the end of the 1950s, interest in family research and theory shifted to family treatment. Gregory Bateson and Don Jackson formed family institutes on the West Coast. Ackerman was on the East Coast, and Carl Whitaker emerged as a practitioner–teacher in the Midwest. Each training group had its own particular interest.

Carl Whitaker was particularly innovative, introducing multigenerations in the therapy sessions. He was most interested in the experiential opportunity with the extended family members, and actively engaged them and challenged them to interact and to have fun with each other. He modeled being humorous, creative, absurd, open, and warm.

Virginia Satir had a profound influence on the early training of many family therapists. She traveled extensively around the country training younger professionals, and she wrote two works often used to teach the practice of family therapy: *Conjoint Family Therapy* (1968) and *Changing with Families*, with Richard Bandler and John Grinder (Bandler, Grinder, & Satir, 1976). Her interest was in the process of the experience of being a family member. The method is to explore carefully the patterns of their communications, and then learn ways to change the dysfunctional communications. She focused on the practical and taught ways for family members to feel increased self-worth by saying directly more of what they felt, leading to more congruent behavior.

Yet another model emerged in the late 1960s based on work done with juvenile delinquents. Structural family therapy is described in a popular textbook as:

> . . . based on a systems theory that was developed primarily at the Philadelphia Child Guidance Clinic, under the leadership of Salvador Minuchin . . . distinctive features are its emphasis on structural change as the main goal of therapy, which acquires preeminence over the details of individual change, and the attention paid to the therapist as an active agent in the process of restructuring the family. (Colapinto, 1991, p. 78)

A significant innovation included challenge with support. The challenging stance of the therapist provoked the family difficulties and created a crisis in the therapy room. This was a critical move away from the more supportive and contained strategies used previously. The disorganization that emerged in the therapy session could be used to open opportunities to explore options for new ways to behave with each other. Since the family is viewed as an "open system," the assumption is that the challenge

of understanding the problem leads to accommodation, and the need for modification leads to change.

Out of the structural family work, combined with general systems theory, came the strategic therapy developed by Jay Haley in the late 1970s. He envisioned the therapist as actively intervening into the family system to initiate alternative ways of viewing and understanding the issues of the family. Goals are clearly set and behavioral changes are defined by the therapist, including "homework" assignments. The therapist involves each member of the family in the change process. The therapist is very directive.

Haley's wife and colleague at the Philadelphia Child Guidance Center, Chloe Madanes, moved their theories further by introducing the idea of the defined patient in the family as carrying symptoms as a metaphor that can both mirror and disguise the real, often hidden, serious issues that family avoids facing. Madanes (1981) made it very clear that "... directives are deliberately planned, and they are the main therapeutic technique" of the therapist (p. 24).

So the movement in family therapy became increasingly behavioral and focused on problem redefinition, combined with new learning approaches that were often therapist-driven. This led to several social learning models, including assorted parent training and child management systems. Family therapy and behavioral therapy merged into popular techniques that are familiar to us, like the concept of "time out" for children who are out of control, "contracts" for work to be accomplished between family members, and behavior "point systems."

Over time, out of each of the emerging theoretical approaches to individual psychotherapy, practitioners have developed concomitant approaches to each of the group therapies, including family therapy and couple therapy. Some of what would be observed in the family therapy session is common to those using a given theoretical approach in individual therapy. However, some of what would be observed in a family session is essentially the same regardless of defined theoretical assumptions. Most family therapists will typically adhere to the following basic understandings:

1. They will see the complete family together for the first session.
2. Each family member will be given equal respect and opportunity to speak.
3. Scapegoating of a family member will not be tolerated.
4. No physical violence will be allowed.
5. Definition, assessment, and goal setting will involve the whole family.
6. Efforts will be made to conduct the therapy with the whole family.

How these basic tenets will be carried out will vary depending on the orientation and style of the psychotherapist.

Some family therapists will only meet with the entire family at all times. Other therapists will meet with whichever family members show up for the appointment. Certain therapists will invite subgroups of the family to do some sessions; for example, the children may meet with the therapist for a session separate from the adults, or the parents may do some couple work separated out from the children. Grandparents or other significant adults may be invited to a session, both to stimulate feelings of inclusion and to gain their observations. The use of multiple families in a group session together also has drawn some attention in the past decade.

Special Issues in Family Therapy

Divorce

In the past twenty years, therapists trained in the area of family psychology have been increasingly called on to work with family members who are facing divorce. Psychologists, social workers, and family counselors are the professionals most often contacted to work with families who are struggling painfully as they go through the complex of issues that emerge during the divorce process.

In 1980, psychologists Judith Wallerstein and Joan Kelly wrote the seminal book on children in the divorce situation, *Surviving the Breakup*. They followed families from the time parents made the decision to separate, through choices about money, property, and child planning, to postdivorce experiences of each member of the family unit. Extensive questionnaires and interviews were used before, during, and after the final divorce arrangements were made, covering five years. In 1989, Judith Wallerstein and Sandra Blakeslee, in *Second Chances*, published their results and observations from a ten-year follow up study of the same population used in the original book.

The Wallerstein findings have become very important to therapists (lawyers and judges, too) for the insights provided into the world of the divorcing family. We are much better prepared to assist families with the foundation of information this research has provided. Among the significant pieces of information, the following stand out to guide our counseling:

1. Couples who consulted family therapists early in the divorce process reported less tension and acrimony.
2. Children who were informed of the basic information as it was unfolding did better than children who were left to wonder and guess about the decisions.
3. Children needed to know how the concrete aspects of their own lives would be affected by the decisions being made. They wanted to know about where they, and each parent, would be living after the divorce. They wanted to know about the specifics of who and what would be in their daily lives, like the pets, the piano, their beds, etc.
4. Children made the easiest adjustment to the divorce when they were exposed to minimal changes during the first year following the divorce of their parents. Those youngsters who could stay primarily in their original physical location, who could attend the same school and/or have the same caretaker, did better than those children who were moved to new, unfamiliar surroundings immediately after the divorce.
5. The youngest of the children made the easiest adjustment to the change. The male preteens exhibited the most difficulty with the divorce changes.
6. Children worried most about the possible loss of a parent as a result of the divorce. Children

do best when both parents continue to be a constant, predictable presence in the ongoing daily lives of the children.

7. Children who were well adjusted before the divorce were usually stabilized after about 18 months. The general psychological condition of the children was very much dependent on the overall quality of life postdivorce, and particularly dependent on the resolution of issues and conflicts between the parents, and on the adjustment of the primary caretaker, who was most often the mother, even with joint custody.

8. Even after five years of postdivorce experience, most children, regardless of age, continued to wish that their parents would be reunited.

It is not uncommon to find couples many years after divorce still questioning the wisdom of their earlier decision. But for every couple who wonder if they should have stayed and worked harder in the first marriage, there is another couple continuing to fight with the first spouse long after the ink has dried on the final divorce papers. The children in these families usually continue to reflect the confusion and discontent of the parents. As the adults are upset, the children carry these problems to school and into the world of their play. These children typically express their fears and distress over these changes that are out of their control by exhibiting regressive behaviors, failing in school, fighting with peers, arguing with family members, and/or withdrawing.

Many of these family members find their way to the offices of family therapists. Depending on the theoretical orientation of the therapist, the child's family of origin may be seen together as a group, or just the child alone will see the therapist, or the parents together or individually will meet with the therapist, or any combination of the family members may be invited into a session.

There are particular challenges for the family therapist consulting with parents living apart. The importance of neutrality is always powerfully present in divorce consultation. Couples who have already separated are most sensitive to felt bias on the part of the therapist. The broken bond of trust is in the room all of the time. The therapist feels its

presence much as the child probably experiences it. Sometimes the therapist becomes the spokesperson for the absent child. The contract between family members and the therapist must be very clear so that fragile trust is not further threatened.

Effective and appropriate family divorce therapy is work in progress. What has emerged thus far is the importance of a knowledge base and training for the the therapist beyond what is required to do individual psychotherapy, group therapy, or general family therapy.

Stepparenting and Blended Family Issues

It is hypothesized that by the year 2000, 50% of the children in the United States will live in stepfamilies. Since most divorced adults remarry within three years of their divorces, it is clear how these projections make sense. While most minor children of divorce continue to live primarily with the parent who did most of the caretaking prior to the parental split, increasingly large numbers of children are in shared physical custody arrangements of some order. With joint custody more the norm, it is understandable that we have ever greater numbers of children spending significant amounts of time in two households.

In Visher and Visher's widely read book about stepparenting (1979) they reported on the limited studies about stepfamily relationships. They do point out several findings that have held up over time and are generally considered common wisdom about stepfamilies:

1. There is a positive correlation between socioeconomic status and stepfamily success.
2. Stepfamilies experience more psychological stress than do intact families.
3. Stepmothers have difficulties with the negative "stepmother" image.

A special issue of the *Journal of Family Psychology* (Levant, 1993) took a varied look at families in transition and reported some stunning data suggesting that large numbers of children will spend at least five years of their lives in a single-parent household headed by the mother. Despite joint custody arrangements, the bulk of the child-rearing responsibility falls to the mother. These mothers most often find themselves experiencing economic difficulties, time pressures, and increased psychological stress.

Where both parents continue to participate actively in the raising of their children postdivorce, or where parents remarry, fewer problems are experienced by most women. As the parents establish new, stable relationships, they are usually better able to let go of the old conflicts with their ex-mates. Understandably, when the divorced parents remarry partners with children, the children face many new situations that cause problems. Often the newly remarried couple feels overly optimistic about the future of the "blended" family. During courtship, the assorted children appear to have fun on joint outings, and conflict with the future stepparent is minimal. In their eagerness to feel renewed, the couple may overlook several realities of the children's experience. Frequently, the parents introduce their new "significant other" to the children too early in the process. Clinical observations support waiting until the adult relationship is clear, strong, and committed before introducing the potential partner to the children. Young children particularly will attach to a new adult. If there are several losses, they learn not to connect and can hold the new stepparent at a distance indefinitely. Wise parents wait to draw in the potential new stepparent, and then introduce him or her gradually into the family system.

There is now significant data (Hetherington, 1993) supporting earlier theories that early adolescents have the most difficult time with parental divorce, remarriage, and adjustment to stepsiblings. Adolescents tend to react more negatively to changes in neighborhood, schools, and parenting styles. Although adolescence is normally a time to begin the process of becoming more individual and separating from the family, the findings suggest that in newly reconstituted families about one-third of the youngsters had disengaged from the family by the age of 15. Where there is a positive adult figure other than the parents, less antisocial peer group involvement is found.

All too often the introduction of a new adult into a family system does cause strain. The introduction of nonrelated children into the family structure triggers stress as well as new rivalries. The previous role of each child is now challenged with the arrival of the "others." These difficulties are particularly pointed when the children are of the same sex and of similar ages. Children will look to their own parents for warmth, support, and clarification. Splitting of the newly forming family unit into "his" and "her" sides is not uncommon. An example of this dynamic from the author's past cases follows:

> When Clara and Henry remarried, each had three children under the age of fourteen. During the courtship time, the youngest boys, who were eight years old, appeared to play easily together. The young teens played games, watched movies, and went on outings with apparent ease. There were some hints of trouble ahead when Henry's oldest daughter rejected the dress for the wedding chosen for the girls by Clara. And Clara's middle son refused to sit at the head table with his siblings, insisting he sit with his grandparents.
>
> Fortunately, the couple was able to buy a new large house to accommodate the large family. But the move did require the younger boys and the younger girls to share rooms. Each of the eldest children were able to have their own bedrooms. Over the first three years every possible problem that could be experienced by adolescents happened to this "blended" family. Each "side" waged war with the opposite parent. Often the youngsters engaged the divorced parent or a grandparent to join in the fight.
>
> As these children grew older and left the family home, the split between Clara's and Henry's children widened and was never resolved. Fortunately, all of these children went on to eventually establish stable relationships of their own. Had the parents been emotionally unstable, overly rigid, lacking in humor, poor, or in ill health, the outcome for this family would not have been so positive.

Part of the challenge to a newly forming family unit postdivorce is time management. With young children frequently needing a different kind of visitation schedule than older children, and school-aged children dividing parts of every week in different households, the calender becomes a chronic source of confusion, debate, and revision. The divorced parents will find that they need to be able to consult regularly in order to meet their own work and social needs, as well as to respond to the particular demands of the children's schedules. Open minds, generous spirits, and an absence of malice are required to make the process work.

There are also particular hazards built into the stepparenting roles. For the woman who has no children of her own but takes on the part of "mother" for her new husband's children, there are all too often unrealistic expectations placed on her by the father. This childless women may come with theories about child rearing and hopes of being a significant influence. A woman with her own children comes to the marriage with fewer and less complex self-expectations. Typically, she just wants to establish a respectful and friendly connection with her husband's youngsters.

Similarly, for the man without his own progeny, there are frequently expectations that he will bring some order and discipline into a household that has been without an active male presence. If his is an easygoing style, he may disappoint his new wife, while winning over the kids. If he attempts to be authoritarian, the kids will fight back with reminders that "You're not my dad, and you can't boss me." When the new husband brings his own children with him into the household, he is apt to focus much more on simple mutual acceptance all around. He wishes for his own children to feel all right with his new mate, wants to demonstrate his ability to include her children, and tends to spend less energy asserting his influence on the stepchildren.

For all "blended" families, there are important issues of loyalties. Loyalty often relates to the culture of the family. How are holidays and birthdays to be celebrated? Who makes meals? What are the expectations about time? Laundry? Pet care? Reporting of information to each family member challenges the family system. At which grandparent's house will we have Thanksgiving dinner? Will half the children attend the synagogue on Saturday morning? Will the other half of the children attend Bible school on Sunday morning? Can Sammy stay at home because he doesn't want to go to any religious service? Who watches TV? Who doesn't have to do homework after dinner and before television?

Additional issues appear as more extended family members are near to the new family. Grandparents care about spending time with their grandchildren, but they may or may not want to take on the responsibilities that go with adjusting to stepgrandchildren. Grandparents also tend to know that the natural parent, though divorced from their offspring, is still an important "player" in the lives of the loved grandchildren. Smart grandparents won't alienate anyone, but thoughtless, uninformed grandparents can create a lot of difficulties for the new blended family.

Emily and John Visher (1979) remind us that with stepfamilies, "... here it is as if one is looking at the process through a microscope. Love and hate are magnified. Rivalry and competition for attention are magnified. Insecurity and the search for identity are magnified.... Remarriage for the adults is a gain of an important adult relationship. For the children remarriage frequently represents a loss of a close parent–child relationship. The child must now share the parent with one or more new individuals...." (p.162).

We see that where blended families can mix the traditions of both original families, and invite all the significant extended family members to join in some family gatherings, then all will benefit from this richness of good will. Where three generations on both sides of the family can be confident and generous of spirit, there is a lot to be gained for everyone. But it is clear that this mixing is a challenge that demands time, information, and energy.

Trends and Future Research Issues

The sum of the current research data (Levant, 1993) clearly points the way to the reality of increased numbers of children in families with steprelatives. The added stressors do have negative effects on children and early adolescents. It will be important to look at long-term outcome studies to assess just what strategies work best for stepparents and which dynamics most positively influence the adjustment of these children in "blended" families.

In just another ten years, we will have more research data added to clinical observations to guide us in our efforts to understand reconstituted families. With less myth and more data, we can anticipate greater effectiveness in evaluating and consulting parents in the postdivorce process.

COUPLE THERAPY

An Overview

The family may experience stress due to several traumatic factors including the following:

- Changes in financial circumstance
- The serious illness and hospitalization or death of a family member
- The mysterious disappearance of a family member
- Any other sudden change in the family environment

The most common stress that affects the family dynamics is significant discord between the parents. Of course, couples also experience distress whether or not they have children.

Couples seeking joint therapy usually have struggled for some time with their problems before seeking professional assistance. Not all of these couples are married, and not all are heterosexual. Some of the couples who come for joint therapy have been together only briefly, others have sustained this one relationship for many years, while still others have had many pairings during their adult years. There are no concise data at the present time to indicate who these couples are demographically.

The most common triggers that motivate couples to consider joint therapy are a threat of divorce by one partner and/or extramarital sexual involvement by one or both parties. Some couples will request joint therapy when they mutually agree that the marriage has chronic issues around sexuality, communication, and power. (These three factors most commonly interact.) Another concern is lifestyle differences. Sometimes the request for couple work is stimulated by the psychotherapy of one of the partners.

Practice Issues

Couple therapy is not conducted in the presence of the children or other family members, but it can take place in a group with other couples. Usually the individual therapist of one party is not the couple therapist to both, but there are exceptions to this model, particularly when both people have already established a positive relationship with the same psychotherapist.

Although some variations among couple therapists are reflections of the theoretical differences we have explored in discussing group psychotherapy, most differences in philosophy and technique have more to do with the personal experience and training of each therapist. Most of the couple therapy being done today tends to reflect the fundamental shift to cognitive-behavioral approaches when working with families.

Basic to all this work is the belief that people do have the ability to change, even in the face of well-established patterns of behavior.

A couple therapist has to establish a trusting, neutral relationship with both parties, and frequently this trust has to be established quickly. When a relationship is in trouble, there is a clear mandate to the therapist to "do something" now. The first session or two may be the only sessions.

One therapist may wish to see each person individually for the first session and bring the couple together for the second session. Another therapist will prefer that the couple always be seen together and so will require that they come in together from the beginning.

The initial session is critical to establishing ground rules for the therapeutic relationship. Most commonly, the therapist explains what the couple can expect, and inquires about their hopes for the process. Some history is gathered. It is a time for both getting acquainted and assessment. There has to be a mutual understanding of what issues will be addressed, and there has to be an agreement regarding commitment to the couple therapy process.

For some couples, agreeing to participate in couple therapy is not a commitment to work at staying together but, rather, a vehicle for defining more openly the differences that will allow for a breakup of the relationship. This clarification most often emerges within the first one to three sessions.

Sometimes one of the partners wants the therapist to hold a secret. That secret most often has to do with an extramarital affair. It is generally accepted practice for the therapist to refuse to enter into this kind of agreement. For constructive therapy to take place, this matter must be brought out in an early session by the client him- or herself.

It might seem that once this information is out and the outside relationship has stopped, the couple could get on with addressing the issues in their relationship. This particular issue is not usually so easily resolved. Humphrey (1987, p. 167) points out: "Such a belief is a great oversimplification, however, for much healing needs to occur before the necessary ingredients for satisfactory sexual/marital interaction can occur.... Therapeutic strategies should be focused ... on behaviors and communications that permit each member of the marital unit to earn the other's trust and respect. Anger must be dissipated, both through cathartic ventilation within the sessions and in the couple's home life. Guilt must be addressed...."

For some couples, an affair is the "symptom" that brings the couple issues to the foreground. For others, this is a way to end the relationship without dealing directly with the issues between them. By considering just this one phenomenon, we begin to see the complexity of learning about couple psychotherapy.

Carlfred Broderick (1983) has conceptualized couple therapy work for traditional marriages in terms of the "therapeutic triangle." He suggests that within this experience we have to consider six important elements that influence this three-way relationship:

1. The husband: his assorted perceptions about himself and his world view
2. The wife: her sense of self, beliefs, and needs
3. The therapist: his or her background of views and experiences
4. The marriage: how each partner views the relationship
5. The therapist's relationship to the man: how he is experienced by the therapist and how he experiences the therapist
6. The therapist's relationship to the woman: how she is experienced by the therapist and how she experiences the therapist

Thus we observe the many psychological levels operating in this therapeutic relationship between the therapist and the couple. A high degree of mutual interest and acceptance will be needed if the couple therapy is to succeed.

Richard Stuart (1980) puts forward a detailed social learning model for conducting behavioral couple therapy. He presents a highly structured format. He explains that his concept of *treatment stages* is like a road map that is used to guide the therapist and the clients in particular directions. Stuart's book is both a description of the step-by-step process of a new learning approach to marriage and a handbook of practical exercises for attaining new goals. From written assignments to communication exercises, we are given the tools to introduce a social learning approach to marital therapy. Therefore, the couple therapy would be clearly orchestrated by the therapist from the very first session to later sessions.

It is more common practice among marriage counselors and therapists, not trained in the Stuart model, to integrate particular approaches devised by assorted trainers and practitioners of repute into a system of behavioral interventions that respond to the existential requirements of the moment. Therapists will draw on many of the following techniques to create an approach that makes sense and seems appropriate to the given situation:

Contracts. With the couple, the therapist articulates expectations. The goal setting may be both short- and long-term, depending on the requested arrangement. Matters of the duration of the therapy, agreements for living together during the therapy, and postponing all talk about divorce would all be part of this task.

George and Anne had been yelling and screaming obscenities at each other for months before coming for their first therapy session. Each had engaged in brief affairs and were able to express their sense of desperation during the initial couple session. They were both hurt and struggling with strong feelings of abandonment. In sharing some family of origin history, they were quickly able to acknowledge that they shared unmet needs to feel special and receive large amounts of attention from the other, due in large part to growing up with parents who were very demanding and self-centered. They readily "contracted" to cut off all contact with past lovers, call "time out" if any discussion felt out of control for either of them, and not use threats of divorce for the next six months while they participated in couple therapy.

"I"-messages. A system that creates more opportunity for openness by restructuring the way feelings and needs are communicated. Clients are taught how to say what they want heard by the other through framing their verbalizations as " I need . . ." or, " I would like . . . " or " I'm concerned about . . . "

When communications begin with "You ought to . . . " or "You always . . . " there is bound to be a defensive response.

Relabeling. Using new and/or different words to describe observations about shared events so that the other person can be open to hearing the communication.

> Karen and Andrew were at an impasse in talking together about Andrew's quiet style. Karen frequently became irritable and pushy when Andrew would not expand on his comments or viewpoint. In their sessions she would call him "withholding" and "passive aggressive." This would usually elicit a silent withdrawing reaction from Andrew. When the therapist helped them to identify that his anxiety was triggered by her verbal "labeling" of his behavior, Karen was then able to practice asking him about his "fears" or "concerns." He was then able to feel less threatened and more "invited" to respond to her.

Reframing. The therapist listens to a complaint and states it from a perspective that is different from that presented by the client. Sometimes the therapist uses a paradox in order to create a shift in an old frozen perception. As the partners experience together this new way of viewing the same old positions, they are able to see alternative ways of dealing with that situation.

Homework. Therapist-directed assignments for the couple to do during the time between sessions. These activities are intended to begin new ways for the couple to be with each other, or to start them thinking and communicating differently than would be their typical pattern.

Pat and Al had been married ten years when they realized that they had stopped being sexual. In their initial therapy session together they were open and talked with each other like good old friends. While they had chosen not to have children, each had very involving careers that engaged each one emotionally, and which they readily discussed together after work hours.

When the therapist inquired about their "fun" time together, there was silence. They acknowledged that the atmosphere they created in their home was quiet and serious, with little to laugh about. While they certainly did have dinner out and attended films, carefully chosen from review lists, they did nothing that was spontaneous or particularly carefree. They were given the "homework" assignment to make two lists each. List One would have at least a dozen activities on it that Pat liked to do for relaxation, and on List Two she would put a dozen activities that to her were sexual "turn-ons" that did not involve sexual intercourse. Al would create the same kind of lists. They would not consult each other when writing their lists. Pat and Al would bring these lists to the next therapy session to be used with the therapist in facilitating communication between the couple. The "homework" would open up new avenues of exploration, in a nonthreatening way, to sharing wishes about contact and intimacy.

Role reversal. In the session, the partners will be asked to exchange places and each speak from the position of the other. The therapist may need to "coach " them to get them started in role-playing the other person. But as they get into this mini-psychodrama, they will begin to have new awareness of the feelings and position of the other that will open up new paths for communication and understanding.

Challenges to Couple Therapy

The wry notion that " if something can go wrong, it will" is certainly a thought to keep in mind as we consider the potential pitfalls for the couple therapist. Purposely placing ourselves into a relationship triangle is in itself bound to be at least uncomfortable, and at worst can feel emotionally dangerous. Let us consider some of the special elements that can create particular difficulties in this therapeutic endeavor.

To be neutral, nonjudgmental, supportive, and fair—while questioning, provoking, teaching, and challenging the couple—demands a lot of the psychotherapist!

Weeks and Hof, in their book *Integrative Solutions* (1995), remind us that many couples come into couple therapy because one or both of the parties are depressed. The authors report on some couples research data indicating that to a high degree women report marital discord as the most common life stressor as a precursor to depression. These depressed women are more likely to have a partner who has a personality disorder or a drug or alcohol problem. The research data reported also suggests that when two depressed spouses do conjoint therapy rather than individual therapy, they show improvement in the depression to the same extent as with individual therapy, and report feeling better about their marriage. Weeks and Hof theorize that a combination of antidepressive drug therapy and conjoint psychotherapy may be shown to be the most effective approach to working with couples dealing with depression.

The fact that depression, drug abuse, physical disabilities, diagnosable thought disorders, suicidal ideation, and other significant conditions do have an impact on the couple experience adds to the complexity of the assessment, treatment issues, and prognosis for successful change. Therapists who leap into the fray lacking experience and/or consultation about these particular issues will wish they had chosen another profession.

Another seemingly straightforward concern, "communication problems," usually covers a wide range of difficult underlying issues that cause the couple to struggle. Many people are initially attracted to each other because of their differences, rather than their commonalities. Thus, the pair does not realize that their communication troubles are less about self-expression and more about differences of background and culture.

We all bring distinctive styles of self-expression from our families and communities of origin into our present settings. Misunderstandings between couples often come out of the inability to speak the same cultural language. The following vignette provides an example from the author's clinical case file:

Joe and Krista maintained a strong sexual attraction for each other through fifteen chaotic years of children, job changes, and moves. They enjoyed theater trips, bridge competitions, and dinners with friends. But they continually argued over child-rearing issues, money, and how to share time. They described their fights as "emotionally exhausting." Joe would talk loudly, expressing strong emotion. He would question Krista's reasoning and debate energetically, putting forth his own position with strength. Krista would first politely explain her concerns and then become more insistent by blaming Joe for the problem. When Joe became more forceful in his verbalizations, even to the extent of using swear words, Krista would back off and either cry or withdraw into silence. This pattern was upsetting to them both.

In therapy they made the discovery that Joe's childhood urban Italian environment taught and encouraged this open, volatile, debate-oriented style of self-expression. Joe enjoyed these stimulating encounters and expected Krista to engage with him in this form of problem solving. Krista, on the other hand, grew up in the outskirts of a small Midwestern city and associated with people who expected children to be "seen and not heard" and females to be soft-spoken. Krista's father had been a dominating bully and rather frightening to her. She learned to be a "good girl" and not offer a point of view that might create any friction. She witnessed her mother manipulate to get her way by withdrawing into coldness. Joe's mother, in contrast, always jumped right into any heated discussion with a clear opinion of her own.

As Joe and Krista came to better understand the "language of culture" of the other, they were able to devise ways to problem-solve that were different from their parents', and could work for them.

Helping people to communicate differently involves a complex of issues that the therapist must be skilled enough to uncover and sort through with the couple. Communication is not just about talking. Communication is also about history and style. Effective interpersonal communication is about inquiring and listening.

Cultural differences can also complicate the relationship between the couple and the therapist. Where the therapist has no framework for understanding the background of the couple, there will be troublesome misunderstandings. If the therapist makes a ready connection with one of the parties but is less at ease with the communication style of the other, the issue of bias will surface. As couple psychotherapists, we have to be keenly aware of our own culture of language and the prejudices about style that come with us into the therapy room. When working with couples, it is all too easy to get tripped up by our own family patterns.

Couples most particularly bring ghosts into the session. All of their past lovers and intimate friends join with parents and siblings to influence and affect the pairing relationship that is in the room. There will likely be three people sitting in the room facing each other during the session, but there will be numerous others whispering their messages, unseen by the therapist.

As with other group therapies, couple psychotherapy requires that the therapist obtain some special training beyond a degree and a class that introduces concepts of family relationships. Most of the major psychotherapy-focused national organizations offer special workshops and training institutes as part of their annual conferences. Several of these same professional organizations publish journals that present updated material on couples issues.

Research and Future Trends

Outcome studies about couple psychotherapy are rare in the clinical literature. A closer look at communication styles, family patterns that influence marriage, and other yet-to-be-identified family-of-origin material will provide a challenge for future study. We would also benefit from a closer look at the dynamics of multiracial, multireligious, and mixed ethnic relationships.

Profound changes in family lifestyles are taking place as this book is being written. As divorce rates level off, people marry at later ages, fewer children per couple are born, and increasingly families are made up of large numbers of unrelated people, we will see shifts in assumptions about "healthy" family dynamics.

Attention will have to be paid to the expanding numbers of adults who choose not to marry. These unmarried adults will be found living alone as well as in long-term relationships. They may share in the raising of their own children or be part-time parent substitutes for a partner's child. Not all couples forming families are heterosexual. Growing numbers of homosexual adults are creating families and sharing, as couples, in the life of the larger community.

The changing patterns of partnerships and the subsequent impact on the rearing of the children will need further exploration, just as the impact of children and in-laws from previous relationships needs more study to illuminate how those dynamics influence the couple.

REFERENCES

Ackerman, N. (1958). *The psychodynamics of family life.* New York: Basic Books.

Ackerman, N. (1984). *A theory of family systems.* New York: Gardner Press.

Bandler, R., Grinder, J., & Satir, V. (1976). *Changing with families.* Palo Alto, CA: Behavior Books.

Barker, P. (1981). *Basic family therapy.* Baltimore: University Park Press.

Bernard, H., & MacKenzie, R. (Eds.). (1994). *Basics of group psychotherapy.* New York: Guilford Press.

Broderick, C. (1983). *The therapeutic triangle.* Beverly Hills: Sage Publications.

Budman, S. (1988). *Theory and practice of brief therapy.* New York: Guilford Press.

Colapinto, J. (1991). Structural family therapy. In A. M. Horne & L. Passmore (Eds.), *Family counseling and therapy.* Itasca, IL: Peacock Publishers.

Cooper-Lonergan, E. (1994). Using theories of group therapy. In H. Bernard & R. MacKenzie (Eds.), *Basics of group psychotherapy.* New York: Guilford Press.

Corey, G. (1990). *Theory and practice of group counseling* (Chapter 14). Pacific Grove, CA: Brooks/Cole.

Dies, R. (1992). *The efficacy and cost-effectiveness of group treatment.* Paper prepared for the AGPA annual meeting.

Durkin, H. (1964). *The group in depth.* New York: International Universities Press.

Hetherington, E. M. (1993). An overview of the Virginia longitudinal study of divorce and remarriage with a focus on early adolescence. *Journal of Family Process* (Special Edition), APA (pp. 39–55).

Humphrey, F. (1987). Treating sexual relationships in sex and couples therapy. In G. Weeks & L. Hof (Eds.),

Integrating sex and marital therapy (pp. 149–170). New York: Brunner/Mazel.

Klein, E. (1992). Contributions from social systems theory. In R. Klein, H. Bernard, & D. Singer (Eds.), *Handbook of contemporary group psychotherapy* (pp. 106–109). Madison, CT: International Universities Press.

Levant, R. (Ed.). (1993). Families in transition. *Journal of Family Psychology* (Special Issue, Vol. 7, No. 1).

Lieberman, M., Yalom, I., & Miles, M. (1973). *Encounter groups: first facts.*New York: Basic Books.

Madanes, C. (1981). *Strategic family therapy* (pp. 23–24). San Francisco: Jossey-Bass.

McKay, M., & Paleg, K. (Eds.). (1992). *Focal group psychotherapy* (Introduction). Oakland, CA: New Harbinger.

Papero, D. (1991). The Bowen theory. In A. M. Horne & L. Passmore (Eds.). *Family counseling and therapy* (pp. 48–75). Itasca, IL: F .E. Peacock.

Polster, E., & Polster, M. (1973). *Gestalt therapy integrated*. New York: Brunner/Mazel.

Powles, W. E. (1983). An overview of group methods. In H. I. Kaplan & B. J. Sadock (Eds.), *Comprehensive group psychotherapy* (pp. 71–73). Baltimore: Williams & Wilkins.

Satir, V. (1968). *Conjoint family therapy*. Palo Alto, CA: Science and Behavior Books.

Schoenholtz-Read, J. (1994). Selections of group interventions. In H. Bernard & R. MacKenzie (Eds.), *Basics of group therapy*. New York: Guilford Press.

Stuart, R. (1980). *Helping couples change*. New York: Guilford Press.

Vinogradov, W., & Yalom, I. (1989). *Group psychotherapy*. Washington, DC: American Psychiatric Press.

Visher, E., & Visher, J. (1979). *Step-families: A guide to working with stepparents and stepchildren*. New York: Brunner/Mazel.

Wallerstein, J., & Blakeslee, S. (1989). *Second chances*. New York: Ticknor & Fields.

Wallerstein, J., & Kelly, J. (1980). *Surviving the breakup: How children and parents cope with divorce*. New York: Basic Books.

Weeks, G., & Hof, L. (1995). *Integrative solutions: Treating common problems in couple therapy*. New York: Brunner/Mazel.

Wolpe, J. (1982). *The practice of behavior therapy*. New York: Pergamon Press.

Yalom, I. (1985). *The theory and practice of group psychotherapy*. New York: Basic Books.

FOR FURTHER READING

Framo, James. (1992). *Family of origin therapy: An intergenerational approach.* New York: Brunner/Mazel. *This is a fine guide to understanding individual, marital, and family problems that includes case studies to illustrate Dr. Framo's point of view about the importance of all the generations in the family.*

James, M., & Jongeward, D. (1973). *Born to win: Transactional analysis with Gestalt experiments.* Menlo Park, CA: Addison-Wesley. *An early, widely read self-help book that is solidly grounded philosophically and includes exercises for self-exploration and understanding of one's family influences.*

CHAPTER 8

BRIEF THERAPY IN CLINICAL PSYCHOLOGY

John F. Cooper

"Brief therapy" simply means therapy that takes as few sessions as possible, not even one more than is necessary, for you to develop a satisfactory solution. (Steve de Shazer, 1991a, p. x)

Brief therapy is best understood as the deliberate use of a limited number of technical and conceptual principles, applied in a focused and purposeful manner. (R. Wells, 1993, p. 5)

At core, brief therapy is defined more by an attitude than by the specific number of treatment sessions. (M. Hoyt, 1990, p. 115)

INTRODUCTION

This chapter on brief therapy (BT) is an orientation to this interesting and challenging area of clinical practice. Individual therapy is emphasized since work with couples and families could easily constitute another chapter. For similar reasons, more detailed descriptions of some of the therapeutic approaches discussed in passing here are available elsewhere in this book. Instead, we will focus on what most brief individual therapies have in common. We will also clarify definitions of brief therapy, introduce literature and research that supports its usefulness for various problems and popula-

tions, discuss models of brief treatment while emphasizing a generic approach, and touch on future trends in the field. This may not seem terribly brief, but as we will discover, the function of time is only one aspect of this approach!

Few subjects in contemporary clinical psychology have generated more passion and controversy than brief psychotherapy. In a recent example, a psychologist publicly resigned from the American Psychological Association because an organization official failed to provide a balanced, scientific perspective on the relationship between brief therapy and managed mental health care (Kalous, 1996). (As a confused Minnesota legislator once said, "sometimes you have to put aside principle and do what's right.") This controversy, both unfortunate in its divisiveness and fertile ground for informed dialogue about effective psychotherapy (Cooper, 1995; Koss & Shiang, 1994), exists for a number of reasons.

First, the concern in the last twenty years, especially by insurance companies and businesses, of providing cost-effective treatment to offset rising health care costs (Broskowski, 1991) has led to a clinical practice style that emphasizes brief forms of psychotherapy, accountability for outcomes, accessibility to treatment by large numbers of people, interaction with medical settings, group practices, and eclectic treatment methods (Bennett, 1988; Johnson, 1995; Sabin, 1991; Shiang & Bongar, 1995). This has forced many reluctant clinicians, typically with longer term psychodynamic backgrounds, to change their practice approaches (Austad & Hoyt, 1992; Budman, 1989; Davanloo, 1979; Hoyt, 1987; Johnson, 1995).

In this connection, brief therapy has become too narrowly and emotionally overidentified with managed mental health care. Indeed, a recent news article announces that with 100 million Americans now insured through managed care: "Gone are the years of examining one's childhood on the psychiatrist's couch. Instead patients are urged to forget the past and focus on the here-and-now. The goal is to develop a practical plan to get functioning again. The briefer, the better" (Meisel, 1995, p. 1E). Although this appears to be generally true, if glibly observed, there is also increasing and counterbalancing awareness among third-party payers and the treatment establishment that "the bulk of mental health treatment cost is consumed by inpatient care and that outpatient treatment, even long-term psychotherapy, is not only salubrious for the patient but far less costly" (Yalom, 1995, p. xi).

A second reason for controversy is that despite an ostensible awareness of cost-efficiency in the everyday practice of psychology, it is not clear that most psychologists have an adequate grasp of what brief therapy is. Although certain authors emphasize brief therapy as the new standard of practice (e.g., Johnson, 1995; Wells, 1993), a recent psychotherapy textbook (Corsini & Wedding, 1995), for example, contains only one specific reference to brief therapy. Additionally, recent surveys give a mixed picture of clinician acceptance of brief therapy. From a sample of California psychologists, Bolter, Levenson, and Alverez (1990) confirmed the estimate of Wells and Gianetti (1990) that only about 30% of therapists actually use brief treatment primarily despite overwhelming evidence of its efficacy (Bloom, 1992). Levenson, Speed, and Budman (1992), on the other hand, found that of 701 psychologists in California and Massachusetts, over 80% used some sort of brief therapy, but only

40% of the time. Thirty percent of this group had no training in brief therapy. Indeed, managed care officials do not even assume that the therapists they contract with know how to do brief therapy (Meisel, 1995) and Koss and Shiang (1994) have advocated for continuing education and training in this area for psychologists.

Of crucial importance to the acceptance of BT is the apparent fact that the attitudes and values that characterize brief therapists are often at odds with what Bloom (1992) calls a "deeply ingrained mental health professional values system" (p. 5). This reflects the belief—research to the contrary notwithstanding—that brief therapy is superficial in its approach to problems and that the longer and "deeper" the treatment, the better (Hoyt, 1987).

Another reason for controversy and confusion about brief therapy lies in the sheer proliferation of types of psychotherapy for every imaginable problem, with relatively few clinicians adhering dogmatically to a single system and with no particular system dominating outcome studies (Norcross & Newman, 1992; Orlinsky & Howard, 1995). Nearly 400 current psychotherapies now exist (Miller, Hubble, & Duncan, 1995), although relatively few methods of psychotherapy, all of them intrinsically brief and most of them cognitive-behavioral (CBT), have actually been proved effective in controlled research (Chambliss, 1996; Kingsbury, 1995; Norcross, 1995). The advantages and merits of brief versus long-term therapy also continue to be debated.

There is confusion about terms often used to characterize and differentiate brief therapies such as *time-sensitive* versus *time-limited*, *short-term*, or even *intermittent* psychotherapy (Budman & Gurman, 1988), as well as the determination of various kinds of brief therapy to separate themselves from an emphasis on doing fewer than a "standard" number of visits (e.g., de Shazer, 1991a). Such exclusive emphasis on the use and role of time in brief therapy loses sight of the fact that few therapies have rigid notions about the number of sessions to be used (e.g., Mann, 1973). Rather, they are mostly concerned with employing certain values, techniques, and relationship stances that make relatively efficient use of time or shorter therapy duration a natural by-product or consequence, not the goal, of treatment (Cooper, 1995).

Furthermore, many therapies, such as CBT or structural family therapy, have qualities, as we shall see, that make them inherently brief, although they are not typically thought of in this way (e.g., Aponte, 1992).

A (VERY) BRIEF HISTORY OF BRIEF THERAPY

It is a little recognized fact that Sigmund Freud, who is typically associated with long-term therapy, actually saw many patients for a few visits. He also had a number of single-session "cures," notably of the famed musician Gustav Mahler's impotency (Bloom, 1992; Messer & Warren, 1995). (It seems unavoidable even in passing not to link Freud and sex!)

Messer and Warren (1995) trace the roots of contemporary brief dynamic psychotherapy to two former students of Freud, Sandor Ferenczi (1920/1960) and Otto Rank (1929/1978) as well as their work together (Ferenczi & Rank, 1925/1986). In essence, Ferenczi and Rank eschewed passive, academic analysis of patients in favor of a more pragmatic, active, emotionally intensive, and focused model with a sensitivity to time limits in therapy. Today, their model would also be seen as having behavioral, integrative, and developmental aspects. For example, in Rank's case, the notion of promoting lifelong growth in a person rather than cure was stressed.

Alexander and French (1946) pioneered shorter term work with large populations adapting techniques from analysis that gave "rational aid to all those who show early signs of maladjustment" (p. 341). Additionally, they began to emphasize the idea of a "corrective emotional experience" that relied heavily on the quality of the therapeutic relationship and the flexibility of the therapist to respond emotionally to the patient, intermittent breaks in therapy to make therapy applications to life, and early goal establishment (Messer & Warren, 1995).

Much of the impetus for brief therapy came from emergency situations, such as treating the trauma of World War II veterans and the classic study on victims of the Coconut Grove nightclub fire trauma (Lindemann, 1944). The significant social turmoil of the 1960s, combined with the Community Mental Health Centers Act under the Kennedy administration, led to the widespread availability of mental health services and substantial patient demand, but with consequent staff shortages. Additionally, theoretical evolution in psychotherapy led to the development of shorter term psychodynamic, behavioral, and pragmatic family-based treatments (Budman & Gurman, 1988; Koss & Butcher, 1986).

Although the past 20 years have seen an enormous expansion of brief therapy, in many ways it is not a new concept. Mahoney (1995), for example, traces some aspects of cognitive therapy to the Stoics and Epicureans. Johnson (1995) has observed with respect to solution-focused therapy that the therapist functions in the manner of the leader described by Lao-Tse—that is, one who helps people think they did the work themselves. Similarly, the notion of elaborating on the intrinsic wisdom within clients via questioning has Socratic roots (Cooper, 1995).

DEFINITIONS

The reader is referred to the quotes at the beginning of this chapter for succinct definitions of BT. It is most important to understand that *brief therapy* is a generic term for treatment that takes many forms. *Short-term therapy* is commonly used synonymously with *brief therapy*, and is usually contrasted with "long-term" therapy along the dimension of treatment duration. However, the concepts of both BT and long-term treatment are too narrowly, if not altogether wrongly, defined only in terms of elapsed calendar time or total number of visits (Cooper, 1995).

For example, some brief therapies can range in the time they plan for treatment from one (e.g., Bloom, 1981, 1992; Talmon, 1990) to 40 sessions (e.g., Malan, 1976). The latter number far exceeds the average number of 6 to 8 visits for therapy of any kind (Garfield, 1978). Many brief therapists (e.g., Norcross, 1995; Koss & Shiang, 1994) would suggest 26 visits as an upper limit for brief therapy on the basis of the criterion of treatment duration alone, in large part because this is where the relative benefits of treatment start to diminish (Howard, Kopta, Krause, & Orlinsky, 1986). However, this whole matter of time and treatment outcome is complicated. We will return to it shortly.

In practice, long-term treatment or treatment in which time is not planfully considered a treatment factor is often episodic. Brief treatments also may be planned as "intermittent" rather than done continuously in the artificial convention of weekly 50-minute sessions (e.g., Kreilkamp, 1989). Brief therapy may even be done for years with challenging problems such as chronic depression or severe abuse and trauma (see, e.g., Dolan, 1991). It is also possible to have few sessions over a long period of time, or many sessions in, say, a period of weeks, or sessions of 20 minutes or 2 hours, and still meet the criteria for brief therapy (Hoyt, 1990; Johnson, 1995). Thus, many brief therapists prefer the term *time-sensitive therapy* to describe BT (e.g., Budman & Gurman, 1988), as this more accurately describes therapy in which time is flexibly and optimally used to meet the demands of a given situation or client.

Finally, there are a group of brief therapies that do in fact set predetermined limits, typically of 10 or 12 visits, and are commonly referred to as *time-limited* (e.g., Time-Limited Dynamic Psychotherapy; Strupp & Binder, 1984; Levenson, 1995). Mann (1973; Mann & Goldman, 1982), for example, sets a rigid limit of 12 visits for every patient in the belief that this facilitates a necessary confrontation with termination and increases focus and motivation for change. At the Mental Research Institute (MRI), therapists adhere to a 10-session model, not so much because it is intrinsic to their theory of practice but for research purposes and convenience. Interestingly, John Weakland of the MRI (see Watzlawick, Weakland, & Fisch, 1974) has confessed to a colleague that this limit tends not to apply in their private practices: "While I am known as a brief therapist, sometimes I do extended brief therapy. I usually blame myself when that happens, but sometimes I can blame the patient" (Johnson, 1995, p. 123).

It is also difficult to distinguish long-term and brief therapies solely on the basis of their structural or technical components. Both share many common processes, including specific therapist activities such as the use of interpretation, confrontation, and nonspecific factors such as support and reassurance (Koss & Butcher, 1986).

Long-term therapy has been defined as "recapitulating one's personal history with a stable figure" (Budman & Gurman, 1988; Budman, Hoyt, & Friedman, 1992). Essentially this means that unlike most brief therapies, long-term therapy places a fundamental emphasis on reviewing, if not reliving, one's past in the presence of a presumably mature and "benevolent" parent figure (alas, not always the case!) who can help correct the presumed contributions of the past to the problems of the present. Additionally, "the passive, vaguely authoritarian approach in some analytic work, its primary emphasis on understanding or resolving internal conflicts not in a patient's awareness, often vague goals and outcome criteria, assumption of resistance and the assumed need for lengthy, frequent, and otherwise rigidly or arbitrarily scheduled treatment are inconsistent with most BT" (Cooper, 1995, p. 8).

SHARED VALUES

Apart from these subtle between-group distinctions, most brief therapies are distinguished from long-term therapy by the intentional use of particular concepts and principles in a focused, purposeful way (Wells, 1993); that is to say, they share a set of clinical features and, perhaps most important, a value orientation that distinguish them from long-term therapy and unite them despite their variety (Pekarik, 1990b).

Budman and Gurman (1988) and Hoyt (1985) have provided a benchmark set of value distinctions for brief therapy from which the following list (adapted from Cooper, 1995) is derived. The shared values of BT include the following:

1. An emphasis on pragmatism, parsimony, and least intrusive treatment versus "cure"; a belief that small changes can set larger changes in motion.

This recognizes that most problems do not require "major surgery" but can be approached practically and conservatively. Even problems that do require significant intervention should generally be considered for conservative treatment first since they may still improve. An interesting illustration of this is the fact that about 15% of people improve between the time they schedule an appointment and the time they are actually seen for mental health treatment! (Howard et al., 1986). The idea of a cure in brief therapy is also less important than the idea that therapy can facilitate change or coping processes that for most people occasionally become derailed or "stuck." In this way, brief therapists can be viewed as much like family doctors, who may see someone periodically over years when care is needed (Johnson, 1995).

2. A recognition that human change is inevitable as opposed to the idea that change cannot occur without therapy. This can be considered an essentially optimistic view of human potential and human nature, insofar as therapy is typically seen as only one of many ways—albeit a good one—of obtaining desirable change. Numerous observers such as Alfie Kohn (1990) have taken psychology to task for the preoccupation of many of its practitioners and researchers, especially those who are analytically inclined, to explain behavior only from self-serving and negative perspectives!

3. A belief that small changes in behavior often will lead to larger ones. This recognizes that the value of therapy generally and BT particularly may be in its catalytic effects (Eckert, 1993).

4. An emphasis on client strengths and resources (versus pathology) and on the legitimacy of presenting complaints. This is not to say that therapists do not explicitly challenge clients' perceptions, goals, or behavior, nor does it suggest that brief therapists necessarily take clients' presentations at face value. However, it is in contrast to the notions that the therapist always knows what is best for clients and that the presenting problem is only a symptom of deeper pathology necessarily

requiring treatment. Brief therapists recognize that most people's lives are their own to manage and that people ultimately have the say about what problems they want to work on. Brief therapy also explicitly searches for ways in which people are coping well or have coped successfully and tries to build on this.

5. Recognition that most change occurs outside of therapy as opposed to happening in session within the necessary presence of a therapist. To paraphrase a saying, "Life happens." Although it appears that the quality of the therapeutic relationship figures preeminently toward a therapeutic outcome (Burns & Nolan-Hoeksema, 1992; Miller, Hubble, & Duncan, 1995; Lambert & Bergin, 1994), it is not the only factor and cannot, practically or even desirably, exist 24 hours a day. As one client explained in canceling her initial appointment: "My husband just died, so I don't need to come in."

6. A commitment to ensuring that a client's outside life is more important than therapy. This suggests quintessentially the willingness for brief therapists to make themselves unnecessary. The fact is, after all, that more than one client has been known, often understandably, to say in some form or another: "I can't pay for the therapy because I'm going to Acapulco."

7. An understanding that therapy is not always helpful. While it is well established that psychotherapy—brief therapy, particularly—is helpful for many people and problems (Lambert & Bergin, 1994; Lipsey & Wilson, 1993), it is relatively rare that psychologists or the popular media acknowledge what is clear every day in clinical practice: Significant numbers of people do not benefit from psychotherapy even over time and may, in fact, deteriorate with treatment (see Lambert & Bergin, 1994, for a partial review). This is true not only for the obvious and egregious cases of sexual impropriety by therapists with clients, but in the course of well-established and well-intended treatments (e.g., Ogles, Lambert, & Sawyer, 1993) or ordinary

therapeutic transactions and impasses (Omer, 1994; Sachs, 1983). LeShan (1990) also observes that psychology has not met the great challenges of the human condition, such as poverty, war, racism, pollution, or other forms of self-destructive behavior. This suggests that therapy has been oversold as a solution to many problems.

8. A belief that therapy should not be "timeless" or unending. This tenet suggests that therapists and clients should always have in mind an answer to the question: How will we know when therapy is done? Additionally, to illustrate the idea that nothing happens in therapy over years that could not happen in much shorter periods, Michael Hoyt tells a story of visiting Malan's (1963) famous Tavistock Clinic in London, where he was told: "Here at Tavistock we allow trainees 35 to 40 sessions. It allows for wasting time and making mistakes." Hoyt's reply: "Well, in America we're more efficient. We find that we can waste time and make mistakes in 12 sessions!" (Hoyt, 1990, p. 120). Although the whole enterprise of studying time limits is full of challenges (see Koss & Shiang, 1994), some research supports the idea that explicitly defining time limits is therapeutic (e.g., Sledge, Moras, Hartley, & Levine, 1990), while other research finds no difference in outcomes between time-limited and time-unlimited therapy (e.g., Luborsky, Singer, & Luborsky, 1975), arguing implicitly for the former.

A survey of 222 randomly selected psychologists by Bolter et al. (1990) lends support to the idea that brief and long-term therapists can indeed be distinguished by their assumptions regarding behavioral change principles. These researchers found that short-term therapists valued an awareness of time limits more than long-term therapists, who supported the idea of "timelessness" as an important therapy quality. Moreover, short-term therapists tended to see that change was possible in a short period, whereas long-term therapists emphasized the more immutable aspects of personality. The groups did not differ on a number of qualities, however, including the importance of major goal definition, focusing on weaknesses or strengths of patients, perceptions of change, or the importance of therapy.

With respect to experienced clinicians, at least, when therapists become more accepting of these values, their effectiveness with clients can actually increase as measured by lower dropout rates, recidivism, and clinical improvement (Burlingame, Fuhriman, Paul, & Ogles, 1989).

BRIEF THERAPY: TECHNICAL FEATURES

In addition to a unifying set of values, most brief therapies share a number of technical features (Bloom, 1992; Cooper, 1995; Koss & Butcher, 1986; Koss & Shiang, 1994; Pekarik, 1990b; Wells, 1993):

1. Determining and maintaining a clear, specific focus. As the saying goes, "If you don't know where you're going, you'll wind up somewhere else." Commonly, clients do not necessarily know what they want out of therapy, or they may have many concerns, often ill defined. A good brief therapist will help organize these in understandable language with recognizable outcomes. Multiple problems are given priorities, and changes in focus are negotiated so as not to lose track of progress. Any confusion or misunderstanding about the purpose and methods of the therapy is immediately addressed.

2. Conscientious and (generally) flexible use of time. Rather than assuming that all clients need or want weekly 50-minute visits for an indefinite period—an odd convention when one thinks about it apart from scheduling convenience—this principle means that time is used to meet the demands of a given situation (see Hoyt, 1990, for a discussion). Thus, the length, frequency, or intensity of session can vary considerably in BT. Someone initially in crisis might be seen twice a week for a couple of weeks or for a lengthy single session and then taper to biweekly or triweekly to allow for practice effects or homework to be implemented. Phone contacts may be used episodically or contacts of shorter than an hour for maintenance and review purposes. Some therapists (e.g., Butler, Strupp, & Binder, 1992; Horowitz et al., 1984; Mann, 1973) limit visits at the outset for motivational reasons or

to facilitate the resolution of transference issues. Other therapists (e.g., Budman & Gurman, 1988; 1992) advocate setting or negotiating time limits beforehand to facilitate focus; others do this more implicitly by suggesting early and regular evaluations of progress (Johnson, 1995). Additionally, many disorders (e.g., panic disorders and unipolar depression) have been shown to respond specifically to structured, time-limited interventions, typically falling within a 12- to 18-visit range in empirical studies for CBT (see Barlow, 1993) and interpersonal therapy. Many people wrongly think BT is treatment that is rushed or pressured but this simply describes poorly done counseling. Importantly, the matter of limited visits by insurers for cost reasons is dubious, if not counterproductive in its effects, and should not be confused with therapeutic time limits. Finally, it should also be noted that the part of the value of negotiating time expectations and limits with clients is to avoid the finding of Pekarik and Finney-Owen (1987) that therapists significantly overestimate how much therapy patients want. An illustration of this follows:

Irving Yalom (1989), a highly regarded existential therapist with a long-term "depth" orientation, tells the story of his encounter with "Penny," a woman disturbed about significant losses in her life. She wishes to see him in the three months he has before he takes a sabbatical. Against his better judgment, since he believes three months of regular visits are inadequate for "decent" therapy, Yalom sees her. Despite a good outcome and a satisfied patient, Yalom remains dissatisfied regarding the depth of therapy he has achieved as insufficient to manage "death anxiety." He sees the patient's rapid progress as exceptional, rather than examining further how he helped her accomplish results in a comparatively short time. In other words, Yalom seems unable to reconcile the patient's experience with his own expectations and needs (Cooper, 1995, p. 30).

3. Limited goals with well-defined outcomes. It is difficult to imagine psychotherapy of any kind that doesn't have some kind of objective. Even if clients want to achieve world peace through psychotherapy, it would have to be accomplished in some stepwise fashion. In BT, goals are overtly negotiated with clients and defined specifically within problem areas. For example, a therapist would ask: What would world peace look like? How would we know it was improved? What exactly would be different? The importance of achievable, observable, behaviorally defined outcomes is in part to increase optimism about and recognition of success for clients and to justify to insurance reviewers why treatment is necessary and effective. Significantly, the very act of establishing and working purposively toward objectives appears to have salutary effects on people (see Csikszentmihaly, 1990, and Myers, 1992, for a discussion).

4. A focus on present stresses and symptoms. Just as most brief therapists do not assume the need for "depth" or historical recapitulation in therapy, neither do they necessarily ignore these as factors in problem development or resolution. However, BT emphasizes making relatively quick transitions from past to the present, because once we know "why," we are still left with "now what?" It also recognizes that many people tend to be satisfied with "symptom relief" and to leave treatment when they get it (e.g., Pekarik, 1983).

5. Rapid initial assessment and integration of assessment to treatment. This therapeutic stance has been characterized as "ready, fire, aim" by O'Hanlon and Weiner-Davis (1989, from Peters and Waterman, 1982). When enough information to justify a working diagnosis or hypothesis about problems is available, trial interventions are discussed and attempted, thus creating a continuous process of diagnosis through action (Wells, 1993). This is not done hastily or carelessly, however. This concept benefits from therapist experience, confidence, skill (Stein & Lambert, 1995), and a willingness to make adjustments if one is "wrong."

6. Routine review of progress and abandonment of ineffective interventions. Consistent with the idea that a failed intervention is simply another opportunity to define better solutions, a good brief therapist will rigorously track the usefulness of the

therapy, through both subjective and objective inquiry. Many clinicians also track the quality of the therapeutic relationship because this appears to be such a significant contributor to outcome (e.g., Burns & Nolan-Hoeksema, 1992; see also Miller et al., 1995).

7. A high level of client–therapist activity. Therapists collaboratively and actively strive to engage clients in a change process. Questioning, educating, clarifying, problem solving, and hypothesis testing are common interactional components of BT. The typical therapist stance of BT in this regard is captured in Eric Berne's question: "What can I do to cure this patient today?" (quoted in Hoyt, 1990). Clients are typically assigned "homework" (something specific to do or think about) to facilitate progress between sessions.

8. The creation of a safe and comfortable environment for emotional expression. Some brief therapists, particularly some psychodynamic ones (e.g., Davanloo, 1979, 1988; Sifneos, 1992; and to some extent Malan, 1963, 1986a, 1986b), are deliberately evocative of affect as a "curative" factor. Other clinicians may place greater emphasis on cognitive or behavioral contributions to change. The forceful, authoritarian stance of these styles, particularly Davanloo's, has come under criticism (see Messer & Warren, 1995, for a review) and does not reflect general brief therapy practice. Almost all brief therapists, however, try to establish an atmosphere of collaboration, understanding, and compassion, which allows for appropriate emotional expression by clients.

9. A practical and eclectic use of treatment techniques. Bloom (1992) has observed that Wolberg, for example, incorporates "teaching, relaxation tapes, hypnosis, homilies, direct suggestion, psychoactive drugs, catharsis, faith, counting on good luck, dream interpretation and crisis intervention" (p. 42). Essentially, however, this principle means that technique does not define brief therapy but is used in service of it. Although the use of manualized treatments and technical purity appears to have re-

search and therapeutic value (Chambliss, 1996), technique contributes less to outcome than do relationship factors such as interpersonal skills and therapist attitudes of warmth and genuineness (Stein & Lambert, 1995; Miller et al., 1995; Lambert & Bergin, 1994; also see Rubin & Niemeier, 1992), which, of course, in themselves involve technique (Mahoney & Norcross, 1993; also see Sachs, 1983). More to the point, familiarity with a broad range of current research and practice allows therapists to tailor treatment more efficiently, confidently, and competently to the individual needs of patients.

CLIENT SELECTION FOR BRIEF THERAPY

Some clinicians (e.g., Shiang & Bongar, 1995), especially those with a psychodynamic inclination (for discussions, see Bloom, 1992; Messer & Warren, 1995; Wells & Gianetti, 1990) emphasize the importance of client selection or exclusion as a distinguishing technical component of BT. Typically, these exclusions include such treatment-resistant conditions as antisocial personalities (see Lykken, 1995), lack of reality testing as in schizophrenia, a history of unsuccessful and presumably competent prior treatment or trial interventions, inadequate motivation for change, and difficulty forming relationships (Donovan, 1987; Ursano, Sonnenberg, & Lazar, 1991). However, as Bloom (1992) correctly observes, these exclusions from brief treatment, broadly and integratively considered, appear grounded in theory rather than empirical evidence. For example, Donovan (1987) expands the applicability of brief dynamic psychotherapies to larger populations of patients by shifting the treatment focus to "pathogenic beliefs" (see Weiss, Sampson, & the Mount Zion Research Group, 1986) rather than the Oedipal conflicts usually associated with dynamic thinking, but the justification for doing so is experiential and theoretical rather than empirical.

Further, there is little if any evidence that psychotherapy of any kind works with the difficult conditions just mentioned (Kingsbury, 1995; Maxmen & Ward, 1995) and as Cooper (1995) notes, if treatment involving these conditions does work, it is likely to involve not only essential relationship factors but "the use over time of such BT hallmarks as establishing treatment priorities; focusing; taking small, concrete steps; regular evaluations of progress and the use of adjunctive support" (p. 11).

WHY PRACTICE BT?

It is probably wise to remember the words of Disraeli when considering the use of data to support a particular position: "There are three kinds of lies: lies, damned lies, and statistics." With respect to the data that follows, however, we can fall back on the comforting thoughts of yet another Minnesota legislator: "These are not my figures I'm quoting, they're the figures of someone who knows what they're talking about."

1. Data supporting the overall efficacy of individual, family, and marital therapy across clients with a variety of presentations is, in fact, research of unplanned, time-unlimited "unacknowledged" brief treatment with patients of less than 20 visits (Budman & Gurman, 1988; Koss & Shiang, 1994).

2. All of the empirically validated treatments to date are intrinsically brief. There are no empirically validated studies of "long-term" treatments. Despite over 400 current psychotherapies (Miller et al., 1995), relatively few methods of psychotherapy have actually been proved effective in controlled research (Norcross, 1995; Kingsbury, 1995). Of the 47 empirically validated treatments identified so far, most are cognitive-behavioral, three are psychodynamic, and one experiential (Chambliss, 1996). Svartburg and Stiles's (1991) meta-analysis of dynamic brief therapy outcomes actually favored CBT treatment but may have had methodological problems (see Messer & Warren, 1995, for a review and critique). Although the bulk of empirical evidence could be seen as favoring treatment with cognitive-behavioral components (see Lambert & Bergin, 1994; Shapiro & Shapiro, 1982), more recent meta-analyses of brief dynamic and/or interpersonal variant therapies (Crits-

Christoph, 1992; Digueur et al., 1993) and comparative studies with respect to depression (e.g., Shapiro et al., 1994) have found dynamic brief therapies as effective as other treatments. In summary, the following may be concluded about what we know at this time regarding individual psychotherapy effectiveness (Kingsbury, 1995, p. 8):

> Behavioral and cognitive behavioral therapies have more consistent and lasting effects than the medications in the treatment of panic disorder, agoraphobia, simple phobias and, to a lesser extent, social phobias. Medications and behavioral techniques are equally effective in obsessive-compulsive disorder, post-traumatic disorder, and generalized disorder. Behavioral therapies of the kind originally developed by Masters and Johnson are more effective than medications in the treatment of sexual dysfunction.
>
> Medications are only temporarily helpful for insomnia, which is more effectively treated with behavioral therapy. In the treatment of major depression without psychotic features, behavioral, cognitive behavioral and interpersonal psychotherapies are as effective as antidepressant drugs. Psychodynamic therapies are less useful but better than placebo.

3. BT corresponds to most patients' (not necessarily most therapists'!) use and expectations of treatment. Most patients average between 5 and 8 visits for therapy regardless of other factors (Garfield, 1986, 1994; Phillips, 1985), corresponding to their own estimates of needing 6 to 10 visits to finish treatment (Garfield, 1978; Pekarik & Finney-Owen, 1987). Recent analysis of the National Medical Expenditures Survey (Olfson & Pincus, 1994), HMO patient data (Craven, 1996; DeLeon, VandenBos, & Bulatao, 1991), and general populations (Taube, Goldman, Burns, & Kessler, 1988) suggests that the vast majority, perhaps up to 85%, of patients are seen for fewer than 11 visits and the modal number of outpatient visits may be as few as one (Garfield, 1986; Hoyt, Rosenbaum, & Talmon, 1992; National Institute of Mental Health [NIMH], 1981). Interestingly, Pekarik and Finney-Owen (1987) found that therapists believed patients needed three times the number of sessions that patients themselves estimated,

a finding that may have roots in consistent data showing that a relatively small number of patients, who are likely to be more memorable to therapists, consume therapy resources disproportionately (Taube et al., 1988).

4. The greatest proportion of treatment gain is obtained early in treatment, perhaps in 6 to 8 sessions (Smith, Glass, & Miller, 1980). Significant clinical relief or return to normal functioning has been found to occur in less than 5 visits for over 50% of people and in 14 sessions for chronic distress, apart from character considerations (Kopta, Howard, Lowry, & Beutler, 1994). According to Howard et al.'s (1986) dose–effect meta-analysis, 62% of people can be expected to significantly improve by 13 visits, with increasing effort required for small increments of change up to, and particularly beyond, 26 visits.

5. Most outcome data indicate that planned BT is at least as effective as long-term treatment. Koss and Butcher (1986) found few studies directly comparing short-term and long-term therapy, and these had equivalent outcomes, implicitly favoring the latter as treatment of choice (Wells, 1993). It should be noted, however, that the comparability of outcomes is disputed for reasons including the use and comparison of averaged data to unique individuals and situations (Beutler, 1991; LeShan, 1990; Persons, 1991). With respect to dose–response studies that suggest "more therapy is better," the confounding of chronological time with time spent in sessions is commonplace (Koss & Butcher, 1986).

The most frequently referenced study in favor of long-term treatment is the meta-analysis of Howard et al. (1986), who found a steady increase in therapy benefits over time. However, this research is criticized by Pekarik (1990b) for using studies employing "nonstandard" therapy practices and median visits considerably exceeding the norm, emphasizing therapist-rated outcomes— which are notoriously incompatible with patient perceptions, the use of "unusual" settings, and the exclusion of CBT approaches. More recently, a

large-scale "naturalistic survey" (Seligman, 1995) found that patients did better the longer they were in therapy, although data appear grouped by chronological time rather than by number of visits. This research, though not necessarily incompatible with the implementation of BT as we have discussed it, has also come under substantial criticism. Jacobson (1996), for example, notes the small size of the responses in relation to the sample, and suggests it favors the more responsive "worried well" and relies on highly inaccurate retrospective memory and self-reports. Individual studies are mixed on this issue. For example, in a controlled study of family therapy, Smyrnios and Kirby (1993) found that families receiving relatively less therapy had the best outcomes, perhaps enhanced by an attitude of therapist confidence in their coping.

6. "Medical offset" literature suggests that even one therapeutic interview, let alone a planned course of BT, can substantially reduce the use of medical services by patients for a period of years (see Bloom, 1992, for a partial review).

7. BT appears to attenuate many of the factors associated with early dropouts insofar as intervening actively, concretely, and positively in the intake has a desirable effect on patient satisfaction and retention (Adams, Piercy, & Jurich, 1991; Mohl, Martinez, Ticknor, Huang, & Cordell, 1991; Sledge et al., 1990). Further, although dropouts or premature termination is a complex phenomenon with multiple, probably interactive variables (Garfield, 1986, 1994), the fact that patients drop out of therapy or finish before their therapists think they should does not necessarily mean patients are dissatisfied with treatment or have not made progress (Bloom, 1992; Pekarik, 1983, 1990a). A conscientious brief therapist still follows up with dropouts, however.

8. Increasingly, third-party payers and regulatory agencies are demanding efficiency, effectiveness, and outcome-supported interventions—all of which are compatible with brief treatment principles (Craven, 1996; Meisol, 1995).

9. BT is ethically consistent with the health care principles of patient autonomy, informed consent, and beginning with the least intrusive treatment (Pekarik, 1990a; 1990b).

THE LIMITS OF BRIEF THERAPY

Why is an awareness of psychotherapy applications and limitations important to brief therapy? Cooper (1995) has suggested that for any therapy to be effective, let alone efficient, the essential ingredients are a reasonably motivated client, a problem amenable to treatment, and a capable therapist. In the absence of these factors, or—this is most important—a therapist's failure to recognize their absence, psychotherapy will not only fail, but may even become, to paraphrase Hobbes's view of life, "nasty, brutish, and long."

This is not to say that despite initial misgiving, one should not try psychotherapy for most patients who request it. For the brief therapist, however, it does mean becoming educated about what kinds of people are most likely to benefit at what time from what kind of treatment with what kind of clinician, conscientiously monitoring progress, and being willing to say when treatment is not working.

We have already observed that many authors consider brief therapy inappropriate for severe psychopathology, including such conditions as some personality disorders, a lack of reality testing, a history of unsuccessful prior treatment or trial interventions, or poor or inadequate motivation for change. Other authors (e.g., Bloom, 1992; Cooper, 1995) have suggested, however, that this describes the limits not simply of brief treatment, but of any psychotherapy. With regard to antisocial behavior and personalities, for example, despite a patently rich descriptive understanding of these enormous problems, there is no known "cure" for them (Gibbs, 1995; Lykken, 1995; Vachss, 1993). Similarly, such problems as schizophrenic spectrum disorders (Shriqui & Nasrallah, 1995) and manic-phase bipolar illness (Maxmen & Ward, 1995) are not yet fundamentally amenable to any non-pharmacological treatments, although adjunctive psychotherapy can certainly be helpful (Kingsbury, 1995).

Regarding personality disorders, some brief therapists (e.g., Pekarik, 1990a) consider treating personality as immaterial to treating specific patient complaints, especially since there is little evidence supporting personality change in therapy. Nevertheless, Winston et al. (1994) report success with various personality disorders in a controlled study using two dynamic approaches that are debatably "brief" (40-session). Similarly, other psychodynamic authors (e.g., Lazarus, 1982; Leibovich, 1981) report success treating severe personality disorders, perhaps because help is offered in concrete, limited, "respectful" ways (Donovan, 1987). Cognitive-behavioral therapy (e.g., Beck, Freeman, et al., 1990) focuses on personality change indirectly, through attention to other specific problems related to personality, such as self-efficacy, that may facilitate broader personality changes. Linehan (Linehan & Kehrer, 1993) has developed an empirically validated "metaparadoxical" approach with borderline personality disorder that is compatible with BT principles and incorporates dynamic, strategic, CBT, and interpersonal elements. Similarly, Budman and Gurman (1988) illustrate an integrated way of dealing briefly with personality disorders that "intrude" in therapy.

A word is also in order here regarding the issue of substance abuse, which is another typical exclusion from BT. Compelling arguments exist (e.g., Budman & Gurman, 1988; Dubovsky, 1993; Gitlin, 1990, 1996) for not doing therapy with active substance abusers, highlighting, for example, the difficulty of separating depression from the effects of excessive alcohol intake. However, good examples of productive work with substance abusers in cognitive (Beck, Wright, & Newman, 1992; McCrady, 1993) and solution-focused or strategic (Berg & Miller, 1992b; Johnson, 1995; Miller & Berg, 1995; Todd & Selekman, 1991) ways have been published. As Cooper (1995) observes, these approaches "emphasize accurate assessment of motivational levels for any behavior change (see Prochaska, 1992), cooperatively engaging patients to use their strengths at the level they are willing to change, and capitalizing on these successes to move toward recovery" (p. 10).

AN OVERVIEW OF VARIOUS BT APPROACHES AND CRISIS THERAPY

A fuller discussion of many of the therapies discussed next can be found in Chapter 6. The reader is encouraged to think of many of the models mentioned here, especially the dynamic approaches, not simply as longer approaches done in shorter time, but as distinctive in themselves. Table 8.1 compares some aspects of various forms of BT.

As noted earlier, several hundred psychotherapies exist, and a good share of these appear to be at least intrinsically brief. Koss and Butcher (1986) listed over 50 forms in their review, but this is clearly a substantial underestimate.

Despite the use of manuals to try to achieve technical purity of application for various therapies, and despite apparent theoretical differences in approaches, the extent to which these differences are "purely" applied in practice is unclear. It has been shown, for example, that therapists applying the same treatment can have quite different outcomes (Luborsky, McClellan, Woody, O'Brien, & Auerbach, 1985).

Moreover, there is a good deal of cross-fertilization across therapies. Donovan (1987), for instance, expands the applicability of brief dynamic therapy by challenging clients' "pathogenic beliefs," which he calls closer to a personality structure than a cognitive function, but which is nonetheless easily seen as cognitive. Bloom (1992) notes that most dynamic therapies are now more interpersonal than intrapersonal. Similarly, a cognitive therapist, Mahoney (1993, 1995) acknowledges this approach's increasing recognition of the importance of "unconscious" (note the dynamic overtones), constructivist (i.e., reality is in the eyes of the viewer), and interpersonal processes. Quick (1995) combines the emphasis of strategic brief therapy on clarification of a problem and interruption of what does not work, with solution-focused brief therapy's emphasis on amplifying exceptions to the rule of a behavior. Johnson and Miller (1994) link solution-

Table 8.1 Comparison of Selected Brief Therapies

APPROACH	CLIENT ACCEPTANCE RATE[a]	BASIC TREATMENT FOCUS	KEY TECHNIQUES
Dynamic			
Mann	Low	Separation anxiety	Transference interpretation
Davanloo	Low	Pre-Oedipal; Oedipal conflicts	Confrontation; interpretation
Gustafson	Low to moderate	"Faults" produced from early trauma	Empathic companionship; interpretation
Wolberg	Moderate to high	Presenting complaint	Flexible; interpretation
Sifneos	Low	Oedipal conflicts	Confrontation; interpretation
Interpersonal	Moderate to high	Interpersonal role disputes, transitions, deficits; grief	Communication and decision analysis; expansion of options
Cognitive-Behavioral			
Beck	High	Cognitive distortions	Collaborative empiricism; cognitive restructuring
Ellis	Moderate to high	Irrational beliefs	Rational disputation; homework
Strategic			
Erickson	High	Presenting problem	Direct, indirect suggestion
Solution-focused	High	Intrinsic solutions to presenting problems	Strategic questioning; use of exceptions

Source: Adapted from Cooper (1995). Adapted in part from Donovan (1987).
[a]Estimated rates are based on authors' clinical reports, other commentaries, or available selection criteria.

focused treatment of depression to Seligman's model of learned helplessness (e.g., Seligman, 1990).

These integrative tendencies notwithstanding, Peake, Borduin, and Archer (1988) differentiate brief therapies broadly along the lines of their dominant psychodynamic, cognitive, or strategic-structural features, while Bloom (1992; see also Jones & Pulos, 1993) suggests that most BT forms can be accounted for by either psychodynamic or cognitive-behavioral theory. In this context, interpersonal psychotherapy (IPT) (Klerman, Weissman, Rounseville, & Chevron, 1984; see also Weissman & Markowitz, 1994) is seen as a middle ground. (IPT is an empirically validated treatment, particularly for depression—see Elkin, 1995; Glick, 1995—that places explicit emphasis on the role of interpersonal processes in change and attempts to link interpersonal problems to current client symptoms.)

As BT evolves, strategic-structural and cognitive-behavioral approaches appear arguably to be gaining favor over dynamic approaches (Lambert & Bergin, 1994; Wells, 1993). Apart from issues of empirical validation, this may be because brief dynamic therapies place greater emphasis on the selection of motivated, functional patients, capable of insight and relationship formation, thus limiting their applicability (Cooper, 1995).

Brief Psychodynamic Approaches

In addition to the emphasis on patient selection and exclusion already noted, brief dynamic therapy also emphasizes the importance of transference and countertransference; confrontation and interpretation of focal, intrapsychic conflict; and, in most instances, the psychological importance of ending treatment (Ursano, Sonnenberg, & Lazar, 1991). As Goldberg (1975, p. 342) notes:

> For psychotherapy to enable an individual to come to terms with the meaning of his existence, he must come to grips with the reality of non-existence. Psychotherapy . . . is a process of termination rather than consolidation of relationship and proliferation of time.

A detailed elaboration of the distinguishing features of a number of brief dynamic approaches can be found elsewhere (e.g., Bloom, 1992; Crits-Christoph & Barber, 1991; Donovan, 1987; Messer & Warren, 1995), and the reader is referred to these as well as to original sources for clinical examples. The following is simply meant to give an impression of the variety that exists in brief approaches.

Malan's (1963, 1976, 1992) emphasis on working with limited treatment goals, identifying a focal conflict, and the "correct" selection of appropriate patients has been a pervasive influence in dynamic BT. His notion of "brief," however, is upwards of 40 sessions. On the other hand, Mann's (1973, 1991) approach adheres strictly to a 12-session limit in order to facilitate the patient's confrontation of "reality" and the process of separation–individuation. A recent randomized controlled study (Shefler, Dasberg, & Ben-Shakhar, 1995) has provided support for the effectiveness of this approach, with improvements being maintained for at least one year.

Strupp and Binder's (1984; Levenson, 1995) time-limited dynamic psychotherapy (TLDP) has also received empirical support. It focuses in a time-limited fashion on cyclical, maladaptive patterns of behaviors, relationships, and expectations and is increasingly integrative. According to Messer and Warren (1995), this approach captures most closely the dimensions of a relational model of psychotherapy. In contrast to drives and structural conflicts, the quality of affective states and the therapeutic relationship and interaction is emphasized. The process of a session is more important than its content, and the accurate reconstruction of the past is less important than the meaning patients give it.

Some brief approaches are clearly drawn from traditional views of Freud's drive model of behavior, utilizing the concepts noted at the beginning of this section. Davanloo (1979, 1988), for example, relentlessly pursues transference interpretations in a way that tends to provoke anger in patients but presumably limits "transference neurosis." He considers his approach applicable even to severe pathology, as does Sifneos (1992) of his "anxiety-provoking therapy." Sifneos challenges Oedipal issues without interpreting defenses first as Davanloo and Malan would (Messer & Warren, 1995), thus giving rise to the anxiety-provoking dimension of his method since defenses are, in effect, challenged without warning.

The approaches of Wolberg (1965, 1980) and Gustafson (1986), the latter of whom views treatment as a series of first sessions but is limited by working mostly with university students, are both flexible and technically eclectic.

Cognitive-Behavioral and Strategic Approaches

In contrast to dynamic brief therapies, cognitive-behavioral theories emphasize assessment and relief of current problems caused by faulty learning and maladaptive habits, the use of empirically based techniques to achieve collaboratively defined goals, and efforts to increase self-efficacy or self-mastery (Orlinsky & Howard, 1995; Peake et al., 1988). Currently, these approaches are moving toward a constructivist rather than strictly empirical view of treatment; that is, treatment effectiveness is enhanced by working within the reality of personal meanings that people create (Mahoney, 1993, 1995; Dobson & Shaw, 1995; see Held, 1995, for a review and critique of this movement).

The inherently brief cognitive therapies of Beck (1976; Beck & Weishaar, 1995) and Ellis (Ellis, 1992, 1995a, 1995b; Ellis & Grieger, 1977) attempt to change problematic thinking. As it has become evident that an exclusive focus on either cognitions or behavior (e.g., Wilson, 1995) is insufficient to change many kinds of problems, cognitive and behavioral therapies have increasingly merged into "cognitive-behavioral" approaches (see Barlow, 1993; Freeman & Dattilio, 1992; Hawton, Salkovskis, Kirk, & Clark, 1989; Hollon & Beck, 1994; Lehman & Salovey, 1990; Mahoney, 1995). These approaches share a systematic yet flexible incorporation of cognitive, behavioral, and social-learning paradigms; attention to objective documentation of symptoms and progress; the use of hypothesis-testing; and increased emphasis on the therapeutic relationship. CBT has been validated for a host of problems.

Strategic therapy may be broadly thought of as referring to specific, usually therapist-generated interventions for specific problems. It is another compelling and popular general approach to brief therapy, which has been of considerable utility in marital and family treatment (see Gurman & Kniskern, 1981; 1991) but which suffers, as does the family therapy field generally, from lack of rigorous empirical studies and research limitations (Alexander, Holtzworth-Munroe, Jameson, 1994).

Strategic therapy can be substantially traced to Gregory Bateson (e.g., Broderick & Schrader, 1981) and Milton Erickson (e.g., Cade & O'Hanlon, 1993; Fisch, 1990; Lankton, Lankton, & Matthews, 1991; Zeig, 1982). Erickson deemphasized pathology and could be quite directive (but often indirect and metaphorical) in his style. His work is further elaborated in Jay Haley's (1980, 1991) "problem-solving" approach. Haley, in turn, has connections to Salvador Minuchin (Aponte, 1992; Minuchin & Fishman, 1981), whose "structural" approach to family problems emphasizes intervention in the transactional processes that both reveal and maintain problems.

The MRI approach (e.g., Fisch, Weakland, & Segal, 1982; Segal, 1991; Watzlawick, Weakland, & Fisch, 1974; Weakland & Fisch, 1992) (to which Haley, Bateson, and Erickson also have connections) differs from structural therapy in that, even though problems are viewed as interactional and systemic, the resolution of the presenting complaint is done by narrowing the treatment focus to specific behaviors. How a behavior is seen as a problem, by whom, and what has been tried to fix it become important, as does working within the client's reality, considering how the problem is maintained by efforts to solve it, and reframing the problem (Cooper, 1995, p. 22).

Other variations of this family of treatment approaches include single-session therapy's (SST; Hoyt et al., 1992; Talmon, 1990) "metatheoretical" perspective: "1. How is the patient stuck (what is maintaining the problem)? 2. What does the patient need to get unstuck? 3. How can the therapist facilitate or provide what is needed?" (Hoyt et al., 1992, p. 62). These authors suggest that this kind of flexible framework is particularly useful for the numerous clients that only come for a single therapeutic contact. At the most disingenuously simple level, Yapko (1992) emphasizes the commonality to all psychotherapy of hypnotic paradigms, pattern interruption, and rebuilding more functional patterns.

A popular variation of strategic therapy, solution-focused brief therapy (Berg & Miller, 1992a, 1992b; Cade & O'Hanlon, 1993; de Shazer, 1985, 1988, 1991b; O'Hanlon & Weiner-Davis, 1989; Walter & Peller, 1992), has emphasized building on exceptions to the presenting problem (that is, what factors allow a problem not to be present all the time in the same degree) and making transitions rapidly to the identification and development of solutions intrinsic to the client or problem.

Budman and Gurman (1988, 1992) emphasize an integrated developmental approach with interpersonal and existential elements focused on the treatment question "Why come to therapy now?" and which has recently incorporated aspects of control mastery theory of the Mount Zion Group. Basch (1995) articulates another integrative/developmental approach of fewer than 20 sessions applicable even to significantly impaired persons by intervening in one of five areas: affect/reason, attachment, psychosexuality, autonomy, or creativity. Reid (1990) has proposed an integrative model utilizing problem-solving, dynamic, behavioral, cognitive, and structural components.

Crisis Therapy

Crisis and brief therapy share many qualities and are often viewed synonymously, although this is simplistic. In general, crisis therapies are provided to people under extreme and often specific stress for the purpose of restoring them to their presumed adequate level of functioning before the crisis (see Shiang & Bongar, 1995). Although this implies that crises are self-limiting (Caplan, 1964), some therapists argue that crisis therapies can and do have the function of providing even more adaptive functioning than before the crisis (Ewing, 1990). Ewing (1990) also suggests that crisis therapies are by definition time-limited, apply widely to human problems, are present-focused and reality-oriented, and require considerable therapist

flexibility with interventions that may include advocacy or education.

Eclectic BT/Prescriptive BT

An important trend in brief therapy is integrationism, which is more reconciliatory than eclecticism. (The reader is referred to the chapter on treatment in this book for additional information.) This trend involves the customized application of specific treatment for specific problems and people at specific times, or what Norcross (1995) has called "prescriptive brief therapy" (also see Norcross & Goldfried, 1992; Norcross & Newman, 1992; and Prochaska, Norcross, & DiClemente, 1994) or "systematic eclectic therapy" (Beutler, Consoli, & Williams, 1995). This brief approach is becoming particularly viable as the range of validated treatment possibilities or "cells" suggested by these interactions, which at one time were prohibitive in number, have become more consolidated (Held, 1995). Moreover, it is inclusive of the promising research and practice emphasis on "common factors" in psychotherapy (Norcross & Newman, 1992) as a welcome antidote to the continued mushrooming of unproved therapies with little new to offer (Miller et al., 1995; see also Orlinsky & Howard, 1995).

This sophisticated approach to therapy tends to reflect informed actual practice and takes into account the obscured differences and subtle interaction effects between clients, therapists, and treatments that are a function of normative or meta-analytic research (Beutler, 1991; Persons, 1991). Aptitude-by-treatment interactions are an emerging field in which evidence suggests, for example, that reactant or oppositional clients may do better with paradoxical or nondirective treatments, whereas impulsive or poorly socialized clients may do better in CBT or directive therapy (Beutler et al., 1995; Lambert & Bergin, 1994; Norcross, 1995, 1996).

BRIEF THERAPY
PROCEDURAL OUTLINE

This section illustrates a largely descriptive and task-oriented model of BT (adapted and portions excerpted from Cooper, 1995) that is as generic as possible to give the reader an idea of how a "typical" brief therapy session might proceed. It leans toward the cognitive-behavioral and strategic schools of thinking but nevertheless has much in common with dynamic structure. The emphasis on a first session is deliberate, as brief therapy in many ways may be seen as a series of first sessions, linked gently but firmly (not rigidly) by a treatment focus. A sample intake note follows for reference and comparison to other approaches in this book.

Preintake Tasks

A brief therapist might gather as much history as possible beforehand by the use of questionnaires or checklists. Although these often do not provide much useful information about the process of therapy, they can help a therapist form preliminary questions and useful hypotheses. Other brief therapists (e.g., O'Hanlon & Wilk, 1987) suggest lying down until the urge to form a hypothesis goes away, since sometimes therapists are unable or unwilling to notice information contrary to their hypotheses once these are formed. Nevertheless, some useful history questions about referral source, past treatment, medications, substance use, suicidality, focal symptoms, and reasons for coming in at this time save time in session.

Similarly, it may be useful for a brief therapist to check the congruence of observable client behavior, say in the waiting room or by phone contact, with their known or stated concern, as this may facilitate an intervention. An obviously anxious client, for example, might benefit from at least implicit efforts at reassurance or calming.

Patients may also be given or sent written information about what to expect in useful treatment, and this should be discussed early on. The therapist might also educate clients by modeling, for example, being on time for the appointment and ending promptly. This conveys a work-oriented tone and an expectation that the time and relationship with the client are valuable and are to be treated as such.

First-Session Tasks

Although this model suggests a sequential direction, it is not rigidly implemented. Also, tasks may overlap or serve multiple purposes, as in an empathetic restatement of a client's problem that conveys understanding (important to relationship building) but also serves to clarify a potential treatment focus.

1. Form a positive working relationship.

Good brief therapists learn how to do this rapidly (and continuously). They recognize that they may only get a limited chance to make a positive impression and that a positive impression is essential to successful therapy. Here are some techniques for forming a positive working relationship:

- Do some mutual therapy education—that is, discuss mutual expectations of treatment, the process of therapy, and such factors as time, cost, or treatment options. This starts to generate an atmosphere of collaboration.
- Use active listening, empathy, and language in a way that demonstrates an understanding of, and respect for, each client's point of view. Having clients believe it when a therapist says "I can see why you feel (or think) that way" is a worthy goal.
- Generally, conveying an air of confidence about achieving a reasonable outcome may have a salutary effect on actual outcome (Beutler, Crago, & Arizmendi, 1986). By inducing hopefulness and an expectation of improvement, salutary placebo effects may be engaged (Beier & Young, 1984; Frank, 1974; Goleman, 1993; Lambert, Shapiro, & Bergin, 1986). On the other hand, unrealistic expectations are not encouraged.
- The therapist's stance is that of a consultant with a desire to be helpful, not a miracle-worker or know-it-all (unless the client requests this—and then the therapist can show off!).
- Find something to like or respect about each client or their coping and call attention to it. Similarly, it is helpful to avoid arguments by finding at least something about client statements or positions with which to be empathic.

2. Find a treatment focus.

Focus is developed collaboratively with patients and is related to the concepts of assessment and diagnosis and refined by asking: What is it that we are going to do something about, or what is it that you want to be different? If multiple problems are identified, they are ranked in the order of importance to the client. Because many clients have difficulty articulating treatment goals, this is most productively treated as confusion that needs to be approached creatively rather than as denial or "resistance." This latter view risks setting up an unnecessarily adversarial relationship (Bischoff & Tracey, 1995).

Formal diagnoses are typically associated with focus in medical or "pathological" models of treatment and are therapist-derived. In BT, on the other hand, it is important to develop diagnostic skills while working within a client's perception of a problem. Most patients do not come in saying, "My Generalized Anxiety Disorder and Avoidant Personality features are being exacerbated by conflicts with my wife." They say instead: "My wife is bumming me out, so I'm going to the bar until things cool off."

As an important aside, Shaffer (1986) and Meehl (1973) have observed problems endemic—some might say epidemic—as a result of poorly formed diagnoses. Shaffer delineates six levels of diagnostic sophistication: (1) no diagnosis is made, leading to "rote meetings" between client and therapist; (2) a differential diagnosis is made but the therapist treats everyone the same way; (3) a DSM diagnosis is made based on an interview with perhaps some testing, but these are not reconciled or replicable; (4) an explicit diagnosis is formed linking a presenting problem to a treatment that has some researched validity; (5) sophisticated case management decisions are made from the outset based on outcome research and revised as necessary in light of therapeutic developments; (6) nothing is assumed about client readiness for change; therapists utilize other sources of information to help assess and challenge or modify "defenses" or interactive styles in the context of the previous levels, such as spouses, cultural contexts, and so forth. A good brief therapist operates at the upper levels of this hierarchy.

To return to a general strategy for achieving focus with clients: Therapists may look for overly rigid and unhelpful cognitive, behavioral, and affective coping patterns of clients. Often these may be grouped into a SORC paradigm (Giles, 1992).

- *Situations* (e.g., losses, illness)
- *Organic causes* (e.g., mitral valve prolapse as a contributor to panic)
- *Responses* (interpersonal or intrapersonal reactions)
- *Consequences,* especially those that may inadvertently strengthen symptomatic behavior and complaints

Other ways to find focus:

- Ask what has brought clients to treatment *now* rather than earlier or later.
- Determine specifically at the outset what would be tangibly different for clients at the end of successful treatment.
- Sometimes a "rule" about client behavior can be formulated collaboratively that can serve as a focus for intervention. For example, a "rule" governing a young man's unhelpful criticism of his girlfriend is formulated in this way: "If I criticize her often enough, she'll do things perfectly." Interventions can then be devised to challenge this belief or behavior.
- Find out how the presenting complaint is a problem for clients, and get agreement about the nature of the problem. It is important to determine the meaning or significance of a problem to a client. For example, the young woman above thinks that her boyfriend's infidelity means that something must be wrong with her. This perception then can become a potential treatment focus.

3. Negotiate criteria for a successful outcome.

Once problems have been identified, goals or solutions are negotiated with clients through sensitive questioning and the exchange of information about what we know is effective for certain kinds of problems or patients.

Goals are generally set in positive, specific, achievable, and measurable terms. This contributes to and reinforces a sense of control for clients. For example, if clients say they are depressed and a goal is to "not be depressed anymore," asking what will be different when they're not depressed any more suggests a positive focus. Clients might say then they will be "happier," which meets the criterion of positive focus but lacks specificity. If clients say they are "depressed," therapists ought to find out exactly what this means to them and how it is a problem. Fatigue, lack of pleasure, and sadness are more manageable than "depression," and treatments can be targeted at these problems that can be measured even by rudimentary scaling. The unquestioned acceptance of broad, vague terms (e.g., *anxious* or *low self-esteem)* or of popular terms such as *co-dependency* may be subject to the Barnum effect (Logue, Sher, & Frensch, 1992) and is to be avoided.

4. Distinguish clients from nonclients.

Because not everyone who appears in therapy is necessarily interested in changing his or her behavior, and the active involvement of patients is heavily related to outcome (see Miller et al., 1995), the concept of *customers, complainants,* and *visitors* (e.g., de Shazer, 1988; see also Berg & Miller, 1992b; Johnson, 1995) is useful in determining "real" client status, particularly as it emphasizes working optimally with different stages of client motivation for change.

Clients or "customers" are people who acknowledge that there is a problem and indicate a genuine willingness to work on it. "Complainants" will say a problem exists but do not see themselves as part of a solution. They can be challenging because, despite apparent distress, they convey a sense of helpless and often anger since they see the solutions to their problems as lying outside of themselves. Family members trying to change alcoholics and many depressed patients, possibly owing to cognitive distortions or lack of energy, fit into this category. "Visitors" do not acknowledge that there is a problem. They often come at someone else's request or under pressure. The treatment of choice here is for the therapist to respect the patients' belief that their lives are sufficiently in order.

5. Identify clients' motivational levels, and tailor interventions accordingly.

These questions are useful to consider in this regard:

- Who is (most) willing and able to change?
- What are they willing to do to change or to accept matters?
- Can strategies be devised for nonclients?

Additionally, the five stages of change in addictive behavior provide a framework for evaluating motivation in psychotherapy (Prochaska, 1992; Prochaska et al., 1994):

- *Precontemplation:* No serious intent to change in the foreseeable future is apparent.
- *Contemplation:* Patients think seriously about change but debate the pros and cons of doing so.
- *Preparation:* Patients intend to take action in the next month and have unsuccessfully taken action in the past year.
- *Action:* Patients actively modify behavior, experiences, or environment.
- *Maintenance:* Patients work to consolidate gains.

These last three stages correspond to having a genuine client, while stage 2 roughly corresponds to the complainant and stage 1 to the visitor. A different kind of intervention is required for each stage of change, and failure to recognize this may result in inefficient and ineffective treatment. Table 8.2 clarifies the general relationship of interventions to these levels of motivations and client status. Preferred strategies for intervening with clients thus reflect their relative degree of participation in the change process.

6. Do something that makes a difference today.

At a minimum, a good brief therapist will listen actively and empathetically to clients. Noticing and allowing if not encouraging affective expression may be helpful, but since it is usually insufficient for change, immediate, active interventions are a significant art of BT. These may include determining and building on past positive coping with similar problems, role-plays, problem solving, education, normalization of behavior, relaxation training, directives, and appropriate confron-

Table 8.2 The Customer Status–Task Matrix

Status	Do you have a problem?	Are you willing to work hard to solve it?	Appropriate Tasks or Responses
Customer	Yes	Yes	Reframing, homework, confrontation, interpretation; the patient is asked to change his views of the problem and his behavior.
Complainant	Yes (but . . .)	No	Give client compliments and ask him to observe (but not change) own behavior for coping strategies and what works best, or to observe others' behavior for times when the problem is absent or not so much a problem. Ask whether the client can predict those times when problem is absent. Changing of views is implied, not explicit.
Visitor or guest	No	No	Emphasize positive relationship; give compliments about strengths and abilities; perhaps warn about the danger of change and recommend no change "for now" and engage in pleasant conversation. Look for the "hidden customer" by asking how the referring person/agency would know when the client no longer needs to come to therapy.

tation or interpretation. Discussing the process of obtaining desired solutions and defining or redefining the roles of therapy and client may be necessary, particularly if clients are not sufficiently motivated to do what is necessary to change a problem.

A universal activity in brief therapy is to conceptualize or reframe problems in ways that suggest solutions. Reframing is a desirable change in perspective that often leads to corresponding changes in attitude and behavior (e.g., Watzlawick et al., 1974; Weeks & Treat, 1992). In reframing, the strategically minded brief therapist looks especially for positive intentions behind problematic behavior, the positive function of symptoms, or their positive unintended consequences—whatever can genuinely be considered an alternative view of a problem (Johnson, 1990). As an example,

a couple's fighting, subjectively distressful but not otherwise harmful, is reframed as a form of

intimacy and trust-building. Or, to distressed parents: "Your son may have the belief that only by acting up can he be assured of your love." In these cases, the behavior is reframed, accurately (this is important) and more desirably, as a component or a test of intimacy and love. (Cooper, 1995, p.47)

7. Negotiate homework.

The idea of assigning or negotiating homework during and after sessions is not to punish clients but to keep treatment focused and to help people use time productively between sessions. This also is consistent with evidence that goal-directed activity is essential to feelings of well-being (Csikszentmihalyi, 1990). *Homework* refers to some effort, cognitively or behaviorally, to acquire skills, test assumptions, or change established patterns in which clients are stuck (Johnson, 1992, 1995). Homework may include standard cognitive-behavioral techniques, symbolic or ritualistic tasks (which can have particular advantages in multicultural therapy), or even the whimsical (see Levy & Shelton, 1990), such as flipping a coin or asking a people-pleasing client to poll all his friends about what he should do regarding a problem (Johnson, 1992). Clients may be asked to change roles in family disputes or to alter the frequency, intensity, duration, or place of a symptom that seems out of their control (e.g., Ascher, 1989; Madanes, 1981; O'Hanlon & Wilk, 1987). Homework in BT is tailored to be consistent with client goals, values, abilities, levels of motivation, and interests.

8. Charting and documenting outcomes.

Documenting sessions in brief therapy is not particularly different from the documentation that should accompany good therapy of any kind. It is one—though not necessarily an infallible—measure of the integrity of the therapy and a way to communicate this to other professionals. Note that for the example in Table 8.3, details are included primarily as they concern the immediate problem or enable others to see why the diagnoses or treatment plans were made. Thus, lengthy family histories or detailed descriptions of events usually are not necessary and may even obscure more important data or foci. It is especially important to note details consistent with BT principles: the current concern, patterns of coping, objectives in seeking treatment, exceptions to the problem's occurrence, client strengths, and specification of how possible solutions are going to be implemented.

Subsequent session documentation would, of course, be much shorter, focusing on the most salient features of the session and emphasizing how an intervention and subsequent homework are consistent with goals already established or modified. Progress and outcomes of treatment should be continuously monitored in well-done BT, using subjective and objective instruments that are congruent with the problem and objectives of treatment (see Ogles, Lambert, & Masters, 1996). The quality of the therapeutic relationship should also be regularly assessed (Burns & Nolan-Hoeksema, 1992). It is generally unnecessary, if not contrary to brief treatment principles, to do routine testing (especially personality testing) in therapy that does not add in-

cremental validity to an interview or advance the therapy in some tangible way (Cooper, 1995).

SUBSEQUENT-SESSION TASKS

The principles of first-session tasks are consistent throughout treatment, although their form and emphasis may change as treatment demands. Follow-up tasks include reviewing homework from previous sessions, establishing or reestablishing a focus for the present session, working collaboratively toward at least one tangibly useful intervention or interaction, negotiating new homework consistent with progress and goals, and assessing the helpfulness of the session and the quality of the therapeutic relationship. It may be helpful to plan for and rehearse responses to "relapses," and the attentive brief therapist is especially concerned with finding ways to motivate clients.

As noted earlier, some brief therapists see the formal ending of treatment as crucial because of the presumed importance to the patient of the therapist. Other therapists believe the strict establishment of time-limited treatment facilitates treatment outcome and separation from the therapist. Many clinicians, however, expect that patients may come in periodically over time when they get "stuck." The idea of terminating a patient from this perspective is irrelevant (Johnson, 1995). In any case, if therapeutic progress toward clearly defined and mutually understood goals has been regularly noted, the ending of a course of treatment is typically self-evident. This is likely to be so even if the number of therapy visits has not been predetermined.

WORKING WITH FAMILIES, COUPLES, AND GROUPS

For a detailed look at treating families and groups, the reader is referred to Chapters 7 and 9 of this book. However, the BT assumptions, principles, and approaches outlined here are readily extended to the realm of family, couples, and child treatment (e.g., Alexander et al., 1994; Bloom, 1992; Budman & Gurman, 1988; Budman et al., 1992; Cooper, 1995; Gurman & Kniskern, 1991; Hudson & O'Hanlon, 1992; Johnson, 1995; Kreilkamp, 1989; Scheidlinger, 1984; Selekman,

Table 8.3 Sample Intake Notes

Identification: Emma Howe is a divorced Caucasian female, 35, employed as a secretary. She has a 13-year-old son, Brian, who lives with her and has minimal paternal contact. The patient was referred by Dr. Zoe Loft of this clinic.

Presenting problem: "I've been depressed all my life." Ms. Howe also reports more acute depressive and anxiety symptoms staring 3 months ago, when her son left for a month to visit his father and she was left to "confront" her relationship with her "noncommittal" boyfriend of 3 years, Bubba. Dr. Loft placed her on Zoloft 150 mg and Klonopin 0.5 mg at night, to which she has been only partially responsive. Her general treatment goal is "to feel happier."

Problem history: Ms. Howe cannot remember an extended period of euthymia. She notes prior episodes of depression during her divorce 4 years ago and 2 years ago when her current boyfriend left her for a time. They have reunited, but he remains uncommitted to marriage, which the patient wants. Her current symptoms include being "sad all the time," though she rates her mood about a "4" on a 10-point scale. She notes "I don't enjoy anything," and has "little appetite," with a weight loss of about 5 lbs initially, now stabilized. She reports guilt about being an inadequate mother and partner, expectations of being punished for no reason, harsh self-criticism, difficulty making decisions, and fatigue secondary to "waking up a lot." She has occasional nightmares but wakes a few times a week with palpitations, in "cold sweats," and with feelings that she just wants "to quit everything and get away." She has started to avoid going out with her closer friends because she does not expect to have a good time.

Ms. Howe notes that she has a historic difficulty saying "no" to people, taking great pains not to hurt them and avoiding conflict. Examples include wearing clothes "that aren't me" to please Bubba, letting a man whom she likes at work kiss her even though she was uncomfortable with it, and "spoiling" her son because she couldn't spend enough time with him.

Ms. Howe believes she would be happier if (1) she were married to someone who accepted her as she was and was more "sociable"; (2) she were in her own home rather than an apartment; (3) she could make a decision about whether to move on in her relationship; (4) she did not worry so much about money; and (5) she spent more time and set better limits with her son.

Her previous helpful coping has consisted of exercising, dressing as she likes, and spending "quality" time with her son and friends. It was observed with her that she appears to have considerable resilience and a clear idea of what is important to her in spite of her confusion.

Previous treatment: None.

Medical history: Noncontributory.

Chemical use history: Drinks moderately in social context. Has stopped caffeine intake, which was moderate.

Family history: Positive for paternal and fraternal alcoholism. The patient's mother has apparently been treated with antidepressants. The patient's parents divorced when she was 9. She has an ambivalent relationship with her father but feels close to her mother though she doesn't "see her enough."

Mental status exam: Pt. was alert, oriented, and cognitively intact at the interview. She was prompt and neatly groomed. She was easily engaged with fair eye contact. Psychomotor status normal though she appeared physically tense. Speech occasionally halting but otherwise normal. Mood: sad and somewhat apprehensive. Affect: constricted. Denies suicidal or homicidal thinking or intent. Intelligence, insight, and judgment appear roughly in the average range.

Assessment and diagnosis:

Axis 1: 300.4 Dysthymic Disorder, probable early onset
296.31 Major Depression, Recurrent, Mild (Provisional)
300.01 Panic Disorder Without Agoraphobia (Provisional)
Rule out 300.02 Generalized Anxiety Disorder

Axis II: 301.90 Personality Disorder NOS (Provisional), dependent and avoidant features.

Axis III: None

Axis IV: Single parent; limited finances; conflicts with boyfriend

Axis V: Current GAF: 55
Highest GAF last year: 70

Plan: Continue medication per Dr. Loft. Treatment goals: (1) improvement and stabilization of mood; (2) increased assertiveness skills; and (3) establishing a sense of personal control over her life. Patient ideas for feeling better are noted in HPI and will serve as functional goals. Pt. agreed to homework of spending Saturday afternoon with her son, dressing one day as she wished this week, and/or walking for 30 minutes three times a week to see what a difference these things made to her mood.

Source: J. F. Cooper, *A Primer of Brief Psychotherapy* (New York: Norton, 1995).

1991; Todd & Selekman, 1991; Weeks & Treat, 1992; Wells & Giannetti, 1990, 1993).

As with individual treatment, significant therapeutic change can occur and persist in children and families in much less time than is commonly thought necessary (e.g., Smyrnios & Kirby, 1993) and includes the possibility of treating a family via one person (Szapocnik, Kurtines, Perez-Vidal, Hervis, & Foote, 1990). Moreover, the most clearly validated treatments for couples and families, such as the work of Neil Jacobson and José Szapocznik, are inherently brief (see Alexander et al., 1994, and Johnson, 1995, for discussions).

With respect to groups, there appear to be no clear exclusions (such as seriously disturbed or chronically mentally ill clients) for brief group treatment that would not apply to longer term models provided that goals, structure, and therapist interventions are appropriately tailored to the group (Klein, 1985). In general, BT groups are distinguished from other groups by the basic values and common treatment principles outlined earlier in this chapter (see Wells & Giannetti, 1990, for examples).

Potential advantages to brief group therapy include: (1) treating a number of people simultaneously, including couples, who share a similar problem that can serve as organizing focus, and (2) using other group members as assistant therapists (Bloom, 1992). Some people appear to find comfort or benefit in the universality of a group. Groups may be a treatment of choice for some problems, such as depression or social skills deficits in adolescents (e.g., Fine et al., 1989), or for circumscribed problems such as panic disorder that are amenable to inherently time-limited and structured treatment. However, strictly time-limited groups have not been shown to be superior to other formats in some regards (see Wells & Giannetti, 1990, and Yalom, 1995, for partial reviews of brief group approaches). Indeed, the whole field of group research is sufficiently young to prevent unequivocal statements about group treatments, brief or otherwise (Bednar & Kaul, 1994).

MULTICULTURALISM AND BRIEF THERAPY

A more thorough discussion of working with different cultures than is possible here is found in Chapter 15. Although rapidly changing demographics in the United States necessitate attention to this subject (that technically refers to African Americans, Asian Americans, Latino Americans, and Native Americans), the lack of rigorous research and unique methodological challenges (such as separating cultural effects from other factors in treatment) make truly valid statements beyond opinions, anecdotes, and experience about multicultural therapy, including brief therapy, extremely difficult.

A typical response to this dilemma is to recapitulate the obvious call for greater understanding and research effort, particularly with therapy process, and for honest writers to acknowledge that their thoughts are often not empirically based (e.g., Casas, 1995). Thus, not much can be said about working with culturally different clients in brief therapy that could not be said of therapy generally.

Further, current multicultural thinking tends to oversimplify relations between racial and ethnic groups, which from the perspective of history reveal few simple or inviolable patterns (see Sowell, 1994) and from the perspective of sociobiology is an oxymoron (Lykken, 1995). Nevertheless, Triandis (1996) has observed that cultures are likely to have their own psychology, which does not necessarily reflect that of contemporary and indigenously Western points of view.

In their review, Sue, Zane, and Young (1994) find some empirically based suggestions that certain conditions may be related to working effectively with different cultures. These are quite compatible with the sensibilities of BT. They include: (1) ethnic similarity between clients and therapists of some minority groups or individuals; (2) using culturally responsive forms of treatment (presumably when they can be identified); (3) pretherapy intervention and education with prospective clients; (4) therapist training in cultural awareness and the culturally specific manifestations of problems; and (5) therapist sensitivity to the heterogeneity of ethnic minority groups.

Our experience in doing brief therapy with clients representing over a dozen nationalities and the large subcultures in this country is that BT principles are also compatible with the multicultural concepts of credibility and giving (Sue & Zane, 1987). Credibility needs to be achieved rapidly to help ensure treatment continuity. It is accomplished through (1) a congruent understanding of the problem; (2) culturally compatible means of problem resolution (suggesting the need to learn how a problem might typically be handled in a particular culture); and (3) mutually agreed-on goals for treatment. It may be advisable, as with any client, to inquire about the client's familiarity with therapy and comfort-seeking help from someone who may not know much about their culture. An expressed willingness to understand someone better may enhance mutual understanding and lead to productive work or a more appropriate referral (Cooper, 1995).

Giving involves providing some immediate treatment benefit or "gifts," even in the first session. These gifts may include "anxiety reduction, depression relief, cognitive clarity, normalization, reassurance, hope and faith, skills acquisition, a coping perspective, and goal setting" (Sue & Zane, 1987, p. 42). Because brief therapists generally adopt a flexible style, those who work multiculturally might incorporate explicitly into a brief treatment approach the history, rituals, and philosophies of a given culture once it is known to them.

Another way of considering universality in cultural psychology is through an understanding of "cultural syndromes" such as normative "tightness," cultural complexity, activity–passivity elements, a notion of honor, collectivism, individualism, and vertical or horizontal relationship dimensions (that is, hierarchical versus democratic) (Triandis, 1996). A brief therapy stance that reflects this awareness is likely to bear similarities to "technical eclecticism" discussed earlier (Casas, 1995).

FUTURE TRENDS IN BRIEF TREATMENT

Cummings (1995) suggests that economic factors (for better or worse) are likely to continue to shape the delivery of psychotherapy. While there are debates about who is likely to be delivering these services—for example, "cheaper" master's-level therapists versus doctoral-level psychologists (see Humphreys, 1996)—if clinical psychologists continue to perform psychotherapy, it behooves them to learn about empirically validated treatments to justify to third-party payers who are disease-model oriented that they are more than "nice people" trying to help (Bologna & Feldman, 1994; Chambliss, 1996; Johnson, 1995). As we have observed, all of the empirically validated treatments to date are intrinsically brief and are likely to remain so because of their relative ease of study.

The limits of what can be accomplished in shorter-than-expected time will continue to be tested empirically. For example, Craske (1995) describes a 4-session CBT model for panic disorder involving cognitive restructuring, breathing re-

training, and interoceptive exposure that was effective in a controlled study with medical patients. The authors suggest that for this subset of people who may be unwilling to participate in the usual 12- to 16-week CBT treatment, bibliotherapy, homework, and audiotapes might supplement the treatment.

We are in an era of heightened interest in common psychotherapy factors and the selective application of integrated concepts to specific kinds of people and problems (e.g., Norcross & Goldfried, 1992). In other words, there will be increasing emphasis on moving beyond simplistic notions of whether a certain brief therapy works, to greater sophistication and integration in choosing particular kinds of therapies for particular problems and kinds of patients (Norcross, 1995; Orlinsky & Howard, 1995a; b).

Finally, an understanding of brief therapy generally is of considerable contemporary importance, in no small part because, as Koss and Shiang (1994) note:

> In addition to being a clearly viable treatment option, brief therapy is now routinely utilized in research studies examining "psychotherapy." However, this successful evolution into prototype therapy for research should not deter adherents of the brief approaches from continuing to press for greater understanding of those unique elements that define the format in order to contribute to scientific theory about the way people change. (p. 693)

REFERENCES

Adams, J. F., Piercy, F. P., & Jurich, A. (1991). Effects of solution focused therapy's "formula first session task" on compliance and outcome in family therapy. *Journal of Marital and Family Therapy, 17,* 277–290.

Alexander, F., & French, T. M. (1946). *Psychoanalytic therapy: Principles and applications.* New York: Ronald Press.

Alexander, J. F., Holtzworth-Munroe, A., & Jameson, P. (1994). The process and outcome of marital and family therapy: Research review and evaluation. In A. E. Bergin & S. L. Garfield (Eds.), *Handbook of psychotherapy and behavior change* (pp. 595–620). New York: Wiley.

Aponte, H. J. (1992). The black sheep of the family: A structural approach to brief therapy. In S. H. Budman,

M. F. Hoyt, & S. Friedman (Eds.), *The first session in brief therapy* (pp. 324–345). New York: Guilford Press.

Ascher, L. M. (Ed.). (1989). *Therapeutic paradox*. New York: Guilford Press.

Austad, C. S, & Hoyt, M. F. (1992). The managed care movement and the future of psychotherapy. *Psychotherapy, 29*, 109–118.

Barlow, D. H. (1988). *Anxiety and its disorders: The nature and treatment of anxiety and panic*. New York: Guilford Press.

Barlow, D. (Ed.). (1993). *Clinical handbook of psychological disorders* (2nd ed.). New York: Guilford Press.

Barlow D., & Craske, M. (1994). *Mastery of your panic and anxiety—II*. Albany, NY: Graywind Publications.

Basch, M. F. (1995). *Doing brief psychotherapy*. New York: Basic Books.

Beck, A. T. (1976). *Cognitive therapy and emotional disorders*. New York: International Universities Press.

Beck, A. T., Freeman, A., et al. (1990). *Cognitive therapy of personality disorders*. New York: Guilford Press.

Beck, A. T., & Weishaar, M. E. (1995). Cognitive therapy. In R. J. Corsini & D. Wedding (Eds.), *Current psychotherapies* (5th ed., pp. 229–262). Itasca, IL: Peacock.

Beck, A. T., Wright, F. D., & Newman, C. F. (1992). Cocaine abuse. In A. Freeman & F. M. Dattilio (Eds.), *Comprehensive casebook of cognitive therapy* (pp. 185–192). New York: Plenum Press.

Bednar, R. L., & Kaul, T. (1994). Experiential group research. In A. E. Bergin & S. L. Garfield (Eds.), *Handbook of psychotherapy and behavior change* (4th ed., pp. 631–664). New York: Wiley.

Beier, E. G., & Young, D. M. (1984). *The silent language of psychotherapy* (2nd ed.). New York: Aldine de Gruyter.

Bennett, M. J. (1988). The greening of the HMO: Implications for prepaid psychiatry. *American Journal of Psychiatry, 145*, 1544–1549.

Berg, I. K., & Miller, S. D. (1992a). *Dying well: A case presentation of solution-focused therapy*. Audiotape. Milwaukee: Brief Family Therapy Center.

Berg, I. K., & Miller, S. D. (1992b). *Working with the problem drinker: A solution-focused approach*. New York: Norton.

Bergin, A. E., & Garfield, S. L. (1994). Overviews, trends and future issues. In A. E. Bergin & S. L. Garfield (Eds.), *Handbook of psychotherapy and behavior change* (4th ed., pp. 821–830). New York: Wiley.

Bergman, J. S. (1985). *Fishing for barracuda: Pragmatics of brief systemic therapy*. New York: Norton.

Berkman, A. S., Bassos, C. A., & Post, L. (1988). Managed mental care and independent practice: A challenge to psychology. *Psychotherapy: Theory, Research, and Practice, 25*, 449–454.

Beutler, L. E. (1991). Have all won and must all have prizes? Revisiting Luborsky et al.'s verdict. *Journal of Consulting and Clinical Psychology, 59*, 1–7.

Beutler, L. E., Consoli, A. J., & Williams, R. E. (1995). Integrative and eclectic therapies in practice, In B. Bongar & L. E. Beutler (Eds.), *Comprehensive textbook of psychotherapy: Theory and practice* (pp. 274–292). New York: Oxford University Press.

Beutler, L. E., Crago, M., & Arizmendi, T. G. (1986). Therapist variables in psychotherapy process and outcome. In S. L. Garfield & A. E. Bergin (Eds.), *Handbook of psychotherapy and behavior change* (3rd ed., pp. 257–310). New York: Wiley.

Bischoff, M. M., & Tracey, T. J. G. (1995). Client resistance as predicted by therapist behavior: A study of sequential dependence. *Journal of Counseling Psychology, 42*, 487–495.

Bloom, B. (1981). Focused single-session therapy: Initial development and evaluation. In S. Budman (Ed.), *Forms of brief therapy* (pp. 167–216). New York: Guilford Press.

Bloom, B. L. (1990). Managing mental health services: Some comments on the overdue debate in psychology. *Community Mental Health Journal, 26*(1), 107–124.

Bloom, B. (1992). Bloom's focused single-session therapy. In B. Bloom (Ed.), *Planned short-term therapy* (pp. 97–122). Boston: Allyn and Bacon.

Bologna, N. C., & Feldman, M. (1994, May–June). Outcomes, clinical models, and the redesign of behavioral healthcare. *Behavioral Healthcare Tomorrow*, 31–36.

Bolter, K., Levenson, H., & Alvarez, W. (1990). Differences in values between short-term and long-term therapists. *Professional Psychology, 21*, 285–290.

Broderick, C. B., & Schrader, S. S. (1981). The history of professional marriage and family therapy. In A. S. Gurman & D. P. Kniskern (Eds.), *Handbook of family therapy* (pp. 5–38). New York: Brunner/Mazel.

Broskowski, A. (1991). Current mental health care environments: Why managed care is necessary. *Professional Psychology: Research and Practice, 22*(1), 6–14.

Budman, S. (1989, August). *Training experienced clinicians to do brief treatment—Silk purses into sows' ears*. Paper presented at the 97th annual convention of the American Psychological Association, New Orleans, Louisiana.

Budman, S. H., & Gurman, A. S. (1988). *Theory and practice of brief therapy*. New York: Guilford Press.

Budman, S. H., & Gurman, A. S. (1992). A time-sensitive model of brief therapy: The I-D-E approach. In S. H. Budman, M. Hoyt, & S. Friedman (Eds.) *The first session in brief therapy* (pp. 111–134). New York: Guilford Press.

Budman, S. H., Hoyt, M. F., & Friedman, S. (Eds.). (1992). *The first session in brief therapy*. New York: Guilford Press.

Burlingame, G., Fuhriman, A., Paul, S., & Ogles, B. M. (1989). Implementing a time-limited therapy program: Differential effects of training and experience. *Psychotherapy, 26*, 303–313.

Burns, D. D., & Nolan-Hoeksema, S. (1992). Therapeutic empathy and recovery from depression in cognitive therapy: A structural equation model. *Journal of Consulting and Clinical Psychology, 60*, 441–449.

Butler, S. F, Strupp, H. H., & Binder, J. L. (1992). Time-limited dynamic psychotherapy. In S. H. Budman, M. F. Hoyt, & S. Friedman, *The first session in brief therapy* (pp. 87–110). New York: Guilford Press.

Cade, B., & O'Hanlon, W. H. (1993). *A brief guide to brief therapy*. New York: Norton.

Caplan, G. (1964). *Principles of preventive psychiatry*. New York: Basic Books.

Casas, J. M. (1995). Counseling and psychotherapy with racial/ethnic minority groups in theory and practice. In B. Bongar & L. E. Beutler (Eds.), *Comprehensive textbook of psychotherapy: Theory and practice* (pp. 311–336). New York: Oxford University Press.

Chambliss, D. L. (1996, June). Identification of empirically supported psychological interventions. *Clinician's Research Digest* (Supplemental Bulletin), *14*, 1–2.

Cooper. J. F. (1995). *A primer of brief psychotherapy*. New York: Norton.

Corsini, R J., & Wedding, D. (Eds.). (1995). *Current psychotherapies* (5th ed.). Itasca, IL: F. E. Peacock.

Craske, M. (1995). Brief cognitive-behavioral versus non-directive therapy for panic disorder. *Journal of Behavior Therapy and Experimental Psychiatry, 26*, 113–120.

Craven, S. (1996, June 20). Unpublished data presented at UBS Minnesota Provider Partnering Training Meeting, Minneapolis.

Crits-Christoph, P. (1992). The efficacy of brief dynamic psychotherapy: A meta-analysis. *American Journal of Psychiatry, 149*, 151–158.

Crits-Cristoph, P., & Barber, J. P (Eds.). (1991). *Handbook of short-term dynamic psychotherapy*. New York: Basic Books.

Csikszentmihalyi, M. (1990). *Flow: The psychology of optimal experience*. New York: Harper Perennial.

Davanloo, H. (1979). Techniques of short-term psychotherapy. *Psychiatric Clinics of North America, 2*, 11–22.

Davanloo, H. (1988). The technique of unlocking the unconscious: Part 1. *International Journal of Short-Term Psychotherapy, 3*, 99–121.

DeLeon, P. H., VandenBos, G. R., & Bulatao, E. G. (1991). Managed mental health care: A history of the federal policy initiative. *Professional Psychology Research and Practice, 22*(1), 15–25.

de Shazer, S. (1985). *Keys to solution in brief therapy*. New York: Norton.

de Shazer, S. (1988). *Clues: Investigating solutions in brief therapy*. New York: Norton.

de Shazer, S. (1991a). Foreword. In Y. M. Dolan (Ed.), *Resolving sexual abuse*. New York: Norton.

de Shazer, S. (1991b). *Putting difference to work*. New York: Norton.

Diguer, L., Luborsky, L., Singer, B., Luborsky, E., Dickter, D., & Schmidt, K. A. (1993, June). *The efficacy of dynamic psychotherapy versus other psychotherapies*. Paper presented at the meeting of the Society for Psychotherapy Research, Pittsburgh, Pennsylvania.

Dobson, K. S., & Shaw, B. F. (1995). Cognitive therapies in practice. In B. Bongar & L. E. Beutler (Eds.), *Comprehensive textbook of psychotherapy: Theory and practice* (pp. 159–172). New York: Oxford University Press.

Dolan, Y. M. (1991). *Resolving sexual abuse*. New York: Norton.

Donovan, J. M. (1987). Brief dynamic psychotherapy: Toward a more comprehensive model. *Psychiatry, 50*, 167–183.

Dubovsky, S. L. (1993, September). *Treatment resistant depression: Psychotherapy and pharmacology*. Paper presented at annual meeting of Park Nicollet Medical Center, Minneapolis, Minnesota.

Eckert, P. (1993). Acceleration of change: Catalysts in brief therapy. *Clinical Psychology Review, 13*(3), 241–253.

Elkin, I. (1995). Initial severity and differential treatment outcome in the National Institute of Mental Health Treatment of Depression Collaborative Research Program. *Journal of Consulting and Clinical Psychology, 63*, 841–847.

Ellis, A. (1992). Brief therapy: The rational-emotive method. In S. H. Budman, M. F. Hoyt, & S. Friedman (Eds.), *The first session in brief therapy* (pp. 36–59). New York: Guilford Press.

Ellis, A. (1995a). Rational emotive behavior therapy. In R. J. Corsini & D. Wedding (Eds.), *Current psychotherapies* (5th ed., pp. 162–197). Itasca, IL: Peacock.

Ellis, A. (1995b). *Better, deeper and more enduring brief therapy*. New York: Brunner/Mazel.

Ellis, A., & Grieger, R. (Eds.). (1977). *Handbook of rational-emotive therapy* (Vol.1). New York: Springer.

Epperson, D. L., Bushway, D. J., & Warman, R. E. (1983). Client self-terminations after one counseling session: Effects of problem recognition, counselor gender, and counselor experience. *Journal of Counseling Psychology, 30*, 307–315.

Ewing, C. P. (1990). Crisis intervention as brief therapy. In R. A. Wells & V. J. Giannetti (Eds.), *Handbook of the brief psychotherapies* (pp. 277–297). New York: Plenum Press.

Ferenczi, S. (1920/1960). The further development of an active therapy in psychoanalysis. In J. Richman (Ed.), (1960), *Further contributions to the theory and techniques of psychonalysis* (pp. 198–216). London: Hogarth.

Ferenczi, S., & Rank, O. (1925/1986). *The development of psychoanalysis*. Madison, CT: International Universities Press.

Fine, S., Gilbert, M., Schmidt, L., Haley, G., Maxwell, A., & Forth, A. (1989). Short-term group therapy with depressed adolescent outpatients. *Canadian Journal of Psychiatry, 34*, 97–102.

Fisch, R. (1990). The broader interpretation of Milton Erickson's work. In S. Lankton (Ed.), *The Ericksonian monographs, No. 7. The issue of broader implications of Ericksonian therapy* (pp. 1–5). New York: Brunner/Mazel.

Fisch, R., Weakland, J., & Segal, L. (1982). *The tactics of change: Doing therapy briefly*. San Francisco: Jossey-Bass.

Fisher, S., & Greenberg, R. P. (1993). How sound is the double-blind design for evaluating psychotropic drugs? *Journal of Nervous and Mental Disease, 181*, 345–350.

Frank, J. D. (1974). *Persuasion and healing*. New York: Schocken.

Freeman, A., & Dattilio, F. M. (Eds.). (1992). *Comprehensive casebook of cognitive therapy*. New York: Plenum Press.

Garfield, S. L. (1978). Research on client variables in psychotherapy. In S. L. Garfield & A. E. Bergin (Eds.), *Handbook of psychotherapy and behavior change* (2nd ed., pp. 271–298). New York: Wiley.

Garfield, S. L. (1986). Research on client variables in psychotherapy. In S. L. Garfield & A. E. Bergin (Eds.), *Handbook of psychotherapy and behavior change* (3rd ed., pp. 213–256). New York: Wiley.

Garfield, S. L. (1994). Research on client variables in psychotherapy. In A. E. Bergin & S. L. Garfield (Eds.), *Handbook of psychotherapy and behavior change* (4th ed., pp. 190–229). New York: Wiley.

Gibbs, W. W. (1995, March). Seeking the criminal element. *Scientific American*, pp. 100–107.

Giles, T. R. (1992). Brief therapy. *Strategies and Solutions, 1*, 10–12.

Gitlin, M. J. (1990). *The psychotherapist's guide to psychopharmacology*. New York: Free Press.

Gitlin, M. J. (1996). *The psychotherapist's guide to psychopharmacology* (2nd ed.). New York: Free Press.

Glick I. D. (Ed.). (1995). *Treating depression*. San Francisco: Jossey-Bass.

Goldberg, A. (1975). Narcissism and the readiness for psychothrapy termination. *Archives of General Psychiatry, 32*, 695–699.

Goldfried, M. R., & Norcross, J. C. (1995). Integrative and eclectic therapies in historical perspective. In B. Bongar & L. E. Beutler (Eds.), *Comprehensive textbook of psychotherapy: Theory and practice* (pp. 254–274). New York: Oxford University Press.

Goleman, D. (1993, October 17). Placebo more powerful than was thought, study finds. *Minneapolis Star Tribune*, p. 17E.

Gurman, A. S., & Kniskern, D. P. (Eds.). (1981). *Handbook of family therapy* (Vol. 1). New York: Brunner/Mazel.

Gurman, A. S., & Kniskern, D. P. (Eds.). (1991). *Handbook of family therapy* (Vol. 2). New York: Brunner/Mazel.

Gustafson, J. P. (1986). *The complex secret of brief psychotherapy*. New York: Norton.

Haley, J. (1980). *Leaving home*. New York: McGraw-Hill.

Haley, J. (1991). *Problem-solving therapy* (2nd ed.). San Francisco: Jossey-Bass.

Hawton, K., Salkovskis, P. M., Kirk, J., & Clark, D. M. (Eds.). (1989). *Cognitive behaviour therapy for psychiatric problems: A practical guide*. Oxford: Oxford University Press.

Held, B. S. (1995). *Back to reality*. New York: Norton.

Henry, W. P., Strupp, H. H., Schact, T. E., & Gaston, L. (1994). Psychodynamic approaches. In A. E. Bergin & S. L. Garfield (Eds.), *Handbook of psychotherapy and behavior change* (4th ed., pp. 428–467). New York: Wiley.

Hollon, S. D., & Beck, A. T. (1994). Cognitive and cognitive-behavioral therapies. In A. E. Bergin & S. L.

Garfield (Eds.), *Handbook of psychotherapy and behavior change* (4th ed., pp. 428–467). New York: Wiley.

Hollon, S. D., DeRubeis, R. J., Evans, M. D., Wiemer, M. J., Garvey, M. J., Grove, W. M., & Tuason, W. B. (1992). Cognitive therapy and pharmacotherapy for depression: Singly and in combination. *Archives of General Psychiatry, 49*, 774–781.

Horowitz, M. J., Marmar, C., Krupnick, J., Wilner, J., Kaltreider, N., & Wallerstein, R. (1984). *Personality styles and brief psychotherapy*. New York: Guilford Press.

Howard, K. I., Kopta, S. M., Krause, M. S., & Orlinsky, D. E. (1986). The dose–effect relationship in psychotherapy. *American Psychologist, 41*, 159–164.

Hoyt. M. F. (1985). Therapist resistance to short-term dynamic psychotherapy. *Journal of American Academy of Psychoanalysis, 13*, 932–112.

Hoyt, M. F. (1987). Resistance to brief therapy. *American Psychologist, 42*, 408–409.

Hoyt, M. F. (1990). On time in brief therapy. In R. A. Wells & V. J. Giannetti (Eds.), *Handbook of the brief psychotherapies* (pp. 115–145). New York: Plenum Press.

Hoyt, M. F., Rosenbaum, R., & Talmon, M. (1992). Planned single-session psychotherapy. In S. H. Budman, M. F. Hoyt, & S. Friedman, *The first session in brief therapy* (pp. 59–86). New York: Guilford Press.

Hudson, P. O., & O'Hanlon, W. H. (1992). *Rewriting love stories: Brief marital therapy*. New York: Norton.

Jacobson, N. (1996, January–February). Does therapy work? *The Family Therapy Networker*, 12–14.

Johnson, L. D. (1990). *Using language for change*. Unpublished manuscript.

Johnson, L. D. (1992). *Homework assignments*. Unpublished monograph.

Johnson, L. D. (1995). *Psychotherapy in the age of accountability*. New York: Norton.

Johnson, L. D., & Miller, S. D. (1994). Modification of depression risk factors: A solution-focused approach. *Psychotherapy, 31*, 244–253.

Jones, E. E., & Pulos, S. M. (1993). Comparing the process in psychodynamic and cognitive-behavioral therapies. *Journal of Consulting and Clinical Psychology, 61*(2), 306–316.

Kalous, T. D. (1996, February). Managed care is here to stay [Letter to the editor]. *APA Monitor*, p. 3.

Kingsbury, S. J. (1995, September). Where does research on the effectiveness of psychotherapy stand today? *The Harvard Mental Health Newsletter*, p. 8.

Klein, R. H. (1985). Some principles of short-term group therapy. *International Journal of Group Psychotherapy, 35*, 309–329.

Klerman, G. L., Weissman, M. M., Rounsaville, B. J., & Chevron, E. S. (1984). *Interpersonal therapy of depression*. New York: Basic Books.

Kohn, A. (1990). *The brighter side of human nature*. New York: Basic Books.

Kopta, S. M., Howard, K. I., Lowry, J. L., & Beutler, L. E. (1994). Patterns of symptomatic recovery in psychotherapy. *Journal of Consulting and Clinical Psychology, 62*, 1009–1016.

Koss, M. P., & Butcher, J. N. (1986). Research on brief therapy. In S. L. Garfield & A. E. Bergin (Eds.), *Handbook of psychotherapy and behavior change* (3rd ed., pp. 627–670). New York: Wiley.

Koss, M. P., & Shiang, J. (1994). Research on brief therapy. In A. E. Bergin & S. L. Garfield (Eds.), *Handbook of psychotherapy and behavior change* (4th ed., pp. 664–700). New York: Wiley.

Kreilkamp, T. (1989). *Intermittent time-limited therapy with children and families*. New York: Brunner/Mazel.

Lambert, M. J., & Bergin, A. E. (1994). The effectiveness of psychotherapy. In A. E. Bergin & S. L. Garfield (Eds.), *Handbook of psychotherapy and behavior change* (4th ed., pp. 143–190). New York: Wiley.

Lambert, M. J., Shapiro, D. A., & Bergin, A. E. (1986). The effectiveness of psychotherapy. In S. L. Garfield & A. E. Bergin (Eds.), *Handbook of psychotherapy and behavior change* (3rd ed., pp. 157–211). New York: Wiley.

Lankton, S. R., Lankton, C. H., & Matthews, W. J. (1991). Ericksonian family therapy. In A. S. Gurman & D. P. Kniskern (Eds.), *Handbook of family therapy* (Vol. 2, pp. 239–283). New York: Brunner/Mazel.

Lazarus, L. W. (1982). Brief psychotherapy for narcissistic disturbances. *Psychotherapy, 19*, 228–236.

Lehman, A. K., & Salovey, P. (1990). An introduction to cognitive-behavior therapy. In R. A. Wells & V. J. Giannetti (Eds.), *Handbook of the brief psychotherapies* (pp. 239–259). New York: Plenum Press.

Leibovich, M. (1981). Short-term psychotherapy for the borderline personality disorder. *Psychotherapy and Psychosomatics, 2*, 57–64.

LeShan, L. (1990). *The dilemma of psychology*. New York: Dutton.

Levenson, H. (1995). *Time-limited dynamic psychotherapy: A guide to clinical practice*. New York: HarperCollins.

Levenson, H., Speed, J. L., & Budman, S. (1992, June). *Therapist training and skill in brief therapy: A survey of Massachusetts and California psychologists.* Paper presented to the Society for Psychological Research, Berkeley, California.

Levy, R. L., & Shelton, J. L. (1990). Tasks in brief therapy. In R. A. Wells & V. J. Giannetti (Eds.), *Handbook of the brief psychotherapies* (pp. 145–163). New York: Plenum Press.

Lindemann, E. (1994). Symptomatology and management of acute grief. *American Journal of Psychiatry, 101,* 141–148.

Linehan, M. M., & Kehrer, C. A. (1993). Borderline personality disorder. In D. Barlow (Ed.), *Clinical handbook of psychological disorders* (2nd ed., pp. 396–442). New York: Guilford Press.

Lipsey, M. W., & Wilson, D. B. (1993). The efficacy of psychological, educational, and behavioral treatment: Confirmation from meta-analysis. *American Psychologist, 48*(12), 1181–1209.

Logue, M. B., Sher, K. J., & Frensch, P. A. (1992). Purported characteristics of adult children of alcoholics: A possible "Barnum effect." *Professional Psychology: Research and Practice, 23,* 226–232.

Luborsky, L., McClellan, A. T., Woody, G. E., O'Brien, C. P., & Auerbach, A. (1985). Therapist success and its determinants. *Archives of General Psychiatry, 32,* 995–1008.

Luborsky, L., Singer, B., & Luborsky, L. (1975). Comparative studies of psychotherapies. *Archives of General Psychiatry, 32,* 995–1008.

Lykken, D. T. (1995). *The antisocial personalities.* Hillsdale, N.J: Erlbaum.

Madanes, C. (1981). *Strategic family therapy.* San Francisco: Jossey-Bass.

Mahoney, M. J. (1993). Theoretical developments in the cognitive psychotherapies. *Journal of Consulting and Clinical Psychology, 61,* 187–193.

Mahoney, M. J. (Ed.). (1995). *Cognitive and constructive psychotherapies: Theory, research and practice.* New York: Springer.

Mahoney, M. J., & Norcross, J. C. (1993). Relationship styles and therapeutic choices: A commentary on the preceding four articles. *Psychotherapy, 30,* 423–426.

Malan, D. H. (1976). *The frontier of brief psychotherapy.* New York: Plenum Press.

Malan, D. H. (1986a). Beyond interpretation: Initial evaluation and technique in short-term dynamic psychotherapy: Part 1. *International Journal of Short-Term Psychotherapy, 1,* 59–82.

Malan, D. H. (1986b). Beyond interpretation: Initial evaluation and technique in short-term dynamic psy-

chotherapy: Part II. *International Journal of Short-Term Psychotherapy, 1 ,* 83–106.

Malan, D. H. (1992). *Psychodynamics, training, and outcome in brief psychotherapy.* Oxford: Butterworth-Heineman.

Malan, J. (1963). *A study of brief psychotherapy.* London: Tavistock.

Mann, J. (1973). *Time-limited psychotherapy.* Cambridge, MA: Harvard University Press.

Mann, J. (1991). Time-limited psychotherapy. In P. Crits-Christoph & J. P. Barber (Eds.), *Handbook of short-term dynamic psychotherapy* (pp. 17–44). New York: Basic Books.

Mann, J., & Goldman, R. (1982). *A casebook in time-limited psychotherapy.* New York: McGraw-Hill.

Massad, P. M., West, A. N, & Friedman, M. J. (1990). Relationship between utilization of mental health and medical services in a VA hospital. *American Journal of Psychiatry, 147*(4), April.

Maxmen, J. S., & Ward, N. G. (1995). *Essential psychopathology and its treatment* (2nd ed.). New York: Norton.

McCrady, B. S. (1993). Alcoholism. In D. Barlow (Ed.), *Clinical handbook of psychological disorders* (2nd ed., pp. 362–395). New York: Guilford Press.

Meehl, P. (1973). Why I do not attend case conferences. In P. Meehl (Ed.), *Psychodiagnosis* (pp. 225–302). New York: Norton.

Meisol, P. (1995, October 31). The therapy shrink. *The Baltimore Sun,* p. 1E.

Messer, S. B., & Warren, C. S. (1995). *Models of brief psychodynamic therapy: A comparative approach.* New York: Guilford Press.

Miller, S. D., & Berg, I. K. (1995). *The miracle method: A radical new approach to problem drinking.* New York: Norton.

Miller, S., Hubble, M., & Duncan, B. (1995, March–April). No more bells and whistles. *The Family Therapy Networker,* 53–63.

Minuchin, S., & Fishman, H. C. (1981). *Family therapy techniques.* Cambridge, MA: Harvard University Press.

Mohl, P. C., Martinez, D., Ticknor, C., Huang, M., & Cordell, L. (1991). Early drop-outs from psychotherapy. *Journal of Nervous and Mental Disease, 179,* 478–491.

Myers, D. G. (1992). *The pursuit of happiness.* New York: Avon.

National Institute of Mental Health. (1981). *Provisional data on federally funded community mental health centers 1978–79.* Report prepared by the Survey and Reports Branch, Division of Biometry and Epidemiology. Washington, DC: U.S. Government Printing Office.

Norcross, J. C. (1995, September). *Brief prescriptive psychotherapy: Customizing psychological treatments and therapeutic relationships.* Presentation sponsored by Walk-In Counseling Center, Minneapolis, Minnesota.

Norcross, J. C. (1995). Dispelling the dodo bird verdict and the exclusivity myth in psychotherapy. *Psychotherapy, 32,* 500–504.

Norcross, J. C., & Goldfried, M. R. (Eds.). (1992). *Handbook of psychotherapy integration.* New York: Basic Books.

Norcross, J. C., & Newman, C. F. (1992). Psychotherapy integration: Setting the context. In J. C. Norcross & M. R. Goldfried (Eds.), *Handbook of psychotherapy integration* (pp. 3–46). New York: Basic Books .

Ogles, B. M., Lambert, M. J., & Masters, K. S. (1996). *Assessing outcome in clinical practice.* Boston: Allyn and Bacon.

Ogles, B. M., Lambert, M. J., & Sawyer, D. (1993, June). *The clinical significance of the NIMH Treatment of Depression Collaborative Research Program data.* Paper presented at the annual meeting of the Society of Psychotherapy Research, Pittsburgh.

O'Hanlon, W. H., & Weiner-Davis, M. (1989). *In search of solutions: A new direction in psychotherapy.* New York: Norton.

O'Hanlon, W. H., & Wilk, J. (1987). *Shifting contexts.* New York: Guilford Press.

Olfson, M., & Pincus, H. A. (1994). Outpatient psychotherapy in the United States: II. Patterns of utilization. *American Journal of Psychiatry, 151,* 1289–1294.

Omer, H. (1994). *Critical interventions in psychotherapy.* New York: Norton.

Orlinsky, D. E., & Howard, K. I. (1995a). *Comprehensive textbook of psychotherapy: Theory and practice.* New York: Oxford University Press.

Orlinsky, D. E., & Howard, K. I. (1995b). Unity and diversity among psychotherapies: A comparative perspective. In B. Bongar & L. E. Beutler (Eds.), *Comprehensive textbook of psychotherapy: Theory and practice* (pp. 3–24). New York: Oxford University Press.

Peake, T. H., Borduin, C. M., & Archer, R. P. (1988). *Brief psychotherapies: Changing frames of mind.* Beverly Hills, CA: Sage Publications.

Pekarik, G. (1983). Improvement in clients who have given different reasons for dropping out of treatment. *Journal of Clinical Psychology, 39,* 909–913.

Pekarik, G. (1990a). *Brief therapy training manual.* Topeka, KS: Washburn University.

Pekarik, G. (1990b, January). *Rationale, training, and implementation of time-sensitive treatments.* Presentation to Executive Directors, MCC Companies, Inc. Minneapolis, Minnesota.

Pekarik, G., & Finney-Owen, G. K. (1987). Psychotherapist's attitudes and beliefs relevant to client drop-out. *Community Mental Health Journal, 23*(2), 120–130.

Pekarik, G., & Wierzbicki, M. (1986). The relationship between expected and actual psychotherapy duration. *Psychotherapy, 23,* 532–534.

Persons, J. B. (1991). Psychotherapy outcome studies do not accurately represent current models of psychotherapy. *American Psychologist, 46*(2), 99–106.

Peters, T., & Waterman, R. (1982). *In search of excellence: Lessons from America's best run companies.* New York: Harper & Row.

Phelps, P. A. (1993). The case of oppositional cooperation. In R. A. Wells & V. J. Giannetti (Eds.), *Casebook of the brief psychotherapies* (pp. 287–303). New York: Plenum Press.

Phillips, E. L. (1985). *Psycotherapy revisited: New frontiers in research and practice.* Hillsdale, NJ: Erlbaum.

Prochaska, J. O., DiClemente, C. C., & Norcross, J. C. (1992). In search of how people change: Applications to addictive behaviors. *American Psychologist, 47,* 1102–1114.

Prochaska, J. O., Norcross, J. C., & DiClemente, C. C. (1994). *Changing for good.* New York: Avon.

Quick, E. (1995). *Doing what works in brief therapy: A strategic solution-focused approach.* Orlando, FL: Academic Press.

Rank, O. (1929/1978). *Will therapy.* New York: Norton.

Reid, W. J. (1990). An integrative model for short-term treatment. In R. A. Wells & V. J. Giannetti (Eds.), *Handbook of the brief psychotherapies* (pp. 55–77). New York: Plenum Press.

Rubin, S. S., & Niemeier, D. L. (1992). Non-verbal affective communication as a factor in psychotherapy. *Psychotherapy, 29,* 596–602.

Sabin, J. E. (1991). Clinical skills for the 1990's: Six lessons from the HMO practice. *Hospital and Community Psychiatry, 42*(6), 605–608.

Sachs, J. S. (1983). Negative factors in brief psychotherapy: An empirical assessment. *Journal of Consulting and Clinical Psychology, 51*(4), 557–564.

Scheidlinger, S. (1984). Short-term group therapy for children: An overview. *International Journal of Group Psychotherapy, 34,* 573–585.

Segal, L. (1991). Brief therapy: The MRI approach. In A. S. Gurman & D. P. Kniskern (Eds.), *Handbook of family therapy* (Vol. 2, pp. 171–199). New York: Brunner/Mazel.

Selekman, M. D. (1991). The solution-oriented parenting group: A treatment alternative that works. *Journal of Strategic and Systemic Therapies, 10*(1), 37–50.

Seligman, M. E. P. (1990). *Learned optimism.* New York: Pocket Books.

Seligman, M. E. P. (1995). The effectiveness of psychotherapy: The Consumer Reports Study. *American Psychologist, 50(12)*, 965–974.

Shaffer, W. F. (1986). Diagnosis as a sham and a reality. *Journal of Counseling and Development, 64*, 612–613.

Shapiro, D., Barkham, M., Rees, A., Hardy, G. E., Reynolds, S., & Startup, M. (1994). Effects of treatment duration and severity of depression on the effectiveness of cognitive-behavioral and psychodynamic-interpersonal psychotherapy. *Journal of Consulting and Clinical Psychology, 62*, 522–534.

Shapiro, D. A., & Shapiro, D. (1982). Meta-analysis of comparative outcome studies: A replication and refinement. *Psychological Bulletin, 92*, 581–604.

Shefler, G., Dasberg, H., & Ben-Shakhar, G. (1995). A randomized controlled outcome and follow-up study of Mann's time-limited psychotherapy. *Journal of Consulting and Clinical Psychology, 63*, 585–593.

Shiang, J., & Bongar, B. (1995). Brief and crisis psychotherapy in theory and practice. In B. Bongar & L. E. Beutler (Eds.), *Comprehensive textbook of psychotherapy: Theory and practice* (pp. 380–405). New York: Oxford University Press.

Shriqui, C. L., & Nasrallah, H. A. (1995). *Contemporary issues in the treatment of schizophrenia.* Washington, DC: American Psychiatric Press.

Sifneos, P. S. (1992). *Short-term anxiety-provoking therapy: A treatment manual.* New York: Basic Books.

Sledge, W. H., Moras, K., Hartley, D., & Levine, M. (1990). Effect of time-limited therapy on patient drop-out rates. *American Journal of Psychiatry, 147*, 1341–1347.

Smith, M. L., Glass, G. V., & Miller, T. I. (1980). *The benefits of psychotherapy.* Baltimore: Johns Hopkins University Press.

Smyrnios, K. X., & Kirby, R. J. (1993). Long-term comparison of brief versus unlimited psychodynamic treatments with children and their parents. *Journal of Consulting and Clinical Psychology, 61*, 1020–1027.

Sowell, T. (1994). *Race and culture: A world view.* New York: Basic Books.

Stein, D. M., & Lambert, M. J. (1995). Graduate training in psychotherapy: Are outcomes enhanced? *Journal of Consulting and Clinical Psychology, 63*, 182–196.

Strupp, H. H., & Binder, J. L. (1984). *Psychotherapy in a new key: A guide to time-limited dynamic psychotherapy.* New York: Basic Books.

Sue, S., & Zane, N. (1987). The role of culture and cultural techniques in psychotherapy. *American Psychologist, 42*(1), 37–45.

Sue, S., Zane, N., & Young, K. (1994). Research on psychotherapy with culturally diverse populations. In A. E. Bergin & S. L. Garfield (Eds.), *Handbook of psychotherapy and behavior change* (4th ed., pp. 783–817). New York: Wiley.

Svartberg, M., & Stiles, T. C. (1991). Comparative effect of short-term dynamic psychotherapy: a meta-analysis. *Journal of Consulting and Clinical Psychology, 59*, 704–714.

Szapocnik, J., Kurtines, W. M., Perez-Vidal, A., Hervis, O. E., & Foote, F. H. (1990). One person family therapy. In R. A. Wells & V. J. Giannetti (Eds.), *Handbook of the brief psychotherapies* (pp. 493–513). New York: Plenum Press.

Talmon, M. (1990). *Single-session therapy: Maximizing the effect of the first (and often only) therapeutic encounter.* San Francisco: Jossey-Bass.

Taube, C. A., Goldman, H. H., Burns, B. J., & Kessler, L. G. (1988). High users of outpatient mental health services: Definitions and characteristics. *American Journal of Psychiatry, 145(1)*, 19–24.

Todd, T. C., & Selekman, M. D. (1991). *Family therapy approaches with adolescent substance abusers.* Needham Heights, MA: Allyn and Bacon.

Triandis, H. C. (1996). The psychological measurement of cultural syndromes. *American Psychologist, 51*, 407–415.

Ursano, R. J., Sonnenberg, S. M., & Lazar, S. G. (1991). *Concise guide to psychodynamic psychotherapy.* Washington, DC: American Psychiatric Press.

Vachss, A. (1993). Sexual predators can't be saved. *Star-Tribune*, January 7, p. 21A.

Walter, J. L., & Peller, J. E. (1992). *Becoming solution focused in brief therapy.* New York: Brunner/Mazel.

Watzlawick, P., Weakland, J., & Fisch, R. (1974). *Change.* New York: Norton.

Weakland, J. H., & Fisch, R. (1992). Brief therapy—MRI style. In S. H. Budman, M. F. Hoyt, & S. Friedman (Eds.), *The first session in brief therapy* (pp. 306–324). New York: Guilford Press.

Weeks, G. R., & Treat, S. (1992). *Couples in treatment: Techniques and approaches for effective practice.* New York: Brunner/Mazel.

Weiss, J., Sampson, J., & the Mount Zion Psychotherapy Research Group. (1986). *The psychoanalytic process: Theory, clinical observations, and empirical research.* New York: Guilford Press.

Weissman, M. M., & Markowitz, J. A. (1994). Interpersonal psychotherapy: Current status. *Archives of General Psychiatry, 51,* 599–606.

Wells, R. A. (1993). Clinical strategies in brief psychotherapy. In R. A. Wells & V. J. Giannetti (Eds.), *Casebook of the brief psychotherapies* (pp. 3–17). New York: Plenum Press.

Wells, R. A., & Giannetti, V. J. (Eds.). (1990). *Handbook of the brief psychotherapies.* New York: Plenum Press.

Wells, R. A., & Giannetti, V. J. (Eds.). (1993). *Casebook of the brief psychotherapies.* New York: Plenum Press.

Wilson, G. T. (1995). Behavior therapy. In R. J. Corsini & D. Wedding (Eds.), *Current psychotherapies* (5th ed., pp. 197–229). Itasca, IL: Peacock.

Winston, A., Laikan, M., Pollack, J., Samstag, L. W., McCullough, L., & Muran, J. C. (1994). Short-term psychotherapy of personality disorders. *American Journal of Psychiatry, 151*(2), 190–194.

Wolberg, L. R. (1965). The technique of short-term therapy. In L. R. Wolberg (Ed.), *Short-term psychotherapy* (pp.127–200). New York: Grune & Stratton.

Wolberg, L. R. (1980). *Handbook of short-term psychotherapy.* New York: Thieme-Stratton.

Yalom, I. (1989). *Love's executioner & other tales of psychotherapy.* New York: Harper Perennial.

Yalom, I. (1995). Foreword. In I. D. Glick (Ed.), *Treating depression.* San Francisco: Jossey-Bass.

Yapko, M. (1992). Therapy with direction. In S. H. Budman, M. F. Hoyt, & S. Friedman (Eds.), *The first session in brief therapy* (pp. 156–180). New York: Guilford Press.

Zealberg, J. J., Santos, A. B., & Puckett, J. A. (1996). *Comprehensive emergency mental health care.* New York: Norton.

Zeig, J. (Ed.). (1982). *Ericksonian approaches to hypnosis and psychotherapy.* New York: Brunner/Mazel.

Zimet, C. N. (1989). The mental health care revolution: Will psychology survive? *American Psychologist, 44,* 703–708.

FOR FURTHER READING

Bloom, B. L. (1992). *Planned short-term psychotherapy: A clinical handbook.* Boston: Allyn and Bacon. *A comparative review with good references and examples of clinical work.*

Budman, S. H., & Gurman, A. S. (1988). *Theory and practice of brief therapy.* New York: Guilford Press. *A classic reference emphasizing the authors' "I-D-E" approach and now somewhat outdated, but with useful information nevertheless.*

Budman, S. H., Hoyt, M. F., & Friedman, S. (Eds.). (1992). *The first session in brief therapy.* New York: Guilford Press. *An engaging casebook-like reference comparing different approaches across the first session. With editorial commentaries and interviews.*

Johnson, L. D. (1995). *Psychotherapy in the age of accountability.* New York: Norton. *A readable, entertaining perspective of doing brief therapy in an era of managed care by a highly skilled, funny, and opinionated therapist.*

Koss, M. P., & Shiang, J. (1994). Research on brief therapy. In A. E. Bergin & S. L. Garfield (Eds.), *Handbook of psychotherapy and behavior change* (4th ed., pp. 664–700). New York: Wiley. *A definitive overview of the subject.*

Messer, S. B., & Warren, C. S. (1995). *Models of brief psychodynamic therapy: A comparative approach.* New York: Guilford Press. *This detailed review is refreshingly grounded in research.*

Shiang, J., & Bongar, B. (1995). Brief and crisis psychotherapy in theory and practice. In B. Bongar & L. E. Beutler (Eds.), *Comprehensive textbook of psychotherapy: Theory and practice* (pp. 380–405). New York: Oxford University Press. *Another useful overview and summary with some unique thinking relating, as the title suggests, theory to practice.*

Wells, R. A., & Giannetti, V. J. (Eds.). (1990). *Handbook of the brief psychotherapies.* New York: Plenum Press. *More theoretically based than its companion book below.*

Wells, R. A., & Giannetti, V. J. (Eds.). (1993). *Casebook of the brief psychotherapies.* New York: Plenum Press. *Illustrations (not all of which are successes) of actual cases.*

CHAPTER 9

ASSESSMENT AND TREATMENT OF CHILDREN AND ADOLESCENTS

Gary Geffken

INTRODUCTION

History of Child Psychology

At the beginning of the twentieth century, Freud developed his theory of personality, which emphasizes the importance of early childhood development. Freud's psychoanalytic perspective on child development is evident in his well-known analysis of the case of little Hans, a little boy whose phobia of horses Freud attributed to the oedipal complex (Freud, 1959). Despite this emphasis, the recipient of Freud's psychoanalysis remained the adult patient. Lightner Witmer is credited with establishing the first psychology clinic for children in 1896 (Routh, 1994). His early cases involved treating educational problems in children. During this era, in an effort to differentiate retarded from nonretarded children in the French school system, Binet and Simon developed the Binet-Simon scale, which became the forerunner of contemporary intellectual testing with children (Sattler, 1992).

Children became a focus of intervention and treatment in the early 1900s. At the turn of the twentieth century, personal hygiene was discovered as a source of the spread of disease. This was general-

ized from the physical realm to the mental realm, which spawned the development of mental hygiene clinics and child guidance clinics. There was such an impetus to develop these clinics that by 1914 almost every city had such a clinic, as the theory was that treating children early may prevent the need for future institutionalization. In the 1920s Freud's psychoanalytic approach was modified by his student Melanie Klein and his daughter Anna Freud to address the treatment of children. Early behaviorism was introduced to child psychology in 1920, when Watson and Rayner described the case of Little Albert. They demonstrated that it was possible to condition behaviorally a fear response to a white rat. Despite an emphasis on children in the development of theory, most of the initial growth of clinical psychology focused on adults, as outlined in subsequent chapters.

In 1949 the Wechsler Intelligence Scale for Children was published. It represented a downward extension of the adult intelligence scale. In 1968 Erikson published *Identity, Youth and Crisis*, in which he described the eight stages of psychosocial development. The American Psychological Association (APA) established sections on clinical child psychology and pediatric psychology, thus further emphasizing the importance of studying, assessing, and treating children.

As mentioned earlier, the real growth of clinical psychology focused on adults. Many of the personality theories and assessment methodologies did not account for the developmental nature of childhood. Hence, while early clinicians were studying and writing about the psychological nature of childhood, the growth of child psychology as a scientific enterprise did not take place until much later.

Overview of This Chapter

This chapter is divided into three main sections: assessment, intervention, and special issues dealing with children.

The section on assessment begins with a statement on the value of assessment for children and the need for attention to developmental considerations. This is followed by a review of psychometric issues, including the standardization of measures for children, various types of standardized scores, and important considerations regarding reliability and validity. These technical issues will form the background for a review of measures commonly used with children and adolescents. Broad categories of measures will include intellectual measures, achievement measures, adaptive behavior scales, personality tests, and parent report measures. The section on assessment will conclude with a case report illustrating child assessment.

The next section of this chapter will focus on intervention. The section will begin with a review of major theoretical systems, including behavioral models, the cognitive-behavioral model, the psychodynamic model, the family systems model, and play therapy. Additionally, a sampling of empirically validated treatments for children will be reviewed in the context of the DSM-IV. The section on intervention will conclude with a case report of an intervention with a child.

The final major section of this chapter will deal with special issues related to the assessment and treatment of children and adolescents, including a review of ethical issues such as competence, confidentiality, test security, and professional relations.

There will also be a review of special issues in the diagnosis of the mental retardation and learning disabilities. Ethnic minority issues, sexual and physical abuse, and pediatric psychology will also be addressed. Future trends for the field of clinical child psychology will also be discussed.

ASSESSMENT

The Value of Assessment

What advantages does a clinical psychologist have over a lay person when sizing up a child or adolescent? Clinical psychologists' special expertise in child assessment lies in their knowledge of how to ask questions or conduct a clinical interview, their background in psychopathology, their background in child and adolescent development, and their psychometric expertise in measurement. These sources of expertise are factors in the decisions of school guidance counselors, pediatricians, neurologists, and child psychiatrists to refer youngsters to clinical psychologists for evaluation.

The APA and an overwhelming majority of state psychological associations maintain that a doctoral degree in psychology and state licensure is necessary to practice clinical psychology. A doctoral degree should include basic training in the core areas of psychology, including courses in development, psychopathology related to both children and adults, and courses in assessment covering objective and projective assessment techniques and behavioral assessment techniques. The doctoral program that trains a clinician to be proficient in the psychological assessment of children requires practicum experiences with both children and adults. Courses in measurement or research design that emphasize the constructs of reliability and validity, together with statistics classes, allow the clinical psychologist to evaluate psychological tests that may be used to select the most psychometrically sophisticated tests from the array of available tests. After finishing a doctoral program, psychology trainees must complete a one-year internship before being awarded a doctoral degree. In addition, after obtaining their doctoral degree, most states require a year of postdoctoral supervision by a licensed psychologist before taking a state licensing exam. Hence, with this brief review of qualifications, one gets a sense of the special expertise that clinical psychologists have in conducting psychological assessments of children and adolescents.

Development

Developmental theories such as Freud's theory of psychosexual development, Piaget's theory of cognitive development, and Erikson's psychosocial theory of development have historically played a critical role in conceptualizing child psychology. They have also provided the groundwork for more contemporary empirically based developmental models. An introduction to the psychological assessment and treatment of children would not be complete without emphasizing issues related to child development. Psychology trainees at both the graduate and undergraduate levels are exposed to coursework in child development. Those who find this area particularly interesting and relevant may opt to concentrate their studies and become developmental psychologists.

Knowledge related to a child's level of development allows the psychologist to tailor therapeutic interventions to a developmentally appropriate level. The competent clinical psychologist is aware of developmental issues, genetic and hereditary influences, and influences occurring during the prenatal period and birth process. The child psychologist needs to be familiar with numerous developmental milestones a child is expected to achieve in areas, including learning of motor skills, language skills, cognitive development, emotional development, intellectual development, and sexual development. It is important for psychologists both to be aware of and to inquire about the timing and attainment of these developmental milestones, as they may have significant impact on further growth. Growth is also influenced by the family and significant others, such as school and peers; thus, clinical psychologists also assess and monitor these influences as they relate to the child. Taken together, these influences are part of an empirical body of knowledge understood as developmental psychology.

Psychometric Issues

When conducting an assessment, clinical psychologists must select instruments from a broad array of psychological tests. These decisions are based on psychometric issues including technical expertise, statistical knowledge, research design, and ethical behavior. How does the clinical psychologist choose from the array of the intellectual tests, achievement tests, and personality tests? Certainly one factor should be the psychometric properties of the test, including how reliable the test is or how consistently the same results are obtained with the same child. It is also important to consider the validity of the test or the degree to which the test can be demonstrated actually to measure the characteristics that it is intended to measure. In addition, one must consider the normative basis of the test, or the group to which a child's scores are compared.

Standardization

The standardization of a test refers to a process by which a test is administered, in identical fashion, to a normative sample of subjects. This allows for the comparison of a particular child to a reference group of children who share similar characteristics, such as age, grade, gender, and/or race. Standardization samples for tests vary enormously. The Wechsler Intelligence Scale for Children, Third Edition (WISC-III; Wechsler, 1991), is a test that was designed with a relatively superior standardization process. In developing the WISC-III, emphasis was placed on developing precise administration procedures, which are specified in the manual for the test. Typically a clinician can administer the WISC-III in 90 to 120 minutes. These administration procedures were followed with a standardization sample of children between the ages of 6 and 16, with approximately 100 boys and 100 girls at each one-year age interval. The sample represents a cross-section of recent U.S. census data, with proportionate numbers based on ethnicity, socioeconomic status, geographic location, and other relevant variables. Children and adolescents who are administered this test are compared to this standardization sample.

For the reasons described earlier, clinicians frequently select the WISC-III as an intellectual assessment tool when a question arises about the intellectual development of a particular child. There are numerous psychological tests that are not comparable to the WISC-III for a variety of issues related to psychometrics. Often, when tests are developed, not as much care is taken in developing a standardization sample that is as representative of the U.S. census data, and also administration procedures are not as carefully described.

Types of Scores

Once a youngster has taken a test, the examiner must score the test. There are numerous types of scores that are important to know about in understanding psychological tests. Some are described next.

Raw scores. Generally, the child's responses on a psychological test are summed to obtain a raw score. On an ability test, the raw score represents correct responses to test items, whereas on a personality or behavior rating scale the raw score is indicative of responses consistent with the construct that the test is measuring. These raw scores do not tell the examiner how the child performed in relation to other children with similar characteristics (e.g., age-related comparison group); thus, the informative value of raw scores to the examiner is quite limited. For example, if one were scoring an arithmetic test, the same raw score or number of correct items would have a very different meaning for a child of 5 who received a score of 15 out of 20 correct compared to a child of 15 who got 15 out of 20 correct. To account for such discrepancies, the raw scores are converted to standardized scores.

Standardized scores. Once a raw score has been converted to a standardized score, the examiner may compare a child's performance to the standardization sample. Using the foregoing example, a 5-year-old child taking an arithmetic test could have his performance compared to other 5-year-old children, while the 15-year-old could have his performance compared to other 15-year-old children.

There are numerous types of standardized scores. In this chapter there is a review of deviation scores, percentiles, T-scores, age equivalents, and grade equivalents.

Deviation scores. Deviation scores are typically used to refer to a child's performance on ability tests, such as IQ tests or achievement tests. Deviation scores are appropriately used on tests that are normally distributed—that is, where the distribution of scores approximates a bell-shaped curve. Using the Wechsler Intelligence Scale for Children, Third Edition, as an example, the mean or average performance on the test is defined by a score of 100. A child scoring 100 has performed at the 50th percentile and has scored better than half the children his age. The standard deviation is a measure of the variability of the scores of the reference group. On the WISC-III the standard deviation is 15. Hence, if a child scores one standard deviation below the mean, we know that a deviation IQ of 85 means they scored at the 16th percentile, regardless of their age. Likewise, if a child scores two standard deviations below the mean, his or her performance is at the 2nd percentile, meaning that the child scored better than only 2% of children of the same age.

Percentile rankings. Percentile rankings are another form of standardized score. Percentile ranks range from a fraction of the first percentile to the 99+ percentile rank. Using percentile rankings, a youngster's score may be described in reference to an appropriate comparison group. A percentile rank represents the percentage of the comparison sample that the child's performance surpassed. Thus, using the WISC-III as an example, a child's IQ score of 100 would be at the 50th percentile, meaning that the child scored better than 50% of the children in the reference group. Similarly, if a child obtained a score of 130 on WISC-III, this would correspond to the 98th percentile, meaning the child scored better than 98% of the children in the appropriate comparison group.

T-scores. T-scores are an alternative form of standardized scores, which are similar to deviation scores and are also related to percentile rankings.

One of the more popularly used personality tests for youngsters that utilizes T-scores is the Minnesota Multiphasic Personality Inventory for Adolescents (MMPI-A). The mean or average score is equivalent to a T-score of 50. This means that a child who obtains a T-score of 50 has scored at the 50th percentile relative to the scale the child's self-report was being measured on. If one desired to look at a child's score on the Depression scale of the MMPI-A, one would know that a T-score of 50 meant that the child endorsed a typical or average amount of items, and generally would not be considered depressed. The standard deviation on the T-score distribution is 10. Therefore, a score of 70 would be two standard deviations above the mean. In terms of percentile rankings, a score of 70 indicates that the child endorsed items with a positive loading onto this scale more often than 98% of his or her appropriate comparison group. If a child were to receive a T-score of 70 on the depression scale of the MMPI-A, he or she would generally be considered depressed.

Age-equivalent scores. Age-equivalent scores are commonly used on children's achievement tests or tests of academic abilities. An age-equivalent represents the average performance of a child at a particular age in the normative sample. For example, if a child received an age-equivalent score of 8 years on a reading achievement test, this would mean that the child performed at the level of the average 8-year-old in the normative sample. Age-equivalent scores are not dependent on the child's actual chronological age; thus an age-equivalent score of 8 years could be obtained by a 5-year-old or a 15-year-old. Parents are typically unfamiliar with the meaning of standardized scores, such as deviation scores and *t*-scores. Thus, the age equivalent score can be a means of communicating a child's achievement to a parent.

Grade-equivalent scores. Grade-equivalent scores are similar to age-equivalent scores and represent another form of standardized scores. Like age-equivalent scores, grade-equivalent scores are frequently used to describe results on achievement tests for youngsters. A grade-equivalent score rep-

resents the average performance of a child at particular grade level in the reference group. Therefore, a grade-equivalent score at the third-grade level would mean that a child's performance was similar to that of the average third-grade child, or at the 50th percentile for the children in third grade. As with the age-equivalent score, this is independent of the actual grade in which the child taking the test is currently enrolled. Hence, a child in the twelfth grade who obtained a third-grade equivalent score would be similar in performance to a child in the first grade who also obtained a third-grade equivalent score. Like age-equivalent scores, grade-equivalent scores may facilitate communication about a child's performance with the child's parents.

Standard error of measurement. Standard error of measurement is a term used to describe the range of scores in which the child's true score likely falls. The standard error of measurement is a confidence interval formed around a child's obtained score. For example, on the WISC-III, if a child obtains a score of 100 with a standard error of measurement of ±6 at the 95% level of confidence, this would indicate that the child's true score would fall between 94 and 106, 95% of the time. Alternatively, if a child was administered the test 100 times, 5 times by chance alone his or her true score would fall outside the range of 94 to 106.

Reliability. As mentioned earlier, reliability and validity of the psychological instruments are also important considerations when choosing a test for administration. When a clinical psychologist administers a test to a child, he or she needs to eliminate as many sources of error as possible in order to assess accurately the child's true score on the measure. There are numerous factors that affect the reliability of a test, or factors that may contribute to the error in a test score. Sattler (1992) has described four factors affecting reliability: test length, test–retest interval, guessing, and variation in the test situation.

In general, if a test is well constructed, a longer test will be more reliable than a shorter one. *Test–retest interval* refers to the time that has elapsed between two separate testing occasions; in general, the longer the interval between test-taking occasions, the more likely it is that other factors such as ability or degree of psychopathology would change. Guessing is another factor affecting the reliability of scores. Guessing by an examinee introduces error into the examinee's score. The final factor that is described by Sattler (1992) is variation in the test situation. This refers to a variety of variables that may have an impact on the examinee's performance, including examiner errors in administration, distracting noise outside the testing room, lack of sleep, hunger, and illness. All of these factors may introduce error into the examinee's score. Various methods for assessing the reliabilty of a test include test–retest reliability, interrater reliability, internal consistency, and alternate form. These were reviewed in Chapter 3 of this book, with the exception of alternate-form reliability, which will be considered next.

Alternate-form reliability refers to the degree of consistency between two different versions of the same test. Most of the tests discussed in this chapter will not have alternate-form reliability. The Woodcock Johnson Tests of Achievement—Revised (WJ-R) does have alternate-form reliability. In alternate-form reliability, two versions of the same test are administered to a large group of children, and the degree of association or relationship between the two different forms of the test is calculated. The advantage of administering a test that has high alternate-form reliability is that it provides the opportunity to re-administer the test to a child, by using a different version. Thus, if the child recalls items from the first form of the test, this recall will not be a factor affecting his or her score in a retesting situation using the alternate form of the test.

Validity. Validity is another important psychometric aspect of a test. It is defined as the extent to which a test measures what it is intended to measure. A test cannot be valid unless it is reasonably reliable; however, tests need more than reliability to be valid. As with reliability, there are several types of validity including: face validity, construct validity, criterion validity including both predictive and concurrent validity, and content validity. These have been reviewed in Chapter 3 of this book. Validity in a test-taking situation can be affected by numerous different factors. These include the degree to which the examinee understood the test instructions, mastery of the language in which the test is administered, and educational experience which differs significantly from the standardization sample (Sattler, 1992). When testing children with certain handicaps such as visual impairment, hearing impairment, or motor impairment, it is important to consider the effects these handicaps will have on the validity of the tests, particularly when the test involves these skills. Likewise, acute emotional disruption or physical illness may adversely affect the validity of test results. Perhaps one of the more common factors affecting the validity of an assessment is an uncooperative child or a child whose attention is so poor as to leave the test invalid. In general, the child to be tested must be similar to the children represented in the standardization sample for the test to be valid.

Measures for Children and Adolescents

This section will review a number of measures frequently used with children and adolescents. Some of the most popular examples of each type of measure will be described. These will include intellectual tests, achievement tests, adaptive behavior scales, personality measures, and parent report measures. This section will conclude with a case report using some of the measures described.

Intellectual Measures

The assessment of intelligence and cognitive abilities is important for children and adolescents. Classifications like gifted, learning-disabled, and retarded are strongly affected by assessments of cognitive abilities. In school, children typically participate in group-administered cognitive ability tests as a means of assessing strengths and weaknesses. Frequently, children are separated early in school based on cognitive ability. This continues throughout high school, college, and professional training and has many controversial societal ramifications (Herrnstein & Murray, 1994).

The Wechsler scales. The Wechsler scales are a prototype of psychological tests for children and adolescents. They have superior standardization, reliability, and validity. There are three Wechsler Scales of Intelligence that may be used with children and adolescents. The Wechsler Preschool and Primary Scale of Intelligence—Revised (WPSSI-R) (Wechsler, 1989b) is used with children age 3 years, 0 months to 7 years, 3 months (see Table 9.1). The Wechsler Intelligence Scale for Children—Third Edition (WISC-III) (Wechsler, 1991) is used with children 6 years, 0 months through 16 years, 11 months. The Wechsler Adult Intelligence Scale—Revised (WAIS-R)* (Wechsler, 1989a) is used for older adolescents beginning at age 16 years, 0 months and extending into adulthood. The Wechsler scales provide a means for assessing intellect through an individually administered test. In most areas of the country, intellectual testing is required for children to receive special educational services. These special services include placement in gifted classes, placement in classes where services are geared toward various levels of retardation, and classification for dropout intervention programs. When intellectual testing is done in conjunction with achievement testing, psychologists can provide schools with classifications of specific learning disabilities. While administering an individually administered achievement test, the examiner has the opportunity to ensure that the child gives sufficient effort to yield a reliable and valid assessment of his or her abilities. This is a distinct advantage over the group-administered cognitive ability testing done regularly in school systems.

The Wechsler scales have certain commonalities that make it easier for the examiner to learn to administer them. Generally they all take between 90 and 120 minutes to administer. Each comprises 11 to 13 subtests or separate tasks of different types of intellectual abilities. Taken together, these subtests yield a global or composite scale score referred to as the Full Scale Intelligence Quotient or FSIQ. The FSIQ is a deviation score or IQ, as referred to in the earlier section on types of scores. It has a mean of

Table 9.1 Subtests and Typical Items on the WPPSI-R

SUBTEST	TYPICAL ITEMS
Object Assembly	Arrange pieces to fit into a form board or assemble jigsaw puzzles.
Geometric Design	Select a matching design; copy a design shown on a printed card.
Block Design	Arrange 3 or 4 blocks to reproduce designs.
Picture Completion	Identify the essential missing part in a picture.
Animal Pegs	Place colored pegs matched with corresponding animals into the appropriate holes.
Information	Includes questions similar to: "How many eyes do you have?" "What color is the sky?" "Tell me the name of a fruit."
Comprehension	Includes questions similar to: "Why do people need to wear clothes?" "Why do we need to keep ice in the freezer?"
Arithmetic	Includes questions similar to: "How many apples are 2 apples and 3 apples?" "Sally has 3 books. She loans 2 of them to her friend. How many books does she have left?"
Vocabulary	Includes questions similar to: "What is a fork?" "What is a flower?" "What does *catch* mean?"
Similarities	Includes questions similar to: "How are green beans and potatoes alike?" "How are a quarter and a dime alike?"
Sentences	Repeat a sentence verbatim. "The big cat ran after the mouse."
Mazes	Find the way through a simple maze.

*As this book was going to press, the WAIS-R was revised and is now the WAIS-III. See Chapter 3 for a description of this revision.

100 set at the 50th percentile, with a standard deviation of 15, which allows the examiner and others who view the results of the testing to understand the child's score in relation to the normative performance of a child the same age. The Full Scale IQ for the Wechsler scales has high reliability and has demonstrated strong correlations with other well-respected measures of intelligence (Sattler, 1992).

All of the Wechsler scales also comprise a Verbal IQ (VIQ) and Performance IQ (PIQ) as secondary indices of the child's intellectual ability. The VIQ is a measure of the child's understanding of verbal expression and comprehension. The PIQ is a measure of the child's perceptual organizational and visual spatial abilities. Factor analysis on the three Wechsler scales supports the existence of separate verbal and performance scales at all ages (Sattler, 1992).

Stanford-Binet Intelligence Scale, Fourth Edition (Thorndike, Hagen, & Sattler, 1986). The Stanford-Binet Intelligence Scale, Fourth Edition (SB: FE) is a descendent of the first popularized measure of intellectual ability, the Binet-Simon Scale of 1905, used in France. Like the Wechsler scales, the Stanford-Binet is a well-respected measure of intellectual ability. It can be administered to individuals between the ages of 2 and 21 years. It is similar to the Wechsler scales in terms of administration time, and it also provides a global composite measure of intellectual functioning. As on the Wechsler scales, the mean of the global composite score is 100; however, the standard deviation is 16 rather than 15.

The Stanford-Binet also yields secondary measures of intellectual ability, which include a verbal score similar to the Wechsler VIQ, an abstract and visual reasoning score similar to the Wechsler PIQ, a quantitative reasoning score that is not paralleled on the Wechsler scales, and a short-term memory scale that is somewhat analogous to a freedom-from-distractibility score, which can be calculated for the Wechsler scales. The Stanford-Binet is not as psychometrically sound as the Wechsler scales. Psychometric problems are especially evident on the 15 tests that contribute to the composites and the secondary indices of intellectual functioning.

Achievement Testing

Achievement testing refers to the assessment of children's abilities related to cognitive skills and information typically acquired in schools. Although some achievement testing is conducted with adults, it is more commonly used with children and adolescents. Most achievement tests yield scores in reading, arithmetic, and spelling. Although a number of different skills and abilities are assessed in achievement testing, this depends on the specific achievement test. Achievement tests are required for the diagnosis of learning disabilities according to Public Law 94-142. The achievement tests described will include the Woodcock Johnson Tests of Achievement—Revised, the Wechsler Individual Achievement Test, and the Wide Range Achievement Test—Third Edition.

Woodcock Johnson Tests of Achievement—Revised (Woodcock, 1977). The Woodcock Johnson Tests of Achievement—Revised (WJ-R) are one of three parts of the Woodcock Johnson battery, which also includes tests of cognitive ability and tests of interests. The WJ-R are extremely well standardized and psychometrically sophisticated tests of achievement. They are applicable to a broad age range extending from 3 years to 90 years.

The WJ-R have 18 different subtests, 9 on a standard battery and 9 on a supplemental battery. The standard battery yields scores in letter–word identification, passage comprehension, calculation, applied problems, dictation, writing samples, science, social studies, and humanities. The supplemental battery has many useful tests for further diagnostic work. Subtests on the standard battery yield composites for reading, arithmetic, and written language.

Wechsler Individual Achievement Test (Wechsler, 1992). The development of the Wechsler Individual Achievement Test (WIAT) is a recent advance in achievement testing with children. There are eight subtests on the WIAT, including basic reading, reading comprehension, spelling, listening comprehension, oral expression, written expression, mathematics reasoning, and numerical reasoning (see Table 9.2). Like the Wechsler Intelligence Scales, the WIAT is also well standardized. At the time of this writing, as with any new test, psychologists are awaiting more extensive research on its reliability and validity.

The WIAT is a unique achievement test as data were collected with the same sample of children on the three Wechsler Intelligence Scales and the WIAT. As a result, the discrepancy formulations of learning disability (described later in this chapter under "Special Topics") are empirically determined. When the administered IQ and achievement test do not share the same standardization sample, assumptions of learning disability are based on a less empirically supported conceptual model rather than being derived empirically (as described later in the chapter).

Wide Range Achievement Test—Third Edition (Jastak & Wilkinson, 1984). The Wide Range Achievement Test (WRAT) is currently in its third edition. Earlier versions of the WRAT-III were criticized for psychometric problems related to standardization. In the development of the WRAT-III, many of the psychometric criticisms were addressed; thus the current edition has advantages not evident in its predecessor. The WRAT-III is a brief test covering the basic areas of numerical calculations, spelling, and basic reading without considering reading comprehension.

Adaptive Behavior Scales

Adaptive behavior scales rate an individual's level of personal independence and social responsibility at different age ranges. Typically, adaptive behavior scales are used with youngsters suspected of having developmental delays or for the classification of mental retardation.

Vineland Adaptive Behavior Scales (Sparrow, Balla, & Cicchetti, 1994). The Vineland Adaptive Behavior Scales (VABS) are a well-developed means of evaluating adaptive behavior. The scales are well standardized with reasonable stratification, and the test has adequate psychometric properties. The VABS consists of three versions: the Expanded Form, the Survey Form, and the Classroom Edition. The Expanded Form and the Survey Form are administered through a parental interview, and the Classroom Edition is designed to be completed by the child's teacher. In cases of institutionalized children, this test would be administered to a caretaker who knows the child well.

The Vineland consists of four basic domains: communication, socialization, daily living skills, and motor skills. These domains are combined to yield an overall adaptive behavior composite score. Additionally, the Expanded and Survey Forms contain a rating scale for maladaptive behavior.

Each of the domains includes several subdomains designed to provide a finer grain of analysis.

Table 9.2 Subtests and Skills Measured on the WIAT for a 5-Year-Old Child

SUBTEST	EXAMPLE OF SKILLS MEASURED
Basic Reading	Reading ability; use of decoding strategies
Mathematics Reasoning	One-step addition; knowledge of the value of coins; reading charts and bar graphs
Reading Comprehension	Sequencing; drawing conclusions; comparing and contrasting
Numerical Operations	Adding rows and columns of three one-digit addends; subtracting two two-digit numbers
Listening Comprehension	Using picture clues; recognizing stated detail, cause and effect; sequencing
Oral Expression	Giving detailed descriptions; directions; explaining steps logically
Written Expression	Development of ideas, organization and unity of writing; grammar, usage, capitalization, punctuation
Spelling	Basic spelling ability

For communication, the subdomains are receptive, expressive, and written language. For daily living skills, the subdomains are personal, domestic, and community behavior. The socialization domain consists of subdomains for social interactions, leisure time, and responsibility. In the motor skills domain there are subdomains for gross and fine motor development, although it should be noted that this scale is only applicable to children up to age 6.

Personality Measures

Personality measures used with children and adolescents differ from the measures previously described in that they focus less on ability and more on psychopathology or problematic characteristics of the individual. They also describe behaviors and emotions displayed by the child or adolescent. Personality measures may be classified as either objective or projective measures. Scoring of objective measures requires less interpretation by the scorer, and they tend to be more face-valid. Projective measures are generally the least psychometrically sound of all of the assessment tools reviewed. Additionally, projective measures provide the child with ambiguous testing stimuli. That is, they are not face-valid, and thus are considered less susceptible to social desirability effects. In general, objective measures have stronger psychometric characteristics than projective measures.

Minnesota Multiphasic Personality Inventory for Adolescents (MMPI-A) (Butcher et al., 1992). The MMPI-A is an objective personality test or psychopathology assessment tool for adolescents between the ages of 12 and 18. The MMPI-A contains 478 statements, which adolescents consider in relation to themselves and respond to as either true or false. These items are then scored to determine whether the adolescent has responded in a manner similar to previously identified groups of adolescents with specific types of psychopathology; such types of psychopathology might include depression, psychopathy, or schizophrenia.

The MMPI-A is distinguished from other objective personality inventories in that it contains validity scales. The validity scales give some indication of whether the adolescent has responded in a socially desirable manner, thus possibly minimizing psychopathology. The validity scales are also used to indicate whether or not an adolescent has attempted to "cry for help" or has exaggerated his or her responses as an attempt to indicate more severe psychopathology. The MMPI-A also allows the clinical psychologist to determine if the adolescent has responded to the items in a random manner. The MMPI-A has a reasonably good standardization sample and is in the process of acquiring reliability and validity data.

Revised Children's Manifest Anxiety Scale (RCMAS) (Reynolds & Richmond, 1985). The RCMAS is a self-report anxiety rating scale for children and adolescents between the ages of six and nineteen. This measure gives an indication of a child's perceived level of symptoms of anxiety. As this measure is face-valid, an individual may respond in a manner responsive to perceived social desirability. The standardization of the RCMAS is less sophisticated than that of the previously discussed tests. However, there exist some psychometric data pertaining to reliability and validity that warrant its use for the assessment of anxiety in children and adolescents.

State–Trait Anxiety Inventory for Children (STAI-C) (Spielberger, Edwards, Montouri, & Lushene, 1970). The STAI-C is another self-report measure of anxiety used for younger populations. It is distinctive in that it has ratings for both state anxiety, or short-term anxiety, which is dependent on a specific situation, and trait anxiety, which is less situation-specific and more enduring. The STAI-C's standardization and other psychometric properties are adequate.

The Yale–Brown Obsessive Compulsive Scale for Children (YBOCS-C). The YBOCS-C, developed by Goodman et al. (1986), is a downward extension of the adult version of the Yale–Brown Obsessive Compulsive Scale. It is a specialized measure as it provides a rating form for a specific diagnostic disorder. Psychometric data are still being collected on the YBOCS-C.

Rorschach Ink Blot Technique. The Rorschach is one of several different projective techniques used with children and adolescents. It is categorized as an ink blot projective technique. Historically there was concern regarding the reliability and validity of the Rorschach. Attempts to address many of the psychometric issues are made by John Exner in the Exner Scoring System (Exner, 1974). Although critics of the Rorschach continue to identify problems with this test, it is widely used as a personality test for children and adolescents.

Projective Story Telling Techniques

The Thematic Apperception Test (TAT) (Murray, 1943) is one of several different story-telling projective techniques; others include the Children's Apperception Test (Bellack & Bellack, 1986), the Roberts Apperception Test (McArthur & Roberts, 1982) and the Tasks of Emotional Development (Cohen & Weil, 1971). These tests or techniques involve presenting the youngster with a picture and asking him or her to tell a story about the picture. General instructions for the TAT ask that the child tell a story identifying what is happening in the picture, what led up to the picture, and what will happen after the picture or how the story will end. In addition, the child is asked to specify what any characters in the story may be thinking or feeling. Depending on the child and his or her history, the examiner selects the pictures he or she wishes to use in the assessment.

Stories are analyzed for thematic content, as many of the cards pull for a particular story theme. Murray developed an elaborate scoring system for the TAT; however, the psychometric properties of the story-telling projective techniques have frequently been called into question. Those who utilize this technique may use it as a tool for developing clinical hypotheses about a youngster. These hypotheses can then be verified by gathering subsequent information through interview and other forms of data collection.

Sentence Completion Techniques

Like the previously described projective techniques, there are numerous sentence completion techniques. The sentence completion technique involves providing the youngster with the beginnings of sentences and asking him or her to complete the sentence. There are numerous psychometric problems with this technique. As with the TAT, formal systems for scoring do exist. In clinical practice some clinicians use the sentence completion technique informally to obtain topical information, such as feelings toward family, school, and peer relations.

Projective Drawings

Projective drawings are techniques that require a child to draw specific objects. These techniques include the House, Tree, Person (HTP), the Draw-A-Person (DAP) task, and the Kinetic Family Drawing (KFD). Scoring systems have been developed for projective drawings (Koppitz, 1968), but critics note that the projective drawing techniques do have significant problems with reliability and validity. Like the majority of the projective techniques, clinicians typically use projective drawings to generate hypotheses about the child, which may be verified or rejected by obtaining subsequent clinical information. Projective drawings are considered particularly useful with some children, as many children will spontaneously draw in a clinical situation what they may be having difficulty articulating. Thus, use of projective drawings in therapy or assessment situations for the purpose of generating a hypothesis may have value in the clinical situation.

Parent Report Measures

Parent report measures are important tools in the assessment of children as they provide corroborating information on data collected during the interview or directly from children. There are a number of different parent report measures. Two of the more popular measures will be described next.

Child Behavior Checklist (CBCL) (Achenbach & Edelbrock, 1986). The CBCL is a commonly used parent rating scale for children between the ages of 2 and 18 years. The CBCL has two separate forms; one form for 2- and 3-year-olds and one that is applicable to 4- through 18-year-olds. Normative data are available on both boys and girls at several different age groupings across the age span.

The CBCL has a competence rating portion and a behavior problem rating portion (see Table 9.3). The competence rating portion yields composite scores on social activities, organizational activities, and school competence. Scores are reported both in terms of percentiles and t-scores. Good standardization, reliability, and validity data are available.

The behavior problem rating portion of the CBCL consists of 108 commonly occurring behavior problems. The parent is required to rate each behavior problem on a scale from 0 to 2 where 0 = not at all present, 1 = somewhat true, and 2 = very true. Factor-analytic studies of youngsters grouped by age and sex yield both narrow- and broad-band factors. This means that a child's difficulties may be described on broad-band factors such as internalizing and externalizing, as well as on more narrow-band factors, including depressed mood, anxious mood, somatic problems, social problems, attention problems, and aggressivity. As with the competence rating portion, good standardization and reliability and validity data are available on the CBCL behavior rating portion.

Table 9.3 The Competence and Problem Scales of the Child Behavior Checklist (CBCL Scale)

Competence Scales:
Activities
Social
School
   Total Competence
Problem Scales:
Narrow Band:
   Withdrawn
   Somatic Complaints
   Anxious/Depressed
   Social Problems
   Thought Problems
   Attention Problems
   Delinquent Behavior
   Aggressive Behavior
   Sex Problems
Broad Band:
   Internalizing
   Externalizing
      Total Problems

Personality Inventory for Children (PIC) (Lachar, 1982). The PIC is a 300-plus-item measure consisting of statements to which the parents respond with either true or false ratings with regard to their child. As with the MMPI-A, validity scales are available on the PIC, which assist clinicians in evaluating whether the parent has exaggerated or minimized child psychopathology. Factor-analytic studies have yielded empirically derived factor scales and clinical scales. The factor scales include: Undisciplined/Poor Self-Control, Social Incompetence, Internalization/Somatic Symptoms, and Cognitive Development. Clinical scales include: Achievement, Intellectual Screening, Development, Somatic Concern, Depression, Family Relations, Delinquency, Withdrawal, Anxiety, Psychosis, Hyperactivity, and Social Skills. Parent responses result in a T-score on each scale indicating the degree to which the description of the child is similar to response patterns characteristic of groups of children who have been described with different personality features. The PIC has psychometric issues that are of some concern to the clinician, but it still provides useful parent report data in assessing children.

Psychological Assessment—Case Study

Reason for Referral

Nancy Brown is a 17-year-3-month-old African American female who was referred by Adolescent Psychiatry for an intellectual and psychological evaluation. Nancy was diagnosed with insulin-dependent diabetes mellitus (IDDM) in 1993 and in December 1995 began experiencing leg pains as well as depressive symptoms, rapid weight loss, and severe metabolic control problems with her diabetes. She was admitted to the Adolescent Inpatient Psychiatry Unit because of significant lower limb pain without demonstrable organic basis, which reportedly interferes with her ability to eat, attend school, and function socially. Nancy is currently being considered as a candidate for admission to the Diabetes Project Unit, a specialized inpatient pediatric psychiatric unit for youngsters with IDDM.

Background Information

Nancy resides in Trenton, OK, with her mother, father, and 22-year-old brother. Her father works as a bus driver, and her mother was released from a long-term job in a nursing home in December 1995. Nancy was diagnosed with IDDM in 1993 following an illness in which a viral infection damaged her pancreas. She began to lose weight in December 1995 and dropped from 125 pounds to 87 pounds at the time of her admission to the psychiatric unit. Nancy was in the eleventh grade at Oakwood High School in Trenton, OK, this year; however, as a result of excessive absenteeism, she will be repeating the eleventh grade. Additionally, Nancy was retained in third grade for poor academic performance. Nancy relayed that she has missed substantial amounts of school as a result of her pain, and beginning in March she remained home and participated in a homebound school program. However, she indicated that her discomfort was so severe that it was difficult for her to keep up with her work. Nancy remarked that her mother encouraged her to consider her health before her schoolwork and stated that she could always obtain a GED.

Nancy described her mood as "sort of sad." She remarked that she becomes upset when her legs hurt or when she sees her mother cry. When her legs hurt, she typically becomes teary, depressed, and hopeless that her condition will ever improve. Nancy remarked that her mother frequently massages her legs for up to two hours to ease her pain. Nancy described a close relationship with each of her parents, and reportedly was concerned about her mother when she lost her job, as her mother was unhappy. She affirmed that her increased experience of pain occurred around the same time as her mother was dismissed from her work, but Nancy did not seem aware of any relationship between the two events. Nancy indicated that her brother had recently informed the family that he is homosexual. She described disapproving of the people her brother associates with and blames him for upsetting her parents.

Behavioral Observations

Nancy presented as a petite, attractive African American female who was appropriately groomed and dressed. She was pleasant, friendly, and maintained good eye contact throughout the interview and testing. During the interview, Nancy was open but did not elaborate on her responses or offer information that was not requested. During testing, Nancy was diligent, examining the task at hand before attempting to solve the problem. If a task appeared too difficult, she would comment, "I don't think I can do that, it looks too hard," but she would attempt the problem if encouraged. She was oriented in all spheres but demonstrated a fairly restricted range of affect, distancing herself from negative emotions.

Assessment Results

On formal examination of intellectual ability (WAIS-R), Nancy obtained a Full Scale IQ of 92 (30th percentile), which falls in the average range of general intellectual functioning. Her Verbal IQ was 89 (23rd percentile), reflecting low average verbal ability, and her Performance IQ was 98 (45th percentile) suggesting perceptual-organizational ability in the average range (see Table 9.4 for individual subtest scaled scores).

Nancy's scores depict relative weakness in the verbal tasks compared to the performance tasks, suggesting poor scholastic aptitude and limited knowledge acquisition over time, as well as poor verbal comprehension/expression skills. Her WAIS-R subtest scales reveal a considerably high degree of scatter, consistent with distractibility.

Scores from the Woodcock-Johnson Tests of Achievement—Revised indicate that Nancy is significantly delayed in all areas of scholastic aptitude for her age and grade level. However, the results of poor scholastic achievement are fairly congruent with her intellectual abilities; thus she does not meet diagnostic criteria for a learning disability. See Table 9.5 for her general achievement scores.

Personality testing (TAT, Sentence Completion, MMPI-A) suggested that although Nancy attempts to present herself in a positive light, she may be experiencing stressors that are contributing to her experience of depression. Nancy's MMPI-A profile was indicative of significant depression and exaggerated somatic concerns. Data from the TAT and Sentence Completion suggested feelings of depression and emotional immaturity.

Table 9.4 Nancy Brown's WISC-III Subtest Scaled Scores

VERBAL SCALE		PERFORMANCE SCALE	
SUBTEST	SCALED SCORE	SUBTEST	SCALED SCORE
Information	8	Picture Completion	9
Digit Span	6	Picture Arrangement	11
Vocabulary	6	Block Design	10
Arithmetic	6	Object Assembly	10
Comprehension	10	Digit Symbol	6
Similarities	6		

Note. M = 10, SD = 3.

Table 9.5 Nancy Brown's General Achievement Scores

	STANDARD SCORE	AGE EQUIVALENT	GRADE EQUIVALENT	PERCENTILE RANK
Broad Reading	87	12-5 years	7.1	
Broad Math	86	12-3 years	6.9	
Broad Knowledge	86	12-4 years	7.0	
Basic Reading	89	12-1 years	6.5	

Note. Scores are based on Woodcock-Johnson Tests of Achievement—Revised.

Summary and Recommendations

Nancy is a 17-year-3-month-old female who was seen for an intellectual and psychological evaluation. Test results suggest that Nancy is performing significantly below her age and grade placement level in school. However, her scores are consistent with what would be predicted from her measured intellect; thus, she does not meet diagnostic criteria for a learning disability. Additionally, Nancy does not appear to have adequate internal resources for managing the pain she experiences. Her pain expression is associated with secondary gains related to receiving special attention from her parents, distracting her parents from other stressful events, and avoiding attending school. Nancy is also experiencing significant depressive symptomatology, and she and her family have not been able to maintain adequate control over her diabetes, both of which are areas of significant concern. She also has experienced a dramatic weight loss over a short period of time. In light of these findings, we recommend that Nancy be admitted to the Diabetes Project Unit. Here she should receive individual therapy, group therapy, and family therapy. Special attention should be placed on Nancy's school remediation, including working with the school to develop an appropriate strategy for strengthening Nancy's areas of weakness.

INTERVENTION

Major Theoretical Systems

Behavioral Treatments

Behavioral treatments are based on learning theories. In this chapter there will be a review of the principles of several learning theories, including classical conditioning, operant theory, and social learning theory. Therapies based on these major learning theories also will be described.

Classical conditioning. Classical conditioning, also known as respondent learning or Pavlovian conditioning, is a theory of learning that is crucial in the behavioral treatment of multiple problem behaviors in children and adolescents. The problematic behavior is conceptualized using principles of classical conditioning, and these principles are then used to treat the problem. Treatment of anxiety-related problems utilizing these paradigms will be discussed.

Basic terms in the classical conditioning model include *unconditioned stimulus*, *unconditioned response*, *conditioned stimulus*, and *conditioned response*. These terms will be illustrated with the classic example of Pavlov's dog. The unconditioned stimulus is a stimulus that automatically elicits the unconditioned response in an organism. In the case of Pavlov's dog, an unconditioned stimulus, such as meat, will automatically elicit salivation, the unconditioned response; the response of salivation when presented with meat does not require any prior learning. The conditioned stimulus, by contrast, refers to a previously neutral stimulus, or one that does not automatically evoke a response. In this example, a bell (the to-be-conditioned stimulus) is presented. Initially it will not elicit a response from the dog. However, when a bell is presented simultaneously or slightly before the presentation of food, classical conditioning will occur. That is, after repeated presentations, the dog will begin to salivate in response to the bell alone. At this point, the bell has become a conditioned stimulus that elicits the conditioned response of salivation in response to the bell.

The classical conditioning model is particularly applicable to treatment of childhood anxieties and fears. Using the same paradigm, Watson and Rayner (1920) produced fear in a young toddler in the classic case of Little Albert. This was achieved by first presenting a loud noise (unconditioned stimulus), which automatically startled Little Albert (unconditioned response). Learning was not required for the loud noise to evoke the startle response in Little Albert. Watson next paired a white rat (to-be-conditioned stimulus) with the occurrence of the loud noise, and eventually Little Albert came to fear (conditioned response) the white rat. Previously the white rat had not elicited a fear response from Albert; thus the white rat had become a

conditioned stimulus to elicit the conditioned response of fear for Little Albert.

Therapies based on classical conditioning that address phobic or anxious responses attempt to break the learned connection that has previously occurred between the conditioned stimulus and the conditioned response. Hence, if one were treating Little Albert, one would attempt to break the previously learned connection between the white rat and the startle or fear response. This would involve teaching Little Albert how to maintain relaxation or another emotional state inconsistent with fear when presented with the white rat. This treatment paradigm is particularly successful in childhood and adolescent phobias such as dental phobias, pill-swallowing problems, anticipatory nausea in reaction to chemotherapy, and many other anxieties and phobias.

Operant theory. Operant theory is a learning theory that embodies principles also known as instrumental conditioning or Skinnerian learning. Many child and adolescent treatments are based on the principles of operant theory originally popularized by B. F. Skinner (1974).

Key terms in operant conditioning include *positive reinforcement*, *negative reinforcement*, *positive punishment*, and *negative punishment*. These terms describe processes that occur as a result of learning from the consequences of one's behavior. These operant terms are abstractly characterized by the proposition that behavior followed by a consequence will affect the future probability of that behavior.

Positive reinforcement refers to the situation in which a behavior is followed by a stimulus that results in the increased probability of the future occurrence of that behavior. Rewarding a child for a desirable behavior would be classified as using a positive reinforcement to increase the likelihood of the rewarded behavior occurring in the future. An example would be parents praising a child when the child performs a chore such as washing the dishes. Another example would be a parent hugging a child to demonstrate pleasure that a child has brought home a paper with a good grade. Positive reinforcement may also occur when undesirable behaviors are inadvertently responded to in a way that increases the possibility of the future occurrence of that behavior. A common example is a parent responding to a child's misbehavior by nagging the child. If this same child receives very little positive attention or nurturance from the parent, nagging provides contact with the parent and may increase the likelihood that the child will misbehave to receive this attention. Another common example of inadvertent positive reinforcement commonly occurs in department and grocery stores. If a child is begging or whining for some desired object in a store, a parent who originally refused to buy the object may give in and buy it in order to quiet the child. Unfortunately, this positively reinforces the obnoxious behavior, and the child may learn that by behaving in this manner he or she can acquire desired objects.

Negative reinforcement is another contingency whereby a child learns through the consequences of his or her behavior. As with positive reinforcement, the outcome of negative reinforcement is increasing (or reinforcing) the future probability of behavior. Unlike positive reinforcement, however, where a stimulus is applied after the occurrence of behavior, in negative reinforcement a stimulus is removed after the occurrence of a behavior. The removal of this stimulus is associated with an increase in the original behavior. Alternatively stated, the occurrence of that behavior is associated with the removal of the stimulus. Both escape learning and avoidance learning characterize negative reinforcement. In escape learning, the youngster is exposed to a stimulus that the child experiences as aversive; thus, the child learns to avoid that stimulus through an increase in some behavior. For example, if a child who is sensitive to criticism is criticized for not cleaning his room, he will likely increase his room-cleaning behavior in order to avoid receiving criticism. In avoidance learning, the child is cued that the aversive stimulus is about to come, thus she performs the behavior in order to avoid the stimulus. For example, a child who sees a parent frown may clean her room in order to avoid receiving further verbal criticism from the parent.

Punishment is a consequence of behavior resulting in the decreased probability of the future occurrence of that behavior. In *positive punishment*, a child performs a behavior that is followed by a consequence that decreases the likelihood that the child will continue to engage in that behavior in the future. The term *positive* here refers to the addition of a stimulus or consequence. For example, if a child interrupts, his parent may respond by scolding the child for interrupting. If the child is less likely to interrupt in the future, then scolding has served as a positive punishment, which has decreased the interrupting behavior.

Negative punishment, like positive punishment, is a consequence of behavior resulting in a decreased probability of the future occurrence of that behavior. However, in negative punishment there is the withdrawal of a stimulus after the occurrence of a behavior that results in the decreased future probability of that behavior. Restrictions or time out is an example of this contingency. If a child hits a sibling, he may lose television privileges for a specified time. When the loss of privileges has the effect of decreasing the probability that the child will hit his sibling again in the future, negative punishment has occurred.

Social learning theory. Social learning theory was popularized by Albert Bandura (1977). Although this is a broad theory encompassing many issues and principles, this review will concentrate on the processes involved in observational learning or modeling. Observational learning occurs when a child is able to model a behavior after watching another individual perform the behavior. This phenomenon occurs with both desirable and undesirable behaviors. In order for observational learning to occur the child must be attending to the individual modeling the behavior, and he/she must retain and recall the observed behavior. It is also necessary for the child to have an opportunity to practice or rehearse the behavior, and there must be some incentive to actually perform the behavior. Many childhood behaviors, both positive and negative, are acquired through observational learning.

Cognitive-Behavioral Treatment

Cognitive-behavioral therapy is a treatment approach which stems from principles in behavior therapy. This intervention developed when traditional behavioral principles were not sufficiently successful in treating both children and adults. Traditional operant principles did not prove to be as useful in producing long-term, generalized change as had been hoped (Bellack & Hersen, 1977). Also, empirical research has not supported the supposed underlying behavioral principles of several effective techniques (Kazdin & Wilcoxon, 1976). The late 1970s witnessed a resurgence of the mind as psychologists began to reject traditional behavioral approaches that failed to consider an individual's private thoughts. Numerous well-defined, empirically validated cognitive-behavioral interventions emerged (Greenspoon & Lamal, 1978; Jaremko, 1979; Ledwidge, 1978, 1979; Locke, 1979, Mahoney & Kazdin, 1979; Meichenbaum, 1979).

Although there are numerous cognitive-behavioral techniques, the general principle of cognitive-behavioral therapy maintains that emotional and behavioral difficulties stem from maladaptive thinking processes. Thus, the goal of cognitive-behavioral therapy is to alter the maladaptive cognitions, as a change in one's thoughts consequently leads to changes in both behavior and emotions. There are a wide range of therapeutic techniques, including altering irrational beliefs (Ellis, 1970), self-instructional training (Meichenbaum, 1977), and self-control training (Kanfer & Karoly, 1972). The goal of these strategies is to promote generalized behavioral and emotional change—in other words, change that will extend beyond the immediate therapeutic exchange into daily situations and tasks. In contrast with the external control exemplified by traditional behavioral therapy, the focus of cognitive-behavioral therapy is on establishing the individual as the locus of control (Whitman, Burgio, & Johnston, 1984). Cognitive-behavioral therapy is particularly useful in treating children with fear and anxiety disorders, phobias, tics, and depression.

Psychodynamic psychotherapy for children. At some point in their lives, many normal children may experience psychological stressors from various factors such as a divorce, loss of a parent or other loved one, change in health status, or a large number of potential situations that may evoke mild emotional or behavioral problems. Treating such children by psychodynamic therapy does not always imply that the child will undergo psychoanalysis, which traditionally refers to Freudian principles and techniques. Although psychodynamic approaches are based on the broad principles of psychoanalytic theory, psychodynamic psychotherapy generally refers to a wide variety of therapeutic approaches designed to provide understanding of and explanations for various behaviors the child may exhibit (Nichols & Paolino, 1986). Psychotherapy for children makes use of numerous approaches with diverse theoretical orientations as helpful adjuncts to treatment. In fact, it has been estimated that there are well over 230 different kinds of psychological treatment used with children (Kazdin, 1988).

As mentioned at the beginning of this chapter, psychotherapy for children traces its origins back to 1909, when Freud cured 5-year-old "Little Hans" of a phobia of horses. Over a decade later, a female psychoanalyst, Hermine Hug-Hellmuth, furthered the psychoanalytic approach with children, originating the concept of play therapy. The use of play in psychotherapy with children was propelled by the ideas of Melanie Klein (1932) and Anna Freud (1965). Both viewed the free play of children as somewhat akin to the concept of free associations, expressing unconscious fantasies, impulses, or internalized conflicts, and allowing for adult insight into the problems and concerns of children.

Since those initial forges into uncharted territory, a deeper understanding of child psychotherapy has developed. Today, much of child psychotherapy depends on the therapeutic alliance between child and therapist. This relationship provides a supportive environment in which the child is free to reflect on himself and others, with the notion that increased awareness of oneself and one's relationships with others is a prime force in the initiation of psychological changes. In addition to the therapist–child relationship and the ultimate goal of development of awareness, other therapeutic principles at work in child psychotherapy include concepts such as corrective emotional experience, abreaction, suggestion, and maturational pull (Carek, 1979).

Corrective emotional experience refers to the counteraction of experience that may have contributed to the child's distortions. For example, kindness and positive affect may help to counteract in part a child's previous experience of mistreatment. *Abreaction* refers to the expression of harbored emotions that may appear as neurotic symptoms. Psychotherapy attempts to teach the child an effective way to cope with emotions and to express them in a reasonable manner. Suggestion also is basic to the psychotherapeutic process and may appear in sessions as the expression of the therapist's confidence in the child's endeavor to be successful in therapy. Finally, *maturation pull* refers simply to the increasing development of the child to more mature levels. The objective of successful psychotherapy in children, then, is simply to remove the impediments to this natural developmental flow.

These principles of individual psychodynamic psychotherapy constitute the basic operational framework within child psychological treatment and child psychiatry. An effective therapist will likely find that integration of other therapeutic techniques into such a personal approach is likely to be successful when treating childhood disorders.

Play therapy. Play therapy is rooted in the fact that play serves several purposes in the normal course of child development. Play is the child's innate way of expressing himself and communicating to others. Play gives the child an opportunity to reveal fantasies or express strong emotions such as anger, fear, tension, or frustration. Play improves motor functions by exercising body muscles and developing increasing coordination. Play also serves as one of the most important ways in which a child learns. Through play, a child learns social functions such as roles and the development of interpersonal relationships. Play encourages cooperation and rule following. Play also can serve to develop cognitive abilities by increasing concentration and promoting vocabulary growth and the development of problem-solving skills.

Play activity follows a sequence of development that may shift depending on the child's cognitive and language abilities, as well as factors associated with the family, culture, or environment. Piaget (1962) called the beginning stages of play the *sensorimotor period*, extending from infancy to 18 to 24 months of age. During this time, children assimilate new sensory information associated with novel people or objects, and eventually adapt themselves to the world of reality. Meaningful activity occurs as children demonstrate purposeful play with toys. According to Piaget (1962), the second stage of the development of play occurs between the ages of 2 and 6 years. As cognitive abilities increase and language use proliferates, children develop the ability to imitate and pretend, creating symbolic play. This pretend play is often used in therapy either to diagnose or to treat childhood disorders. This can be accomplished though the use of miniature life toys, sand creations, or puppets. The final stage of play begins around age 6, when the child participates in games with rules.

As previously mentioned, play therapy with children had its developmental origins rooted in the work of Hermine Hug-Hellmuth, Anna Freud (1965), and Melanie Klein (1932), who attempted to help children gain psychoanalytic insight into their problems. Besides psychoanalytically oriented play therapy, several major approaches exist, including the Rogerian nondirective play therapy, family play therapy, and fair play therapy (Schaefer & O'Connor, 1983).

Psychoanalytic play therapy views play not as therapeutic in itself but, rather, as one of several means of interpreting the child's inner conflicts, fantasies, and desires. Play should promote the observation of these inner states through the use of materials such as paper, crayons, scissors, Play-Doh, blocks, puppets, dolls, toy guns, or balls. The therapist's function is to observe, interpret, and explain to the child the nature of his or her conflict in order to provide an understanding of the problem and find the appropriate resolution.

Nondirective or client-centered play therapy was developed for children by Virginia Axline (1947) from Carl Rogers's client-centered approach. Therapy may either be directive or nondirective in form. In directive therapy, the therapist guides the child in play activities and makes interpretations. In nondirective therapy, all direction and responsibility are left completely to the child. Axline takes the latter approach, describing nondirective play therapy as "an opportunity that is offered to the child to experience growth under the most favorable conditions" (Axline, 1947, p. 16). It encourages the process of normal growth and development by aiding the child to abandon unadaptive behaviors such as extreme aggression. During play therapy, the child is "given the opportunity to realize this power within himself to be himself" (Axline, 1947, p. 23). The therapist provides only a supportive environment consisting of warmth, acceptance, and understanding. Play materials generally consist of a sandbox, a dollhouse, paper, crayons, scissors, Play-Doh, blocks, puppets, dolls, doctor kits, toy guns, balls, or games.

Family play therapy involves parent(s), child(ren), and therapist together in a preplanned play session in order to emphasize the fact that children exist within the context of a family system (Griff, 1983). Parental education is included as a therapy goal, with parenting skills training and role modeling provided by the therapist.

Fair play therapy is based on the premise that children need to be handled equitably and that children who are denied such experiences are likely to be troubled (Peoples, 1983). The therapist takes a more active role in treatment and creates an environment for the child in which he or she feels approval. This approval, however, is not unconditional, but depends on the child's development and maintenance of appropriate behaviors. The goal is to create conditions in which the child can learn to build interpersonal relationships and to solve problems in an adaptive manner.

As Axline (1947) notes, just as adults in therapy "talk out" their feelings and problems, play therapy allows children an opportunity to "play out" their own difficulties. Combined with the effects of a warm and empathic therapist, play therapy may be of use in the treatment of childhood and family problems.

Family Approaches

Carlson (1990) has outlined issues related to family functioning that clinical psychologists must consider when evaluating and treating a child. Is the child's presenting problem actually a family problem? How are the child's difficulties related to family functioning? If the child's problem is related to family functioning, what is the nature of that relationship and how could a treatment plan address these issues?

The psychologist begins to develop a clinical framework for treating a family by identifying stable patterns of interacting or predictable relationships that constitute the family system. Haley (1987) emphasized an examination of routines and rules that define how family members interact. This frame of reference deems it important to understand where the authority or power lies in the family and to conduct an analysis to determine family hierarchies. In a healthy or normally functioning family, the parents maintain more power than the children. In a functional family, identifiable roles help the family function and foster the individual growth and development of specific family members.

Carlson (1990) describes a model for assessing the family context that involves the examination of family subsystems, which include the sibling subsystem, the parent–child subsystem, the parental subsystem, the marital subsystem, the whole-family subsystem, and the extended-family subsystem. Although there is no measure or test to describe adequately the various facets of these subsystems, a clinician can use observation and clinical interviews as tools to develop a rich conceptualization of these family systems. While many clinicians use these techniques and find they hold particular pragmatic or heuristic value, it is not currently possible to evaluate these methods of conceptualization psychometrically.

Within the frame of reference described here, individual development within a family system and general family functioning are thought to be dependent on the clarity of boundaries or rules regarding family members' participation in different roles. The clarity of boundaries is typically seen as a continuum, with enmeshment at one end and disengagement at the other. Both enmeshment and disengagement are considered pathological, as families that operate with these types of boundaries frequently experience stunted emotional growth and dysfunctional family relations. *Enmeshment* occurs when family boundaries are diffuse or unclear. There is frequently intrusion between family members and subsystems that tend to stifle personal autonomy. Alternatively, *disengagement* is defined by overly rigid boundaries; individuals experience excessive autonomy, which provides for inadequate nurturance and support.

Family roles and family boundaries progress through a developmental sequence. Typically, families significantly alter their relations and functioning in response to events such as divorce, remarriage, chronic illness, death, or moving. The family life cycle theory predicts that a child will manifest symptoms when a family structure is rigid and fails to change in response to major changes. Child-rearing practices must be appropriate to the developmental stage of the child, and the family must be flexible and capable of adjusting to stress mediated by changes in individuals. In sum, conceptualization of the child's presenting problem, as characterized by the parent, often changes when one considers the family system framework. Family therapists believe that the identified patient's problems are in actuality the expression of a dysfunctional family system. Families that lack flexibility often fail to adapt adequately to normal life changes, and individuals within such families may develop behavioral difficulties as a symptom of underlying family dysfunction.

Carlson (1990) reviews three methods of family assessment: interview, observation, and questionnaires. Some clinicians prefer to conduct the initial interview with all family members present, as this provides an opportunity to observe the whole family and to obtain information from multiple sources and with multiple perspectives. A key issue to consider while conducting the interview involves an assessment of the family hierarchy, or the arrange-

ment of power within the family system. In troubled families one sometimes sees an inverted parent-child power hierarchy, which Patterson and Reid (1984) describe as a coercive family process. During the interview it is also important for the clinician to begin formulating hypotheses regarding the relative degree of enmeshment and disengagement within the family system. Enmeshment may be characterized by individuals sharing wardrobes, children sleeping with parents, parents confiding details of their marital relations in their children, or individuals in the family requiring unabated attention. Alternatively, disengagement often manifests as parents not being informed about their child's activities or whereabouts, or parents not responding to a child's successes and failures.

Another problematic process to consider while assessing and treating a family is the presence of pathological triangles. Family triangles occur when there is intolerable tension between two family members, and a third family member diffuses the conflict. Carlson (1990) reviews four types of triangles: triangulation, parent-child coalition, and two types of detoured triangles—attacking detouring and supportive detouring.

Triangulation occurs when both parents vie for the child's attention or loyalty, as is commonly seen in divorce situations. The parent-child coalition occurs when a child allies with one parent against the other, as when a mother and a child rally against an uninvolved father. Detouring triangles involve intense focus on a child as a means of avoiding dealing with conflictual feelings between parents. In *attacking detouring,* the child is scapegoated; rather than deal with marital conflict directly, the parents identify the child as a problem. In the case of a *supportive detouring* triangle, a child may be viewed as sick, providing the parents with a child-centered focus as an alternative to facing their own marital conflict directly. Although the assessment of triangulation is based on observation and interview rather than psychometric evaluation, many child clinicians consider it important in conceptualizing childhood psychological problems and in formulating their treatment.

In sum, the goal of family therapy is to realign the family structure and boundaries so that the family is empowered to resolve their difficulties. In the initial interview and initial stages of therapy, the family therapist alligns with each individual member of the family and makes a conscious effort to gain understanding into each individual's perspective. Simultaneously, the therapist observes the family interactions and begins to develop hypotheses regarding patterns of interactions, boundaries, hierarchies, and overall family structure. A family therapist next attempts to highlight and modify family interactions. Therapy typically entails eliciting family interactions, realigning boundaries by increasing either proximity or distance between family members, changing the relationships of members within subsystems, and challenging the family's assumptions. Family therapists, influenced by both the family's presenting problem and their own theoretical orientation, will use a variety of techniques to treat families.

Empirically Validated Therapies for Children

The *Diagnostic and Statistical Manual of Mental Disorders,* fourth edition (DSM-IV; American Psychiatric Association, 1994) diagnoses many childhood disorders, among them problems such as depression, conduct disorders, eating disorders, and elimination disorders (encopresis or enuresis). Given a multitude of therapies for treating each of the various problems of childhood, a therapist would benefit from knowing which treatments have been shown to be the most effective for particular disorders in children.

Recently, the American Psychological Association Division 12 Task Force on Effective Psychosocial Interventions: A Lifespan Perspective was formed to investigate and identify empirically valid psychosocial interventions relating specifically to children, adolescents, and families. The guidelines for what constitutes an empirically valid treatment were followed according to the recommendations formed by the Task Force on Promotion and Dissemination of Psychological Procedures, Division of Clinical Psychology, American Psychological Association (1995). The task force specified certain

criteria for treatments to meet in order to be considered "well-established treatments" or "probably efficacious treatments." According to these criteria, well-established treatments must have been demonstrated by either (1) two good between-group design experiments conducted by at least two different investigatory teams that have been shown to be superior to either a placebo or another treatment; or (2) a large series of well-designed single-case design experiments that also compare the treatment to a placebo or to another treatment. In addition, treatment must be conducted using treatment manuals and the characteristics of the patient sample clearly defined. The criteria are slightly less stringent for meeting a "probably efficacious" treatment label.

As one example of the process cited here, Houts, Berman, and Abramson (1994) conducted a review of 78 studies examining the effectiveness of psychological and pharmacological treatments for children's nocturnal enuresis. They discovered that both psychological and pharmacological treatments had outcomes superior to those in control groups, although those receiving psychological treatment were more likely to have ceased bedwetting at post-treatment and follow-up. One such treatment involves the use of a pad placed under the sleeping child; when the child wets, a circuit is completed through the pad, which sounds the alarm, creating a situation for classical conditioning to occur. The pairing of the full bladder with the alarm to wake up will result in the child self-awakening rather than wetting the bed while asleep (see Figure 9.1). Their review met the guidelines for establishing psychological treatment for enuresis as an empirically valid treatment benefiting enuretic children. Walter and Gilmore (1973) and Wells and Egan (1988) have also provided well-established evidence for the efficacy of parent training programs for children with oppositional behavior. Therapies meeting the criteria for probably efficacious treatments for children include behavior modification for encopresis (O'Brien, Ross, & Christophersen, 1986), and family anxiety management training for anxiety disorders (Barrett, Dadds, & Rapee, 1996). The identification of empirically

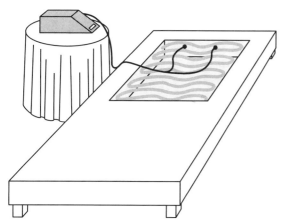

Figure 9.1. The Bell and Pad are regarded as an empirically valid treatment for nocturnal enuresis (bed-wetting).

validated psychological treatments for children is an important process in the development of the field.

Treatment Summary—Case Study

Presenting Problems

Nancy Brown is a 17-year- 3-month-old African American female diagnosed with Insulin Dependent Diabetes Mellitus (IDDM) since the age of 14 years. She was admitted to the Diabetes Project Unit following discharge from the Inpatient Psychiatric Unit. Nancy has experienced significant lower limb pain, poor diabetes control and management, significant school absenteeism, depressive symptomatology, significant weight loss, and interruption in social functioning. Other family stressors include her mother's dismissal from her job, and her 22-year-old brother's recent admission to the family that he is homosexual. Nancy resided on the Diabetes Project Unit for 4 months and 6 days. There she received individual psychotherapy twice weekly, group therapy once weekly, and family therapy every two weeks. Nancy was discharged after successfully completing the program.

Treatment Goals and Progress

Problem 1: Poor diabetes management skills, including poor diet, inconsistent exercise, and skipping injections.

Progress: Nancy demonstrated greatly improved diabetes management skills at the time of discharge. While on the unit she regularly monitored her blood glucose and injected insulin with minimal difficulty. Her knowledge related to diabetes significantly improved as demonstrated by her increased scores on diabetes knowledge tests. She has demonstrated the ability to identify when her blood sugars are low or high and utilizes appropriate techniques to correct irregular blood glucose levels. Nancy's motivation to engage in regular exercise continues to be an area of concern.

Problem 2: Problems with diabetes management by Nancy's family.

Progress: Nancy's parents received ongoing education regarding diabetes management, dietary guidelines, exercise needs, and glucose monitoring each weekend that they visited the Diabetes Project Unit. They appeared highly motivated to learn; however, Mr. Brown failed several of the educational modules and had to retake several of the written tests. Their posttest scores on the Test of Diabetes Knowledge were between 74% and 87%, suggesting they both were able to retain a moderate amount of information related to diabetes management.

Problem 3: Distorted and maladaptive cognitions about eating, which may be related to Nancy's significant weight loss and her relatively slow rate of weight gain.

Progress: Nancy worked on these issues during individual therapy; she expressed frustration with her slow rate of weight gain but appeared to understand the vital role that nutrition and diet play in her diabetes regimen. She expressed some concern regarding her body image (i.e., being too thin), although she gained insight into the reason she had lost 38 pounds prior to being admitted to the hospital. Nancy was also able to develop good meal-planning skills and expressed a desire to continue gaining weight upon her return home.

Problem 4: Difficulties acknowledging interpersonal conflict, especially within the family system. These difficulties result in Nancy's continuing to be extremely dependent on her parents, and interfere with her age-appropriate strivings for independence and autonomy.

Progress: Nancy appeared to develop moderate insight into the role that her family plays in her difficulties in becoming autonomous, and she expressed interest in and some excitement about initiating some age-appropriate activities. However, Nancy had difficulty acknowledging the existence of familial conflict at home, and continued to deny its impact on her emotional health.

In family therapy, Mr. and Mrs. Brown acknowledged their tendency to "overprotect" Nancy but did not develop insight into how their overprotection contributes to her current difficulties in being independent. The Browns also did not recognize patterns of conflict avoidance that maintain these behaviors at home. Individual and family therapy should continue to emphasize the need for conflict resolution and for Nancy to be given opportunities to achieve greater independence within her family system.

Problem 5: Nancy's history of using somatic complaints to receive extra care and nurturance from her family, and to withdraw from activities she does not enjoy.

Progress: Nancy's tendency to use somatic complaints to receive extra care and nurturance was a recurrent theme in individual therapy. Nancy was able to understand the role of negative emotions in her medical complaints; however, she did not develop insight into the operant nature of these somatic complaints. She was reinforced for proper participation in activities, and at the time of discharge this issue remained an area of significant concern warranting further focus in both individual and family therapy.

Problem 6: Nancy and her parents' confusion about the reasons behind Nancy's below-average school achievement, and their questions about school placement options for Nancy once she leaves the Diabetes Project Unit.

Progress: The results of Nancy's psychological, achievement, and educational evaluations were discussed with Nancy and her family. Additionally,

Nancy's high school guidance counselor was contacted and made aware of the extent of her reading difficulties. Nancy will receive extra help from her school in order to remediate these learning difficulties.

Follow-up Recommendations and Planning

1. It is recommended that Nancy continue to be followed by a psychiatrist in her area to manage her antidepressant medication. In addition, she should continue to be followed by an endocrinologist in her area.
2. It is recommended that Nancy enter into individual therapy with a therapist who is familiar with the individual and family issues involved in diabetes management.
3. It is recommended that the Browns continue to receive family psychotherapy to further address family system–related issues.

SPECIAL ISSUES

Diagnosis of Mental Retardation

In the DSM-IV, mental retardation is characterized by significant deficits in both intellectual and adaptive functioning occurring during the developmental period (American Psychiatric Association, 1994). This definition may be broken down into three parts, which are reviewed next.

Significant intellectual deficits are typically diagnosed with an intellectual assessment tool such as one of the Wechsler scales. A significant intellectual deficit refers to overall intellectual functioning that falls two standard deviations below the mean. On the Wechsler scales, this corresponds to a Full Scale IQ score of 69 or lower. This indicates that the individual has scored at or below the 2nd percentile as compared to a normative sample of his or her same-aged peers. Significant deficits in adaptive behavior may be assessed with the Vineland Adaptive Behavior Scales. As with the Wechsler, a significant deficit is defined by a score of 69 or lower, meaning that the individual's adaptive behavior is at or below the 2nd percentile as compared to a normative sample. As discussed in a previous section, the assessment of adaptive behavior involves assessing areas of development related to general daily functioning rather than to intellect. Both significant intellectual delay and adaptive behavioral delay are necessary for the diagnosis of mental retardation. Thus, a child who met only one of these two criteria would not be classified as mentally retarded. The third component of the definition of mental retardation requires that these deficits be evident during the developmental period; in other words, they must be evident prior to age 18. Children and adolescents who receive a diagnosis of mental retardation are entitled to receive special educational services through the school system to address their deficits.

Diagnosis of Learning Disabilities

When children and adolescents appear to be of average or above-average intelligence but do not seem to perform to their potential in school, they are often referred for a learning disability assessment. Prior to our contemporary understandings of learning disabilities, children who appeared to work below their potential might be seen as unmotivated or lazy. Other factors that may explain the failure to perform as expected include the child disliking the teacher or experiencing some recent stressor such as the death of a parent, divorce, or a recent move. These stressors may affect children's emotional stability and subsequent academic performance, and should not lead automatically to the diagnosis of a learning disability. Children who do receive a diagnosis of a learning disability are entitled to receive special services in school that allow for individualized instructional strategies to help these students maximize their intellectual abilities.

Public Law (P.L.) 94-142 and the National Joint Commission on Learning Disabilities (NJCLD) both provide working definitions of learning disabilities. School systems generally utilize the P.L. 94-142 definition. In his description of P.L. 94-142, Sattler (1992) outlines four components that constitute an understanding of learning disabilities. P.L. 94-142 (*Federal Register*, December 29, 1997) (p. 65083, 121A, 5) reads: "Specific learning disability means a disorder in one or more of the basic psycho-

logical processes involved in understanding or in using language, spoken or written, which may manifest itself in an imperfect ability to listen, think, read, write, spell, or to do mathematical calculations." According to P.L. 94-142, the categorization of a learning disability includes such "conditions as perceptual handicaps, brain injury, minimal brain dysfunction, dyslexia, and developmental aphasia." Exclusionary criteria are outlined in the third component of the definition: "the term does not include children that have learning problems which are primarily the result of visual, hearing, or motor handicaps, of mental retardation, of emotional disturbance, or of environmental, cultural or economic disadvantage." Finally, P.L. 94-142 indicates that the designation of learning disabilities should be applied to children who have a severe discrepancy between achievement and intellectual ability.

Although the definition of learning disability as reported above may be criticized, as will be suggested, it does provide a basis for diagnosis that is currently in use. The Wechsler Individual Achievement Test and the Woodcock Johnson Tests of Achievement—Revised are commonly used assessment tools in identifying problems in the abilities described in understanding or using language in the first component of the definition. Terms such as *minimal brain dysfunction* used in the second component of the definition are rarely used today to describe children. The exclusionary criteria, though conceptually important, are somewhat problematic. Given a particular child, it is often difficult to ascertain whether his or her learning problems are due to emotional disturbance or environmental handicap, which would technically exclude them from a diagnosis of a learning disability. For example, a child who met the fourth criterion of having a significant IQ–achievement discrepancy would be technically excluded from the definition if it was determined that his learning disability was as a direct result of his low-SES background and family problems. The question is whether one can assume that the low-SES background and family problems caused the lower achievement scores. If one assumes this to be true, the child would not qualify for the diagnosis and would not receive special educational services. The final criterion, a significant difference between IQ and achievement scores, is a crucial component in operationally defining the diagnosis of learning disability.

Sattler (1992) reviews a second definition of learning disability put forth by the National Joint Commission on Learning Disabilities (NJCLD). Though similar to P.L. 94-142, the NJCLD definition does not exclude mental retardation, nor does it require that the child have an average IQ. To diagnosis a child with a learning disability, a clinician must consider criteria from the DSM-IV and results from individually administered IQ and achievement tests. Although this assessment is fairly costly, it increases the reliability and validity of the diagnosis by following stringent psychometric criteria.

Sattler (1992) outlines several methods by which a significant discrepancy between a child's ability and achievement can be identified. These include the following: (1) the child's achievement is a fixed number of grades behind grade placement; (2) the child's achievement is a graduated number of grades behind placement; (3) a standard score formulation; and (4) a regression equation.

The first method—pertaining to the requirement that the child's achievement is a fixed number of grades behind the child's actual grade placement— is the least sophisticated method of determining a significant discrepancy. For example, a child who is in the third grade must score at a first-grade level on an achievement test to qualify for a learning disability diagnosis. This procedure fails to consider the child's intellect, or whether the child is very bright or very dull. For example, if a child is in the twelfth grade and his achievement scores are at the tenth-grade level, this is much less of a discrepancy than a third grader functioning at the first-grade level.

The second, or graduated method, attempts to account for this problem (Sattler, 1992). The graduated method involves considering the child's current grade placement as a factor in determining the size of a significant grade discrepancy for a diagnosis of a learning disability. When a child is in grades 1 through 3, a one-year discrepancy between achievement and actual grade would be considered significant. However, for a child in grades 4 or 5, 1.5 grades behind may be used as a criterion to be con-

sidered for a learning disability. Likewise, for a child in grades 6 through 8, a criterion of two years behind may be considered; and youngsters in grades 9 through 12 might be required to be three years behind to be considered learning disabled. This process of identifying a discrepancy is an improvement over the first method, but it also does not consider the child's intellectual level.

The standard score formulation of an IQ–achievement discrepancy addresses some of the problems with the grade-based achievement discrepancy methods described. Both intellectual measures, such as the Wechsler scales, and achievement measures, such as the Woodcock Johnson Tests of Achievement, were normed with a mean of 100 and a standard deviation of 15. A comparison of scores on these two measures takes into account both a child's intellectual and achievement level. For example, if a child of 15 has an IQ of 110 and a reading achievement standard score of 88, one can see that there is a significant discrepancy (22 points) between the child's IQ score and achievement scores. In contrast, a 15-year-old child in grade 11 with a measured IQ of 88 and an achievement standard score of 88 might be performing several grade levels behind actual grade placement, although this child would actually be scoring exactly where predicted on the basis of IQ. Thus, this child would not meet criteria for a learning disability when intellect is taken into consideration.

The regression equation formula is the most sophisticated means of identifying a significant discrepancy between IQ and achievement. This method takes into account the regression-to-the-mean effect or, more specifically, the fact that a child who is below average on one measure will likely perform better on a second measure, and a child who is above average on one measure will likely perform worse on a second measure. IQ and achievement tests are not perfectly correlated with one another, and this increases the likelihood of regression to the mean. The regression equation can take this into account. Using two measures that were standardized on the same sample of children, such as the Wechsler Intelligence Scales and the Wechsler Individual Achievement Test, is preferable, as this deals with many psychometric issues and assumptions at stake when using an IQ and achievement test not normed on the same sample. Thus in order to define a learning disability, a clinician who has administered these two tests can look up the two scores in the WIAT manual to determine if the achievement scores are significantly below what would be predicted based on the measured IQ. This method of determining a significant discrepancy is empirically supported rather than hypothetically derived.

Issues in Assessing Children with Ethnic Minority Backgrounds

There is much dispute regarding the appropriate use of current intellectual assessment tools with children from ethnic minority backgrounds. Some consider intelligence tests to have a cultural bias favoring white Anglo-Saxon children (Sattler, 1992). In support of this position is the fact that ethnic minority groups tend to have a lower mean score on intelligence tests than the standardization sample. Specifically, African Americans have repeatedly been found to have scores nearly a standard deviation below the mean of the standardization sample, and Hispanics also have been found to differ significantly from the standardization sample (Sattler, 1992).

Critics of IQ testing have argued that the norms of the standardization sample, which comprise a national, socially stratified group of youngsters, are inappropriate for minority children. Those who favor this position argue that the life experience of minority children is significantly different from the experience of the standardization group (Sattler, 1992). Some critics have argued for the use of pluralistic norms, which involves comparing a child to norms measured on his or her own ethnic group.

Other critics have argued that minority children have problematic test-taking skills that may manifest as test-taking anxiety, thus affecting their performance. Some suggest that white examiners may depress the scores of ethnic minority children, as most examiners in psychological testing situations are white. The difference in ethnic background has been proposed as a factor that may depress or lower the scores of ethnic minority children. It also has been argued that test results of intellectual assessment result in minority children receiving inferior educational placements. Some critics hypothesize that black children would achieve at a higher level if they were allowed to remain in their regular classes.

Sattler (1992) has reviewed research to refute the arguments against the use of intellectual assessment tools with ethnic minority children. Addressing the first criticism, that intelligence tests have a cultural bias, Sattler (1992) describes studies that demonstrate that socioeconomic status (SES) accounts for most of the variance in the differences between ethnic minorities, scores on intellectual tests and the standardization sample. These data show that when SES is controlled, the mean difference between these two groups of children is generally less than 5 points. Hence, it can be argued that SES, as opposed to race, accounts for most of the difference between the ethnic minority group and the standardization sample.

Further data have supported the use of intellectual tests with ethnic minorities, as they are found to be equally predictive of academic achievements when comparing Caucasian and African American children. Further, factor-analytic studies on different ethnic groups produced comparable results, suggesting that the structure of intelligence is similar for Caucasian, African American, and Hispanic American children.

The argument that minority children have deficient test-taking skills is primarily a rhetorical argument, as there are few data demonstrating that factors such as motivation and anxiety have a demonstrable effect. Sattler (1992) has collected data on 29 studies that examine the effect of a white examiner on an African American child's performance. In 25 of the 29 studies, no differences were found when children of ethnic minority backgrounds were tested by white versus African American examiners. Finally, Sattler (1992) rebutted the argument that the results of intellectual tests lead to inferior educational placements of ethnic minority children. Intellectual assessment by individually administered IQ test is not routinely done with any population. To receive an intellectual assessment, a referral must be made, and such a referral would indicate or suggest that a child is already having problems. These policies argue against any mass discrimination against minority groups. Intellectual testing is conducted when a problem has been previously identified, and classification occurs for the purpose of obtaining special services regardless of a child's ethnic background.

Sattler (1992) concludes that while the research he has reviewed does not appear to indicate that intellectual testing with ethnic minority children is unfair, it is paramount that in any assessment the examiner carefully builds rapport and follows testing protocols. Regardless of a child's ethnic background, difficulty with rapport may develop and must be appropriately addressed, as it may influence a child's performance. Special consideration must be given to testing a child whose primary language is not English. Care must be taken to ensure that the child can both adequately express himself and understand English to guarantee that comparison to an English-speaking standardization group is appropriate. Assessing a child with inadequate English skills using an English version of an IQ test for an educational placement would result in a biased, inappropriate assessment.

Sexual and Physical Abuse in Children

The term *child abuse* refers to the physical or sexual abuse or neglect of a child under the age of 18 by the parent or other person responsible for the welfare of the child. A recent report by the U.S. Department of Health and Human Services (1995) reported that in 1993, approximately 1 million children were the victims of abuse and that over 1,000 children died that year as a result of abuse or neglect.

The laws defining child abuse vary from state to state, as do the reporting laws. All states have mandatory child abuse reporting laws requiring individuals to report any cases of suspected abuse. Mandated reporters include physicians, dentists, psychologists, teachers, and others in professions that come into contact with children. This mandatory reporting is assumed to be an act in good faith, with suspicion, not necessarily proof, of child abuse as the motivating factor.

Without such recognition of abuse and subsequent family intervention, many children are injured and even die every year from physical abuse. A diagnosis of physical abuse is based on physical examination findings, along with a history of how the injury occurred. Parents and children should be interviewed separately regarding specific histories of family conflict resolution and child disciplinary methods (Kaplan, 1996). The physical examination also is a vital element in the diagnosis of child abuse. Inflicted bruises often occur at typical sites (such as buttocks, cheeks, neck, earlobes, genitals, and inner thighs) and may fit a recognizable patterns, (e.g., hand marks, bite marks, strap marks, or other unidentifiable strange marks). Often the child may also have inflicted burn, bone, head, or abdominal injuries as well.

Abused children face increased risks for serious emotional, behavioral, developmental, and learning difficulties. Often such children are referred for psychotherapy, where they may learn to deal with their emotional problems resulting from the abuse, and importantly, to redirect their own emotional growth processes in order to disrupt the cycle of abuse that often occurs among generations of families (Kaplan, 1996). Many treatment programs for child abuse cases also focus on the abusive parent. Parental treatment involves providing the abusive parent with emotional support and positive parenting models in addition to effective, nonpunitive child-rearing techniques (Kaplan, 1996).

It is also important for child care professionals to be aware of the signs and symptoms of child sexual abuse. Sexual abuse may be defined as sexual activity with a child under the age of 18 by an adult caretaker, either intrafamilial or extrafamilial. Sexual abuse may range from fondling and voyeurism to intercourse and forcible rape. In 90% of cases, the victim is a young girl under the age of 12 (Schmitt, 1984). Most often the perpetrator is a male. For nearly half of the victims, sexual abuse is a repeated incident occurring over a number of years (Green, 1996).

Often a child is too young to verbalize what is happening to her or him. Usually the reasons for not telling largely outweigh the reasons to report abuse. Children may realize the social stigma attached to being sexually molested. Perhaps they feel they will not be believed, or fear they will be blamed or even abandoned (Burgess & Holstrom, 1975). In some cases, the perpetrator is a family member valued by the child, and the child fears rejection.

Although a large majority of child sexual abuse cases lack evidence of physical signs, if present, these greatly assist in identifying incidents of sexual abuse. Physical symptoms due to sexual abuse include perineal bruises, tears, or venereal diseases. While physical signs may clearly indicate sexual abuse, other signs may manifest as another type of child dysfunction (Faller, 1988). In younger children, one might find sleep disturbances, sex play, loss of toileting skills, depression, and problems in school. Older children, nearing adolescence, may turn instead to drugs and alcohol, crimes, promiscuity, or even suicide attempts (see Asher, 1988, for a review).

Assessment of childhood sexual abuse first involves determining the credibility of the allegation of abuse. This may be accomplished by a skillful investigative interview (see Sgroi, 1983). The allegation of child abuse must be approached with certain clinical assumptions (Faller, 1988). Inclusion of explicit details of sexual behavior thus increases the credibility of a child's accusation. Likewise, most sexual abuse involves a progression of incidents over time, each increasingly more intimate than the previous one. Usually there is the presence of an element of secrecy between the victim and the perpetrator, along with elements of power or pressure. An interviewer experienced with child sexual abuse can then assess the child's credibility on the basis of the responses elicited during the interview. Sgroi (1983) is careful to note that although physical signs of sexual abuse are helpful when present, the lack of any physical evidence does not necessarily weaken the complaint.

An examination of mental status is also needed. Although it is rare, some children may be severely depressed or suicidal and may need immediate psychiatric/psychological evaluation. In addition, the therapist must obtain a detailed history from the child to assist in determining treatment planning.

To provide effective treatment for the sexually abused child, the therapist must be aware of and understand the enormous impact of these issues for the victim (Sgroi, Blick, & Porter, 1983). These issues may include feelings of guilt, fear, depression, low self-esteem, poor social skills, inability to trust, and role confusion, among others, as well as the issue of being "damaged goods." Although no evidence exists for any one treatment method as the method of choice in treating child sexual abuse, several common themes in treatment should emerge. Therapists should encourage the child to identify and express guilty feelings and fears. The therapist should always convey the message that the child was not responsible for the abuse and had a right to disclose the secret of abuse. Family therapy is possible in incestuous cases where the family is willing to take responsibility for the sexual abuse that occurred, and the nonabusive parent for the lack of protection the child received. Individual and group therapy may also be used, as well as play therapy, role modeling, role playing, peer support, and positive peer pressure. The goal of treatment is a strengthening process intended to improve the child's self-image; diminish guilt; and increase trust, self-esteem, and feelings of security.

Pediatric Psychology

Within the realm of psychology, the role of the pediatric psychologist is a relatively recent development, yet the number of pediatric psychologists who can be found working within medical settings has multiplied greatly over the past 20 years. As early as a century ago, Lightner Witmer (1896), the founder of clinical psychology, foresaw the need for psychologists and physicians to integrate their interests in children and to provide care to both children's medical and their psychological problems. As psychologists and physicians have become aware of the large role that biopsychosocial factors play in chronic or acute childhood illness, an active collaboration between the two has been established and is still developing as pediatric psychology continues to defines itself and the role it plays in the health and disease of children.

Logan Wright (1967) formally introduced the term *pediatric psychologist* in his article "The Pediatric Psychologist: A Role Model." Wright saw the pediatric psychologist as a psychologist who delivered clinical services to children in a nonpsychiatric medical setting. A more recent and encompassing definition by Roberts, Maddux, and Wright (1984) state that "pediatric psychology as a field of research and practice has been concerned with a wide variety of topics in the relationship between the psychological and physical well-being of children including behavioral and emotional concomitants of disease and illness, the role of psychology in pediatric medicine, and the promotion of health and the prevention of illness among healthy children" (pp. 56–57).

According to Tuma (1975), the primary feature that distinguishes the role of the pediatric psychologist from that of the clinical psychologist is the setting where the psychological services are provided. The pediatric psychologist is likely to be found in medical and health care settings such as hospital inpatient units, outpatient services, clinics, developmental centers, private pediatricians' offices, and health maintenance organizations, where he or she typically will engage in research, practice, and consultation. As Roberts and Lyman (1990) note, this consultation role includes consults not only to medical professionals but also to parents, nursing staff, educators, welfare agencies, and other social service and health agencies.

Practicing within the demands of the medical system presents some unique challenges to pediatric psychologists. The pediatric psychologist must be able to function effectively in a multidisciplinary setting, maintain and often facilitate effective communication with all necessary parties, and be sensitive to the needs of the medical staff and aware of the pressure placed on them as well (Drotar et al., 1982). Each pediatric patient can expect to spend an average of 13 minutes with the pediatrician (Bergman, Dassel, & Wedgwood, 1966), and often children are admitted only for a short time. This makes it necessary for the pediatric psychologist to conduct rapid assessment and quickly diagnose the problem and its resolution. Implementation of psychological interventions, then, must also be fairly brief and short-term (Roberts & Wright, 1982). In addition, the pediatric psychologist must be careful not to disrupt the physician–patient relationship while delivering services to the child and his or her family (Drotar et al., 1982).

A final challenge for the psychologist working in a medical setting is the conflict between the acute illness model (Drotar, 1982), wherein physicians prescribe treatments to cure the physical problem within the child, and the psychologists' psychoso-

cial perspective, which involves longer assessments and treatments, as well as family, school, and community interventions (Kurz, 1987). In addition, pediatric psychologists are often oriented to the prevention of social, cognitive, affective, or physical problems of childhood even before they develop (Peterson & Ridley-Johnson, 1983; Roberts & Peterson, 1984).

The role that psychological factors play in contributing to the maintenance of health or to medical problems is a complex one. In addition, the illness itself may have a psychological impact on children. Children with chronic physical disorders have been shown to experience an increased risk for overall adjustment problems. In the case of a child with IDDM (insulin-dependent diabetes mellitus), adjustment may have significant implications for health status. In a review of the literature, Geffken and Johnson (1994) found that maladjustment may lead to poor compliance and diabetes control in some cases, and that in other cases, poor control could result in an anxious and depressed child.

Children diagnosed with cancer also face significant adjustment problems such as hair loss, weight loss or gain, fatigue, and other physical side effects that contribute to the risk of psychosocial problems. In addition, invasive medical procedures such as surgery, lumbar punctures, and venipuncture are a source of significant distress and have been shown to differ in impact according to the age of the child. The research suggests that distress levels of pediatric cancer patients under the age of 7 undergoing bone marrow aspirations are 5 to 10 times higher than those of patients over the age of 7 (Jay & Elliot, 1983).

For the child with spina bifida, a birth defect resulting from the failure of one or more of the vertebrae to close completely, social isolation is common and depression frequent (Dorner, 1976). Self-esteem for this group is also significantly reduced when compared to normal age and sex matched children (Hayden, Davenport, & Campbell, 1979). Wallander, Varni, Babani, Banis, and Wilcox (1988) investigated 270 chronically ill and handicapped children and reported that children with spina bifida experience a higher level of psychological adjustment problems when compared to healthy children, although it was no different from the levels exhibited by children with other chronic problems such as diabetes, hemophilia, or cerebral palsy. Their adjustment, however, was better than that of children who were referred to mental health clinics.

Pediatric psychologists must familiarize themselves with the disorders and treatments of childhood in order to provide effective consultation. Collaboration between the physician and the pediatric psychologist is imperative to this discipline, as is the psychologists' commitment to providing quality services (Roberts & Lyman, 1990). The result of such services will be to enhance opportunities for research and practice in the rapidly growing and evolving field of pediatric psychology. As Kurz (1987) notes, the psychological and physical health of future generations will depend on the quality of our pediatric psychologists today.

CONCLUSION AND FUTURE TRENDS

The psychological assessment and treatment of children and adolescents is a broad area. This chapter has provided a sample of assessments and treatments for youngsters. New psychological tests for children in this age group are constantly being developed, and old tests are frequently updated with newer content, materials, and improved norms. As suggested in the section on empirically validated treatments, research is constantly being produced to evaluate treatments for specific conditions and to identify those that are efficacious. Psychologists, as well as the many insurance companies paying for clinic visits, want to identify treatments for children and adolescents that have been proved to work and are cost-effective. In addition, the increasing penetration of the health care field with companies providing managed care subjects the treatments provided by psychologists to frequent utilization review. Clinical psychologists working with children and adolescents must keep up with developments in the field to be able to use the more psychometrically sophisticated assessment techniques and the most efficacious treatments for specific conditions.

As child clinical psychologists must keep abreast of developments in the field, they must also be aware that at times limited scientific data will be available on some assessment techniques and for the treatment of some conditions. Child clinical psychologists will have to use their knowledge of development, psychopathology, and other areas of psychology to make judgments about how to proceed in some clinical situations. Child clinical psychologists must have specialized knowledge to deal with sexual and physical abuse, and they must be aware of the regulations in their state that govern the professional conduct related to this important problem. With the increasing ethnic diversity in the United States, child clinical psychologists must make judgments about when it is appropriate to use particular measures and when their use is deemed inappropriate.

As reviewed in the section on pediatric psychology, the role of clinical child psychology is rapidly expanding into primary and tertiary health care. This occurs as the general principles of psychological assessment and treatment have been found not only to be applicable but also to be efficacious regarding the behavioral and psychosocial aspects of children in the pediatric setting. The opportunities for growth in this exciting area are excellent.

Clinical child psychologists are working in a challenging profession, and the change and development in the field is unyielding. Work in the area will test these psychologists long after they have formally received their doctorate. At the same time, opportunities in the realm of clinical child psychology are very broad, and the likelihood for reward is evident in the progress in the area and in the daily work of the child clinical psychologist.

REFERENCES

Achenbach, T. M., & Edelbrock, C. S. (1986). *Child Behavior Checklist and Youth Self-Report.* Burlington, VT: Author.

American Psychiatric Association. (1994). *Diagnostic and statistical manual of mental disorders* (4th ed., revised). Washington, DC: Author.

Asher, S. J. (1988). Effects of childhood sexual abuse: A review of the issues. In L. E. A. Walker (Ed.), *Handbook on sexual abuse of children.* New York: Springer.

Axline, V. (1947). *Play therapy.* Cambridge, MA: Riverside Press.

Bandura, A. (1977). *Social learning theory.* Englewood Cliffs, NJ: Prentice-Hall.

Barrett, P. M., Dadds, M. R., & Rapee, R. M. (1996). Family treatment of childhood anxiety: A controlled trial. *Journal of Consulting and Clinical Psychology, 64,*333–342.

Bellack, L., & Bellack, S. S. (1986). *Children's Apperception Test.* Larchmont, NY: C.P.S. Inc.

Bergman, A. B., Dassel, S. W., & Wedgwood, R. J. (1966). Time–motion study of practicing pediatricians. *Pediatrics, 38,* 254–263.

Burgess, A. W., & Holstrom, L. L. (1975). Sexual assault of children and adolescents: Pressure, sex, and secrecy. *Nursing Clinics of North America*, 551–563.

Butcher, J. N., Williams, C. L., Graham, J. R., Archer, R. P., Tellegen, A., Ben-Porath, Y. S., & Kaemmer, B. (1992). *Minnesota Multiphasic Personality Inventory for Adolescents: Manual for administration, scoring and interpretation.* Minneapolis: University of Minnesota Press.

Carek, D. J. (1979). Individual psychodynamically oriented therapy. In S. Harrison (Ed.), *Basic handbook of child psychiatry* (pp. 35–57). New York: Basic Books.

Carlson, C. (1990). Assessing the family context. In C. R. Reynolds & R. W. Kamphaus (Ed.), *Handbook of psychological and educational assessment of children: Personality, behavior & content* (pp. 546–575). New York: Guilford Press.

Cohen, H., & Weil, G. R. (1971). *Tasks of emotional development test.* Lexington, MA: D. C. Heath.

Dorner, S. (1976). Adolescents with spina bifida: How they see their situation. *Archives of Disease in Childhood, 51,* 439–444.

Drotar, D. (1982). The child psychologist in the medical system. In P. Karoly, J. J. Steffen, & D. J. O'Grady (Eds.), *Child health psychology* (pp. 1–28). New York: Pergamon Press.

Drotar, D., Benjamin, P., Chwast, R., Litt, C., & Vajner, P. (1982). The role of the psychologist in pediatric outpatient and inpatient settings. In J. Tuma (Ed.), *Handbook for the practice of pediatric psychology* (pp. 232–265). New York: Wiley.

Ellis, A. (1970*). The essence of rational psychotherapy: A comprehensive approach to treatment.* New York: Institute for Rational Living.

Erikson, E. H. (1968). *Identity, youth and crisis.* New York: W. W. Norton.

Exner, J. (1974). *The Rorschach: A comprehensive system.* New York: Wiley.

Faller, K. C. (1988). *Child sexual abuse: An interdisciplinary manual for diagnosis, case management, and treatment.* New York: Columbia University Press.

Freud, A. (1965). *Normality and pathology in childhood.* New York: International University Press.

Freud, S. (1959). Analysis of a phobia in a five-year-old boy. In E. Jones (Ed.), *Collected papers, 3,* 149–289. New York: Basic Books.

Geffken, G., & Johnson, S. B. (1994). Diabetes: Psychological issues. In R. A. Olsen, L. L. Mullen, J. B. Gillman, & I. M. Chaney (Eds.), *A sourcebook of pediatric psychology.* Boston: Allyn and Bacon.

Goodman, W. K., Rasmussen, S. A., Ridde, M. A., Price, L. H., & Rapoport, J. L. (1986). *Children's Yale–Brown Obsessive Compulsive Scale.* Gainesville, FL: Author.

Green, A. H. (1996). Overview of child sexual abuse. In S. J. Kaplan (Ed), *Family violence: A clinical and legal guide.* Washington, DC: American Psychiatric Press.

Greenspoon, J., & Lamal, P. A. (1978). Cognitive behavior modification—Who needs it? *Psychological Record, 28,* 343–351.

Griff, M. D. (1983). Family play therapy. In C. E. Schaefer, & K. J. O'Connor (Eds.), *Handbook of play therapy* (pp. 65–75). New York: Wiley.

Haley, J. (1987). *Problem-solving therapy* (rev. ed.). San Francisco: Jossey-Bass.

Hayden, P. W., Davenport, S. L. H., & Campbell, M. M. (1979). Adolescents with myelodysplasia: Impact of physical disability on emotional maturation. *Pediatrics, 64,* 53–59.

Herrnstein, R., & Murray, C. (1994). *The bell curve: Intelligence and class structure in American life.* New York: Free Press.

Houts, A. C., Berman, J. S., & Abramson, H. (1994). Effectiveness of psychological and pharmacological treatments for nocturnal enuresis. *Journal of Consulting and Clinical Psychology, 62,* 737–745.

Jaremko, M. E. (1979). Cognitive behavior modification: Real science or more mentalism? *Psychological Record, 29,* 547–552.

Jastak, S., & Wilkinson, G. S. (1984). *Wide range achievement test: Administration manual* (rev. ed.). Wilmington, DE: Jastak Associates.

Jay, S. M., & Elliot, C. H. (1983). Psychological interventions for pain in pediatric cancer patients. In G. B. Humphrey (Ed.), *Adrenal and endocrine tumors in children.* Boston: Martinus Nijhoff.

Kanfer, F. H., & Karoly, P. (1972). Self-control: A behavioristic excursion into the lion's den. *Behavior Therapy, 3,* 398–416.

Kaplan, S. J. (1996). Physical abuse of children and adolescents. In S. J. Kaplan (Ed.), *Family violence: A clin-*

ical and legal guide. Washington, DC: American Psychiatric Press.

Kazdin, A. E. (1988). *Child psychotherapy: Developing and identifying effective treatments*. New York: Pergamon Press.

Kazdin, A. E., & Wilcoxon, L. A. (1976). Systematic desensitization and nonspecific treatment effects: A methodological evaluation. *Psychological Bulletin, 83*, 729–758.

Klein, M. (1932). *The psycho-analysis of children*. New York: Norton.

Koppitz, E. M. (1968). *Psychological evaluation of children's human figure drawings*. New York: Grune & Stratton.

Kurz, R. B. (1987). Child health psychology. In G. C. Stone, S. M. Weiss, J. D. Matarazzo, N. G. Miller, J. Rodin, C. Belar, M. Folick, & J. G. Singer (Eds.), *Health psychology: A discipline and a profession* (pp. 285–301). Chicago: University of Chicago Press.

Lachar, D. (1982). *Personality Inventory for Children: Revised format manual supplement*. Los Angeles: Western Psychological Services.

Ledwidge, B. (1978). Cognitive behavior modification: A step in the wrong direction? *Psychological Bulletin, 85*, 353–375.

Ledwidge, B. (1979). Cognitive behavior modification or new ways to change minds: Reply to Mahoney and Kazdin. *Psychological Bulletin, 56*, 1050–1053.

Locke, E. A. (1979). Behavior modification is not cognitive and other myths: A reply to Ledwidge. *Cognitive Therapy and Research, 3*, 119–125.

Mahoney, M. J., & Kazdin, A. E. (1979). Cognitive behavior modification: Misconceptions and premature evaluation. *Psychological Bulletin, 86*, 1044–1049.

McArthur, D. S., & Roberts, G. E. (1982). *Roberts Apperception Test for Children manual*. Los Angeles: Western Psychological Services.

Meichenbaum, D. H. (1977). *Cognitive-behavior modification*. New York: Plenum Press.

Meichenbaum, D. (1979). Cognitive behavior modification: The need for a fairer assessment. *Cognivive Therapy and Research, 3*, 127–132.

Murray, H. A. (1943). *Thematic Apperception Test*. Cambridge, MA: Harvard University Press.

Nichols, M. P., & Paolino, T. J. (1986). *Basic techniques of psychodynamic psychotherapy*. New York: Gardner Press.

O'Brien, S., Ross, L. V., & Christophersen, E. R. (1986*)*. Primary encopresis: Evaluation and treatment. *Journal of Applied Behavior Analysis, 19*, 137–145.

Patterson, G. R., & Reid, J. B. (1984). Social interaction processes within the family: The study of moment-by-moment family transactions in which human social development is embedded. *Journal of Applied Developmental Psychology, 5*, 327–362.

Peoples, C. (1983). Fair play therapy. In C.E. Schaefer & K. J. O'Connor (Eds.), *Handbook of play therapy* (pp. 75–94). New York: Wiley.

Peterson, L., & Ridley-Johnson, R. (1983). Prevention of disorders in children. In C. Walker & M. C. Roberts (Eds.), *Handbook of clinical child psychology* (pp. 1174–1197). New York: Wiley.

Piaget, J. (1962). *Play, dreams, and imitation in childhood*. New York: Norton.

Reynolds, C. R., & Richmond, B. O. (1985). *Revised children's manifest anxiety scale manual*. Los Angeles: Western Psychological Services.

Roberts, M. C., & Lyman, R. D. (1990). The psychologist as a pediatric consultant. In A. M. Gross & R. Drabman (Eds.), *Handbook of clinical behavioral pediatrics* (pp. 11–27). New York: Plenum Press.

Roberts, M. C., Maddux, J. E., & Wright, L. (1984). The developmental perspective in behavioral health. In J. D. Matarazzo, N. E. Miller, S. M. Weiss, J. A. Herd, & S. M. Weiss (Eds.), *Behavioral health: A handbook of health enhancement and disease prevention* (pp. 56–68). New York: Wiley-Interscience.

Roberts, M. C., & Peterson, L. (1984). Prevention models: Theoretical and practical implications. In M. C. Roberts & L. Peterson (Eds.), *Prevention of problems in childhood: Psychological research and applications* (pp. 1–39). New York: Wiley.

Roberts, M. C., Quevillon, R. P., & Wright, L. (1979). Pediatric psychology: A developmental report and survey of the literature. *Child and Youth Services, 2*, 1–9.

Roberts, M. C., & Wright, L. (1982). Role of the pediatric psychologist as consultant to pediatricians. In J. Tuma (Ed.), *Handbook for the practice of pediatric psychology* (pp. 251–289). New York: Wiley-Interscience.

Routh, D. K. (1994). *Clinical psychology since 1917: Science, practice and organization*. New York: Plenum Press.

Sattler, J. M. (1992). *Assessment of children* (revised and updated 3rd ed.). San Diego, CA: Author.

Schaefer, C. E., & O'Connor, K .J. (Eds.). (1983). *Handbook of play therapy*. New York: Wiley.

Schmitt, B. D. (1984). Clinical diagnosis of physical abuse. In R. G. Sanger & D. C. Bross (Eds.), *Clinical management of child abuse and neglect: A guide for the dental professional* (pp. 25–36). Chicago: Quintessence.

Sgroi, S. M. (1979). The sexual assault of children: Dynamics of the problem and issues in program development. In *Sexual abuse of children: Implications from the Sexual Trauma Treatment Program of Connecticut.* New York: Community Council of Greater New York.

Sgroi, S. M. (1983). *Handbook of clinical intervention in child sexual abuse.* Lexington, MA: D.C. Heath.

Sgroi, S. M., Blick, L. C., & Porter, F. S. (1983). Treatment of the sexually abused child. In S.M. Sgroi (Ed.), *Handbook of clinical intervention in child sexual abuse.* Lexington, MA: D.C. Heath.

Skinner, B. F. (1974). *About behaviorism.* New York: Vintage Books.

Sparrow, S. S., Balla, D. A., & Cicchetti, D. V. (1994). *Vineland Adaptive Behavior Scales: Survey form manual.* Circle Pines, MI: American Guidance Service.

Spielberger, C. D., Edwards, C. D., Montouri, J., & Lushene, R. (1970). *State–trait anxiety inventory for children.* Palo Alto, CA: Consulting Psychologists Press.

Task Force on Promotion and Dissemination of Psychological Procedures. (1995). Training and dissemination of empirically validated psychological procedures. *The Clinical Psychologist, 48,* 3–23.

Thorndike, R. L., Hagen, E. P., & Sattler, J. M. (1986). *Stanford-Binet Intelligence Scale—Fourth Edition: Technical manual.* Chicago, IL: Riverside.

Tuma, J. M. (1975). Pediatric psychology? . . . Do you mean clinical child psychology? *Journal of Clinical Child Psychology, 4,* 9–12.

U.S. Department of Health and Human Services, National Center on Child Abuse and Neglect. (1995). *Child maltreatment 1993: Reports from the states to the National Center on Child Abuse and Neglect.* Washington, DC: U.S. Government Printing Office.

Wallander, J. L., Varni, J. W., Babani, L., Banis, H. T., & Wilcox, K. T. (1988). Children with chronic physical disorders: Maternal reports of the psychological adjustment. *Journal of Pediatric Psychology, 13,* 197–212.

Walter, H. I., & Gilmore, S. K. (1973). Placebo versus social learning effects in parent training procedures designed to alter the behavior of aggressive boys. *Behavior Therapy, 4,* 361–377.

Watson, J. B., & Rayner, R. (1920). Conditioned emotional reactions. *Journal of Experimental Psychology, 3,* 1–14.

Wechsler, D. (1989a). *Manual for the Wechsler Adult Intelligence Scale—Revised.* San Antonio, TX: The Psychological Corporation.

Wechsler, D. (1989b). *Manual for the Wechsler Preschool and Primary Scale of Intelligence—Revised.* San Antonio, TX: The Psychological Corporation.

Wechsler, D. (1991). *Manual for the Wechsler Intelligence Scale for Children—Third Edition.* San Antonio, TX: The Psychological Corporation.

Wechsler, D. (1992). *Wechsler Individual Achievement Test manual.* San Antonio, TX: The Psychological Corporation.

Wells, K. C., & Egan, J. (1988). Social leaning and systems family therapy for childhood oppositional disorder: Comparative treatment outcome. *Comprehensive Psychiatry, 29,* 138–146.

Whitman, T., Burgio, L., & Johnston, M. B. (1984). Cognitive behavioral interventions with mentally retarded children. In A. W. Meyers & W. E. Craighead (Eds.), *Cogntive behavior therapy with children* (pp. 193–227). New York: Plenum Press.

Witmer, L. (1896). The common interest of child psychology and pediatrics. *Pediatrics, 2,* 390.

Woodcock, R. W. (1977). *Woodcock-Johnson Psycho-Educational Battery: Technical report.* Allen, TX: DLM Teaching Resources.

Wright, L. (1967). The pediatric psychologist: A role model. *American Psychologist, 22,* 323–325.

FOR FURTHER READING

Bellack, A. S., & Hersen, M. (1977). *Behavior modification: An introductory textboo*k. Baltimore, MD: Williams & Wilkins.

Petersen, L., & Harbeck, C. (1988). *The pediatric psychologist: Issues in professional development and practice.* Champaign, IL: Research Press.

Reynolds C., & Kamphaus, R. (Eds.). (1990). *Handbook of psychological and educational assessment: Intelligence and achievement.* New York: Guilford Press.

Reynolds C., & Kamphaus, R. (Eds.). (1990). *Handbook of psychological and educational assessment: Personality, behavior, and context.* New York: Guilford Press.

Roberts, M. (1995). *Handbook of pediatric psychology* (2nd ed.). New York: Guilford Press.

Sattler, J. M. (1992). *Assessment of children* (revised and updated ed.). San Diego, CA: Author.

CHAPTER 10

TREATMENT RESISTANCE

Salvatore Cullari

INTRODUCTION

The concept of treatment resistance has been around for thousands of years and probably extends back to the earliest human attempts at healing. In looking at medical care throughout the centuries, we see that a number of practicing physicians have described patients who either actively or passively disregarded their advice. Of course, given the poor efficacy of medical treatment before the twentieth century and the fact that the cure was often more lethal than the ailment, innumerable people were probably better off being resistive.

From a rational point of view, treatment resistance does not make much sense. Spending a lot of time and money in order to improve a medical or psychological condition and then not cooperating seems totally inconsistent with logic. However, this concept appears to be recognized universally, and healers of all types have attempted to minimize its effects. In both scientific and folk medicine it is indisputable that virtually all practitioners have understood and used the power of expectation, persuasion, and status to help maximize cooperation and treatment compliance.

Treatment resistance appears to be a complex process involving many diverse factors. For example, from an evolutionary and biological perspective, all species seem to have two predisposing and conflicting properties. The first is a propensity toward change. Through maturity and exposure to different environmental stimuli, we are constantly reaching new levels of development. Both mentally and biologically, we are never exactly the same person we were the day before. On the other hand, we also appear to have a drive or inclination to remain the same. Depending on the environment, either of these drives may promote or hamper survival. When long-term conditions are harmonious and remain fairly stable, organisms that are relatively unchanging are favored. In a rapidly changing environment, however, those that are steadfast are not likely to survive. The notorious dinosaurs may serve as an example of both of these extremes. For millions of years, they reigned supreme on earth, but they disappeared when swiftly changing environmental conditions overtaxed their capability to change.

In a different context, these two conflicting forces appear to be the backbone of treatment resistance as well. Resistance may be seen as the outcome of conflicts or ambivalence associated with simultaneous attempts at self-transformation and self-preservation. Very simply, treatment resistance can be defined as any factor that prevents or delays therapeutic change. It may be construed as similar to a governor that prevents changes from being made too quickly or too extensively. After all, change is always associated with something unfamiliar, and the unknown is often frightening. Following this viewpoint, resistance should be seen as a healthy adaptive function that needs to be understood rather than an enemy that needs to be defeated. In addition, as many writers have pointed out, resistance should be considered a useful form of communication to the therapist and perhaps to clients themselves.

SIGMUND FREUD

In terms of psychotherapy, Sigmund Freud was the first to formally explore the notion of treatment resistance. His initial thoughts about this concept were formed through his work with Fraülein Elisabeth Von R. (Freud, 1895/1955), whose symptoms included unexplained chronic pain in her legs that made it difficult to walk. Freud started treating this young woman in 1892 while he was still refining the method of free association. The prepsychoanalytic approach he used with Elisabeth was called the "pressure technique." It involved pressing his hands on her forehead and having her report any images or ideas that came to her mind. He found that at times Elisabeth said she was not able to come up with anything, although her facial expressions suggested otherwise. Further, when Freud insisted that she share what she was thinking, or repeated the process, she inevitably did have something to report. From these seemingly inconspicuous observations, Freud began to develop his theory of resistance, which later became the cornerstone of psychoanalytic theory.

Freud's concept of resistance is inseparably linked to his notion of repression. According to psychoanalytic theory, repression is an unconscious ego defense mechanism that blocks or diverts highly threatening or anxiety-producing ideas, insights, urges, images, or affect from conscious awareness. Once this material is repressed into the unconscious, a strong counterforce is set up that prevents it from becoming conscious again. This counterforce results in resistance. As Freud (1895/1955) stated: "Thus a psychical force . . . had originally driven the pathogenic idea out of association and was now opposing its return to memory" (p. 269).

The notion of repression is similar in some ways to that of the "fight-or-flight" response. For example, we defend ourselves from physical harm by fighting or fleeing from whatever danger confronts us. In an analogous manner, the ego automatically defends itself from emotional threats by driving pathogenic ideas out of conscious awareness. This includes anything that arouses shame or intense fear, or that is unbearable to think about. Although the threatening material itself in a sense disappears, the emotional energy associated with it remains in the unconscious and demands some expression. Thus, a great deal of energy must be expended to keep everything under control, and this is why eventually these conflicts must be addressed. However, we are not consciously aware of any of these operations.

Freud saw resistance and repression forming two of the three major components of neurotic disorders. The third entailed the symptoms themselves. Freud came to his conclusions about the origins of neurotic symptoms while working with patients with hysteria. Now called a conversion disorder, this condition results in physical symptoms that appear without any known physiological cause. According to the theory, symptoms, which are fully conscious to the individual, are symbols or substitutes for the repressed pathogenic ideas. As long as the symptoms are present, the repressed material can be avoided and anxiety is minimized. This results in an adaptive, though dysfunctional, solution to the dilemma.

Typically, there is not a one-to-one correspondence between pathogenic ideas and symptoms. For example, in one of Freud's famous cases, he speculated that the symptom of uncontrollable hand jerking was related to three repressed childhood memories: being struck in the hand by a schoolteacher, being startled while playing the piano, and being forced to message the back of an uncle whom the patient greatly feared. With repeated cases such as these, Freud came up with a revolutionary notion: that a mental activity can at times be converted into a physical symptom.

To complete the circle, if the repressed ideas can be made conscious, the symptoms may disappear. However, the counterforce of resistance attempts to prevent this and therefore blocks therapeutic progress. From an unconscious point of view, the ego views recovery as dangerous and perhaps as a threat to its very existence. Although the symptoms themselves may be very uncomfortable, they pale in comparison to the dread associated with the repressed material. In a sense, the ego chooses the lesser of the two evils. In this case, the drive behind resistance is protection.

Although Freud continued to make revisions on his theory of resistance throughout his lifetime, his most influential ideas are presented in the 1926 work entitled *Inhibitions, Symptoms and Anxiety* (Freud, 1926/1959). Here Freud outlined five types of unconscious resistance, each originating from the id, ego, or superego (see Table 10.1). The first of these, *repression resistance*, has already been described. In sum, on a conscious level, the client would like to get better, but the ego instinctively clings to its protective function.

The second type is called *transference resistance*. Here, the perceptions that the patient has about the therapist or others are determined by previously significant interpersonal interactions. For example, since the therapist is customarily an authority figure, patients may unconsciously respond to this person in a manner shaped by early experiences with their parents. The basic idea behind transference is that we bring to new relationships the same emotions, fears, wishes, and anxieties that have been shaped in previous ones. However, this transference is unconscious and, of course, may be inappropriate in the new circumstance.

Freud spent a great deal of time discussing transference in his writings because he felt it was one of the most important elements of psychotherapy. He believed that the significant aspects of transference that are played out in therapy mirror the specific conflicts that undermine the patient's neurotic symptoms. For example, in his first introduction of transference resistance (1895/1955, p. 302), Freud illustrated a case of a female patient whose hysterical symptoms stemmed from an incident she had experienced as a child. While talking with an older man, this young girl secretly wished that he would take hold of her and kiss her. She did not initially remember this experience in therapy because it had been repressed. During analysis, however, she had the same impulse about Freud and the same frightened affect associated with it. According to Freud, this had the effect of emotionally immobilizing her. Once these thoughts and feelings were uncovered and worked through, however, they were able to make progress again. Thus, Freud concluded that the operations of both transference and resistance may serve as markers for topics that should be fully explored and worked through in therapy.

In the same publication, Freud described circumstances in which transference resistance is most

Table 10.1 Freud's Primary Types of Unconscious Resistance

TYPE	ORIGIN	EXAMPLE
Repression	Ego	Patient's ego blocks repressed thoughts and emotions from conscious awareness.
Transference	Ego	Behaviors and emotions directed at the therapist are based on patient's previous interpersonal relationships.
Secondary gain	Ego	Patient derives indirect benefits from symptoms by being able to avoid or escape major responsibilities.
Id	Id	Patient refuses to give up childish impulses or behaviors such as extreme self-centeredness or wanting immediate gratification.
Superego	Superego	Patient has an unconscious need for self-punishment that prevents any therapeutic improvement.

likely to occur. These include situations in which patients feel neglected or insulted, feel they are becoming too dependent on the therapist, or become aware of strong feelings toward the analyst. As an example, patients who have been abused or neglected by their parents may be prime candidates for transference resistance because of the mixed approach–avoidance feelings and expectations that they have toward caregivers, which may then be transferred to the therapist.

The third type of resistance described by Freud is now called *epinosic* or *secondary gain*. These are the added benefits that accompany the sick role, such as the ability to escape work, school, or other interpersonal responsibilities. In this case, making a recovery means losing these advantages. This type of resistance also includes what is sometimes called *compensation neurosis*. For example, a patient may demonstrate epinosic resistance if he is receiving disability or workmen's compensation. Note that this is not the same as malingering, in which individuals are faking a psychological disorder.

The fourth type of resistance is called *id resistance*. This relates to childish wishes and needs that might interfere with treatment. These include being dependent on the therapist or others, being self-centered and demanding immediate gratification, making unreasonable demands, or refusing to experience the pain or frustration that usually accompanies successful therapy.

The last type of resistance is called *superego resistance* and, according to Freud, may be the most difficult to recognize. Here the individual unconsciously refuses to get better because of guilt feelings or a need for punishment; such a patient may seem to take one step forward and two steps back. In a sense, some patients feel most gratified when they are miserable.

FREUD'S CONTEMPORARIES

Many of Freud's original ideas about resistance have survived almost intact to this day, but his followers have made some important adjustments to his theory. For example, Edward Glover (1955) clarified the idea of *obvious* versus *unobtrusive*

types of resistance. The obvious type includes behaviors that are overt and easy to identify—for example, overt silence, skipping therapy sessions, or dropping out completely. The unobtrusive type may be more difficult to recognize because it is subtle and often hidden under a facade of compliance and cooperation. Unobtrusive resistance frequently becomes more obvious when a long period of time has elapsed and the client has not made any progress.

Aside from Freud, Ralph Greenson (1967) has written more about resistance than any other psychoanalyst. One of the notions he explored was that of *screen defenses*. Here the client will recall certain material (e.g., screen memories) that averts other more painful recollections. For example, a client may remember that her brother committed suicide when she was a teenager, but not that he did so after they were caught having sexual intercourse.

Another concept that Greenson investigated was the distinction between *ego-alien* and *ego-syntonic* resistance. Ego-alien resistance results in thoughts or behaviors that are out of character for clients and are typically recognized as being illogical. Because the individual tends to be consciously aware of these, they are usually easy to work through. On the other hand, ego-syntonic resistant behaviors appear to be rational and useful to clients even when they are not. For example, a patient may find it difficult to form a trusting relationship with anyone, but may not recognize this as a problem. Similar to Wilhelm Reich's idea of character resistance, these idiosyncrasies represent long-established habitual patterns of protective thoughts or behaviors. Because clients do not recognize the defensive aspect of these motives, they are easily rationalized and thus very difficult to address.

A number of other modifications to Freud's theory of resistance have been made over the years. These are summarized by Sandler, Holder, and Dare (1970; see also Sandler, Dare, & Holder, 1973). To Freud's original five categories, they add the following:

1. Resistance related to therapeutic changes that may disrupt a patient's important relationships. For example, a housewife may avoid

becoming more assertive because doing so might jeopardize her marriage.

2. Resistance due to the potential loss of the therapist when the client leaves therapy. This is especially strong when the client and therapist have developed a strong therapeutic relationship, or when the client lacks strong relationships in the outside world.

3. Resistance related to threats to the client's self-esteem. For example, a patient may avoid some topics because of feelings of shame. This is related to superego resistance.

4. Resistance that results from the therapist's use of faulty procedures or inappropriate treatment methods. This is often an adaptive type of resistance. For example, a client may be noncompliant if she feels the therapist is incompetent.

5. Resistance due to strong traits and characteristics that form the core structure of the individual's personality. This is sometimes called *character resistance* and results from clients' defensive coping strategies that have become fixed behavior patterns through their lifetime. For example, an individual may be chronically offensive in order to avoid close interpersonal relationships. Clients typically do not recognize their qualities as offensive, and thus this type of resistance may be among the most difficult to overcome. It appears that many of these types of character resistances relate to interpersonal processes and may be detected or understood through the client–therapist relationship.

As further modifications in psychoanalytic theory were made, resistance was seen less as a total intrapsychic biological force and more as an interpersonal and social phenomenon. This change paralleled the movement in psychoanalysis from an almost complete emphasis on the id and instinctual drives to the equally important role of the ego. Leading this transition was Heinz Hartmann (1958). Although he died in 1970, his ideas about resistance are remarkably current. For example, he suggested that individuals can never be totally separated from their social contexts. In this case, the

person's ethnic or economic background may determine what resistances are brought to therapy and how they are expressed. Along the same lines, he suggested that each person's resistive patterns are unique and thus therapists must match their treatment styles to the characteristics of the individual. This sounds very similar to the current notion of eclecticism.

In addition to the individuals already cited, other psychoanalytic writers addressing the concept of resistance include Karl Menninger (1973), Robert Langs (1981), Reuben Fine (1982), Roy Schafer (1983), Herbert Strean (1990), and Martha Stark (1994). The interested reader is referred to these references and to the recommended reading list at the end of the chapter for further information.

NONPSYCHOANALYTIC APPROACHES TO RESISTANCE

Nonpsychoanalytic approaches to psychotherapy have not emphasized the importance of resistance as much as Freud and his followers have. There are several reasons for this. One is a general backlash against Freud and his theory on the grounds that it is speculative and unscientific. In this case, the central role of resistance in psychoanalysis made it a frequent target for critics. A second reason for the discounted role of resistance is the importance afforded to the function of free will, which complemented the rise of phenomenological theories. Generally speaking, the ideas of resistance and free will are incompatible. A third factor is the diminishing importance of the role of the unconscious and intrapsychic conflicts in understanding human behavior. In the traditional psychoanalytic view of resistance, it is construed as being both intrapsychic and unconscious.

Despite these trends, the topic of resistance has enjoyed a rebirth recently, and many orientations are giving it much more consideration. The following section briefly explores the topic of resistance in relation to nonpsychoanalytic theories.

Phenomenological Approaches

Carl Rogers did not discuss the issue of resistance to any great extent. In general, he saw it as a mechanism for clients to protect their self-concept, and believed it is often expressed through an unwillingness to self-disclose. For example, in the early stages of therapy, many clients attempt to maintain their distorted ideal self-image through avoidance of their "real" self. By minimizing self-disclosures, experiences that are incongruent with their inflexible ideal self-concept can be averted. In this respect, Rogers suggested that resistance may result when therapists attempt to make changes too quickly or force clients to open up too soon. In general, Rogers maintained that through the use of appropriate client-centered therapeutic techniques, resistance can be greatly reduced or prevented.

Existentialists such as Rollo May and J. F. T. Bugental hold an analogous view and suggest that resistive behaviors help clients control the pace of therapy and postpone experiencing certain types or intensities of emotions. Similar to Rogers, Bugental notes that resistance represents a client's fear of meeting his or her own real or authentic self. In this sense, clients are often in the classical approach–avoidance conflict of wanting to change while at the same time galvanized to avoid change. As in psychoanalytic theory, Bugental maintains that the resistive behaviors clients display in therapy mirror the neurotic processes that dominate their lives. He also notes, however, that simple cognitive insights are not sufficient to make any real or lasting changes in clients. He maintains that significant awareness of the resistance must be directly and fully experienced.

Fritz Perls and other early Gestalt theorists initially saw resistance much as Freud did. In effect, they agreed that its general purpose was self-protection. Eventually, however, Perls modified his view and concluded that human behavior is the outcome of self-regulation and balance rather than conflicts. He believed that neurotic reactions result from the loss of both internal and external awareness, which in turn disturbs the process of self-regulation. In this model, resistance is seen as an outcome of initially accommodating personality structures that are used to block threatening aspects of the self or environment from awareness. Later, however, these may harden into fixed patterns of neurotic behaviors. For example, a person's chronic denial of anger may lead to a problematic level of nonassertiveness. Nonetheless, this "resistance to awareness" is considered to be an adaptive function rather than an adversary. In other words, if a client is being resistive, there must be a good reason for it, at least from the client's unconscious point of view.

Perls believes that both symptoms and resistance operate to help clients achieve some goal for which they lack any alternative methods. In this case, one of the functions of therapy should be to help individuals become aware of why they need their resistance. One way of doing this is to help clients try out new behaviors or experience avoided aspects of their personality within the confines of a safe therapeutic environment (Breshgold, 1989). Ultimately, Gestalt therapy requires that clients experience the painful feelings or awareness they have so actively avoided. According to Gestalt theory, this is the only way that closure and eventual healing can occur. As Breshgold describes it, "destruction of an old figure is required for the emergence of a new one" (1989, p. 86). The ultimate goal of Gestalt therapy is the integration of every part of oneself, including those that we fail to recognize.

Collectively, proponents of phenomenology do not see resistance as a strong impediment to therapy. In fact, in many ways the term *resistance* is incompatible with the basic tenets of these orientations. For example, the label of resistance denies the client's perception of reality and replaces it with the value judgments of the therapist. In addition, the concept of resistance implies something that occurs in isolation, which is inconsistent with the idea of a dynamic, interrelated social and living environment. In other words, rather than coming out of the blue, resistance is a healthy protective function that clients need, at least at that point in time. Similarly, concordant with the notion of free will, resistance is seen as an option rather than an uncontrollable compulsion. Therefore, the general rule is to work with it rather than against it.

Behaviorism

In the past, behaviorists have not dealt extensively with the notion of resistance, for several reasons. First, the treatment focus tends to be on environmental rather than intrapsychic factors. For this reason, interventions may not be done directly with clients, and thus there may not be direct exposure to resistance. Second, behaviorists generally do not endorse concepts such as the unconscious or repression, which are the backbone of the traditional view of resistance. Nevertheless, as behaviorists (at least those in private practice) have moved away from strictly operant procedures to a more cognitive and eclectic stance, they have written a great deal more about this subject. For example, some behavior therapists consider resistance to be either noncompliance with treatment methods (e.g., Shelton & Levy, 1981) or a result of the inability of the therapist to design an effective treatment program. Speaking of the latter, Lazarus and Fay (1982) suggest that "The concept of 'resistance' is probably the most elaborate rationalization that therapists employ to explain their treatment failures" (p. 115). They suggest (p. 120) that seven factors are responsible for most treatment nonsuccess:

1. There is inappropriate therapist–patient matching or lack of rapport.
2. The therapist fails to conduct an accurate assessment.
3. The therapist fails to deal with the client's social network.
4. The therapist uses incorrect techniques.
5. The therapist lacks training, is inexperienced, or uses appropriate techniques incorrectly.
6. The client has extreme biological or psychological deficits.
7. The desired outcome is not valued by the patient.

In general, they conclude that if the client is not getting better, it is largely (though not entirely) the therapist's fault.

Another view of resistance that many behaviorally oriented therapists endorse is succinctly summarized by Munjack and Oriel (1978). They divide resistance into five distinct types. In Type I, the patient lacks an understanding of the purpose of the intervention or how to carry it out. This would include clients who are unsophisticated or concrete thinkers. In this case, the therapist should be careful to explain his or her expectations on a level that the client can understand.

Type II resistance results from skill deficits. An example would be a person who does not comply with a homework assignment because of poor reading ability, or a person who lacks certain interpersonal skills.

Type III resistance is characterized by a lack of motivation. Basically, the person does not want to change, does not believe change is necessary, or does not believe he or she has the ability to change.

Type IV resistance results when the therapy makes the client feel overly anxious or guilty. This would include a client's reluctance to discuss embarrassing material.

Type V resistance results from secondary gains or positive reinforcement resulting from the symptoms. These would include insurance or disability payments, additional social attention, the ability to avoid work, and similar outcomes.

As would be expected, behaviorists tend to deal with resistance in a manner consistent with their views of human behavior, which include working with observable and measurable behaviors. They use techniques such as behavioral contracting, reinforcement or response cost, relaxation training, and self-monitoring. Most of these techniques are designed to promote treatment compliance, which will be considered separately in this chapter.

Cognitive Models

Cognitive therapists have viewed resistance in various ways depending on their particular theoretical orientation. For example, Albert Ellis (1985) believes that one of the strongest and most basic types of resistance is low frustration tolerance or what he terms "discomfort anxiety." This involves a basic opposition to change and a desire to maintain the status quo despite the fact that the client's condition may be uncomfortable or very painful (p. 11). Ellis suggests that humans have a general tendency to succumb to the "pleasures of the moment" rather than consider long-term negative effects of their behaviors. Thus, many people fall prey to the meshes of immediate gratification or are unwilling to experience the distress or discomfort associated with change. This is a theme that can be found among many other psychotherapeutic approaches as well. Ellis also points out that therapists can often play a major role in contributing to the client's resistance and therefore need to explore how they influence or may even be the main cause of the client's resistance.

Another theme of resistance in cognitive theory is the idea of a defensive and perpetuating self-system (Liotti, 1987; Mahoney, 1991). The following is a brief explanation of this model.

Through experience, individuals organize perceptions of themselves and the world into cognitive structures called *schemas*. For example, our schema of professors may include the generalization that they are absent-minded, intelligent, liberal, and so on. In our lifetime we form thousands of different schemas. Once these are formed, they are very difficult to change, even if reality suggests they are no longer valid. According to some theorists (e.g., Mahoney, 1991), this stabilizing force may be due to survival-enhancing hereditary factors that are related to our need to understand and predict life experiences. On the other hand, the process of psychotherapy often introduces ideas that are inconsistent with some of these preestablished schemas. This is especially true for those related to the self, which may be the most resistant to change. In this case, an internal drive for cognitive consistency may lead to a rejection of schema-incompatible ideas, which then may be interpreted as resistance. For example, some depressed individuals see themselves as worthless and inept. Although these descriptions typically are not true, people often cling to these inaccurate yet accustomed self-images rather than accepting alternatives. Even if we are not comfortable with our current state of affairs, they are at least predictable and less anxiety-provoking than change.

A third variation of resistance in cognitive theory is the notion of reactance. Originally described by Brehm (1966), *reactance* is an individual's attempt to restore lost or threatened freedom of choice whenever he or she feels others are trying to control him or her. This may occur even when people realize that the advice given is for their own good. In a

therapy setting, reactance may be expressed through noncompliance or possibly by a client's doing the exact opposite of what is prescribed. The difference between this and other cognitive models is that what is being resisted is the influence rather than change itself.

Individuals seem to differ in their sensitivity to reactance. Those with high levels of this attribute may need to be treated with special procedures such as paradoxical techniques (see Dowd & Trutt, 1988). On the other hand, clients who are low on this dimension may benefit more from therapy that is highly structured or directive. Interestingly, some therapists believe reactance may be due to both interpersonal and intrapersonal influences (Arkowitz, 1996). In other words, at times we may react negatively to our own internal directives.

Communication, Strategic, and Systems Theories

The contributors to this large class of orientations are too numerous to list completely. They include Gregory Bateson, Jay Haley, Don Jackson, John Weakland, Milton Erickson, Steve de Shazer, and a multitude of family therapists. Like other multifaceted theories, the concept of resistance within this group varies depending on the particular variation one adopts. In general, however, these theories view reality from a circular rather than a linear (cause-and-effect) perspective. For example, in the traditional linear model, the client is seen as a separate entity who acts and is acted on by the therapist or the environment. In this case, there is a dichotomy between the client and the therapist, which often results in a perception of opposition. Circular reality is distinguished by an interactive model, where there is constant feedback and adjustment between all members of the system. From this viewpoint, resistance does not originate from the client but, rather, from the relationship between client, therapist, and other system components.

Another central concept related to resistance within this philosophy is the idea of homeostasis. This notion is especially pertinent in family therapy and relates to a process that attempts to maintain a system's stability. Any effort to change the system or anything that can cause an imbalance is met with resistance. A similar theme is the idea that resistance is the system's attempt to protect one or all of its members. Because all of the members are interconnected, any change in one person will affect everyone else and thus destabilize the system.

Advocates of these orientations often deal with resistance through the use of paradoxical techniques. One of the advantages of paradoxical techniques is that they allow the therapist to make use of the resistance rather than trying to overcome it. Another advantage is that this approach often changes the perceived reality of the client, which then makes dealing with resistance or the problem behavior much easier.

Haley (1987, pp. 80–84) summarizes the general stages of paradoxical interventions as follows:

1. A working relationship is established that is designed to bring about change.
2. The problem is clearly defined.
3. Exact goals are specified.
4. A plan to deal with the problem is offered.
5. The current authority on the problem is disqualified. By this, Haley means that there is usually someone in the target person's family who is in charge of "curing" the client of the problem, but is probably instrumental in maintaining it. The situation must be set up so this person or the system itself does not become upset when the problem disappears.
6. The paradoxical directive is given.
7. The therapist observes the results and continues to encourage the problem behavior.
8. As the client makes changes and improves, the therapist does not take credit for it. For example, Haley suggests that the therapist should be puzzled by the improvement.

Relabeling, reframing, and symptom prescription are some of the more popular paradoxical techniques. Relabeling and reframing involve changing the meaning of a problem, event, or situation to a more therapeutically useful perspective. For example, a child's disruptive behavior may be relabeled as a means to keep the family together. To be effective, this process must cause the client to see the problem differently than she did before, but in a way that is consistent with her way of thinking or view of the world.

In a similar manner, one of the ways reframing can be used is by finding the positive aspects of a problem. For example, a couple's constant arguments may be reframed as a way to give each other a lot of attention. What seems to make reframing effective is that its aftermath is irreversible. That is, once this technique is used, you cannot easily return to your previous view of the problem.

Symptom prescription involves instructing or encouraging clients to maintain or exaggerate their problem behaviors or symptoms. The advantage of this technique is that if it is successful, clients learn that their symptoms are controllable rather than autonomous. On the other hand, if clients are reactant, they must reduce or eliminate their symptoms in order to go against the therapist. For example, a client might be asked to increase the daily number of "uncontrollable" angry outbursts he has toward his spouse.

A procedure that is similar to symptom prescription is restraining. This is a technique whereby the therapist discourages or prohibits the client from changing or suggests that change occur very slowly. It is an especially useful technique with clients who are highly reactant because the only way to resist the therapist is to change. For example, you might inform clients who have been noncompliant that changing their behaviors will be very difficult and that they may want to proceed even slower than usual.

Although all of these techniques have been found to be very useful with clients who resist change, they should be used only by experienced or specially trained therapists.

Summary

The preceding section has looked at resistance from the perspective of different treatment paradigms. Although resistance appears to be universally conspicuous across all therapy orientations, its perceived meaning and the way it is handled vary greatly, for a number of reasons. One relates to the theoretical differences between the various orientations themselves. For example, it is not unusual that cognitive theories would pay much more attention to resistance manifested by faulty cognitions or that behaviorists would tend to focus on overt compliance or environmental issues. This is what these therapists are trained to do. Similarly, there appear to be various forms of resistance that lend themselves more readily to different orientations. For example, resistance may relate to behaviors, cognitions, or emotions, and different orientations tend to pay more or less attention to each of these factors.

Another reason that various orientations view resistance differently relates to schemas and paradigms. Once we adopt a certain view of the world, our perceptions and memories are very much slanted by that perspective. As Rosenhan (1973) clearly demonstrated in his famous study, we often see what we expect to see. This is true in the therapy room as well. If we believe that resistance develops primarily from repression, we will attend to and recall most vividly those instances that confirm this expectation. In this way, our beliefs about resistance become self-validating and self-perpetuating.

In a similar manner, the specific techniques used in distinct orientations may result in different resistive patterns. For example, the marked neutrality or "blank screen" orientation seen in some psychodynamic procedures may promote transference reactions more than a cognitive-behavioral approach. On the other hand, the greater emphasis placed on homework assignments by behaviorally oriented therapists might make noncompliance much more salient, and nondirective therapists may be less likely to see or elicit reactance. Table 10.2 summarizes the various ways each orientation conceptualizes resistance and how it is generally treated.

AN INTEGRATED MODEL OF RESISTANCE

Although each treatment model deals with resistance in a different manner, several common themes are seen in virtually all of these views. These include the ideas of protection or defensiveness, conflict, ambivalence, and communication. In a similar manner, the behaviors that are typically

Table 10.2 How Different Treatment Orientations View Resistance

ORIENTATION	SOURCE	FUNCTION	MANIFESTED BY:	TREATMENT	IMPORTANCE OF CONCEPT	VIEWED AS:
Psychoanalytic	Intrapsychic conflicts or impulses	Protective	Repression	Insight	Very high	Negative; needs to be overcome
Client-centered	Self-concept	Protective	Lack of self-disclosure	Rogerian techniques	Low	Due to inappropriate pace or treatment techniques
Behavioral	Client, therapist, or environment	Feedback	Non-compliance	Contracting; behavioral techniques	Medium to high	Therapist incompetence; lack of client skills or understanding
Gestalt	Client	Protective	Lack of awareness	Experiential	Low	Incompatible with current theory
Systems	Family or system	Homeostasis	Protection of system or members	Paradoxical techniques	Low	Natural component of change process
Cognitive	Client or therapist	Protection of self-system	Reactance; ambivalence	Paradoxical or cognitive techniques	Medium to high	Natural component of change process
Existential	Client	Protective	Lack of awareness	Self-awareness or none	Low	Legitimate self-expression; generally incompatible with theory

considered to be resistive in nature are fairly common across all orientations. Table 10.3 lists a number of behaviors that may be interpreted as resistive in nature (although their expression may be due to other factors). Although this is not an exhaustive list, it does include the common types of behaviors that many therapists view as resistance. It is important to note, however, that resistance does not necessarily imply inappropriateness and that it does not always emanate exclusively from the client.

All of the treatment orientations described here have contributed greatly to our understanding of resistance. Because of the divergent views of resistance, however, the concept remains ill defined and generally difficult to deal with in a therapeutic setting. The following section is an attempt to integrate the many ideas surrounding resistance into a unified model that may be easier to conceptualize and process. The basic assumptions of this model are as follows:

1. Treatment resistance involves intrapersonal, interpersonal, and extrapersonal factors.

Table 10.3 Common Resistive Behaviors In Psychotherapy

Acting out	Making extra demands on the
Ambivalence	therapist
Antagonism	Missing therapy sessions
Argumentativeness	Noncompliance
Avoidance	Nondisclosure
Blaming others	Not being fully truthful
Blocking	Not paying for therapy
Censoring	sessions
Changing the topic	Not putting any effort into
Constant cynicism	changing
Constantly responding,	Not taking responsibility for
"I don't know"	change
Defensiveness	Passivity
Defiance	Passive-aggressiveness
Demanding	Rigidity (inflexibility)
Discounting	Regression
Disproportionate sense	Reluctance
of entitlement	Sarcasm
Dropping out of therapy	Seductiveness
Evasiveness	Silence
General	Skepticism
uncooperativeness	Symptom substitution
Inappropriate anger/	Talking too little or too much
hostility	Tardiness
Intellectualization	Withdrawing
Limit testing	

2. At the intrapersonal level, it includes both state and trait variables. In other words, resistance may be due to specific temporary occurrences in the treatment session or may be related to more global character traits manifested in the client.

3. Treatment resistance is an important form of communication that has both purpose and meaning.

4. There appear to be some advantages to viewing resistance as a continuous rather than a discrete variable. This means that rather than being either present or nonpresent, resistance varies along a continuum from very low to very high levels. Human behavior is rarely, if ever, entirely one-sided, and this appears to be the case for resistance as well. Accepting resistance as a continuous variable implies that therapists may be willing to work with it instead of trying to defeat it. Further, the argument may be made that, as with anxiety, lower levels of resistance may be more advantageous than a zero level.

5. Treatment resistance includes behavioral, affective, and cognitive components. The behavioral aspect generally involves noncompliance or behaviors that interfere with reaching treatment goals. The cognitive aspect includes ambivalence toward change, resistance to self-awareness, and a reluctance to change core beliefs about the self. These may also include irrational beliefs about the self or others. At the affective level, the individual may attempt to avoid painful memories, feelings, or emotions associated with traumatic events or may fear the change process itself. It is assumed that there is great overlap between these three variables and that at times they may operate virtually simultaneously.

6. The label of treatment resistance always involves a subjective evaluation and judgment. It has been suggested that the classification of treatment resistance be limited to situations where an appropriate diagnosis has been made and effective treatments are used. Although conceptually this is an important distinction, in practice it may be difficult,

if not impossible, to evaluate this realistically, and thus this discrimination may serve no useful purpose. A differentiation also might be considered between treatment resistance and a resistant disorder (e.g., schizophrenia). Again, conceptually, this may be meaningful, but pragmatically it may be difficult to separate the two. The point here is that if one does not accept a pejorative connotation to treatment resistance, the label does not matter much. Ultimately, regardless of what we call the situations described here, they need to be evaluated and addressed. A more inclusive definition of treatment resistance appears to offer the most benefits in terms of treatment effectiveness. Table 10.4 summarizes these points.

In attempting to deal with resistance, it is important to take a proactive rather than a reactive approach. For example, the therapist should try to prevent certain types of resistance from occurring in the first place. This is especially important in this era of managed care and brief forms of therapy because there simply will not be enough time to act on resistance in the traditional manner.

To deal effectively with resistance, it is important to identify its general source. The way we address resistance usually depends on this. At times, the source of the resistance may be connected to the reason that the client is referred for therapy. For example, in certain types of personality disorders, the characteristics of the disturbance itself may be the prime reason for the resistance. At other times, the referral problem and source of resistance are independent.

The origins of resistance fall into three broad categories, although these are not mutually exclusive. In fact, there is likely to be a lot of overlap among them. Likewise, the resistance may be due to more than one primary source. The following section describes these influences in more detail (see Table 10.5).

Intrapersonal Factors

These encompass the conscious and unconscious intrapsychic factors described by Freud and others, such as repression, transference, or a resistance to self-awareness. This category also includes other characteristics that generally stem from the individual, such as values, beliefs, guilt, shame, character traits, or idiosyncratic types of resistance resulting from the client's personality or other established patterns of behavior. For example, reactance would be included in this category, as well as individuals who are chronically defensive, angry, or uncooperative. The client's cultural background or level of acculturation is also a potential source of resistance. Other intrapsychic factors include resistive behaviors resulting from secondary gains or malingering (see Cullari, 1996b, Appendix C, for a discussion of resistance and malingering).

This category also includes various psychological disorders that contribute to resistance in therapy, such as the lack of motivation often seen in major depression or schizophrenia or the interfering aspects of various personality disorders. Similarly, it includes resistance that results from lack of appropriate client skills or other prerequisites for change.

It is important to distinguish between character or trait forms of resistance, which are likely to be repeated throughout therapy, and the state or transient forms of resistance that may occur in response to a particular stimulus. For example, a client may find a particular topic extremely painful or may be more resistive during a particular stage of therapy. Of course, there may be a positive correlation between the occurrences of state and trait types of resistance, but some types of resistance may be due

---

Table 10.4 Basic Assumptions of an Integrative Model of Resistance

1. Treatment resistance involves intrapersonal, interpersonal, and extrapersonal factors.
2. At the intrapersonal level, it includes both state and trait variables.
3. Treatment resistance is an important form of communication that has both purpose and meaning.
4. Treatment resistance should be treated as a continuous rather than discrete variable.
5. Treatment resistance includes behavioral, affective, and cognitive components.
6. Treatment resistance always involves a subjective evaluation and judgment.
7. Therapists should take a proactive rather than a reactive approach to dealing with resistance.

Table 10.5 Potential Sources of Resistance in Psychotherapy

I. Intrapersonal factors:
    a. Repression or suppression
    b. Reactance
    c. Transference
    d. Resistance to self-awareness
    e. Guilt, shame, or denial
    f. Personality traits or established patterns of behavior
    g. Strong habits or values
    h. Secondary gains or malingering
    i. Client's skill level or other prerequisites for change
    j. Psychological disorders
    k. State characteristics
    l. Client's cultural background or level of acculturation

II. Interpersonal factors:
    a. Client–therapist relationship
    b. Client's social system
    c. Client's interpersonal coping styles

    d. Countertransference
    e. Incompatibility between client's current stage of change and treatment interventions
    f. Cultural or racial differences between client and therapist

III. Extrapersonal factors:
    a. Characteristics of the therapist, such as personality, training, experience, or treatment orientation
    b. Misdiagnosis or ineffective interventions
    c. Treatment-setting variables such as behavior of support staff, scheduling, or distance to office
    d. Factors related to insurance, managed care, or cost of therapy
    e. Environmental factors such as a lack of resources (e.g., financial, transportation, baby sitting), living in poverty, chronic effects of racism or other aversive societal influences on the client

primarily to the client's or therapist's having an off day or other temporal factors in each person's environment.

Interpersonal Factors

A prime example of this category involves the relationship between the client and the therapist. In other words, resistance may be due to an incompatibility between the two or may simply be the outcome of this social exchange. The effects of countertransference are included here as well. In addition, this category includes resistance that results from the function of outside social systems, such as families or friends, and issues such as co-dependency. Likewise, it includes the interpersonal coping styles or patterns the client uses with others, which may or may not be the target of the therapy.

At a different level, this category also includes resistive behaviors related to the incompatibility between the client's current stage of change and treatment interventions. Recently, there has been a great deal of interest in matching treatment interventions with the client's prevailing stage of change (see Prochaska & DiClemente, 1986).

At times, clients coming from different cultures or ethnic groups may be perceived to be resistive when in fact much of their behavior may be the result of techniques that they do not understand or that are inconsistent with their view of the world.

For example, some cultures have great difficulty with the concept of a "talking cure," which is the basis of Western psychotherapy. To reduce this type of resistance, clinicians should try to learn as much as they can about different cultures before initiating psychotherapy and should modify their treatment strategies accordingly (see Chapter 15).

Extrapersonal Factors

This category includes various characteristics of the therapist, such as training, experience, treatment orientation, bias, values, social skills, and other personality factors. It also includes resistance resulting from a misdiagnosis or ineffective treatment interventions. Likewise, it includes resistance that results from the therapist's choice of intervention, as well as procedural factors such as intrusiveness. Of course, there is likely to be a lot of overlap between this category and interpersonal sources.

In some cases, resistance may be due to nontreatment variables such as insurance, managed care, cost of therapy, distance to the office, behavior of support staff, scheduling, and similar factors. Environmental factors such as a lack of resources (e.g., money, transportation, child care), living in poverty, chronic effects of racism, or other aversive societal influences on the client should also be considered.

FUNCTION AND AWARENESS OF RESISTANCE

With resistance that is primarily intrapsychic in nature, it is useful to identify the general function of the resistance. To some extent, intrapsychic resistance is always adaptive in nature and represents the individual's best attempt to deal with a difficult situation as best as he can. Therefore, it is very useful for the therapist to gain an idea of why clients need their resistance. Often it involves wanting to avoid something negative or not wanting to give up something positive or safe (at least from the client's perspective). For example, resistance may represent an attempt to avoid painful memories or emotions or the hard work that usually accompanies meaningful change. In a similar manner, its purpose may be to maintain a familiar, though dysfunctional, lifestyle. For instance, the client may not want to give up the immediate gratification associated with drugs, alcohol, or other addictive behaviors. At times, the client may not know what the function of the resistance is or may not want to share it, but it is often helpful to assess this. In addition, it is advantageous to see how the treatment resistance fits in with the client's overall personality or lifestyle. Often there are important overlaps in these areas that may be utilized in developing treatment interventions.

Another important piece of information is an estimation of the client's level of awareness of the resistance. Contrary to the psychoanalytic point of view, the assumption here is that awareness of resistance varies between the two extremes of total awareness and total lack of awareness. In this case, it may occur at the unconscious level, or, at the other extreme, clients may be fully aware of their resistance. However, as with other attributes falling within the normal curve, it is likely that most cases will turn out somewhere in between.

Once therapists assess the origin, function, and awareness of the resistance, they will be in a better position to design a strategy to address it. Consistent with the general theme of this book, it is recommended that resistance be mediated with an integrative therapeutic approach that is matched to a particular client's need. Although it is beyond the scope of this chapter to address the treatment of resistance in length, the following example will serve as a case in point. In addition, the next section will address the frequently encountered behavioral aspects of resistance.

Case Illustration

The following example of resistance is based on a true case, although some of the details have been changed for confidentiality and illustrative purposes. It demonstrates the complexity of resistance as well as the importance of seeking its source. It is also illustrates the concept of transference and the importance of a strong therapeutic relationship.

A 20-year-old married female was referred for therapy because of depression and drug abuse. In addition to the aforementioned conditions, she presented with a mixed diagnostic picture including symptoms of anxiety, a personality disorder, an eating disorder, and a possible dissociative disorder. Compounding her problems were chronic feelings of low self-esteem.

The client had been abusing drugs for a number of years. Both of her parents were alcoholics, and she grew up in a chaotic environment. She denied being sexually or physically abused while growing up, but she was often neglected. Despite her history, she described her childhood as "normal." However, when she was a teenager, her father would often bring home pornographic videotapes and they would sit together in the living room and watch them. She did not see anything in particular wrong with this behavior and reacted almost as if it were a normal family activity. It was apparent that her mother was often absent or incapacitated and that she was dependent on her father for her emotional needs.

During the initial therapy sessions, she was withdrawn, guarded, and emotionally flat, but often seductive. Although she was superficially cooperative, very little progress was being made. It was evident that she was trying to detach herself from her feelings. She hardly ever spoke about her husband or mother, and it appeared that her father was still the center point of her life.

The roots of her resistance seemed to involve

Case Illustration *Continued*

both intrapersonal and interpersonal factors. Her seductive behaviors were obvious attempts to manipulate the therapist and the therapy session. Observations outside of the therapy sessions indicated that this was a typical strategy that she used in her interactions with others as well. It was also clear that she was actively avoiding some topic areas and was trying to sidestep the treatment process in general.

Although the therapist held a cognitive-behavioral orientation, he decided to largely use a Gestalt approach with this client, including extensive use of the "empty chair" technique. Through this process, she gradually became aware of some intense feelings of unexpressed anger she had toward her mother and of many unresolved issues. She also became less defensive and began accepting more responsibility for her actions.

During the fourth session, she admitted to prostituting herself in order to get money for drugs. Nevertheless, she said that she did not do this on a "regular" basis. Her husband, who also abused drugs, was aware of the situation and though verbally disapproving, allowed it to continue. While engaging in prostitution, she took on the persona of someone she called Joni (pronounced "Johnny"). She claimed that she was able to

change her "personality" at will and was consciously aware of these "alters." However, she did not fit the classic pattern of a multiple personality disorder, and no dissociative episodes were observed during therapy.

During subsequent sessions, progress was slow. Nevertheless, as her self-awareness increased and the therapeutic relationship began to develop further, she became more trusting and disclosing. Finally, during the tenth session, she casually announced that Joni had had sexual intercourse with her father about two months before initiating therapy. She reported that this was the first time that this had occurred, but it was not entirely clear who had initiated the encounter. She initially described the details of this incident in a matter-of-fact way, without any emotional involvement. Her father, who was also aware of her prostitution, gave her $50 afterwards.

The next few sessions proved to be the turning point of her therapy. She was gradually able to make a connection with her feelings and at one point cried almost the entire session. She also approached therapy with an entirely new attitude. Gradually, she was able to make significant progress with all of her symptoms and she left treatment in a very much improved condition.

TREATMENT ADHERENCE

Treatment adherence covers a broad collection of behaviors, including attending therapy on a regular basis, cooperating with the treatment process, taking prescribed medications, completing "homework" assignments, not engaging in self-destructive behaviors, and many others. Although the words *adherence* and *compliance* are often used interchangeably, some writers maintain that *compliance* indicates a passive role on the part of the client and prefer to use the term *adherence,* which suggests a more active cooperation between client and therapist. This convention will be generally used in this section.

It is important to note that the main reason we want clients to adhere to treatment programs is to

improve their condition. This assumes that the interventions we propose will be effective, which is not always the case. As Achterberg-Lawlis (1982) and Davidson (1982) have suggested, perhaps we are putting the cart before the horse by developing compliance technologies before perfecting treatment regimes. Although it is clear that clients need to adhere to treatment regimes in order to improve, it is also important to note that therapists have an ethical obligation to provide interventions that have the best chance for success.

Previous research suggests that adherence tends to decrease in the later stages of therapy, especially when progress is slow. This highlights the importance of early treatment successes and the benefits of keeping therapy brief when possible. It also appears that clients are more likely to comply when they are required to learn new behaviors as opposed to changing old ones. For example, in treating an eating disorder, it may be easier to get clients to use a new exercise program as opposed to changing their established eating habits. Correspondingly, clients are least likely to adhere to programs that attempt to eliminate entrenched behavior patterns or habits such as smoking or substance abuse. In addition, clients are less likely to adhere to a treatment program when they have a chronic rather than an acute condition or when the benefits of the intervention are not immediately obvious to them. An example of the latter is a prevention program or an intervention that requires an extended period of time.

As with resistance, it is best to view adherence as a continuous rather than a discrete variable, as it can vary from complete lack of cooperation to near full cooperation. Correspondingly, adherence may fluctuate widely during the course of therapy. In this regard, it is useful to view adherence as an active, ongoing process rather than a static one. Like resistance, adherence is a complex phenomenon that involves a number of interrelated variables that often change over time, and thus it needs to be assessed and addressed continuously.

It is important to differentiate facilitating of adherence from reducing nonadherence. Each may have different causes and operate independently from the other. For example, not knowing how to carry out the treatment program usually leads to nonadherence, but complete understanding of the program does not necessarily lead to compliance. In this case, the two may need to be addressed separately, and a different intervention may be needed for each. In addition, adherence behaviors are multidimensional in the sense that clients may adhere to some parts of the treatment program but not to others. It is rare to find a client who is totally cooperative or totally uncooperative with every step of the intervention. Often, clients adhere to programs just enough to maintain some comfort or discomfort level that they can accept.

In a related manner, a distinction should be made between intentional and nonintentional nonadherence. In the latter, clients may want to cooperate but may not be able to for reasons that are largely beyond their control. For example, they may not understand what they are supposed to do, or they may lack necessary prerequisite skills or may have psychological conditions that prevent them from carrying out the treatment program. In intentional nonadherence, clients do understand the program and have the skills for completing it, but they do not do so for reasons that are largely voluntary in nature. These include factors such as secondary gains, projecting blame elsewhere, or not really wanting to change.

For nonadherence, it is also important to distinguish between clients who resist some aspect of the intervention as opposed to other treatment conditions. DiMatteo and DiNicola (1982) label these two categories the *process* and *content* of influence. The content portion of influence generally includes factors that are related to the intervention, whereas the process type includes variables such as qualities of the therapist or the client–therapist relationship. For example, a treatment plan that is too difficult to carry out would be related to content, whereas reactance would be related to process. Clients who react negatively to content may remain in therapy but not make any gains because of nonadherence. By contrast, clients who have difficulty with the process of therapy are more likely to skip treatment sessions or drop out.

It is obvious that there is potentially a great deal of overlap between treatment resistance and nonadherence. In fact, some therapists see the two as being essentially equivalent. Many behaviorists believe that nonadherence is due to either ineffectual treatment plans or other observable factors that can be manipulated and controlled. Indeed, they see the term *resistance* as unnecessary because it does not offer any additional explanatory advantages over *nonadherence*. However, not everyone agrees with this conclusion. As we have already seen, the psychoanalytic notion of resistance contends that it is largely unconscious and involuntary. Here, an analogy is that nonadherence functions in similar fashion to a fever that is due to an underlying infection (which represents the resistance). In this case, resistance may be expressed through nonadherence, but it may be expressed in other ways as well. For example, a client may express resistance by being overly compliant. According to this theory, dealing simply with the overt features of nonadherence would have little effect on the fundamental causes of resistance. Unfortunately, most treatment orientations have not addressed this question to any great extent, and thus there is no general consensus in the field.

There is no simple or satisfactory answer to the relationship between resistance and noncompliance because the answer depends on how one defines each of these constructs. If one accepts the broadest possible definition of both nonadherence and resistance, then the two may in essence overlap entirely. However, there appear to be both theoretical and practical advantages to maintaining a distinction between the two. From a theoretical perspective, it is not clear that the two are in fact equivalent. Although strong empirical evidence is lacking, many clinical signs point in the direction of two distinct entities. From a practical orientation, it is possible and perhaps even common for a client to adhere to a treatment program yet be resistive (or vice versa). For example, an individual might comply fully with interventions for depression yet fail to report a substance abuse problem. A possible compromise is to use the term *resistance* when describing the overall process of therapy and *nonadherence* when dealing with specific procedures or interventions. Although this may not be a perfect solution, it appears to be a viable alternative for the present time.

Assessing Adherence and Nonadherence

There are a number of ways to measure treatment adherence (DiMatteo & DiNicola, 1982; Masek, 1982; Meichenbaum & Turk, 1987). The most commonly used methods are self-reports, self-monitoring, therapist or clinical ratings, biochemical indicators (such as blood tests for lithium, antiseizure, or other medications), record of broken appointments, direct observation, and clinical outcome. Each of these methods has various drawbacks. For example, self-reports or self-monitoring may be inaccurate or unreliable because of poor memory or

imprecise measurement, or because the client may not be telling the truth.

Dunbar (1979) points out that clients tend to underreport poor adherence and overreport good compliance. She suggests that the therapist should create an accepting and nonthreatening atmosphere for reporting nonadherence. She emphasizes that it is important to tell clients what behaviors should be monitored and to provide training when necessary. In addition, any recommended recording materials should be easy to use.

The use of clinical outcome measures to assess adherence appears logical, but this falsely assumes a direct relationship between treatment adherence and improvement. This process may be inadequate because the intervention may not be effective or because generalization did not occur. Similarly, some clients improve despite being nonadherent, and others do not improve even though they follow the program religiously. Overall, using outcome as an indication of adherence appears to be unreliable.

Other methods of measuring adherence also have some drawbacks. Subjective ratings of clients' compliance behaviors by therapists have not been found to be very dependable. It appears that therapists overestimate the amount of compliance by clients and cannot predict accurately when or which clients are compliant. Direct observation may be an option, but it can be time-consuming and is typically not cost-effective. Therefore, despite their own shortcomings, self-report methods and/or direct questioning by the therapist appear to be the most suitable ways to gauge adherence.

Factors Responsible for Adherence and Nonadherence

As discussed previously, there is a great deal of overlap between nonadherence and resistance. In fact, the sources of both are similar and may involve intrapersonal, interpersonal, or extrapersonal factors. Table 10.6 summarizes the major reasons for nonadherence in psychotherapy.

Among the most important intrapsychic reasons for both adherence and nonadherence is the client's *belief system,* a complex variable that involves clients' assumptions and attitudes about themselves,

Table 10.6 Major Factors Associated with Treatment Nonadherence

1. The client misinterprets or does not understand the treatment program, or it is too complex.	16. The client's symptoms are maintained by strong secondary gains and/or he or she feels comfortable maintaining the "sick role."
2. The treatment plan is ineffective and/or the client has multiple problems and the wrong one is being addressed.	17. Clients have progressed to a point where they are uncomfortable with or fear additional change, or do not desire further progress.
3. The client does not like the therapist, or there is a poor client–therapist relationship.	18. The client does not want to change, is not ready for change, or is not convinced that change is important or necessary.
4. The client lacks the required skills or resources to carry out part or all of the plan.	19. The client has an ulterior motive for being in therapy.
5. The client disagrees with the plan or is not satisfied with treatment.	20. The client forgets to use the treatment procedure.
6. The client has nondiagnosed disorders (e.g., drug and alcohol abuse) that interfere with the program.	21. The client has low expectations (self-efficacy) for success or believes treatment goals are unreachable.
7. The client's attitudes or belief system (rational or irrational) interfere with carrying out the program. For example, the client believes in "fate" or expects a "higher power" to take care of the problem.	22. The treatment plan or process is inconsistent with the client's racial, ethnic, or economic background.
8. The client's symptoms or physical and sensory impairments (anxiety, depression, hopelessness, psychosis, problems with memory, etc.) interfere with compliance.	23. The treatment plan interferes with the client's interpersonal relationships. 24. The therapist fails to monitor the treatment plan or gives insufficient feedback.
9. The client's family, environment, or social system interferes with or prevents the individual from adhering to the program.	25. The therapist fails to explain adequately the rationale of the intervention or how it is to be carried out.
10. The client gives in to immediate gratification despite negative long-term consequences.	26. The client has had previous treatment failures or poor experiences in psychotherapy.
11. The client perceives the treatment's "costs" to outweigh its benefits.	27. The treatment causes aversive side effects (e.g., side effects of medications).
12. The treatment plan is too difficult to carry out, too aversive, too time-consuming, or too disruptive to the client's lifestyle.	28. Another family member requires a lot of attention or assistance.
13. Treatment takes much longer than the client expects or desires.	29. The therapist is too demanding or not demanding enough.
14. The client is engaging in self-handicapping behaviors.	30. The client lacks insight or does not fully understand the disorder or its course.
15. The therapist fails to supervise the treatment program properly or make appropriate adjustments to the plan.	31. The therapist has not learned enough about the client to make appropriate recommendations.

their disorder, and the treatment process. A client's belief system comprises the individual's notions about causation, insight and motivation for improvement, self-efficacy and acceptance of the diagnosis, anticipation of success, understanding of what will occur if the disorder is not treated, anticipation of the difficulty of treatment, and perception of having contributed to the treatment process. Obviously, the client already will have established some of these beliefs before beginning therapy. The therapist may be able to modify some of them, but others are likely to be entrenched. It is thus important for the therapist to have a general idea of the beliefs clients bring to therapy and to attempt to tailor the treatment intervention accordingly. Because of the relatively short duration of treatment that is currently in vogue, it also makes sense to use pre-

therapy training or similar procedures. Specific treatment interventions and recommendations associated with client belief systems are reviewed by Cullari (1996b), Meichenbaum and Turk (1987), and Becker and Maiman (1980).

Moving on to interpersonal factors, a significant determinant of treatment adherence is the client's level of satisfaction with treatment (DiMatteo & DiNicola, 1982). Most studies are consistent in showing that clients who are satisfied with the treatment process are more likely to comply with recommendations. Conversely, those who are not satisfied tend to skip therapy sessions or to drop out altogether. The important components that contribute to client satisfaction include the setting, quality, and effectiveness of treatment interventions, and, perhaps most significant, the client–therapist relationship. The latter has been addressed extensively in the psychotherapy literature and thus will be reviewed only briefly in the next section.

Despite the obvious importance of client satisfaction, it is surprising how often it is not addressed by therapists. For example, a recent study by Cullari (1996a) shows that only 20% of psychotherapists conduct client satisfaction surveys with their clients. This is unfortunate because such surveys are relatively easy to carry out and can provide crucial information for the clinician. Measures of client satisfaction usually involve some type of rating scale or face-to-face inquiry. Some considerations for client satisfaction evaluations are to conduct them with every client and to do them early enough in treatment so that appropriate modifications can be made. In addition, open-ended questions should be used, as they have been found to be more reliable and informative than simple rating scales.

Another consequential interpersonal component related to adherence is the client's social system. The many ways that networks can improve adherence are summarized in Table 10.7. Despite the potential usefulness of family and friends, they can also interfere with treatment. For example, they may have their own psychological problems that need attention, or they may not want the client to change for various reasons. Thus, these systems must be evaluated in terms of how they can both help and hinder the therapy process, and the intervention should be modified appropriately when necessary.

Methods for Increasing Adherence in Psychotherapy

The following section briefly describes procedures that can increase the level of adherence in psychotherapy. The assumptions here are that treatment adherence is in the best interest of the client and that the most appropriate and effective interventions have been selected. Of course, the way clinicians approach adherence in therapy is directly linked to their treatment orientation. For example, the concept of adherence is in some ways inconsistent with the theoretical underpinnings of client-centered, existential, or Gestalt theories of treatment. It is therefore not surprising that these orientations have not developed an extensive technology to address it.

On the other hand, adherence is a focal point of behavioral or cognitive-behavioral treatment, and these therapists have developed the most extensive procedures to deal with this potential problem. Nearly all behaviorally oriented therapists believe that the crucial factors associated with adherence relate to antecedents, consequences, and expected consequences. Therefore, the techniques used to increase adherence center around these variables. The following are the most frequently used behavioral techniques to promote adherence: self-monitoring (Dunbar & Agras, 1980), behavioral contracting (Kanfer & Gaelick-Buys, 1991; Litt, Salovey, & Turk 1986), goal setting (Ford, 1992; Meichenbaum & Turk, 1987; Pervin, 1991), self-efficacy

---

Table 10.7 How the Client's Social Network Can Improve Adherence

The client's social network can:
1. be used to reinforce, encourage, or assist the individual in adhering to treatment interventions, and to provide feedback concerning the changes that are being made.
2. contract with the therapist to supervise or in some cases implement the treatment plan (for both adults and children).
3. provide negative feedback to the client for nonadherence.
4. Prompt or remind the client to follow the treatment plan.
5. provide the therapist with information concerning possible factors that may interfere or prevent client adherence.
6. offer the therapist recommendations that may increase adherence or indicate reasons why adherence may be a problem.
7. assist with data collection.
8. make environmental changes that support adherence (buying special supplies or equipment; joining the client in certain activities, etc.).
9. support the client in times of a crisis and act as a buffer to reduce environmental stress.
10. encourage the client to attend therapy and ensure that he or she does not drop out.
11. remind the client to take medications.
12. have positive expectations for treatment effectiveness.
13. provide support services such as transportation or baby-sitting.
14. report relapse or prodromal signs of deterioration.
15. assist with maintenance after treatment is completed.

(Bandura, 1977), reinforcement and response cost (Kanfer & Goldstein, 1991), and relapse prevention (Chiauzzi, 1991; Marlatt & Gordon, 1985).

Along with the behaviorists, communication and strategic theorists and family therapists also have developed an extensive array of paradoxical techniques to deal with adherence, although these are usually described under the heading of resistance. Because these have already been described, they will not be repeated here. The interested reader is referred to Anderson and Stewart (1983), Ascher (1989), Weeks and L'Abate (1982), de Shazer (1988), or Bergman (1985) for more detailed information about these techniques.

Perhaps the factor that influences adherence the most and cuts across all theoretical orientations is the client–therapist relationship. A myriad of complicated factors influence this relationship, but the following seem to be the most important, at least as they relate to adherence:

1. The therapist's general interpersonal skills and ability to put the client at ease

2. Clients' perceptions that they are treated with respect and as individuals

3. Clients' perceptions that they are actively involved in the treatment plan

4. The degree to which clients feel their expectations are being met in therapy or their satisfaction with treatment

5. The therapist's level of enthusiasm and ability to motivate the client

6. The degree to which clients feel that they can trust the therapist

7. Client's perception of the therapist's expertise

8. The therapist's ability to address adequately the potential fears the client brings to therapy

9. The quality and clarity of communication between the client and the therapist

10. Clients' perception of feeling safe and secure and having the ability to self-disclose without repercussions

The client–therapist relationship has been discussed extensively in the literature by a number of writers, including Frank (1961, 1982); Luborsky,

---

Table 10.7 Increasing Adherence in Psychotherapy

1. Each client should be allowed to make significant contributions to the treatment plan.
2. An adherence history should be conducted when appropriate to find out what has been done in the past, what procedures were successful, and what obstacles prevented carrying out previous programs.
3. Clients should be allowed to make choices among alternative procedures whenever possible.
4. Treatment goals should be realistic and match the resources of the client.
5. Brief forms of therapy should be used when possible.
6. When appropriate, the client's social system should be enlisted to help with the treatment intervention.
7. The treatment intervention should be adapted to the client's ethnic or social background.
8. The client should be allowed to play devil's advocate against the intervention in order to get some ideas of potential problems.
9. Clients should reverse roles with the therapist and explain the intervention in their own words to make sure they really understand the plan.
10. Homework assignments made in the early stages of therapy should be brief and relative easy to carry out.
11. Clients should be given plenty of feedback and encouragement, and the treatment plan should be adjusted as necessary.

12. Clients should explore the costs, benefits, and side effects of the treatment. What will happen to them if they do or do not follow the intervention?
13. Client and therapist should explore and identify the potential signs that the treatment is or is not effective. An expected time frame should be discussed.
14. The time commitments of the intervention should be stacked up against the client's family, occupation, or related responsibilities.
15. The intervention should be consistent with the client's core beliefs about causation and treatment.
16. The treatment intervention should be weighed against the client's other immediate needs (for housing, social services, etc.) so that the two do not conflict.
17. Additional physical or mental disorders that may interfere with completing the intervention (e.g., anxiety, poor memory, organic disorders) should be identified.
18. Clients' satisfaction with the intervention and treatment in general should be assessed throughout therapy.
19. Treatment generalization, maintenance, and relapse potential should be addressed.
20. Clients' beliefs that they can be successful should be maintained and strengthened through therapy.

Crits-Christoph, Mintz, and Auerbach (1988); Sexton and Whiston (1994); and Cullari (1996b). Learning to build a strong relationship with clients, however, is largely an art form that needs to be accomplished and developed through experience.

Table 10.7 presents a number of recommendations that can be used to increase adherence in psychotherapy. These are not based on any single orientation and can be used with a variety of different clients and treatment goals.

FUTURE TRENDS

The history of treatment resistance is as old as the field of psychotherapy itself. Yet, as I hope this chapter has demonstrated, we still have a lot to learn about this puzzling concept. Until recently, the notion of treatment resistance was closely entwined with psychoanalytic theory. Other treatment orientations either ignored it altogether or addressed it only superficially. This state of affairs is rapidly changing. Treatment resistance has recently received a great deal of professional attention, and as the field of psychotherapy continues to become more integrative, this trend is sure to continue.

A number of questions remain to be answered about resistance. These include its relationship to nonadherence, a more definitive knowledge of the factors that produce it, and procedures that can be used to address it effectively in psychotherapy. Along the same lines, the future will, I hope, produce a definition of treatment resistance that can be accepted across theoretical paradigms. In the future, unlike the past, our knowledge of resistance will be based on research methods that are less subjective, yet designed to have practical value to therapists working in the field.

REFERENCES

Achterberg-Lawlis, J. (1982). The psychological dimensions of arthritis. *Journal of Consulting and Clinical Psychology, 50*, 984–992.

Anderson, C. M., & Stewart, S. (1983). *A practical guide to family therapy*. New York: Guilford Press.

Arkowitz, H. (1996). Toward an integrative perspective on resistance to change. *In Session, 2*(1), 87–98.

Ascher, L. M. (1989). *Therapeutic paradox*. New York: Guilford Press.

Bandura, A. (1977). Self-efficacy: Toward a unified theory of behavioral change. *Psychological Review, 84*, 191–215.

Becker, M. H., & Maiman, L. A. (1980). Strategies for enhancing patient compliance. *Journal of Community Health, 6*, 113–137.

Bergman, J. S. (1985). *Fishing for barracuda*. New York: Norton.

Brehm, J. W. (1966). *A theory of psychological reactance*. New York: Academic Press.

Breshgold, E. (1989). Resistance in Gestalt therapy: An historical theoretical perspective. *The Gestalt Journal, 12*(2), 73–102.

Chiauzzi, E. J. (1991). *Preventing relapse in the addictions: A biopsychosocial approach*. New York: Pergamon Press.

Cullari, S. (1996a). Psychotherapy practice questionnaire. *The Independent Practitioner*, 16(3), 140–142.

Cullari, S. (1996b). *Treatment resistance: A guide for practitioners*. Boston: Allyn and Bacon.

Davidson, P. O. (1982). Issues in patient compliance. In T. Millon, C. Green, & R. Meagher (Eds.), *Handbook of clinical health psychology* (pp. 417–434). New York: Plenum Press.

de Shazer, S. (1988). *Clues: Investigating solutions in brief therapy*. New York: W. W. Norton.

DiMatteo, M. R., & DiNicola, D. D. (1982). *Achieving patient compliance: The psychology of the mental practitioner's role*. New York: Pergamon Press.

Dowd, E. T. & Trutt, S. D. (1988). Paradoxical interventions in behavior modification. In M. Hersen, R. M. Eisler, & R. E. Miller (Eds.), *Progress in behavior modification* (pp. 96–130). Newbury Park, CA: Sage Publications.

Dunbar, J. M. (1979). Issues in assessment. In S. J. Cohen (Ed.), *New directions in patient compliance* (pp. 41–57). Lexington, MA: Lexington Books.

Dunbar, J. M., & Agras, W. S. (1980). Compliance with medical instructions. In J. M. Ferguson & C. B. Taylor (Eds.), *The comprehensive handbook of behavioral medicine* (Vol. 3, pp. 115–145). New York: Spectum Publications.

Ellis, A. (1985). *Overcoming resistance.* New York: Springer.

Fine, R. (1982). *The healing of the mind* (2nd ed.). New York: Free Press.

Ford, M. E. (1992). *Motivating humans: Goals, emotions, and personal agency beliefs*. Newbury Park, CA: Sage Publications.

Frank, J. D. (1961). *Persuasion and healing*. Baltimore: John Hopkins University Press.

Frank, J. D. (1982). Therapeutic components shared by all psychotherapies. In J. H. Harvey & M. M. Parks (Eds.), *Psychotherapy research and behavior change* (pp. 9–37). Washington, DC: American Psychological Association.

Freud, S. (1955). Studies on hysteria (with Josef Breuer). In J. Strachey (Ed. & Trans.), *The standard edition of the complete psychological works of Sigmund Freud* (Vol. 2). London: Hogarth Press. (Original work published 1895).

Freud, S. (1959). *Inhibitions, symptoms and anxiety.* Standard Edition (Vol. 20, pp. 77–178). (Original work published 1926).

Glover, E. (1955). *The technique of psychoanalysis.* New York: International Universities Press.

Greenson, R. R. (1967). *The technique and practice of psychoanalysis.* New York: International University Press.

Haley, J. (1987). *Problem-solving therapy* (2nd ed.). San Francisco: Jossey-Bass.

Hartmann, H. (1958). *Ego psychology and the problem of adaptation.* New York: International Universities Press.

Kanfer, F. H., & Gaelick-Buys, L. (1991). Self-management methods. In F. H. Kanfer & A. P. Goldstein (Eds.), *Helping people change* (pp. 305–360). New York: Pergamon Press.

Kanfer, F. H. & Goldstein, A. P. (1991). *Helping people change.* New York: Pergamon Press.

Langs, R. (1981). *Resistances and interactions.* New York: Jason Aronson.

Lazarus, A. A., & Fay, A. (1982). Resistance or rationalization? A cognitive-behavioral perspective. In P. Wachtel (Ed.), *Resistance* (pp. 115–133). New York: Plenum Press.

Liotti, G. (1987). The resistance to change of cognitive structures: A counter proposal to psychoanalytic metapsychology. *Journal of Cognitive Psychotherapy: An International Quarterly, 1,* 87–104.

Luborsky, L., Crits-Christoph, P., Mintz, J., & Auerbach, A. (1988). *Who will benefit from psychotherapy?* New York: Basic Books.

Mahoney, M. J. (1991). *Human change processes: The scientific foundations of psychotherapy.* New York: Basic Books.

Marlatt, G. A., & Gordon, J. R. (1985). *Relapse prevention: Maintenance strategies in the treatment of addictive behaviors.* New York: Guilford Press.

Masek, B. J. (1982). Compliance and medicine. In D. M. Doleys, R. L. Meredith, & A. R. Ciminero (Eds.), *Behavioral medicine: Assessment and treatment strategies* (pp. 527–545). New York: Plenum Press.

Meichenbaum, D., & Turk, D. C. (1987). *Facilitating treatment adherence.* New York: Plenum Press.

Menninger, K. A. (1973). *Theory of psychoanalytic technique* (2nd ed.). New York: Basic Books.

Munjack, D. J., & Oziel, L. J. (1978). Resistance in the behavioral treatment of sexual dysfunctions. *Journal of Sex and Marital Therapy, 4,* 122–138.

Pervin, L. A. (1991). Self-regulation and the problem of volition. In M. L. Maeher & P. R. Pintrich (Eds.), *Advances in motivation and achievement* (pp. 1–20). Greenwich, CT: JAI Press.

Prochaska, J., & DiClemente, C. (1986). The transtheoretical approach. In J. C. Norcross (Ed.), *Handbook of eclectic psychotherapy* (pp. 163–200). New York: Brunner/Mazel.

Rosenhan, D. L. (1973). On being sane in insane places. *Science, 179,* 250–258.

Sandler, J., Dare, C., & Holder, A. (1973). *The patient and the analyst.* New York: International Universities Press.

Sandler, J., Holder, A., & Dare, C. (1970). Brief psychoanalytic concepts: V. Resistance. *British Journal of Psychiatry, 117,* 215–221.

Schafer, R. (1983). *The analytic attitude.* New York: Basic Books.

Sexton, T. L., & Whiston, S. C. (1994). The status of the counseling relationship: An empirical review, theoretical implications and research directions. *The Counseling Psychologist, 22,* 6–78.

Shelton, J. L., & Levy, R. L. (1981). *Behavioral assignments and treatment compliance: A handbook of clinical strategies.* Champaign, IL: Research Press.

Stark, M. (1994). *Working with resistance.* Northvale, NJ: Jason Aronson.

Strean, H. S. (1990). *Resolving resistances in psychotherapy.* New York: Brunner/Mazel.

Turk, D. C., Salovey, P., & Litt, M. D. (1986). Adherence: A cognitive-behavioral perspective. In K. E. Gerber & A. M. Nehemkis (Eds.), *Compliance: The dilemma of the chronically ill* (pp. 44–72). New York: Springer.

Weeks, G. R., & L'Abate, L. (1982). *Paradoxical psychotherapy: Theory and practice with individuals, couples and families.* New York: Brunner/Mazel.

FOR FURTHER READING

Arkowitz, H. (1996). Resistance to change in psychotherapy. *In Session, 2*(1). New York: John Wiley. *This is a special issue devoted entirely to treatment resistance.*

Bugental, J. F. T. (1987). *The art of psychotherapy.* New York: Norton. *This is an excellent book that covers many topics in psychotherapy, including resistance, from an existential-psychoanalytic point of view.*

Cullari, S. (1996). *Treatment resistance: A guide for practitioners.* Boston: Allyn and Bacon. *This book greatly expands on most of the areas presented in this chapter.*

Howe, D. (1993). *On being a client.* London: Sage. *This book looks at psychotherapy from a client's perspective and describes what clients hope to gain from treatment.*

Kottler, J. A. (1986). *On being a therapist.* San Francisco: Jossey-Bass.

Kottler, J. A. (1992). *Compassionate therapy.* San Francisco: Jossey-Bass.

Kottler, J. A., & Blau, D. S. (1989). *The imperfect therapist: Learning from failure in therapeutic practice.* San Francisco: Jossey-Bass. *This series of books from Kottler cover many aspects of being a psychotherapist and are recommended for everyone entering the field of clinical psychology.*

CHAPTER 11

BIOLOGICAL FOUNDATIONS OF CLINICAL PSYCHOLOGY

Clifford N. Lazarus

INTRODUCTION

To appreciate fully the breadth and depth of the biological underpinnings of clinical psychology and human phenomenology, it is helpful to consider the origins of consciousness itself. This chapter begins with a brief overview of the development of human consciousness—an evolution that starts before the dawn of time and leaves off at the present moment with you, our readers, accomplishing a feat that is nothing less than wondrous: perceiving and intellectually processing the words on this page. You, like all people, are biophysiologic beings—countless quadrillions of atoms arranged in such a way as to be self-perpetuating, self-regulating, self-aware, living, breathing entities of matter and energy. Fundamentally, we are chemical consciousness and, perhaps, the way the universe has come to know of itself.

The next part of this chapter will focus on the primary organ of consciousness, the brain, its evolution, development, structure, and function. Then we will explore research and diagnostic methods used in neuroscience and how dysregulation of various brain systems can lead to symptoms of psychopathology. Next, the importance of differential diagnosis will be discussed (i.e., discriminating between true psychological disturbances and medical conditions that can masquerade as psychological disorders). The remainder of the chapter will address the topics of health psychology and behavioral medicine.

THE EVOLUTION OF CONSCIOUSNESS: FROM THE BIG BANG TO THE BIG BRAIN

Atomic and Molecular Evolution

According to the most current theories of cosmology and astronomy, the universe is between 10 and 20 billion years old and was born out of a cataclysmic event called the Big Bang (Hawking, 1988; Krauss, 1995). Before the Big Bang, all the matter and energy in the universe was contained in an infinitely dense, polydimensional point that, for some unknown reason, exploded outward and began expanding at the speed of light toward eternity, releasing in its wake the very fabric of the universe—energy, matter, space, and time. In the first micromoments following its violent birth, the nascent universe consisted of protomatter: a variety of subatomic, fundamental, or elementary particles (i.e., quarks, leptons, and bosons, entities that may be the ultimate, irreducible constituents of matter and energy). These gave rise to larger subatomic structures such as protons, neutrons, and electrons, which in turn gave rise to atoms, the smallest units of the elements that make up all coherent matter and substance in the universe. Since the Big Bang, atoms have condensed out of the universal expansion for unimaginable millennia following a sort of thermodynamic and molecular evolution that eventually led to the formation of all celestial bodies from the largest superclusters of galaxies to the smallest motes of interstellar dust. Among the products of this cosmic evolution are countless solar systems like our own, which contain planets that have, in at least the case of our Earth, spawned life.

The Origins of Consciousness: From Single Cells to Conscious Organisms

In much the same way that atomic and molecular evolution produced the stars, planets, and eventually life, it is not difficult to imagine a similar evolutionary process, driven by the forces of chemistry, physics, and natural selection, leading to increasingly complex microorganisms and ultimately to all present-day life forms. Although the question of just when life actually sprang into existence cannot be confidently answered, some sort of time scale has been established that places the first microorganisms on the Earth about 3.4 billion years ago. Evidence for this assertion is based on the discovery of microfossils, resembling present-day bacteria and algae, in flintlike rocks that, according to radioactive dating, are 3.4 billion years old (Curtis, 1979; Postlethwait & Hopson, 1995). Thus, life began very early, perhaps within the first billion years of the Earth's history, since current best estimates place the age of our planet at approximately 4 to 5 billion years.

It is hypothesized that a variety of factors led to the proliferation of increasingly complex living systems and the current-day diversity of life forms. The first living entities were probably extreme *heterotrophs* (from the Greek for "other feeder")—organisms that cannot synthesize all their needed organic compounds and so must feed on organic materials found in the external environment. (Organic compounds are those that contain carbon atoms and make up the majority of biomolecules. Biomolecules are things like proteins, carbohydrates, and fats, substances vital for life that make up living organisms.) These primitive microorganisms, and their similarly primitive current-day descendants, lacked a nucleus and are referred to as *prokaryotes* (meaning "before" + a "nut" or "kernel," because these entities lack the membrane-bound intracellular structures that look like small nuts or kernels under magnification). As the numbers of prokaryotic heterotrophs increased, they began to use up the rich supply of available organic molecules on which their existence depended and which took many millions of years to accumulate. This factor, then, set the stage for another Darwinian competition—cells that could make efficient use of the limited resources were more likely to survive than cells that could not.

Over the ensuing ages, cells evolved that were able to assemble more and more of the organic molecules they needed out of simple inorganic materials like water and carbon dioxide. Thus, the *autotrophs* (from the Greek for "self-feeder") emerged—microorganisms that are able to synthesize all the organic molecules they need for survival from inorganic substances and some form of energy such as sunlight. Indeed, the most successful of the autotrophs were those that evolved a method that allowed them to make direct use of the sun's energy, the process of photosynthesis.

With the advent of photosynthesis, the flow of energy in the biosphere came to resemble its present-day form—light energy from the sun powering photosynthetic autotrophs, which in turn serve as the center of the food web to nourish all other forms of life. With the appearance of photosynthetic cells, another important factor was introduced into the developing biosphere—the steady accumulation of atmospheric oxygen. This in turn provided the impetus for the evolution of organisms that produced most of their energy by the process of cellular respiration—the oxygen-requiring, water- and carbon dioxide–liberating, breakdown and release of energy from fuel molecules.

The next evolutionary step was the advent of eukaryotic microorganisms, a transition second only to the origin of life itself in terms of biological significance. *Eukaryotes* (meaning "good" + a "nut" or "kernel," because these entities have membrane-bound intracellular structures that look like small nuts or kernels under microscopy) are relatively large cells that contain various *organelles* ("little organs"), including a nucleus, that are separated from the cell's cytoplasm by special membranes (to be discussed). Exactly how eukaryotes originated is a topic of much debate. One plausible explanation is that larger and more complex cells resulted from symbiotic associations among prokaryotes. According to this theory, some prokaryotic cells merged with or took up residence inside other prokaryotes. Such associations must have conferred certain adaptive advantages (perhaps nutrients and protection for the smaller cells and new energy sources for the larger cells) that led to the success and proliferation of these new cellular organisms. Eventually, the symbionts evolved into the cellular organelles we see in eukaryotes today.

Now that we have traced the evolution of eukaryotic cells, we will provide a quick overview of their structure and function. This will provide an important foundation on which much of neuroscience rests because an adequate understanding of neurobiology requires a general knowledge of cellular physiology. For the remainder of this chapter, when we mention cells we will be referring to eukaryotic animal cells unless specifically stated otherwise.

Cells are tiny membrane-bound masses of protoplasm that form the fundamental units of living matter. They are the smallest structures capable of maintaining life and reproducing. The branch of science that studies cells is called *cytology*.

The most conspicuous structural feature of a cell is its membrane. Cellular membranes form both the outer boundary of the cell itself and the boundaries of most of its internal structures. The current view of cellular membranes is called the *fluid mosaic model*, which depicts the membrane as a dynamic, fluid-like entity instead of a static, solid structure. The fluid mosaic model postulates that two layers (i.e., a bilayer) of phospholipid molecules (mole-

cules that contain phosphate atoms and fats or lipids) form the inner and outer skin of the membrane, and that various proteins are scattered throughout it in all possible positions, on the outer and inner surfaces, partially penetrating the outer and inner surfaces, and extending completely through the membrane (see Figure 11.1). This arrangement is the natural consequence of the dual nature of phospholipids, which have *hydrophilic* ("water-loving") phosphate heads and *hydrophobic* ("water-fearing") fatty acid tails. As a result they position themselves so that the water-loving heads face the extracellular and intracellular fluids, while the water-fearing tails point away from both the fluid outside the membrane and the fluid inside the cell. Hence, the phosphate heads become packed together like the tiles in a mosaic, the fatty acid tails associate in the *anhydrous* ("without water") layer between the phosphate heads, and a wide assortment of diversely positioned proteins diffuse across the bilayer.

Cell membranes perform a wide range of vital functions. They serve as boundaries between the external and internal cellular environments, anchor many biologically crucial molecules (like receptors and ion channels), and transport substances into and out of the cell. Indeed, a constant flow of chemical traffic moves continually in both directions through cell membranes—an endless procession of water molecules, nutrients, gases, waste products, and many kinds of ions. Some of these transportation processes (e.g., osmosis and diffusion) are termed *passive* because they are driven by forces that do not depend on the cell's own energy and therefore rely on concentration gradients to power them. Other transportation mechanisms are referred to as *active* because the energy that drives them comes from chemical reactions taking place inside the cell. Unlike passive transport, which can only move molecules from areas of high concentration to areas of lower concentration, active-transport processes can move materials against concentration gradients. Most active transport involves the participation of energy donating molecules like adenosine triphosphate (ATP). In addition to their molecular transport functions, cell membranes also help maintain the cell's structural integrity and contain many of

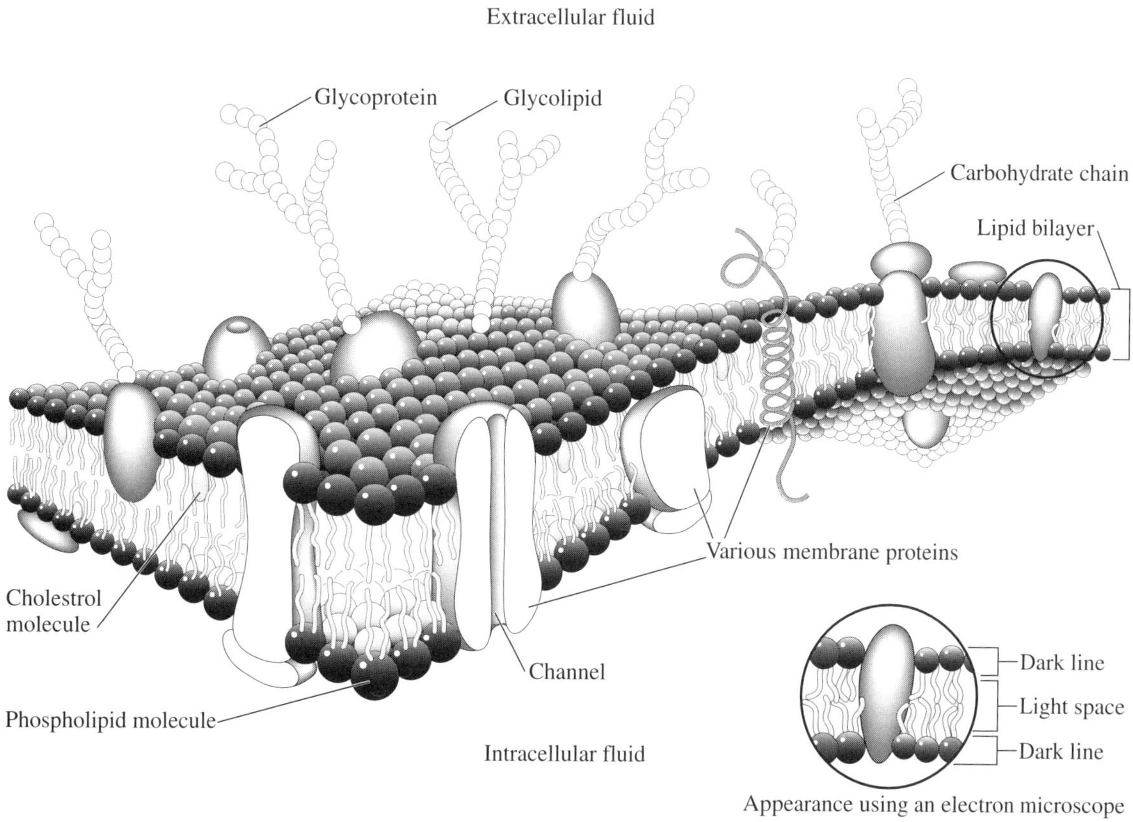

Extracellular fluid

Glycoprotein   Glycolipid

Carbohydrate chain

Lipid bilayer

Various membrane proteins

Cholestrol molecule

Channel

Phospholipid molecule

Intracellular fluid

Dark line

Light space

Dark line

Appearance using an electron microscope

Figure 11.1. The fluid mosaic model of cellular membranes.

the receptors for chemical messengers such as neurotransmitters and hormones.

Surrounded by the cellular membrane is the *protoplasm*, a special kind of matter that composes all cells. Protoplasm is a complex organization of thousands of biomolecules, amazingly formed out of only two dozen elements—mostly hydrogen, oxygen, carbon, and nitrogen, which account for more than 99% of the atoms in protoplasm. Together with phosphorus and sulfur, these elements make up protoplasm's major compounds—water, proteins, carbohydrates, lipids, and nucleic acids—which, except for water, are all unique to it. Indeed, by far the most abundant compound in protoplasm, as well as in the inanimate world, is water. Basically, protoplasm can be thought of as a richly complex mixture of water and organic substances that performs the countless, yet finely coordinated and integrated, biochemical reactions that give rise to and maintain life.

Similar to protoplasm is *cytoplasm,* which can be thought of as all of a cell's protoplasm except its nucleus. In other words, cytoplasm is the part of a cell between its outer membrane and its nucleus. As can be clearly seen in Figure 11.2, far from the homogeneous fluid it was once thought to be, cytoplasm contains a rich assortment of small structures called *cytoplasmic organelles*, the little organs of the cell. These include the endoplasmic reticula, Golgi bodies, ribosomes, mitochondria, lysosomes, centrosomes, nucleus, and nucleolus, each of which will be described in turn. In addition to housing the organelles, cytoplasm contains an internal scaffold aptly called a *cytoskeleton,* made up of microscopically thin protein threads, fibers, and tubules called microfilaments, intermediate fibers, and microtu-

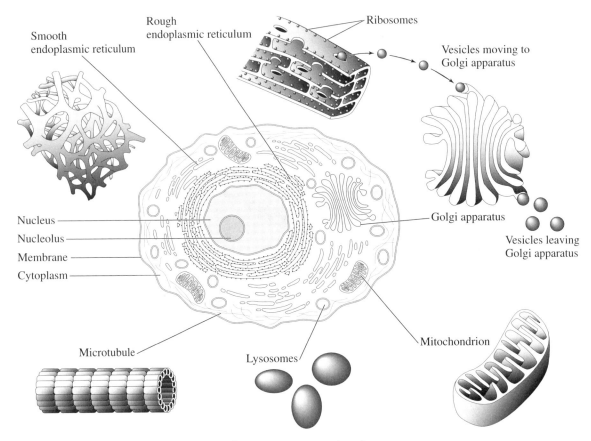

Figure 11.2. Anatomy of a cell.

bules, respectively. These function to help the cell keep its shape, anchor its organelles, direct the flow of internal chemical traffic, and in some cases aid in motility.

The endoplasmic reticulum (*endoplasm* means the cytoplasm near the center of the cell, and *reticulum* means netlike formation) is a network of interconnecting flattened sacs, tubes, and channels once thought to be limited to the deep interior of the cell but now known to be distributed widely beyond the endoplasm. Two types have been described—rough endoplasmic reticulum (RER) and smooth endoplasmic reticulum (SER). RER is densely studded with ribosomes (to be discussed) on its outer surface, which under magnification appear as innumerable small granules and impart its "rough" appearance. RER is involved in the synthesis, modification, and transportation of proteins. Not sur-

prisingly, cells that produce a lot of proteins have an abundance of RER. SER lacks the ribosomes that dot the surface of RER, hence its designation as "smooth." Cells that synthesize a lot of lipids—such as gland cells that make steroid hormones—have lots of SER. It is also conspicuous in liver cells, where it appears to be involved in various detoxification processes.

Golgi bodies are small groups of flattened membrane-bound sacs stacked loosely on one another and surrounded by tubules and vesicles. Their main function is to modify, package, and distribute secretory products as well as to distribute and recycle the cellular membrane.

Ribosomes are the most numerous of the cells organelles. Made up of a special type of RNA and specific proteins, they are sites where amino acids are assembled into polypeptides. Ribosomes can be found either free floating in the cytoplasm or associated with rough endoplasmic reticula.

Another important organelle is the *mitochondrion* (plural: *mitochondria*), a relatively large, abundant, and variously shaped organelle which is the principal site of ATP production. ATP (adenosine triphosphate), is a vital cellular energy molecule that powers many biochemical reactions. Indeed, the greater the energy requirement of the cell, the more mitochondria it is likely to have. Mitochondria can thus be thought of as the cell's power plants.

Lysosomes are essentially membranous bags of destructive enzymes that are usually formed in the Golgi bodies. They are involved in the catabolic activity (breaking down large molecules into smaller ones) of many cells. Although they are capable of breaking down all the major biomolecules of the cell—except, it seems, the vesicle that encases them—they more often protect than destroy cells. For example, some types of white blood cells engulf harmful substances, which are then digested by the lysosomes' catabolic enzymes.

Centrosomes, as their name suggests, are organelles located near the center of the cell, adjacent to the nucleus. They are a pair of small tubular masses lying at right angles to each other and contain structures called *centrioles,* which are made up of nine triplet bundles of microtubules. Centrosomes seem to play an important role in distributing chromosomes during cell division.

Perhaps the most important and largest cytoplasmic organelle is the *nucleus,* which usually occupies the central portion of the cell. The nucleus is surrounded by its own special membrane, which contains pores at frequent intervals through which materials pass between the *nucleoplasm* (the nucleus's cytoplasm) and the cellular cytoplasm. The nucleus carries the cell's hereditary information—DNA packed into dense, tightly coiled structures called *chromosomes*. In essence, the nucleus stores, duplicates, transfers, and transcribes genetic information and thereby orchestrates and conducts the myriad, integrated, highly coordinated biochemical symphonies of all living processes.

The final organelle we will mention is the *nucleolus* (plural: *nucleoli*). Nucleoli are small spherical structures found within the cell's nucleus. They function to synthesize ribosomal RNA and assemble ribosome subunits. The proteins that are part of the ribosomes are manufactured in the cytoplasm and migrate into the nucleoli, where they combine with the RNA to form the ribosomal subunits. The subunits then leave the nucleoli and move into the cytoplasm, where they couple to form the completed ribosome. As described earlier, after assembly, many ribosomes associate with rough endoplasmic reticula or remain free floating in the cytoplasm, where they participate in protein synthesis.

According to the best available fossil evidence, the first eukaryotes evolved approximately 1.6 billion years ago (Curtis, 1979), almost 2 billion years after the origin of their prokaryotic progenitors. Once that milestone was reached, the subsequent 1.5 billion years witnessed a continuously expanding evolutionary explosion, which has culminated to date in countless species of astonishing complexity, diversity, and specialization. The driving force behind this continuing evolution and species diversity is the ongoing process of natural selection. Organisms that are well suited to take advantage of their environments survive, reproduce, and continue to evolve, whereas those that are not perish and become extinct. In a manner believed to be similar to that which produced eukaryotes from prokaryotes, adaptive symbiotic associations among eukaryotic microorganisms led to cellular aggregates that became the forerunners of simple tissues and primitive multicelled organisms.

Over the hundreds of millions of years that followed, this basic process continued to operate, leading to increasingly complex multicellular organisms and eventually to the origin of the modern animal kingdom. Currently, at the pinnacle of the animal kingdom sit the most highly evolved of all organisms, the vertebrates—animals with backbones and many kinds of specialized tissues, including elaborate sensory and neuromotor systems. At the apex of the vertebrates reside the mammals, with, their unique, large, convoluted brains, and at the summit of the mammals dwell human beings: *Homo sapiens,* "wise man," who possesses the most complex brain of all extant animals. It is a brain certainly large enough to know of itself and seek to understand its origin and purpose—an organ that has been evolving out of the cosmic expansion for 10 to 20 billion years and is, perhaps, the way that the universe has come to know of and begin to understand itself.

THE BRAIN

Evolution of the Human Brain: Part One—Basic Life Support

The brain's function is to initiate, integrate, and coordinate the countless biological processes that maintain the life of the organism. It does this by way of an elaborate network of signaling tissues that reach out to various targets throughout itself and the body and communicate specific messages by way of chemical transmitters. In much the same way that increasingly complex multicellular animals are believed to have evolved from simpler single-celled organisms, the human brain is thought to have undergone a similar evolutionary history (Carpenter, 1996; Curtis, 1979). The coordination of a single-celled organism like an ameba is passively chemical. Its brain is its nucleus, which acts in conjunction with its other organelles by chemical and molecular diffusion. Similarly, even in some multicellular organisms communication among cells may be passive and chemical, whereby cells in one part may release messengers, hormones, and transmitters that determine what another part does. As size and complexity increase, however, a more active and integrated system of communication among cells becomes necessary, particularly when cells perform specialized functions such as sensation, digestion, secretion, locomotion, and so forth.

Another important factor is speed of signaling. Simple diffusion is a slow process, especially in bigger organisms in which chemicals released at one end might take a long time to reach cells at the other end. If speed of response is not particularly important and there is some kind of fluid circulation that will speed up the dispersion of messengers, this strategy may nevertheless be sufficient even in large organisms. Indeed, our own hormonal control is an example of such a system. Besides its slowness, another limitation of this process is that it is

very imprecise. Consider, for example, that when we are startled the release of stress hormones, like adrenaline, into our blood results in diffuse and indiscriminate reactions throughout our whole body. For rapid and localized responses, we need a signaling system that will release the messenger as quickly as possible and only at the site where it is needed. This function of rapid and localized chemical secretion is precisely what nervous tissue has evolved to do.

Perhaps the ancestors of nerve cells were sensory receptors, cells on the exterior of the organisms that developed sensitivities to chemical, mechanical, thermal, or electromagnetic stimulation. In primitive organisms, activation of these cells probably caused them to release specific chemicals that caused reflexive reactions in populations of other cells, which, in turn, resulted in the organism doing something, such as moving. Eventually, these sensory cells might have formed connections with other entirely internal cells that responded to the chemicals released by the sensory cells by secreting chemicals of their own. Obviously, these processes must have contributed some survival advantages to the organisms that evolved them, and over the ages the system of interconnecting secretory cells became more and more complex.

Because it appears that life was born out of the womb of the primordial seas, it will come as no surprise that the first prototype brains also appeared in the Earth's early oceans. One present-day creature that may provide us with a peek through the keyhole into the distant past of the brain's development is the hydra (Carpenter, 1996). Hydras are small (about one inch long), cylindrical, solitary animals that have tentacles equipped with special stinging cells surrounding their mouths. Although they lack many specialized organs, such as those for respiration and excretion, they do have a network of intercommunicating nerve cells or neurons. This neural net has sensory cells on the animal's surface that respond to mechanical and chemical stimuli, and interconnect with muscle cells and secretory glands. Thus, the hydra's brain is spread diffusely throughout its entire body, with only a slightly greater density around its mouth. Yet it can, nevertheless, generate coordinated and seemingly purposeful behavior (e.g., attaching to an object, stunning prey, and eating). Another contemporary organism that might resemble the first primitive creatures with rudimentary nervous systems is the sea squirt. This animal has a mere 300 nerve cells arranged in a tube that enable it to swim through the water and orient itself to light.

The next step in the evolution of the nervous system probably involved an increase in the size and specialization of sensory organs, such as olfactory (smell) receptors and eyes. It is possible to imagine that if an animal had a typical direction of movement, such organs would tend to develop at its front end, and the extra flow of sensory information through such organs might have resulted in an increased density of signal-receiving cells in the animal's head. This, then, would have led to the development of the first true brain and is best reflected in the present-day planarian or flat worm (Carpenter, 1996). In planarians we find a dense concentration of nerve cells close to the eyes, which gives rise to a pair of nerve cords that run down the body and send off side branches that connect with other cells. Thus, in planarians we see a centralized brain and nerve cords that serve to coordinate complex behaviors like movement and digestion.

The next developmental step in the brain's evolution probably occurred with the advent of segmented aquatic worms, similar to contemporary earth worms. Like planarians, these animals have a centralized concentration of nerve cells in their heads and nerve cords running the length of their bodies, but in addition they have extra clusters of nerves called *ganglia*, one to each segment. Each ganglion is a kind of brain in its own right, which explains why a decapitated earth worm is still capable of many kinds of behavior. In the segmented worms we see the beginnings of structures that resemble our own vertebral column (Carpenter, 1996).

The earliest actual brain that bears more than a superficial similarity to our own probably appeared in the first early fish, which heralded the advent of the vertebrates. According to Curtis (1979), these animals first appeared about 500 million years ago, or about 3.1 billion years after the dawn of the prokaryotes and 4 billion years after the formation of the Earth. In addition to having a much greater number of centralized nerve cells than any previous creature, it is believed that these animals had swellings at portions of their brains where the density of neurons was especially great. But perhaps the most important milestone of neural development that emerged with these organisms was the evolution of insulating sheath around their nerves, which allowed the speed of their signals to increase dramatically. Over the next hundred million years, fish thrived as the Earth's most highly evolved animals.

Evolution of the Human Brain: Part Two—The Dawn of Emotions

So far we have described the development of a brain that functions to coordinate the activities of various cells, tissues, and organs with the single purpose of sustaining life through sensing, moving, eating, digesting, breathing, and reproducing. Then, about 395 million years ago the first amphibians appeared, and 100 million years later the first reptiles evolved (Curtis, 1979). With the advent of amphibians and reptiles, the brain underwent further expansion and developed structures and functions that made survival on land possible. In addition, a unique feature appeared, which we call the reptilian brain and which reached its peak during the age of dinosaurs, between 200 and 65 million years ago. The reptilian brain might have been responsible for the first emotions. Indeed, it is believed that many dinosaurs nurtured their young and thus might have had powerful emotions and biologic drives that stemmed from such complex social behavior (Gould, 1995). As we will explore later, we and all animals that evolved after the dinosaurs have retained this bit of neural architecture in the part of our brain referred to as the *limbic system*.

Evolution of the Human Brain: Part Three—The Emergence of Cognition

During the reign of the dinosaurs, another quantum evolutionary leap took place—the appearance of the first birds and primitive mammals. With the rise of the mammals, the reptilian brain was literally overshadowed by the exceedingly intricate mammalian brain, which evolved a cerebrum wrapped around its reptilian core. The mammalian cerebrum possesses a thin outer layer called the *cortex* (from the Latin for "bark"), which probably allowed for their survival and ascendance in the midst of the dinosaurs' extinction. Whatever the cause of the massive dinosaurian extinction of 65 million years ago (e g., comet strike, catastrophic climate change, etc.), it is clear that various terrestrial environments changed dramatically during that period. Possessing the cerebral cortex, the early mammals were very likely able to "think," learn, and solve problems of survival, which enabled them to adapt to the changing landscape by finding new ways of exploiting the prevailing environment. Thus, with the mammals the brain developed a characteristic that transcended the basic life support, biological drive, and emotive functions of its earlier incarnations—namely, that of cognition.

Over the following tens of millions of years, mammals held dominion on the Earth and continued to thrive and evolve. Then, about 30 million years ago, the apes evolved, and with their emergence the Earth probably saw its first tool users. This development of using tools (presumably, nothing more than sticks and stones) might have catalyzed another dramatic step forward in the development of the brain. Finally, approximately 5 million years ago the cortex appeared in a new type of mammal, early human. Since that time, we have continued to evolve and spread across much of the planet, but the structure and function of our brains has remained more or less unchanged.

As this description of the nervous system's evolution suggests, our brains are actually three brains in one—an amazingly complex origami of tissue folded into a single organ. As can be seen in Figure 11.3, at the base of our brain where it gives rise to the

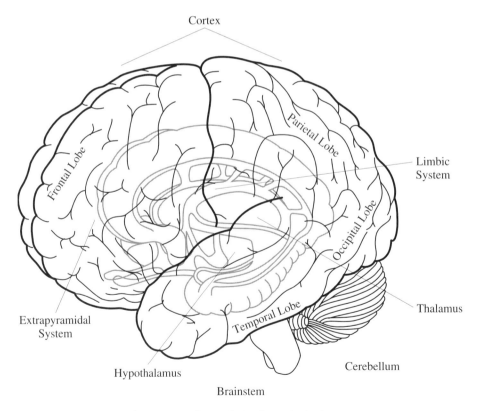

Figure 11.3. A human brain illustrating brainstem, limbic/subcortical structures, and cerebral cortex.

spinal cord is the brainstem, which regulates the basic mechanisms of life support: nonconscious or so-called autonomic processes like breathing, digestion, and circulation. This is the part of our nervous system that we inherited from the earliest true-brained creatures, like ancient fish. Resting on top of and wrapped around our brainstem is the limbic system, which derives its name from the Latin word *limbus*, meaning "border" or "edge." The limbic system is a group of interrelated structures deep within the brain that appear to mediate many biological drives and emotional states. This is the legacy of the reptiles—the reptilian brain that made survival on land possible. But by far the most recent part and literally the crowning glory of our brain is its *cerebral cortex*—the intricately convoluted outer layer of our brain, a mere quarter-inch thick, that gives rise to all the conscious, sensory, and perceptual phenomena we think of as human experience. It is our cortex that allows us to perceive ourselves and the world through our senses; to see, smell, hear, taste, and touch. Perhaps most important, the cortex serves as our thinking cap. It allows us to plan, to learn, to speak, and to behave in a manner that we have come to consider as uniquely human.

Microstructure of the Human Brain: Neurons and Neural Transmission

The human brain is without doubt the most complex organ and perhaps the most complex single structure on the planet. It is a mere three-pound gelatinous blob of tissue we carry around in a bony, spherical container on our shoulders; yet it produces the entire spectrum of conscious human experience—our universe of inner space. Interestingly, when astronomers and cosmologists talk about outer space, they speak in terms and numbers so vast they boggle the imagination—15 billion light years of space-time folded around hundreds of billions of galaxies containing trillions of stars, planets, and other celestial bodies! Similarly, when neuroscientists describe the tissue that gives rise to our universe of inner space, they speak of equally mind-numbing numbers—15 billion transmitting neurons encased in more than 100 billion neurons,

in total creating trillions of interconnections! To help put these numbers in perspective, consider that if you counted at the rate of one per second around the clock, 24 hours a day, 7 days a week, it would take you more than 11.5 days to count to one million. To reach one billion would require counting for more than 31.5 years, and to count up to one trillion you would be counting nonstop for the next 31,688 years!

To reduce this staggeringly complex organ to more manageable terms we will begin with an exploration of a single brain cell. Then we will build upward and outward from that starting point until we have integrated both the microscopic and macroscopic features of the brain into a coherent whole. Before venturing deeper into the territory of the central nervous system, however, it is helpful to define a few basic terms that form the foundation of neuroscience.

Neuron: A nerve cell that receives, integrates, and transmits electrochemical signals. The functional units of the nervous system.

Soma: The cell body containing the nucleus and many other cytoplasmic organelles and the point of origin of the neurofilaments, the dendrites and axon.

Neuroglia: Literally, "nerve glue." Neural cells that support transmitting neurons both physically and nutritionally. There are two main types: (1) *astrocytes,* which are relatively large, star-shaped cells that connect neurons with the brain's blood supply and also anchor them in place, and (2) *oligodendroglia,* which function principally to encase axons in insulating sheaths called *myelin,* which increases the rate at which they can conduct impulses.

Neurotransmitter: A chemical messenger that carries information from one neuron to another at the synapse. (Actually, autotransmission can also occur; this is when a single neuron synapses with itself.) There are three general categories of neurotransmitters: (1) *biogenic amines* like serotonin, norepinephrine, dopamine, and acetylcholine (the term *amine* simply refers to any organic molecule containing a nitrogen atom, usually derived from ammonia, NH_3); (2) *amino acids* like GABA and glutamate; and (3) *neuropep-tides* or small proteins like beta-endorphin.

Synapse: The junction between neurons transmitting and receiving membranes. Usually a physical gap across which neurotransmitters diffuse when released.

Axon and terminal: The transmitting neurofilaments of neurons. Electrochemical impulses called action potentials travel down the axon resulting in the release of neurotransmitters from the terminal area where they are stored in discrete packages called vesicles. The axon terminals are small knoblike swellings, sometimes referred to as *boutons* from the French for "button." The terminal is synonymous with *presynaptic membrane*.

Dendrites: The receptive neurofilaments of neurons, containing receptors where neurotransmitters bind. Also referred to as the *postsynaptic membrane*.

Receptors: Specialized molecular binding sites where neurotransmitters dock, thereby producing physiologic effects. Most receptors are large proteins that span the neural membrane, thus having portions on the exterior of the cell where the neurotransmitters bind, and portions in the cell's interior that subsequently initiate biochemical reactions within the neuron.

Polarization: The state of having opposite qualities or powers. The difference in electrochemical charge that develops between the outside and inside of the neural membrane such that the interior is negatively charged relative to the exterior. For all intents and purposes, polarization is synonymous with a neuron's resting membrane potential.

EPSP: Excitatory postsynaptic potential. A depolarizing stimulus that increases the likelihood that the receiving neuron will "fire" or initiate an action potential.

IPSP: Inhibitory postsynaptic potential. A stimulus that decreases the likelihood that the receiving neuron will fire, usually by hyperpolarizing the cell.

TOE: Threshold of excitation. A critical degree of excitation or depolarization at which the neuron fires in an all-or-none fashion.

Action potential: The chain reaction of events that involves the temporary loss or reversal of polarization at a segment of the axon for a micromoment and initiates the same repeating sequence of events in the immediately adjacent portion of the axon, ultimately resulting in neurotransmitter release from the nerve terminal.

Neurons, also referred to as *nerve cells*, are the functional units of the nervous system. Neurons receive, integrate, and transmit electrochemical impulses via neurotransmitter-dependent, ionic, and/or enzymatic interactions across cellular membranes (Carpenter, 1996; Hyman & Nestler, 1993). Although at first this definition seems dauntingly complex, the elegance of neural structure and function will soon become increasingly clear. Like all nucleated animal cells (i.e., cells having a nucleus or eukaryotes) neurons have the typical complement of organelles but in addition have some unique features that make them especially well adapted to their roles as signal senders and receivers. These unique characteristics are *neurofilaments* (fine threadlike structures) called dendrites and axons and are illustrated in Figure 11.4.

Although it is a slight oversimplification, dendrites can be thought of as the neuron's receptive membrane—the site where most incoming messages are received. A given neuron can have many points on its soma where dendrites originate. Axons are the neuron's transmitting components, the structures that send signals. Although both dendrites and axons may branch out into numerous offshoots, usually the axon originates from a single trunk called the *axon hillock* where it leaves the cell body. Neurons synthesize their neurotransmitters in their cell bodies and, with the help of their Golgi bodies, package them in membranous sacks called *vesicles*. The vesicles protect the neurotransmitter from the enzymatic degradation that would occur if they were free floating in the cell's cytoplasm. After synthesis and packaging, the vesicles of neurotransmitters are delivered to the terminal boutons of the axon, aided by the cytoskeleton, where they await release upon the arrival of an action potential, as will be described (see Figure 11.5). Incidentally, the word *bouton* comes from the French word for

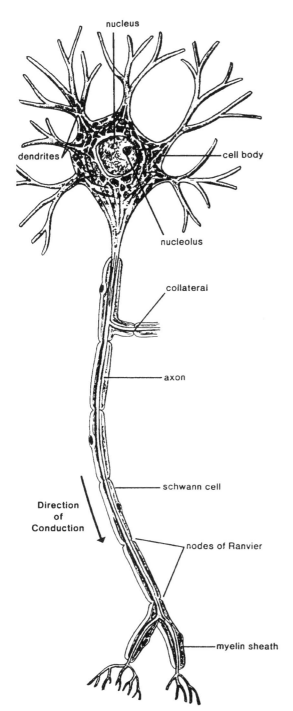

Figure 11.4. A typical neuron illustrating cell body, dendrites, and axon with myelin sheath and unsheathed nodes.

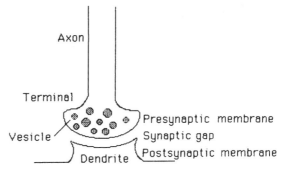

Figure 11.5. Close-up of a synapse indicating axonal terminus with vesiculated neurotransmitter, gap junction, and postsynaptic dendritic membrane.

button because the axon terminals have tiny swellings that resemble buttons when seen under magnification.

When a neuron is at rest (i.e., not "firing" or sending an impulse), a very narrow margin of the axoplasm (axon's cytoplasm) bordering the intracellular membrane is negatively charged. Conversely, a very narrow margin of the exterior fluid surrounding the outer membrane is positively charged. This separation of charge, so that the interior of the neuron is negatively charged relative to its exterior, is termed *polarization* (the state of having opposite qualities or powers). Polarization is due to a property of the cellular membrane called *selective permeability,* which means that the membrane allows some molecules to cross into or out of the cell, but not others. Another important factor that helps to polarize the neuron is an active (ATP-driven), membrane-bound molecular pump that extrudes sodium ions and retrieves potassium ions. Because the pump has binding sites of three sodium atoms, but only two for potassium atoms, for every three sodium ions pumped out of the cell, only two potassium ions are taken in. Because the resting neural membrane is normally impermeable to sodium, a large concentration gradient develops so that the quantity of sodium ions outside the neuron is much greater than the quantity of sodium within it. Because substances tend to seek equilibrium by moving down concentration gradients (i.e., molecules will randomly move by diffusion from areas of high concentration to areas of lower concentration), a significant tension builds, tending to force the sodium into the cell. Similarly, an intracellular concentration gradient develops that favors the movement of potassium ions out of the neuron.

The net result is that the immediate interior of the neuron is negatively charged relative to the immediate exterior. This charge difference, of about 70 millivolts, is called the neuron's resting membrane potential and can be thought of as analogous to a cocked crossbow. See Figure 11.6 for an illustration of this concept. If anything occurs to pull the trigger, the crossbow will fire by suddenly releasing the energy stored in its bow. Similarly, since the sodium and potassium ions are seeking to equalize their distribution across the membrane (they are "cocked"), if anything occurs to increase the permeability of the membrane to them, an immediate rush of sodium into and potassium out of the cell will result. This flipflop of ions—sodium in, potassium out—causes a change in the neuron's polarity so that its interior becomes momentarily positive relative to its exterior. When this happens, as is illustrated in Figure 11.7, the neuron is said to have depolarized.

Certain neurotransmitter–receptor interactions increase membrane permeability to sodium ions, which produces a decrease in the degree of polarization (partial depolarization) because the interior membrane margin becomes less negatively charged as a result of the influx of positively charged sodium ions. This is referred to as an EPSP, or *excitatory postsynaptic potential*, and tends to push the neuron toward firing. Other neurotrans-

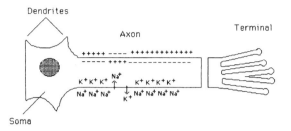

Figure 11.7. Illustration of axonal depolarization showing charge reversal due to sodium influx and potassium efflux.

mitter–receptor interactions produce an increase in the degree of polarization (hyperpolarization) either because of increasing membrane permeability to negative ions like chloride (thus adding additional negative molecules to the already negative intracellular environment) or by further decreasing permeability to positive ions (so that even more accumulate outside the membrane). This is called an IPSP, or *inhibitory postsynaptic potential*, which tends to inhibit the neuron from firing.

At any moment a neuron can be receiving dozens, perhaps even hundreds or thousands, of signals from many other neurons. Some can be EPSPs, while others might be IPSPs. When the amount of excitation from EPSPs crosses a threshold, the *threshold of excitation* or TOE, the neuron fires (Carlson, 1994). This is accomplished by a complete loss and even reversal of polarization of the axon for a tiny fraction of a second, due to the membrane's change in permeability to specific ions, which was triggered by the threshold amount of EPSPs. What happens is a domino effect, as follows: When the TOE is reached, sodium ion channels open, thus increasing the membrane's permeability to sodium, which allows it to rush into the cell down its concentration gradient. This causes the membrane to become more permeable to potassium, which, almost simultaneously with the sodium influx, rushes out of the cell down its concentration gradient. As this is happening, the membrane's sodium ion channels close, restoring its resistance to sodium. Next, the membrane rapidly becomes resistant to potassium ions again. At this point, the sodium–potassium pump removes sodium ions and retrieves potassium ions, thus restoring the membrane's resting potential. This

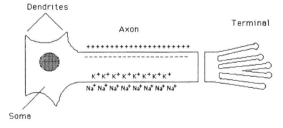

Figure 11.6. Schematic of a neuron's resting membrane potential illustrating the separation of sodium and potassium ions and the resultant charge differential.

complete sequence of events is termed the *action potential* and is initiated at the axon hillock, the conical area of origin of the axon from the nerve cell body.

The occurrence of the action potential at any given point along the axon triggers a similar succession of changes in the immediately adjacent portion of the axonal membrane. As the sequence is replicated there, a similar series of events arises in the next axonal segment and so on down the line. In this manner, the action potential is self-propagated like a wave along the entire length of the axon (Swonger & Constantine, 1983). Most neurons, however, have myelin sheaths covering most of their axons like insulation around an electric cord. Unlike an electric cord's continuous cover, the myelin sheaths surrounding axons have discrete segments called *nodes* where the axon's membrane is unsheathed (refer to Figure 11.4). This allows the action potential to jump from node to node, rather than traversing along the entire length of the axonal membrane, thus increasing the speed that nerve signals can travel. Indeed, according to Sherwood (1993), some large myelinated nerve fibers, such as those supplying skeletal muscles, conduct impulses as fast as 120 meters per second (360 miles per hour), compared with speeds of only a few millimeters per second (2 miles per hour) in small, unmyelinated fibers like those supplying the digestive tract.

When the action potential reaches the terminal portions of the axon, a cascade of events takes place that results in the release of neurotransmitters into the synaptic space—a process called *exocytosis*. Once released, the neurotransmitter diffuses across the synapse, where some of it binds to specific molecular receptors on the postsynaptic membrane. Depending on the type of neurotransmitter and the nature of the receptor, the neurotransmitter–receptor interaction will produce either an EPSP or an IPSP. When the sum of the EPSPs and IPSPs exceeds the TOE, the postsynaptic neuron will fire. This entire process is called neural transmission and is illustrated in Figure 11.8.

In addition to regulating ion channels in the cellular membrane, many neurotransmitter–receptor interactions activate second messenger systems. Although a detailed discussion of second messen-

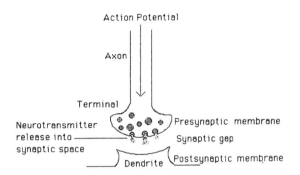

Figure 11.8. Close-up of synapse illustrating arrival of action potential and release of neurotransmitter into synapse.

ger systems is far beyond the scope of this chapter, suffice it to say that second messenger systems involve complex cascades of biological reactions that take place in the cell's interior. In such cases, the neurotransmitter is the first messenger that, upon binding to the receptor, activates or inhibits other chemicals inside the cell, which, then also function as chemical messengers. These second messengers, in turn, initiate a variety of physiologic events, usually involving activation of specific enzymes, that produce additional (third) chemical messengers and biochemical reactions that can ultimately influence the genetic functions of the cell (e.g., Craig & Stitzel, 1994; Hyman & Nestler, 1993).

Neurotransmitters

As described earlier, neurons are specialized cells uniquely adapted to receiving, integrating, and transmitting electrochemical impulses by way of neurotransmitter molecules. To be classified as a commonly accepted neurotransmitter, a substance must satisfy certain criteria. It must be synthesized and packaged in the cell body; be transported to and stored in vesicles at the axon terminals; be liberated via exocytosis into the synaptic gap upon depolarization; bind to specific molecular receptors where it produces a physiologic effect; and be associated with a process for its deactivation such as enzymatic degradation or reuptake. Currently the major types of neurotransmitters that can be classified according to chemical composition or molecular structure are the small-molecule transmitters, which include the biogenic amines and amino acids, and neu-ropeptides. Although a detailed summary of all of the known transmitter molecules is far beyond the scope of this chapter, we will highlight some of the important aspects of each type.

Often students of neurophysiology are eager to know if a given neurotransmitter is excitatory or in-hibitory. The answer to this commonly posed ques-tion can be answered in two words: "It depends." That is, whereas some transmitters (e.g., GABA) are typically described as inhibitory and others (e.g., norepinephrine) as excitatory, whether or not a given neurotransmitter produces an IPSP or an EPSP depends on the receptor it binds to. Most transmitters bind to several subtypes of receptors, not just one. For example, there are at least seven varieties of serotonin receptors, five kinds of dopamine receptors, and several receptors for nore-pinephrine (Hyman & Nestler, 1993). At some receptors, norepinephrine is excitatory (e.g., at most of its targets in the sympathetic nervous sys-tem), while at others it is inhibitory (e.g., at alpha-2 receptors in the locus ceruleus, a brainstem nu-cleus). Thus, there are probably no absolutely exci-tatory nor invariably inhibitory neurotransmitters. Postsynaptic potentials will always depend on the specific transmitter–receptor interaction. Further-more, many neurotransmitters are found all through the body, not only in the CNS, and play many differ-ent roles at these peripheral locations. Serotonin is widely distributed throughout the gut and on the surface of red blood cells. Epinephrine and norepi-nephrine are hormones released from the adrenal gland, and acetylcholine is the transmitter present at all neuromuscular junctions, to name only a few ex-amples.

The best known small-molecule neurotransmit-ters are the biogenic monoamines, which consist of a variety of chemicals including serotonin, norepi-nephrine, epinephrine (also called noradrenaline and adrenaline respectively—hence the terms *noradrenergic* and *adrenergic*), dopamine, acetyl-choline, and histamine. (Incidentally, the term *bio-genic* stems from the word *biogen*, which refers to a number of protoplasmic molecules that continually undergo secretion and absorption; recall that an amine is any molecule containing a substituted

ammonia group—that is, a nitrogen atom with a carbohydrate side chain. Hence, a biogenic mono-amine is a molecule with a single amino group that alternately undergoes secretion and absorption.)

Serotonin has many important functions in the CNS and is thought by some to be the "workhorse" of neurotransmitters, involved in sleep, arousal, motivation, appetite, and sex. Norepinephrine plays a "Paul Revere" role in the brain in that it sounds the alarms that mobilize our fight-or-flight stress response. Both serotonin and norepinephrine appear to be involved in depressive illnesses. Nore-pinephrine's chemical cousin, epinephrine, is not well understood as a neurotransmitter, but it ap-pears to be involved in regulating some autonomic (life support) processes. Dopamine is critically im-portant in mediating extrapyramidal motor control (to be discussed) and, when deficient, results in symptoms of Parkinson's disease. It is also in-volved in regulating the release of some important pituitary hormones, and seems inextricably woven into the processes that underlie psychotic thought disorders like schizophrenia. Acetylcholine's role in the CNS seems related to learning and memory. Alzheimer's disease, a progressive neurodegenera-tive illness whose hallmark is memory loss, appears to involve the degeneration of the brain's major ace-tylcholine-producing structure, the hippocampus. Although it is now known to be a neurotransmitter as well as a ubiquitous chemical outside of the CNS, histamine's function in the brain is not well under-stood.

The amino acid neurotransmitters that have been best elucidated are the predominantly inhibitory transmitters GABA (gamma-aminobutyric acid) and glycine; and glutamate and aspartate, both of which appear to be predominantly excitatory. In ad-dition to monoamines and amino acids, the brain contains an unknown number of peptide (small-protein) neurotransmitters called *neuropeptides*. Two of the most well studied neuropeptides are beta-endorphin, a naturally occurring opiate-like molecule, and substance P, which appears to be im-portant in conveying pain sensations. Many of the peptide transmitters are believed to act as neuro-modulators or neuroregulators by modulating or regulating the binding of other transmitters, like the monoamines and amino acids, at their receptors. They are also thought to exert longer lasting postsynaptic influences than the small-molecule transmitters (Carlson, 1994).

By far the most well studied neurotransmitters are the biogenic amine small-molecule transmitters, especially acetylcholine and norepinephrine, since they occur in high concentrations in the peripheral nervous system and are, therefore, more accessible and more segregated than centrally occurring transmitters. Ironically, despite being so well studied relative to other neurotransmitters, the biogenic amines collectively account for only 5% to 10% of the synapses in the human brain, whereas the amino acid transmitters account for up to 60% of CNS synapses (Kaplan & Sadock, 1991). While only a handful of neurotransmitters have been confidently classified to date, it is believed that as many as several hundred yet-to-be-identified neurotransmitters exist. To make matters still more complex, it is now known that most neurons have co-localized neurotransmitters (Hyman & Nestler, 1993); that is, a single neuron may produce and release more than one neurotransmitter. This recent discovery flies in the face of the long-held Dales hypothesis, which states "One neuron, one neurotransmitter." Indeed, it appears to be the norm that a given neuron can release as many as three different neurotransmitters simultaneously; usually one of each of the three major types—a biogenic amine along with an amino acid and a neuropeptide.

To complicate things even further, there are numerous permutations of synaptic connections (Hyman & Nestler, 1993). Most synapses are axodendritic; that is, the axon of one neuron synapses with the dendrite of another. But there are also axosomatic (axon-to-cell-body) and axoaxonic (one neuron's axon synapses with another neuron's axon) synapses, and dendrites also may make contact with each other in dendrodendritic connections. To introduce yet another layer of complexity, not all neurons communicate at chemical synapses. Some neurons interconnect at what are described as electrical synapses and actually pass ions back and forth directly into each other's cytoplasm (Kandel, Schwartz, & Jessell, 1991). Although it is becoming increasingly clear that electrical synapses play

many important
than a passing mentio
the scope of this chapter.
want to peruse Kandel, Sch
(1991). For our purposes, we will li
neurosynaptic communication to chem
mission only.

Neurons in and of themselves are not especial smart. As we have described, they can do very few things, such as fire or not fire, and communicate with a limited vocabulary of only a few types of chemicals. But put 100 billion of them together in a small area, and let each one "speak" with thousands of other neurons in very specific and precise ways, and a literal brainstorm of activity will take place, resulting in the infinite diversity of human conscious experience. Having outlined the fundamentals of neurophysiology and neural transmission, we will now discuss the brain's development starting in utero and progressing through adulthood.

In Utero Development of the Human Brain: Neurogenesis and Neuromigration

Very early in prenatal development the process of organogenesis begins—the formation of the organs during embryonic and fetal growth in the uterus. As we have described, the brain is by far the most complex organ of the body, so it is not surprising that the central nervous system (CNS) is the first organ system to begin developing, since it needs this head start (no pun intended) to ensure adequate size and function at birth. In fact, well within the first three weeks of development, the CNS is plainly evident as a strip of tissue, the neural plate, which runs down the embryo's back. By the eighteenth day of gestation, the neural plate folds in on itself, forming a neural groove which closes by the end of the first month to form the neural tube. Concurrently with the formation of the CNS, all the other organ systems of the body are also developing, but the process of neurogenesis is unequaled insofar as its rate of cell formation is simply astonishing.

At birth, a neonate has well over 100 billion neurons (for reasons we will describe, many more than it needs) which means that on average it is develop-

CAL PSYCHOLOGY

roles in neurophysiology, more
of them here is far beyond
Interested readers might
wartz, and Jessell
uit the focus of
ical trans-

a
in
ly.)
toge-
p but,
differ-
e of brain
ocation to
roduct is to
te, fetal alco-
devastating ef-
tec. es of neurogen-
esis and i. that alcohol and
many other dru. address of the mi-
grating neurons so tha. ve at the wrong des-
tinations, resulting in the p. sical and intellectual
malformations that are the hallmarks of fetal alcohol syndrome.)

Postnatal Development of the Human Brain: Dendrite Proliferation and Plasticity

These in utero neurodevelopmental phenomena are nothing less than astounding. During the first several years of life, the similarly spectacular neuromaturational processes of dendrite proliferation, neural pruning, and functional plasticity occur. As mentioned earlier, the neonate has many more neurons than it needs. It seems that the brain produces an enormous number of extra neurons because, unlike most other tissues of the body, the brain does not replace worn out or injured cells with new ones. Why this is so is a poorly understood mystery of neurobiology, but it may have to do with the persistence of memory. If the brain were constantly to replace its cells, it might not be able to retain memories since memories probably depend on very specific microstructural and neurochemical relationships among vast clusters of neurons. Replace one or more of the neurons in a cluster, and the entire configuration of synapses may change, since each cell is interconnected with as many as 10,000 other cells. So, not only would the brain cell itself have to be replaced, but every one of its thousands of specific synaptic elements would have be to du-

plicated exactly, too—a rewiring job that is, it seems, far too intricate for the brain to do successfully.

So, instead of replacing cells, the brain starts out with more cells than it ordinarily needs in a lifetime and hopes the organism that houses it won't do anything monumentally stupid like riding a bicycle without a helmet, driving in a car without a seat belt, or getting into a boxing ring. But how does the brain decide which neurons to keep and which ones are dispensable? The answer, in a word, is *experience*. At birth, a neonate emerges into a world of constant stimulation. Bewildering assortments of sights, sounds, smells, tastes, and textures are piped into the CNS, where the sensory data activate huge numbers of neurons in specific regions of the brain. At the same time, the newborn starts to move his or her muscles by breathing, crying, feeding, and generally wriggling around, which sends further information to the motor centers. This continuous bombardment of stimuli entering the CNS initiates a process known as dendrite proliferation. Although it may be true that the brain isn't producing any more neurons, per se, this early stimulation nevertheless fosters an incredible growth of dendrites, which branch out to form vast forests of connections with other neurons. In fact, the word *dendrite* derives form the Greek *dendron,* which means "tree," because under magnification they resemble trees with lots of branches. The more healthy stimulation a newborn receives, the more dendrite proliferation he or she will enjoy and the more intricately interconnected his or her brain will become.

When the connections among neurons are stimulated frequently, they form stable networks and communication pathways that may endure for the life of the individual. Alternatively, when formative neural networks and pathways are not reinforced enough, they decay. This process is called *neural pruning* because many of the elaborate branches of the dendritic trees actually dwindle when they are not fertilized with enough stimulation. Only those interconnections and pathways that are well rehearsed become strengthened and are likely to persist. As the saying goes, "Use it or lose it"—literally. The processes of dendrite proliferation and neural pruning occur throughout the life span but are most active during the first five years of life. Thereafter, far fewer new connections are formed in the brain despite the fact that pruning phenomena continue as a result of natural pathway decay and inevitable cell death. In fact, the proliferation of dendrites in very young brains is so impressive that they have an amazing potential for plasticity—that is, the capacity to adapt to changing circumstances like loss of tissue due to illness or injury.

If a mature adult suffers a catastrophic brain injury, depending on what regions of the brain are affected, he or she may never recover any significant amount of lost function. For example, if a stroke obliterates some of the speech centers in an adult brain, the victim will probably have significant, lifelong speech deficits, because the brain of an adult is not flexible enough to compensate for the damage by assigning new functions to other intact areas. But in the brain of a young child a similar loss of tissue may not have any far-reaching consequences because the child's brain, in the midst of dendrite proliferation, has ample opportunity to reroute vital connections and appoint other regions the function of speech. In essence, we can see from this brief description of dendrite proliferation, neural pruning, and plasticity that a remarkable reciprocal relationship exists between the brain and the environment. The structure and function of our brains determine our experience, and our experience determines the structure and function of our brains. We will now turn our attention to the structure and function of the fully developed adult brain.

Structure and Function of the Adult Human Brain

Because a comprehensive atlas of structural and functional neuroanatomy would fill more than this entire text, we will instead provide an overview of some of the brain's most obvious features. To reiterate an important point, our brains are really three brains in one: a primitive brainstem responsible for basic life support and some aspects of motor integration; a reptilian brain or limbic system responsible for much of our motivation, emotional experiences, and biological drives; and the cerebrum, the seat of our consciousness, intellectual abilities, and voluntary behavior. Refer to Figure 11.9 for an illustration of this structural arrangement and for some important neuroanatomical landmarks.

The brainstem is the portion of the CNS at the very top of the spinal cord at the base of the brain. It consists of two major parts, the *medulla oblongata* (often just called the *medulla*) and the *pons*, as well as an adjacent structure called the *cerebellum*. The medulla lies closest to the spinal cord and contains centers for the regulation of heartbeat, breathing, blood pressure, and muscle tone. It also houses important reflex centers for vomiting, coughing, sneezing, swallowing, and hiccuping. In addition, the medulla gives rise to the reticular formation, one of the oldest structures in the brain, a direct descendant of the primitive nerve nets (recall that *reticular* means "net-like"), which still functions as the nervous system in a creature like the hydra. The reticular formation receives sensory information from various pathways and relays it to the spinal cord, limbic system, and cortex. It plays important roles in sleep, arousal, selective attention, and controlling many of the reflexes mentioned earlier.

The pons is a rather large bulge in the brainstem lying right above the medulla, directly in front of the cerebellum. Like the medulla, it contains a portion of the reticular formation and is similarly important in sleep and arousal. Behind the pons sits the cerebellum ("little brain"), which, as its name implies, resembles a miniature cerebrum. It is covered by a cerebellar cortex and has a cluster of deep cerebellar nuclei that project to its cortex, just as the cerebrum has a set of internal nuclei that project to it. (In neuroanatomy, *nuclei*—plural of *nucleus*—are essentially homogeneous groups of nerve cells in the brain or spinal cord that can be clearly demarcated from neighboring cell groups.) The cerebellum makes it possible for us to stand, walk, and perform highly coordinated movements. It receives information from the cortex about vision, hearing, equilibrium, and individual muscle actions, which it then integrates to exert a balancing and coordinating effect on movements. Indeed, damage to the cerebellum results in abnormal motion patterns such as jerky and poorly coordinated movements.

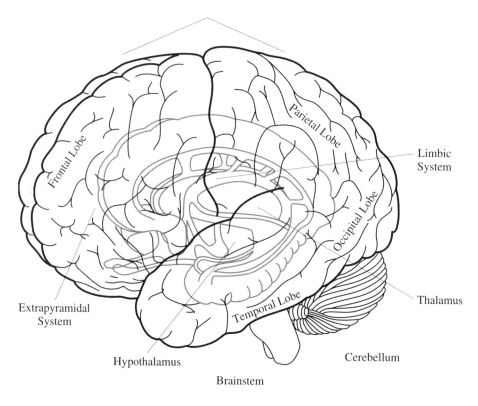

Figure 11.9. A human brain illustrating brainstem, limbic/subcortical structures, and cerebral cortex.

The next portion of the brain we will discuss is the limbic system, a set of interconnected structures lying deep within the brain. It appears that the limbic system originally formed most of the cortical surface of the CNS, but over the course of time was eclipsed by the *neocortex* ("new cortex") which swelled into the modern cerebral hemispheres, completely engulfing the older limbic structures so that they now appear as a curved border (hence the name—a *limbus* is a circular edge or border) deep in the brain's interior. The functions of the limbic system are many and complex. Much of it appears to be dedicated to governing emotion and motivation. It has nuclei that are important in regulating the body's inner environment (e.g., temperature control) and biologic drives like hunger, thirst, and sex. In addition, some of the limbic system is integrally involved with learning and memory.

The largest portion of the human brain is the cerebrum, which is responsible for conscious experience and voluntary behavior. The cerebrum is divided into halves by a deep longitudinal groove producing the right and left cerebral hemispheres, which are joined by a massive bridge of nerve fibers called the *corpus callosum* (see Figure 11.10).

The cerebral hemispheres are dramatically convoluted, which greatly increases their surface area relative to halves of an equally sized smooth brain. The convolutions consist of large grooves called *fissures*, smaller grooves called *sulci* (plural of *sulcus*), and *gyri* (plural of *gyrus*), which are the conspicuous bulges between adjacent grooves. In general terms, the entire cerebrum can be mapped according to its three major functions. First, there are *association areas,* which are believed to produce and control intellectual, creative and artistic,

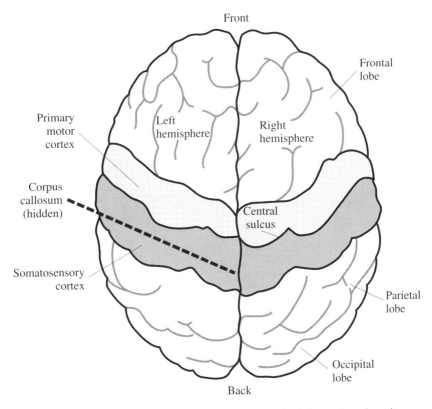

Figure 11.10. Top view of the brain illustrating longitudinal division into the right and left hemispheres and showing the corpus callosum.

learning and memory processes. Second, there are *sensory areas,* which receive afferent (directed toward a central organ or section, such as the CNS) nerve impulses from the sense organs to produce sensory experience. Third, the *motor areas* of the cerebrum initiate voluntary movements by way of efferent nerve impulses that send signals from the CNS to effectors such as muscles.

As shown in Figure 11.11, each cerebral hemisphere is further divided into four lobes, the frontals, parietals, temporals, and occipitals, each of which governs specific aspects of cognitive, sensory, and motor functions. The *frontal lobes* are responsible for much of the higher intellectual processes, including planning, concentrating, language production, complex problem solving, and judgment. In addition, the posterior region of the frontal lobe is the primary motor cortex, which allows us to move our skeletal muscles voluntarily.

Some people have suggested a dichotomy vis-à-vis the different functions of the right and left frontal lobes: The left lobe thinks in words and mediates rational, logical, and analytical operations, whereas the right lobe thinks spatially and governs processes like creativity, intuition, and artistry. Although some data support this division-of-labor model of the brain (e.g., Gazzaniga & LeDoux, 1978), it is generally agreed that the two hemispheres share information by virtue of their interconnectedness via the corpus callosum, and thus think holistically. One true dichotomous aspect of the brain, however, is the fact that as far as motor and sensory functions are concerned, the left hemisphere controls most of the right side of the body and the right hemisphere controls most of the left side of the body (see the discussion of decussation, to come).

The *parietal lobes*, which sit between the frontal and occipital lobes at the top of the brain, contain the

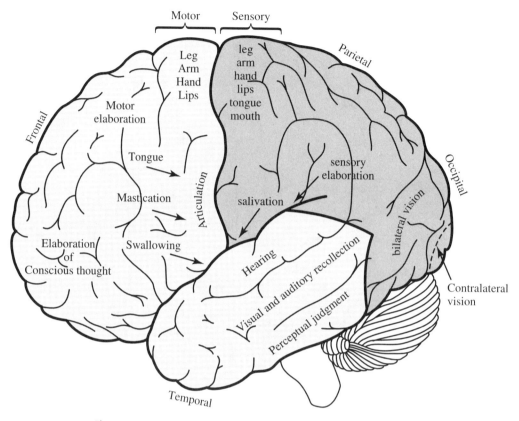

Figure 11.11. Side view of a cerebral hemisphere indicating its four lobes.

somatosensory cortexes that allow us to perceive sensations from our bodies and skin like touch, temperature, pressure, and pain. They also have association areas that function in the understanding of speech, interpretation of sensations, and use of words to express thoughts and feelings. Below the parietal lobes, partially under and behind the frontal lobes, are the *temporal lobes* which have sensory areas responsible for hearing and smell. Their association areas, like the parietals, aid in the interpretation of sensory experiences, especially complex sensory patterns like music and visual memory. The *occipital lobes* are the rearmost lobes of the cerebrum and contain the primary visual cortexes. Here is where the neurophysiological phenomena that give rise to the conscious experience of vision take place. The association areas of the occipital lobes function in visual interpretation and combine visual images with other sensory experiences.

Another crucial function of the brain is the initiation, coordination, and integration of voluntary movement. This aspect of behavior is carried out by the brain's motor systems, some of which we have already touched on, but warrant additional discussion because some drug therapies used in treating various clinical disorders can have dramatic impacts on motor functioning. Voluntary movement is the end product of a complex sequence of neuronal and muscular events involving the three major components of the motor system: the corticospinal tracts, the basal ganglia, and the cerebellum. The corticospinal nerve fibers originate at cell bodies in the motor cortex of the frontal lobe and pass through structures deep in the brainstem before continuing along the spinal cord, hence the name *corticospinal*, and ultimately to their targets at neuromuscular junctions.

Corticospinal nerve tracts *decussate* (cross over

like the arms of an X, X being the symbol for the Roman numeral 10, which derives from the Latin word *decussis*), where they pass through conspicuous, pyramid-shaped structures in the medulla called the *medullary pyramids*. For this reason, the corticospinal tracts are often referred to as the *pyramidal tracts* or the *pyramidal motor system.* Lesions of these fibers result in weakness or even total paralysis of mostly voluntary movement. Decussation of nerve fibers also explains why many sensory and motor functions are controlled by opposite sides of the brain. Sensory and motor fibers originating in the left cerebral hemisphere cross over to innervate corresponding tissues on the right side of the body, and vice versa. Thus, damage to left cerebral sensorimotor tissue results in deficits on the right side of the body, and right-hemisphere damage results in left-side deficits.

Another important motor system is made up of the *basal ganglia*, a group of interrelated structures lying deep in the forebrain. Unlike the corticospinal or pyramidal tracts, motor output from the basal ganglia does not pass through the medullary pyramids, and hence is called the extrapyramidal system. Lesions of this system cause involuntary movements like those seen in patients with Parkinson's disease. Indeed, some psychotropic medications, mainly the typical antipsychotic agents, produce Parkinsonian-like side effects and other so-called extrapyramidal symptoms (EPS) by interfering with dopamine transmission at the basal ganglia.

The last of the major motor systems is the cerebellum, which we have already discussed. Disorders of the cerebellum, are associated with abnormalities in the rate, range, and force of movement. In a healthy individual, the three motor systems work in concert to produce, integrate, refine, coordinate, and execute all voluntary motor behavior.

RESEARCH AND DIAGNOSTIC METHODS IN NEUROSCIENCE

A variety of methods and procedures now exist that allow clinicians and researchers to visualize the living human brain. While newer and more sophisticated imaging tools are constantly being invented, our current technology can provide us with only a mere peek through the keyhole into the marvelous territory of the living brain. Nevertheless, some of the techniques to be described have started a veritable revolution in our understanding of the structural and functional relationships among the brain's tissues and how these processes may relate to conscious experience.

Electroencephalography

One of the oldest and still widely used noninvasive methods of neuroscience is electroencephalography (EEG), which utilizes electrodes placed on the scalp to measure the gross electrical activity of the brain. The actual instrument is the *electroencephalograph,* and the graphic brain wave tracings it produces is the *electroencephalogram*. According to Kaplan and Sadock (1991), EEG wave forms are classified as follows: Delta waves are less than 4 cycles per second (hertz or Hz) and are present usually only during deep sleep. Theta waves fall between 4 and 8 Hz and are also characteristic of sleep. Alpha waves equal 8 to 13 Hz and are normally present in an awake adult whose eyes are closed. Beta waves are greater than 13 Hz and usually replace alpha activity when a person opens his or her eyes or is mentally stimulated. Interpretation of the EEG involves a visual inspection of the frequency (speed) and amplitude (size or height) of the various wave tracings and an inspection for unusual spikes or bursts of activity, which may indicate epileptic or seizure events.

Computed Tomography

Tomography refers to any of several techniques for making X-ray pictures of two-dimensional planar sections of a three-dimensional object by blurring out the images of all the other planes. Computed tomography (CT), also referred to as computerized axial tomography (CAT), is one such technique that utilizes computers to generate images of anatomical slices or even a three-dimensional reconstruction of an entire organ. The more radiation a tissue absorbs, the lighter it appears; the less radiation a tissue absorbs, the darker it appears in the computerized image. In the brain, lesions of 0.5 centimeters (0.39 inches) usually show up well on cross-sectional CT images. CT is useful in a variety of diagnostic considerations, including evaluating patients for dramatic or acute disorders like strokes, traumas, and tumors. It is also useful in the workup of some psychiatric patients who present with dementia; confusion; or mood, movement, or thought disorders of unknown cause. Though an excellent tool for examining bony structures and calcifications, for determining the presence or absence of masses or lesions, and for evaluating the overall architecture of the brain, CT is limited insofar as it cannot discriminate gray matter (cell bodies) from white matter (axons) and reveals little about cerebral metabolism. For these purposes, MRI and PET studies, respectively, are much better.

Magnetic Resonance Imaging

Previously called nuclear magnetic resonance spectroscopy (NMR), and used for many years as a tool in organic chemistry for the identification of organic molecules, magnetic resonance imaging (MRI) has recently become one of the most widely used noninvasive diagnostic tools in medicine and neuroscience. When a powerful magnetic field is applied to the brain or to any soft tissue, the hydrogen nuclei in the tissue's water molecules become aligned in a very precise way and resonate at a specific frequency. When exposed to electromagnetic pulses, the resonating hydrogen nuclei emit characteristic energy patterns that are analyzed by a computer to produce the final image. The pictures produced by MRI are perhaps the most highly resolved and detailed of all brain-imaging techniques. Unlike CT, MRI can clearly delineate gray matter from white matter and is, therefore, excellent in detecting demyelinating lesions like those seen with multiple sclerosis and other demyelinating illnesses. Another advantage of MRI over CT is that it does not expose the patient to X-rays. Because of the strong magnetic field it uses, however, MRI is contraindicated in patients with steel surgical appliances, metal skull plates, and cardiac pacemakers. Though unequaled in providing exceptionally well resolved images of the brain's anatomy, standard MRI pro-

cedures cannot tell us much about what is going on in the brain metabolically. For that, PET is currently the procedure of choice.

Positron Emission Tomography

Unlike CT and MRI, positron emission tomography (PET) allows neuroscientists to assess actual ongoing metabolic activity in cortical and subcortical regions of the brain. PET is an astonishing tool that has literally opened up completely new windows onto the landscape of neurophysiology and is helping to advance our understanding of normal and abnormal brain function like nothing previously imagined. For PET studies, organic molecules—usually glucose—that have been labeled with positron-emitting atoms are administered to the patient or subject (a *positron* is a subatomic particle of the same mass as an electron, but with a positive charge). When the radioactive glucose reaches the brain, it is taken up by neurons where positrons are emitted, which collide with electrons that are normally present in the cell's tissue, producing photons that are detected by the PET camera and assembled by computer into a composite color image. The different colors of the image reflect the degrees of metabolism in the tissues of the brain. Since neurons' glucose utilization is directly proportional to their metabolic activity, the more radioactive glucose they take up, the more photons they will emit and the brighter they will appear on the computer-generated composite. Thus, on a PET scan, the brighter colors (red, orange, and yellow) indicate regions with the most metabolic activity, and darker colors (green, blue, and violet) correspond to less metabolically active areas. From PET data, we can make inferences about what regions of the brain seem to control, mediate, or govern phenomenological and conscious experiences.

Functional MRI

Functional MRI is a new method that combines the excellent anatomical resolution of MRI pictures with information about regional brain metabolism similar to that produced with PET scans. This is accomplished by MRI instruments that image elements other than hydrogen, such as phosphorus nuclei, which have functional and metabolic significance (Kaplan & Sadock, 1991). Another functional MRI methodology measures changes in cerebral blood oxygen levels that occur when neuronal activity induces small changes in the brain's microvasculature (Fogel & Schiffer, 1996). So far, functional MRI has successfully measured metabolism in the visual cortex and in the primary motor cortex.

Cerebrospinal Fluid Neurotransmitter Metabolite Assays

In addition to cortical and subcortical gray and white matter, the brain contains another important feature, the fluid-filled ventricles. The ventricles are a series of hollow, interconnected chambers deep within the brain that are filled with a liquid called *cerebrospinal fluid* (CSF). CSF is produced in the brain from blood by a special vascular structure called the *choroid plexus*. The brain is continuously making CSF, which circulates through the ventricles as well as all around the exterior of the brain and in the central canal of the spinal cord. After circulating for several hours, the CSF is reabsorbed back into the bloodstream. One of the functions of CSF is to bathe the brain in a protective cushion of liquid, which reduces the pressures exerted on it by gravity and inertia, especially at its base. As CSF circulates around and within the CNS, it collects various substances, including neurotransmitter metabolites.

After participating in neural transmission, many neurotransmitters are biochemically transformed (metabolized) by specific enzymes. (As we will describe in the next chapter on psychopharmacology, some of these neurotransmitter-metabolizing enzymes can be intentionally paralyzed to produce clinical improvement. For example, the monoamine oxidase inhibitors, MAOIs, block the activity of the enzyme monoamine oxidase, which normally breaks down monoamine neurotransmitters like dopamine, norepinephrine, and serotonin, and are effective pharmacotherapeutics for depressive illness.) The products of this enzymatic degradation are called *metabolites* and include chemicals that are specific to a given neurotransmitter. For example, dopamine's primary metabolites are DOPAC (dihydroxyphenylacetic acid) and HVA (homovanillic acid); norepinephrine's major metabolite is MHPG (3-methoxy-4-hydroxy-phenylglycoaldehyde); and serotonin's principal metabolite is 5HIAA (5-hydroxyindole acetic acid). By evaluating the concentrations of neurotransmitter metabolites in CSF, one can make inferences about the amount of transmitter activity going on in the brain. As currently practiced, however, CSF neurotransmitter metabolite assays are not very useful in diagnosing psychopathology because metabolites from the spinal cord can significantly contribute to the CSF, and transmitter metabolites from deep brain structures might not reach the CSF efficiently (Kaplan & Sadock, 1991).

Neuropsychological Assessment

Despite their great value in research and diagnosis, the brain-imaging, electrophysiological, and fluid assay techniques outlined here are often inadequate to the task of clinical psychological assessment. Some neurophysiological phenomena that have important clinical manifestations simply cannot be detected, measured, or resolved with even the most sophisticated neuroimaging equipment. In these cases, when it seems likely that a patient is suffering some impairment of brain functioning but nothing turns up on a thorough medical or neurological exam, neuropsychological testing can prove extremely useful. Since we have already introduced the major aspects of neuropsychology in Chapter 3, we will simply reiterate here that the task of neuropsychology is to understand patients whose behavioral, cognitive, emotional, or perceptual difficulties are, or may be, due to cerebral dysfunction. This determination is made by testing the patient with a variety of methods and instruments, mostly question and answer, paper-and-pencil, and object manipulation tests, each of which measures a specific and different dimension of psychological functioning (Lezak, 1983). Depending on the results of the evaluation, localization of impairment, which may be due to an injury or abnormality that was undetectable with neuroimaging, can be inferred. Then a plan can be devised to help the patient compensate for or recover deficits or lost functioning. Some of the most frequently used tests in neuropsychology are the Halstead-Reitan and Luria-Nebraska batteries, as well as many of the Wechsler intelligence and memory scales.

BIOLOGICAL DYSREGULATION AND PSYCHOPATHOLOGY

On the basis of our discussion of the brain thus far—its origins, evolution, development, architecture, and function—it is easy to see why we have described it as perhaps the most intricate single structure on the planet and certainly the most complex organ of the body. As much as we appear to know about this marvelous matter of consciousness, our understanding pales to utter insignificance when compared to the enormity of what we have yet to learn about the brain. Indeed, despite the astounding advancements in technology we are in the midst of enjoying, the enterprise of neuroscience is still in its infancy. Nevertheless, despite our knowledgeable ignorance, we have in recent years been able to glean enough reliable data to make certain guesses and inferences about the brain's normal and abnormal functioning. One thing is very clear: Normal brain function depends on an extremely delicate biochemical balance. Even a slight change in the concentration or activity of a single neurotransmitter can cause a physiologic chain reaction, resulting in profound and far-reaching psychological repercussions.

There is a plethora of material addressing the psychosocial etiology (the science and study of the causes and courses of diseases) of psychopathology dating back well over a century, to the time of Freud. Lately, a similarly growing volume of literature has focused on biologic theories of psychological disorders. Interestingly, some of the more recent biologic studies have shed light on just how false the dichotomy of mind versus body or psychological versus physiological is. Indeed, as this chapter has tried to emphasize, the mind and the body are different sides of the same coin and, as we will explore, the two sides intersect at the level of psychological functioning, where remarkable and

reciprocal influences occur. Thus, while the etiologic theories of psychopathology to be discussed are decidedly biologic, we trust our readers will know that we are presenting just one side of the coin, and it is understood that this reductionistic slant is only a heuristic thread to be woven into the Gestalt of a biopsychosocial tapestry. Given the enormity of the field and the limits of this chapter, only a few representative examples will be presented here.

Major Depression

There are many sources of information that support a biologic theory of causation for depression. These include genetic data, especially monozygotic adoptive studies (identical twins separated at birth and raised in different families), which suggest a profound genetic loading for the illness. PET studies have indicated decreased levels of metabolic activity in the parts of the prefrontal cortex in depressed patients (Baxter, 1991). Assays of CSF from depressed patients have found abnormally low levels of serotonin and norepinephrine metabolites. Sleep EEG studies have indicated abnormal sleep patterns in patients with depression, especially a tendency to enter REM unusually early in the sleep cycle. But perhaps the most compelling evidence in support of a biological etiology of depressive illness is the remarkable effectiveness of the antidepressant medications. These data collectively have led to the development of the biogenic amine, or monoamine, theory of depression, which posits that depressive symptoms are due to a deficiency of either or both serotonin and norepinephrine in crucial structures of the limbic system, especially the hypothalamus.

Recall that the limbic system appears to govern important aspects of mood, memory, and motivation, and that the hypothalamus seems to control many basic physical states and biological drives like sleep cycles, energy, appetite, libido, and pleasure. Interestingly, when people become depressed, the typical symptoms they experience include changes in mood, memory, motivation, sleep patterns, energy, appetite, libido, and pleasure. Clearly, the pathophysiology (alteration in normal function as distinguished from structural defects) of depression involves the processes of the limbic system and its relationships with other brain and body systems. As we will explore in the next chapter, the mechanism of action (MOA) of the best available antidepressant medications involves increasing the amounts of monoamines like serotonin and norepinephrine at central synapses. Thus, when the brain's serotonergic and noradrenergic pathways get a "shot in the arm," the symptoms of depression often remit.

What causes these neurochemical deficiencies in the first place, however, is still unclear. Furthermore, it is possible that depression symptoms are due to alterations in receptor or enzyme functioning rather than changes in neurotransmitter concentrations per se. For example, perhaps there are too few or too many specific monoamine receptors, or too much neurotransmitter-metabolizing enzyme activity. In fact, the observation that synaptic effects (more neurotransmitter in the synapse) of antidepressants are achieved within hours of drug administration, while therapeutic effects (symptom improvement) usually take weeks of continuous drug use, suggests that there is far more to the pathophysiology of depression than mere monoamine deficiencies.

Obsessive-Compulsive Disorder

Once thought to be a rare disorder, obsessive-compulsive disorder (OCD) is now known to be much more common than was once believed, affecting as many as 2% to 3% of the U.S. population (Preston, O'Neal, & Talaga, 1994). The major features of OCD are recurring obsessions (persistent intrusive, anxiety-provoking thoughts, images, or impulses that are recognized by the patient as senseless) and compulsions (repetitive behaviors or rituals that are performed in response to an obsession in an effort to neutralize anxiety, such as excessive checking, washing, counting, or touching). In recent years a number of findings from neurobiology, medication research, and clinical practice have provided convincing evidence for a physiological basis for OCD. Some of these data are based on the fact that OCD tends to run in families and hence

seems to have a genetic loading. More convincing, however, is that in double-blind, placebo-controlled medication research studies, very few OCD patients improve on placebo, whereas a considerable proportion of depressives, panic sufferers, and generally anxious patients do. Even more compelling are data from neuroimaging studies like PET scans that have revealed an abnormally active metabolic circuit in the brains of OCD sufferers that does not appear to be present in the brains of non-psychiatric people. This hyperactive circuit appears to involve the supraorbital (directly above the eye socket) prefrontal lobe, as well as limbic structures like the caudate nucleus and thalamus. Furthermore, it has been demonstrated that when OCD patients are successfully treated with either serotonergic antidepressants or behavior therapy, the hypermetabolic activity normalizes (Baxter et al., 1992).

These observations and data have led to a two-pronged biologic theory of OCD (Preston et al., 1994). The first part is that the frontal lobes normally act to inhibit the emergence of primitive behaviors or instinctual urges related to grooming, nest building, and patrolling territorial boundaries. These primitive and instinctual behavioral routines are common in many species and must confer adaptive or survival advantages to them. In humans with OCD, these rituals probably stem from abnormal neuronal activity in certain limbic nuclei that are not successfully overridden by the frontal lobes. Hence, washing, cleaning, and checking may reflect the excessive breakthrough of once adaptive primal urges that are deeply rooted in the primitive tissues of the brain.

The second aspect of the model holds that similarly ancient and adaptive neuronal mechanisms exist to serve animals in times of potential danger. This model suggests that when danger threatens, the frontal lobes guide and direct sustained mental focus and attention by activating the limbic structures, which feed back to the frontal lobes to maintain alertness and vigilance. Thus, the frontal lobes function as a launching pad for worry, which mobilizes the limbic system, which in turn helps the organism to stay alert until the danger has passed or has been dealt with, at which time the reverberating worry circuit shuts off. In OCD, it is presumed that the automatic worry shutoff fails to stop the neural loop, so that the brain continues viscerally and emotionally to sense danger even when there is cognitive evidence that the threat is over. This causes the person to try to shut off the worry manually by engaging in rituals that are maladaptive efforts to neutralize anxiety. Evidently, activation of serotonergic pathways in the overactive limbic structures has an inhibitory effect on the hyperactive worry circuit, which leads to symptom improvement. This explains why the serotonergic antidepressants are effective treatments for OCD, whereas other types of medications that have more limited effects on serotonin transmission are not. Apparently behavior therapy produces similar effects at the frontal, caudate, thalamic circuit, as evidenced by its great success rate and PET study data (Baxter et al., 1992).

Panic Disorder

Imagine feeling fine, minding your own business, when suddenly out of the blue you're gripped by an overwhelming sense of intense fear. Suddenly you feel dizzy, your chest tightens, and you have trouble catching your breath. Your heart races; you shake, tingle, feel nauseous, and break into a cold sweat.

Sounds like a heart attack, right? Wrong! As surprising as it sounds, we have just described a classic panic attack. Panic attacks are often unpredictable, sudden-onset, usually brief periods of intense fear associated with a variety of frightening physical symptoms. And yes, many panic sufferers do present at the emergency room convinced they have had a coronary or a stroke.

Perhaps the most current and elegant biological model of panic disorder is based on the inappropriate activation of the "hard-wired" neuroendocrine pathways responsible for eliciting the fight-or-flight stress response. In times of actual or perceived danger, the brain triggers a complex, multi-leveled neurochemical and hormonal reaction with the sole purpose of mobilizing the animal to take rapid and vigorous action. This involves the activation of the stress response, which turns off nones-

sential physiological systems (parasympathetically mediated processes like digestion, elimination, and reproduction) and stimulates much needed sympathetic functions like increasing heart rate, blood pressure, and oxygen consumption, which prepare the organism for potentially life-saving action (i.e., fighting to be the diner rather than the dinner, or fleeing to safety if possible). In panic disorder, it seems, this normally adaptive alarm reaction is excessively sensitive and, consequently, fires off false alarms at inappropriate times.

One of the brain structures that seems to play an important role in the pathophysiology of panic disorder is a small cluster of norepinephrine-containing cells deep in the brainstem called the *locus ceruleus* (from the Latin for "blue place" because it appears as a small, bluish area). Amazingly, the locus ceruleus (LC) contains only about 20,000 neurons, but its axons have a remarkably wide distribution throughout much of the cortex and the limbic system. When the cortex perceives danger, it signals the LC to trigger the fight-or-flight response. For this reason, the LC is described by some as the adrenal gland of the brain (e.g., Preston et al., 1994). If for any reason the LC is functioning with a "hair trigger," it will fire off excessive and inappropriate fight-or-flight reactions.

Another hypothesized contribution the LC makes to panic disorder has to do with autoinhibition. In addition to projecting widely throughout the brain, the LC has axons that synapse with its own cell bodies. At these (alpha-2 noradrenergic) autoreceptors, norepinephrine produces IPSPs that reduce the excitability of the LC cell bodies. In panic disorder, however, this inhibitory autoreceptor mechanisms is thought to be dysfunctional so that, once stimulated, the LC continues to fire [false] alarm signals to the limbic system and cortex, uninhibited by the normal braking function of its autoreceptor stimulation.

Psychotropic medications that work well in treating panic disorder include the antidepressants and benzodiazepines (drugs like Klonopin, Valium, and Xanax). The MOA of the noradrenergic antidepressants (e.g., Tofranil) is thought to be mediated by their ability to increase the amount of norepinephrine at the LC inhibitory autoreceptor synapses, thus increasing the braking ability of this mechanism to reduce LC excitation. Similarly, the serotonergic antidepressants (e.g., Prozac) are believed to exert their therapeutic effects by stimulating inhibitory serotonin receptors on LC dendrites and cell bodies. The antipanic effects of benzodiazepines are brought about by these drugs' GABA-ergic activity. Recall that GABA is a predominantly inhibitory amino acid neurotransmitter that hyperpolarizes many neurons by binding to and opening chloride ion channels in the cell membrane, allowing an influx of chloride ions to take place. Since chloride is a negative ion, when it enters a cell, the cell is pushed further away from firing (due to hyperpolarization). Benzodiazepines bind to the same chloride ion channel that GABA binds to, thus potentiating the effects of GABA at its receptors. These drugs probably stabilize the excitation of the LC by facilitating the inhibitory actions of GABA at its cell bodies.

Schizophrenia

Recognized for thousands of years as a clinical syndrome, schizophrenia was described by the Hippocratic school as "dementia," distinct from "mania" and "melancholia." In the late 1800s, Kraepelin described a syndrome he called *dementia praecox* ("premature dementia"). Over the centuries there have been numerous etiologic theories about this tragic and debilitating illness, including religious, social, and psychological explanations. Among all the psychological disorders commonly seen by clinicians, however, perhaps none has as compelling a biological foundation as schizophrenia.

Early evidence for a biologic cause of schizophrenia came from family and twin studies, which indicated a strong genetic component to the illness. More recent evidence comes from neuroimaging studies such as CT scans that reveal structural abnormalities like enlarged ventricles and widened cortical sulci in the brains of schizophrenics. PET studies with schizophrenics have demonstrated decreased activity in the frontal cortex, MRI scans have shown abnormally small hippocampal structures, and CSF assays have found a positive correla-

tion between HVA (a dopamine metabolite) levels and clinical severity (Preston et al., 1994). Furthermore, as is the case with OCD, schizophrenics do not improve on placebos. The final piece of biologic evidence supporting a neurobiological etiology of schizophrenia is the efficacy of the antipsychotic medications, which has led to the dopamine hypothesis.

The dopamine hypothesis postulates that the symptoms of schizophrenia are caused by overactivity of dopamine in a number of different brain regions. In the basal ganglia, for instance, dopamine is crucial to the regulation of motor functioning. In the limbic and brainstem areas, it plays a vital role in emotional control and in filtering stimuli. In the cortex, dopamine is probably involved in a variety of cognitive and perceptual processes. Hence, excessive dopaminergic activity can lead to behavioral agitation (via the basal ganglia), failure to screen stimuli adequately (via brainstem and thalamic nuclei), inappropriate emotional states (via various limbic structures), and disorganization of perception and thought (via cortical areas). This theory is supported by two main lines of evidence. First, as mentioned, there are very effective medications for schizophrenia. All of them, to date, block dopamine receptors in parts of the limbic system and cortex. Second, drugs that potentiate or increase dopamine activity (such as amphetamines) can induce a psychotic reaction that is essentially indistinguishable from paranoid schizophrenia, and, if given to schizophrenics, dopaminergic drugs can intensify psychotic symptoms.

Although the dopamine theory has a lot of merit, it is incomplete insofar as it does not explain why almost 30% of schizophrenic patients do not benefit from traditional antipsychotic drugs. Indeed, recently the characteristics of schizophrenia have been expanding (e.g., Preston et al., 1994) and now include at least three symptom constellations that suggest it is a heterogeneous disorder. There are positive symptoms, which are excesses like hallucinations, delusions, agitation, and bizarre behavior. There are negative symptoms, or deficits, such as lacking pleasure (anhedonia), apathy, reduced emotional range, poverty of thought, and impaired motivation. The third cluster, described as "characterological" symptoms, include social isolation, feelings of inadequacy, and poor social skills. Although positive symptoms respond well to typical, dopamine-blocking antipsychotic drugs, negative and characterological symptoms do not. In the next chapter, we will have more to say about drug therapies for schizophrenia and about psychopharmacology in general.

As compelling as some of these biologic data are, it is very important to consider that correlation does not imply causation. Just because we know that dopamine receptor blockers reduce some of the symptoms of schizophrenia, we cannot state emphatically that schizophrenia is caused by an excess of dopamine. All we can say confidently is that one piece of the schizophrenia puzzle seems to involve excessive dopaminergic activity in the CNS. But whether or not this is a cause-and-effect relationship or merely a correlational finding remains to be determined. It is possible that some other variable is the causative agent responsible for the symptoms of schizophrenia—for example, a virus that results in excessive dopamine synthesis or hyperactive dopamine receptors. Similarly, when explaining the biological underpinnings of depression, OCD, panic—or any clinical condition, for that matter— we must be careful not to conclude prematurely that we have the answer. Remember, while we have accumulated an impressive body of solid scientific data, the discipline of neuroscience is still in the stone ages. In trying to understand the human brain, it is as if we are reasonably intelligent apes attempting to fathom how a computer works by sticking nails in it and then measuring their voltages or by passing electric currents through it and watching how it reacts (or by noting how its function changes when we knock pieces off of it with a hammer, or when we gum up its inner workings with mud, sap, or sand).

DIFFERENTIAL DIAGNOSIS OF COMMON MEDICAL CONDITIONS

Several times throughout this chapter we have referred to the human brain as the most complex single entity in existence (at least on our planet, as far as we know). Perhaps the only thing even more

elaborate than the brain itself is the human organism in toto. Indeed, the brain exists in the ecosystem of the body and participates in a multitude of reciprocal relationships with all of the other organ systems. Just as the brain controls and influences the other tissues of the body, the other organs of the body can influence and affect the brain. Since the brain is the seat of conscious experience and gives rise to thoughts, feelings, and actions, anything that affects the brain can have a profound effect on psychological functioning. Thus, it will come as no surprise to learn that there are a great number of medical illnesses and conditions that can masquerade as psychological disturbances. Clearly, before one can treat a problem, it must first be confidently identified, since the foundation of effective therapy is accurate diagnosis. Therefore, all competent clinicians must be good diagnosticians who are well versed in the science and art of differential diagnosis—that is, in differentiating among a range of possible conditions and systematically excluding them one by one until the most probable diagnosis has been rendered. Again, because many diseases and conditions can present as apparent psychological disorders, it is the job of the mental health providers to shed light on the true nature of the problem so they can confidently treat it with psychological interventions or, if necessary, refer the patient to an appropriate medical specialist.

Good and Nelson (1991) have suggested the useful mnemonic MED'CL to help in categorizing many of the medical conditions that present as or with psychological symptoms. M stands for Metal poisoning; E refers to Endocrine system malfunction; D addresses the many Drug reactions like side effects and toxicity that can occur; C refers to Cancers and malignancies that produce psychological symptoms; and L stands for Lots of others since there is a potpourri of other important medical disorders that mimic psychopathologies.

Some of the more common metal poisonings include lead (most common in children who live in older homes containing lead-based paint), mercury (in people who work in vacuum pump and thermometer manufacturing), aluminum (present in many antacids), manganese (used in the battery-manufacturing industry), arsenic (found in some pesticides), and bromides (found in some old-time medicinal preparations). All of these metals can affect the CNS by binding to crucial metabolic enzymes, thus leading to a host of physical, psychological, and neurological symptoms. Often a simple blood test ordered by a medical doctor can diagnose metal poisoning or intoxication. In some cases, as with lead and mercury, treatment involves chelation therapy. This is when substances called *chelating agents* (pronounced "KEY-late-ing"), like EDTA and dimercaprol, are administered to patients. In the body, chelators pull the metal out of circulation, or away from enzymes, by binding to it, resulting in a metal–chelate complex that can be eliminated in the urine.

There are a variety of endocrinopathies (pathologies of the endocrine systems) that masquerade as psychopathologies, especially thyroid and adrenal disorders. The thyroid gland, located in the front of the neck, is responsible for regulating general metabolism, which it does through its principal hormone thyroxine. If the thyroid produces too little thyroxine, hypothyroidism results and can present as almost identical to depressive illness. In other cases, excessive production of thyroxine, hyperthyroidism, can mimic symptoms of anxiety disorders. Similarly, hypo- or hyperfunction of the adrenal glands (the pyramid-shaped glands that sit atop the kidneys) can lead to a host of psychological symptoms. The outer layer of the adrenals (called the *adrenal cortex*) produces a variety of steroid hormones that participate in many physiologic processes. One of them, *cortisol*, acts on carbohydrate metabolism and influences the nutrition and growth of various tissues. When the adrenals produce too much cortisol, a condition called Cushing's disease might result, which can produce psychological symptoms akin to mania and depression. The opposite condition, adrenocortical hypofunction, can result in a condition called Addison's disease, which can also imitate depression. Thyroid and adrenal function can be assessed easily using standard medical evaluations, including blood tests that measure the amount of circulating hormones, and hormone-releasing or -stimulating factors.

One additional endocrinopathy that warrants mention is a condition called pheochromocytoma.

As mentioned earlier, the adrenal cortex produces and releases steroid hormones like cortisol. The inner portion of the adrenal gland is referred to as the *adrenal medulla* and produces and releases the catecholamines epinephrine and norepinephrine—the same chemicals that function as neurotransmitters in the brain—which are important hormones in the periphery. When a tumor in the adrenal medulla causes great bursts of epinephrine and norepinephrine to enter the bloodstream, it can feel like a panic attack to the patient. Besides mimicking panic symptoms, pheochromocytomas cause discrete episodes of hypertension (elevated blood pressure), which can aid in its diagnosis. In addition to blood pressure monitoring, a 24-hour urine collection test can determine the presence or absence of abnormal catecholamine metabolite levels, which provides a useful "compass" for the diagnostician.

Certain medications, including prescription, over-the-counter (OTC), and "recreational" drugs, are notorious for causing psychological disturbances. Some of the most common offenders are the older antihypertensives (e.g., reserpine and propranolol), which are known to cause depression. As mentioned earlier in our discussion of schizophrenia, amphetamines can lead to psychotic reactions, as can other illicit drugs like PCP. Interestingly, many people think that just because a drug is available OTC, it is safe to use. The truth is that many OTC preparations can be extremely dangerous. For example, OTC diet pills can lead to severe insomnia, nervousness, and even dangerous elevations in blood pressure. Even seemingly innocuous substances like antacids can lead to severe metabolic imbalances if used too frequently. As for recreational drug use, alcohol is a huge contributor to the incidence of depression, and caffeine use is linked to chronic anxiety and acute panic attacks. The list goes on almost endlessly. Just about any drug, or any substance for that matter, if used improperly, can lead to toxicity that can dramatically affect psychological functioning.

Malignancies also can cause changes in mental status, personality, and psychological functioning. Pancreatic cancers frequently cause severe depression, which can be the presenting complaint. Lung tumors can have a dramatic impact on the CNS and lead to psychological symptoms like dementia. And, as mentioned before, pheochromocytomas can produce a clinical picture similar to that seen with panic disorder.

A hodgepodge of other medical conditions can produce or present as psychological problems. These include metabolic disorders like Wilson's disease (a disorder of copper metabolism) and acute intermittent porphyria (the "madness" of King George III) to name only two. There are also hereditary illnesses like Huntington's disease, vitamin deficiencies, electrolyte imbalances, and hard-to-detect seizure phenomena that can all challenge the most skillful diagnostician.

The upshot here is simple. Many people seeking professional attention for a psychological complaint should have a thorough medical evaluation before being treated with either psychosocial or psychotropic interventions. Of course, this doesn't mean that every patient with mild complaints of everyday living, or relationship problems, should be given a complete medical workup before starting psychotherapy. It does mean, however, that psychologists and other nonmedical mental health providers need to beware of the myriad organic causes of psychopathologies. Only then can they intelligently refer to other clinicians for further tests or treatment, and work closely with primary care physicians so that patients can receive the most appropriate and comprehensive services that they may need.

HEALTH PSYCHOLOGY AND BEHAVIORAL MEDICINE

One of the most recent and exciting developments in modern psychological science involves recognition of its increasing confluence with the disciplines of medicine, neuroscience, and biology. For example, the emerging field of psychoneuroimmunology (PNI) has demonstrated that psychological phenomena can affect various nervous system processes that can ultimately have an impact on immune function. In other words, as we have underscored several times in this chapter, in humans, psychology and biology are different sides of the same coin and are inextricably woven together into the complete tapestry of our being. Indeed, the mind and the body influence and determine each other in ways we are only beginning to understand. This far-from-complete understanding of the interactive and mutually deterministic nature of the mental and physical aspects of the human organism has opened windows and doors onto new territories in health science and clinical practice.

One excellent example of this physiology/psychology reciprocal determinism comes from the work of Baxter et al. (1992), as outlined earlier in the section on OCD. Recall that Baxter's PET scan data revealed an abnormally active metabolic circuit in the brains of OCD sufferers that does not appear to be present in the brains of other people. Furthermore, when OCD patients are treated successfully with serotonergic antidepressants, the hypermetabolic activity normalizes. But the astonishing thing is that when OCD patients are successfully treated with behavioral therapy, their brain scans look normal, too! Thus, regardless of the treatment modality—drugs or behavior therapy—similar or possibly even the same curative (or at least palliative) neurobiological changes can be achieved. This means that with many psychological conditions, even ones with profound biological underpinnings like OCD, treatment can involve either *taking* something for the condition (i.e., psychotropics) or *doing* something about it (i.e., behavior therapy). In some cases, both medication and psychological therapy can be undertaken concurrently, which often produces a desirable synergistic effect ("1 + 1 = 3").

In general, we can conceptualize health psychology as an emerging field that capitalizes on the mutual influences of psychological and biological processes, thus promoting mental and physical well-being through methods that involve cultivating healthy lifestyle patterns. Similarly, behavioral medicine can be thought of as any of a number of health-promoting interventions that do not rely on the use of physical medicine. For example, consider the treatment of essential hypertension (high blood pressure without any detectable cause). A person is told by his or her doctor that he or she has hypertension, which can be treated by any one of several antihypertensive medications. Or, he or she is told, a program of lifestyle change involving losing 10 pounds, eliminating extra salt and fats from the diet, getting frequent cardiovascular exercise, and practicing relaxation regularly can also achieve the desired effect. Some people would choose the second approach to avoid the expense and side effect risks of antihypertensives. Others, however, might opt for the seductive quick fix and passive treatment with medication. Or, as we suggested earlier, both approaches can be undertaken simultaneously—medication to produce rapid symptom improvement and lifestyle changes to allow for the reduction or discontinuation of drugs with a minimum of relapse potential. In any case, healthy outcomes can be accomplished by taking something for the condition, by doing something about it, or both.

As the foregoing discussion illustrates, it is inaccurate to dichotomize the mind and the body. Related to this is another false dichotomy that many people tend to endorse, that of nature versus nurture. Are psychological difficulties like anxiety and depression inherited conditions stemming from genetic determinants, or are they largely due to environmental factors such as early childhood or other significant experiences? The answer to this question is: It's probably both. Just as the mind and the body are different facets of the same total entity, nature and nurture, or genetics and environment, are also inextricably intertwined, and both seem to play necessary roles in the development of psychological disturbances and most medical illnesses, too (e.g., Gould, 1995).

The paradigm that seems to offer the most elegant explanation of this issue is the diathesis–stress model of illness. A *diathesis* is a genetically based constitutional predisposition toward a particular disease or disorder. *Stress* refers to any environmental factor or circumstance that may have a negative impact on one's body and thus trigger the disease process. Here is an example that may help to illustrate this idea. Henry and Harry are identical twins and are therefore essentially clones from a purely genetic standpoint. Both men inherited genes that resulted in their developing an abnormally thin mucosal lining in their stomachs. Thus, as a result of inborn genetic factors, both Henry and Harry have less protection against stomach acids

than most other people. This is the diathesis side of the equation. Henry is an English professor who enjoys his job very much and has excellent health habits such as getting regular exercise, eating mostly low-fat foods, avoiding too much alcohol, and rarely using medications like aspirin. Harry is an air traffic controller who finds his job very demanding, eats lots of fast food, drinks alcohol often, and uses aspirin frequently. This, as you probably guessed, is the stress side of the formula. Well, not surprisingly, Harry develops stomach ulcers, while his genetically identical twin, Henry, has no gastrointestinal problems at all.

This same model can be applied to psychological disorders like depression, panic, OCD, and even schizophrenia. That is, people probably inherit various genetic predispositions toward particular neurochemical imbalances. If specific stressful environmental circumstances are experienced, they can trigger the disease process, which will result in manifestations of the condition. Alternatively, despite having a genetic propensity for an illness, if a person can "dodge the bullet" of environmental triggers, he or she will probably never develop any symptoms of consequence. It is the role of health psychologists to help people identify if they may be at risk (by detailed studies of personal and family history) and then to equip them with appropriate psychological armor (lifestyle changes, stress management skills, etc.) to reduce the likelihood or severity of health problems. This requires a broad-based understanding of the interdependent biopsychosocial factors that enter into health, illness, and psychological practice. We hope that this chapter has provided a thorough foundation of some of the important biological processes that are part of the comprehensive clinical picture.

REFERENCES

Baxter, L. R. (1991). PET studies of cerebral dysfunction in major depression and obsessive-compulsive disorder: The emerging prefrontal cortex consensus. *Annals of Clinical Psychiatry, 3*, 103–109.

Baxter, L. R., Schwartz, J. M., Bergman, K. S., Szuba, M. P., Guze, B. H., Marriotta, J. C., Alazvaki, A., Selin, C. E., Feung, H. K., Munford, P., & Phelps, M. E. (1992). Caudate glucose metabolic rate changes with both drug and behavior therapy for obsessive-compulsive disorder. *Archives of General Psychiatry, 49,* 681–689.

Carlson, N. R. (1994). *Physiology of behavior* (5th ed.). Boston: Allyn and Bacon.

Carpenter, R. H. S. (1996). *Neurophysiology* (3rd ed.). New York: Oxford University Press.

Craig, C. R., & Stitzel, R. E. (1994). *Modern pharmacology* (4th ed.). Boston: Little, Brown.

Curtis, H. (1979). *Biology* (3rd ed.). New York: Worth.

Fogel, B. S., & Schiffer, R. B. (Eds.). (1996). *Neuropsychiatry*. Baltimore: Williams & Wilkins.

Gazzaniga, M. S., & LeDoux, J. E. (1978). *The integrated mind*. New York: Plenum Press.

Good, W. V., & Nelson, S. E. (1991). *Psychiatry made ridiculously simple.* Miami, FL: MedMaster.

Gould, S. J. (1995). *Dinosaur in a haystack: Reflections in natural history*. New York: Harmony Books.

Hawking, S. W. (1988). *A brief history of time: From the Big Bang to black holes.* New York: Bantam.

Hyman, S. E., & Nestler, E. J. (1993). *The molecular foundations of psychiatry*. Washington, DC: American Psychiatric Press.

Kandel, E. R., Schwartz, J. H., & Jessell, T. M. (1991). *Principles of neural science* (3rd ed.). Norwalk: Appleton & Lange.

Kaplan, H. I., & Sadock, B. J. (1991). *Synopsis of psychiatry: Behavioral sciences clinical psychiatry* (6th ed.). Baltimore: Williams & Wilkins.

Krauss, L. M. (1995). *The physics of star trek*. New York: Basic Books.

Lezak, M. D. (1983). *Neuropsychological assesment.* New York: Oxford University Press.

Postlethwait, J. H., & Hopson, J. L. (1995). *The nature of life* (3rd ed.). New York: McGraw-Hill.

Preston, J., O'Neal, J. H., & Talaga, M. (1994). *Handbook of clinical psychopharmacology for therapists*. Oakland, CA: New Harbinger.

Sherwood, L. (1993). *Human physiology: From cells to systems* (2nd ed.). St. Paul, MN: West.

Swonger, A. K., & Constantine, L. L. (1983). *Drugs and therapy: A handbook of psychotropic drugs* (2nd ed.). Boston: Little, Brown.

FOR FURTHER READING

Carlson, N. R. (1994). *Physiology of behavior* (5th ed.). Boston: Allyn and Bacon. *Currently in its fifth edition, Neil Carlson's* Physiology of Behavior *has consistently distinguished itself as one of the most important and readable texts on the subject. This book is suitable for undergraduates and graduate students alike and should find a place on the bookshelf of anyone serious about biopsychology.*

Hyman, S. E., & Nestler, E. J. (1993). *The molecular foundations of psychiatry*. Washington DC: American Psychiatric Press. *Hyman and Nestler's book is a small (239 pages) powerhouse of a text on neuroscience and psychiatry. Although many of its concepts are for advanced students and academically oriented clinicians, it is written so that advanced concepts, defined by vertical rules in the left margin, can be skipped without loss of the overall message of the chapters or book.*

Kandel, E. R., Schwartz, J. H., & Jessell, T. M. (1991). *Principles of neural science* (3rd ed.). Norwalk: Appleton & Lange. *Perhaps the definitive text on the subject of neural science. Although it may be beyond the scope of most undergraduates who lack a solid grounding in science, for the serious or advanced reader, it is an extremely valuable reference source.*

Sherwood, L. (1993). *Human physiology: From cells to systems* (2nd ed.). St. Paul, MN: West. *An excellent basic textbook on human physiology that runs the gamut from cellular anatomy through organismic physiology. Packed with hundreds of clear diagrams and useful illustrations, Sherwood's book is a great resource for any student of biological science. Look for the third edition, which was published in 1997.*

Stahl, S. M. (1996). *Essential psychopharmacology: Neuroscientific basis and practical applications*. New York: Cambridge University Press. *This is a clearly written text supplemented by a wealth of high-quality color graphics that are both instructive and entertaining. This book, which explains the neurobiological concepts underlying the drug treatment of psychiatric disorders, is indeed an essential text for students, scientists, psychiatrists, psychologists, and other mental health professionals.*

CHAPTER 12

PSYCHOPHARMACOLOGY FOR CLINICAL PSYCHOLOGISTS

Dan Egli

INTRODUCTION

Psychopharmacology is primarily concerned with the development of new psychoactive or psychotropic drugs that ameliorate psychological or psychiatric disorders. This chapter will discuss the primary psychoactive drug classes for the major psychological and psychiatric disorders.

Within psychopharmacology, two of the most important general principles have to do with pharmacokinetics and pharmacodynamics (Benet, Mitchell, & Sherner, 1990). This chapter does not allow room for getting into an extensive discussion of these two principles, but simply states that *pharmacokinetics* is what the body does to a drug whereas *pharmacodynamics* describes what a drug does to the body (Hansten & Horn, 1990). The four primary phases of pharmacokinetics are absorption, distribution, metabolism, and elimination (Winter, 1988). The pharmacodynamics of a drug depends on drug concentrations at sites of action and includes such things as enzymes and receptors. Knowledge of the various components of psychopharmacology allows prescribers to be more effective in choosing a first-line agent for a specific disorder, and to more effectively prescribe in the presence of other medications, both psychotropic and nonpsychotropic, as well as dealing with other factors that may alter pharmacokinetics such as age or other disease states (Baldessarini, 1985).

In general, psychologists have had relatively little training in the area of psychopharmacology at either the pre- or post-doctoral level. Training in psychopharmacology for psychologists has typically occurred through supervision in continuing education once the psychologist is out of school, and it is only of late that graduate schools in clinical psychology are more actively considering how to integrate psychopharmacology course work into the predoctoral training. With the recent developments within the American Psychological Association that focus in part on developing psychopharmacology training modules for various levels of exposure and experience to psychopharmacology, more and more graduate schools are looking to incorporate psychopharmacology curriculum and more and more state and provincial associations are looking to add continuing education (CE) in the area of psychopharmacology.

In many rural settings across the country, most of the prescribing of psychotropics is done by nonpsychiatric physicians who, often by their own admission, are ill equipped to handle the intricacies of prescribing psychotropics (Beardsley, Gardocki, Larsen, & Hidalgo, 1988). Appropriately trained psychologists are increasingly available to collaborate with prescribers to help them make accurate differential diagnoses and make recommendations or suggestions about adding, decreasing, or discontinuing a specific psychotropic agent (see Table 12.1 for a list of common abbreviations in psychopharmacology).

The various disorders that psychologists treat are becoming increasingly well defined in terms of both diagnostic criteria and treatment from both a psychotherapeutic and a pharmacologic approach (Watsky & Salzman, 1991). Perhaps one of the best examples of this is obsessive-compulsive disorder (OCD), where there is an increasingly homogeneous body of literature supporting the specific behavioral interventions of in vivo exposure (IVE) and response prevention (RP). In addition, with the emphasis on the neurotransmitter serotonin (5-HT), antiobsessional agents have been developed that target OCD symptomatology. Combining these approaches for the OCD patient who has symptoms of at least moderate severity often has an extremely synergistic effect. More studies and investigations are occurring with a variety of other disorders in an attempt to come up with greater specificity of treatments, both pharmacologically and nonpharmacologically. Examples would include the treatment of panic disorder, social phobias, and major depression.

This chapter will discuss the major psychotropic drug classes and, in order of presentation, will focus on the following:

1. Neuroleptics
2. Anxiolytics
3. Hypnotics
4. Mood stabilizers
5. Antidepressants
6. Psychostimulants

NEUROLEPTIC DRUGS

Neuroleptics can be viewed as synonymous with the antipsychotic drugs, which are also called major tranquilizers. The primary indication for these agents is the treatment of acute and chronic psychosis, as well as the prophylactic treatment of schizophrenia. Other indicated conditions include Bipolar Disorder, Tourette's Syndrome, and Organic Aggressive Syndrome (OAS). The neuroleptics were developed in the 1950s, when thorazine was initially being developed in the context of surgery and anesthesia treatment. At that time, Delay and Deniker demonstrated its efficacy with acute psychosis.

Table 12.1 Common Abbreviations in Psychopharmacology

ac	before meals	qod	every other day
aq	water	qid	four times a day
bid	twice a day	tid	three times a day
d	day(s)	IM	intramuscular
Dx	diagnosis	CNS	central nervous system
EPS	extrapyramidal side effects	FDA	Food and Drug Administration
hs	at sleep/at night	h	hour(s)
ng	nanogram	mEq/L	milliequivalents per liter
ml	milliliter	mg	milligrams
TCA	tricyclic antidepressant	5-HT	serotonin
MAOI	monoamine oxidase inhibitor	SSRI	selective serotonin-reuptake inhibitor
HCA	heterocyclic antidepressant	SNRI	serotonin norepinephrine reuptake inhibitor
TD	tardive dyskinesia	DNRI	dopamine norepinephrine reuptake inhibitor
NMS	neuroleptic malignant syndrome	ADD	attention deficit disorder
OCD	obsessive-compulsive disorder	ADHD	attention deficit hyperactivity disorder
GAD	generalized anxiety disorder	BZ	benzodiazepine
pc	after meals	prn	as needed
q	every	GABA	gamma-aminobutyric acid
qp	once a day; daily	Tx	treatment

Since then, numerous double-blind studies have replicated this agent's effectiveness (Carpenter, Hanlon, Heinrichs, Summerfelt, Kirkpatrick, Levine, & Buchanan, 1990).

Currently the neuroleptics can be broken up into the following types (see Tables 12.2 and 12.3): phenothiazines, thioxanthenes, dibenzoxazepines, dibenzodiazepines, butyrophenoes, diphenylbutyrylpiperidines, rauwolfian alkaloids, and a number of investigational/ experimental agents. The underlying theme in terms of mechanism of action among the neuroleptics is their ability to block dopamine receptors (Davis, Kahn, Ko, & Davidson, 1991). The primary concern with the use of these agents is extrapyramidal symptoms (EPS) and Parkinsonian symptoms (Carpenter & Henrichs, 1983). Some of the newer atypical neuroleptics are less likely to cause EPS; these include clozaril and risperdal. A number of investigational new drugs that are close to being approved will also be available in depot (IM) form. These generally last about 2 to 4 weeks and are used as a maintenance type of therapy (Comaty & Janicak, 1987). The main advantage of these for the noncompliant patient is that depot neuroleptics guarantee that the medication is in the patient's system and that a minimum blood level is achieved over a long period of time.

Generally, the newer atypical neuroleptics are viewed as being reserved for use in patients who have a more treatment-resistant form of schizophrenia and where there has been a poor or only partial response to other adequate trials (appropriate dose and appropriate duration of dose) of more typical neuroleptics (Lieberman, Kane, & Johns, 1989; Lieberman, 1996). Some research suggests that the more negative symptoms of schizophrenia (e.g., cognitive impairment, speech impoverishment, and anhedonia) may respond better to the atypical neuroleptics. There are several different types of dopaminergic receptors, often categorized as D1, D2, D3, D4, and D5. Most pharmacologists feel that the typical antipsychotic drugs produce their effects primarily by blocking the D2 subtype, and the newer atypical neuroleptics may be less likely to involve D2 blockade and may have greater 5-HT2 (serotonin receptor) blockade. This may account for the lower incidence of EPS with these agents.

The neuroleptics are fairly heavy in side effects (Pisciotta, 1969), although the benefit-to-risk ratio should always be considered. The side effects from neuroleptics can by broken down into the following categories: temperature regulation; hypersensitivity (e.g., photosensitivity, rashes); ocular changes; endocrine effects; gastrointestinal (GI) effects; anticholinergic effects; central nervous system (CNS), cognitive, and neurological effects; sexual side effects; and cardiovascular effects.

The hypersensitivity reaction of neuroleptic malignant syndrome (NMS) is a potentially fatal side effect unless it is recognized early and the offending agent is discontinued immediately (Levenson, 1985). Therapy of a supportive nature needs to be implemented immediately (typically, fluid and electrolytes), as well as the addition of certain medications. NMS is characterized by rapid heart beat, hyperthermia, altered consciousness, and muscular rigidity. It seems to be more common in cases of rapid neuroleptization, where the antipsychotics are given quickly to a patient who is acutely psychotic and/or manic and in whom the prescribers are trying to achieve a rapid increase in the neuroleptic plasma level. It is estimated that NMS affects approximately 0.5% to 2.4% of patients treated with neuroleptics and is more common in patients who are over 60 years of age. As indicated, the supportive measures need to be instituted immediately and include stopping the offending agent, hydrating the

Table 12.2 Types of Neuroleptic Drugs

TYPE	DRUG NAME
Phenothiazines	
Aliphatic	Thorazine
Piperidine	Serentil
	Mellaril
Piperazines	Prolixin
	Trilafon
	Stelazine
Thioxanthene	Navane
Butyrophenones	Haldol
Dihydroindolone	Moban
Dibenzoxazepine	Loxitane
Dibenzodiazepine	Clozaril
Benzisoxazole	Risperdal
	Zyprexa

Table 12.3 Conventional Antipsychotics

GENERIC NAME	TRADE NAME	TRADITIONAL EQUIVALENTS	DOSE RANGE (mg/d)	EPS POTENTIAL (1–5)
Chlorpromazine	Thorazine	100	30–2,000	2
Thioridazine	Mellaril	100	50–800	1
Mesoridazine	Serentil	50	30–400	1
Fluphenazine	Prolixin	2	0.5–40	4
Perphenazine	Trilafon	8	12–64	3
Trifluoperazine	Stelazine	5	2–40	3
Thiothixene	Navane	4	6–60	3
Haloperidal	Haldol	2	1–100	4
Loxapine	Loxitane	10	20–250	3
Molindone	Moban	10	15–225	3
ATYPICAL ANTIPSYCHOTICS				
Clozapine	Clozaril	50	12.5–900	0
Risperidone	Risperdal	N/A	1–16	0–3
Olanzapine	Zyprexa	N/A	7.5–20	0–1
Experimental				
Sertindole	Serlect	N/A	4–24	0–1
Quetiapine	Seroquel	N/A	100–600	0–1

patient, correcting any electrolyte abnormalities, and cooling the body. Starting the same drug again, but at a lower initial dose, should be done cautiously. The two medications most frequently used to treat NMS are two anticholinergic agents: bromocriptine and dantrolene.

Another concern with the neuroleptics is the development of tardive dyskinesia (TD). This syndrome, consisting of involuntary face, limb, and trunk movements, often arises after long periods of treatment (between 6 and 24 months). It often occurs when neuroleptics are lowered or stopped. Approximately one-quarter of patients develop TD after having been on a neuroleptic for over two years.

In addition to TD, a pseudo-Parkinsonian syndrome can develop. Therefore, anti-Parkinsonian agents are frequently used concomitantly when neuroleptics are being given. The two main types of anti-Parkinsonian agents are those that are anticholinergic and those that are dopaminergic. These anti-Parkinsonian agents are typically used to treat medication induced side effects such as akathisia (restlessness, pacing), tremor and muscular rigidity, dystonia (brief or prolonged contraction of muscles), and akinesia (reduced movements or apathy).

The neuroleptics used frequently in the treatment of Tourette's syndrome are pimozide (Orap) and haloperidol (Haldol). Other indications for neuroleptics besides Tourette's syndrome and schizophrenia include OCD with co-morbid Tourette's syndrome and co-morbid OCD with Axis II schizotypal personality disorder (SPD).

With the newer atypical agent clozapine (Clozaril), one of the main concerns is a higher incidence of agranulocytosis (a decrease in the number of white blood cells). The incidence of this side effect is approximately 1% to 2% of all treated patients. Because of this, it is often not considered as a first-line agent to treat schizophrenia or other psychotic disorders. Weekly white blood count (WBC) tests are required in an attempt to catch the development of this potentially serious blood disorder early. This patient management system was implemented by the manufacturer as part of an attempt to enhance safety through early monitoring. Patients should also report any signs of lethargy, weakness, sore throat, infection, or fever. In addition, there is an increased risk of seizures during treatment, which may be dose-related. However, TD appears to be a less significant risk with Clozaril than with other neuroleptics.

Another antipsychotic medication is risperidone, which belongs to a new chemical class known as the benzisoxazoles. Its mechanism of action is not fully known, but may have a mixed dopamingergic (D2) serotonergic (5-HT2) effect. It also produces fairly little in the way of EPS, at least at typical doses, but can produce a fair amount of sedation. Although TD from this agent can occur with any age group, the elderly are at higher risk. NMS can also occur with this agent. Although risperidone has not been rigorously studied in patients with treatment-resistant schizophrenia, it appears to have a therapeutic role in this patient population. There have not been any studies directly comparing risperidone to clozapine in carefully selected treatment-resistant patients. Risperidone may be used prior to clozapine in view of the fact that it does not cause agranulocytosis.

A wide range of alternative treatments for psychosis and schizophrenia have been used. These include but are not limited to the use of benzodiazepines, the use of mood stabilizers, the use of beta blockers (Koch-Weser, 1981), the use of calcium channel blockers, and a wide range of anecdotal reports that have not achieved formal FDA approval. It should be emphasized that neuroleptics are not addicting and do not cause a withdrawal symptom. In addition, neuroleptics are relatively nonlethal in overdose and are certainly less dangerous than some of the antidepressant classes.

In general, if a patient needs neuroleptic medication, this usually implies the importance of psychiatric care, as most nonpsychiatric physicians are generally very cautious about and hesitant to use these agents because of the problematic side effects, the possibility of the development of NMS or TD, and concerns about drug–drug interactions. Sometimes one might also see the use of a neuroleptic in conjunction with an antidepressant or mood stabilizer in the co-morbid conditions of schizoaffective disorder, delusional disorder, and schizophrenia with bipolar disorder (Donaldson, Glenberg, & Baldessarini, 1983). In these disorders, using only one agent often will address only one clinical syndrome, and an agent for both the mood/affective disorder and the thought disorder is indicated. One can expect the formal approval of several new antipsychotics within the next year or two. Most recently olanzapine (Zyprexa) was approved.

ANXIOLYTICS

Anxiolytics are a group of medicines that can synonymously be termed antianxiety agents or minor tranquilizers. The most common form of anxiolytics includes the barbiturates, the carbamates, noradrenergic agents, and antihistamines.

Generally, the barbiturates and carbamates (specifically meprobamate) are outdated and no longer in use. If someone were to come to a therapist on a barbiturate, one would have to strongly suspect an addiction problem. Similarly, meprobamate is felt by most clinicians to have absolutely no use in present-day psychopharmacologic intervention. The noradrenergic agents are basically represented by the calcium channel blocker clonidine (Catapres) and the beta blocker propranolol (Inderal). This beta blocker is used primarily by noncardiologists for performance anxiety. Specific examples would be pianists who have anxiety playing concerts; singers; and people who shoot archery, pistols, or rifles competitively. The other noradrenergic agent mentioned, clonidine, has moved away from being used as an anxiolytic and tends to be used more frequently as an adjunctive agent in treatment-resistant ADD/ADHD. The antihistamines are rarely used in biologic psychiatry, although they clearly do have some anxiolytic effect.

The majority of anxiolytic focus clearly revolves around the use of the benzodiazepines (BZ). In addition to being indicated for anxiety, these are used for such problems as insomnia (Halcion), preoperative anesthesia, and alcohol withdrawal. One of the subtypes of the BZs is the triazolo-BZ alprazolam (Xanax), which was the first medication formally approved as a panicolytic (antipanic) medication in the United States. This drug is currently off patent and is thus available generically, but it has addictive potential (Ballenger, Burrows, & DuPont, 1988). Newer strategies being used to treat panic disorder marked by panic attacks with or without agoraphobia have moved clinicians away from using the BZ anxiolytics to using antidepressants that have simultaneous anxiolytic efficacy. In fact, some of the newer antidepressants, such as paroxetine (Paxil) and fluoxetine (Prozac), are approved as an indication for panic disorder. It is very likely that within the next year or two, other selective serotonin-reuptake inhibitors (SSRIs) will be approved for such an indication as well. Those SSRIs include sertraline (Zoloft) and fluvoxamine (Luvox). More discussion of these agents will be available in the section on antidepressants.

The benzodiazepine receptors were initially identified in the late 1970s when it was possible to "map" their location within the CNS. These receptors were found to be related to an inhibitory neurotransmitter system in the brain known as gamma-aminobutyric acid (better known as GABA). The primary concern related to the use of these agents is habituation/addiction (Smith & Wesson, 1983). Most physicians avoid these agents altogether because of this, but when they are used, the general rule of thumb is to prescribe the lowest effective dose for the shortest possible time.

Of the BZ anxiolytics, the primary differences have to do with the nature of their metabolism and differences in elimination half-life (Kales, 1982). On the basis of their elimination half-life, BZs can be divided into short-acting, short-to-intermediate-acting, and long-acting. A concern with the short-acting BZs is the interdose breakthrough (or reoccurrence) of symptoms. Also, withdrawal syndromes tend to occur earlier and are more severe (Ulenhuth, DeWit, Balter, Johanson, & Mellinger,

1988). Patients who are trying to taper off short-half-life BZs are often unable to remain drug free for very long and frequently have difficulty getting off the agent altogether. In addition to addiction, other concerns related to the use of the BZs include the withdrawal phenomenon, seizures (especially after abrupt discontinuation), cognitive impairment, state-dependent learning, psychomotor impairment, and disinhibition phenomenon, which are manifested by such things as irritability or aggressiveness (Kales, 1990).

Overdoses resulting in death are fairly rare with this group of agents. BZs that have a longer half-life generally increase the likelihood of daytime "hangover," and this has sometimes been implicated in falls that have occurred in the elderly resulting in broken hips and their various medical sequelae (Greenblatt, Shader, & Abernethy, 1983). Some of the pharmacologic differences of the anxiolytics as well as typical dosage ranges are listed in Table 12.4.

In general, as indicated earlier, the barbiturates and carbamates should be avoided altogether because of their higher risk of addiction than the BZs and because they also have more serious overdose potential. A new class of anxiolytics, known as the azapriones, have one representative agent here in the United States, which is buspirone (BuSpar) (Erickson, Bergman, Schneeweiss, et al., 1980). This is a non-BZ anxiolytic that differs from the BZs in that it is more antidepressant-like in its la-

Table 12.4 Anxiolytics

GENERIC NAME	TRADE NAME	DOSAGE/RANGE (mg/d)	HALF-LIFE (h)	ABSORPTION RATE
BZ Alprazolam	Xanax	0.75–4	14	Intermediate
Chlordiazepoxide	Librium	10–100	24–48	Intermediate
Clonazepam*	Klonopin	1–20	18–50	Intermediate
Clorazepate	Tranxene	7.5–60	60	Rapid
Diazepam	Valium	2–40	40	Rapid
Halazepam	Paxipam	20–160	14	Slow
Lorazepam	Ativan	10–10	12	Intermediate
Oxazepam	Serax	30–120	9	Slow-to-intermediate
Prazepam	Centrax	20–60	60	Slow
Azapirone				
Buspirone	BuSpar	15–60	2–3	Rapid

* BZ anticonvulsant.

tency of onset of action and often takes 2 to 4 weeks for its full therapeutic effect. In addition, it is generally nonsedating, does not impair motor coordination, does not potentiate alcohol, and does produce dependency/addiction. It is not effective for anxiety that requires an immediate effect, does not prevent BZ withdrawal, and is indicated as a panicolytic (antipanic) medication. BuSpar is probably most useful in a patient who has chronic and/or acute anxiety and who has not had previous exposure to a BZ. Patients who are used to the effects of BZs will generally actively resist any attempt to switch over to buspirone. Also, patients need to take BuSpar on a daily basis for at least 2 to 4 weeks before they can expect to see any therapeutic effect.

Other off-label (not FDA-approved) uses of this anxiolytic include using it as a potentiating or augmenting agent in treatment-resistant obsessive-compulsive disorder (OCD). There are mixed data suggesting that there may be a subset of patients who are only partially responsive to an antiobsessional agent; when buspirone is added to that regimen, they get a more robust antiobsessional effect. In addition, a number of clinicians are using buspirone in higher doses for patients who are irritable, angry, or described by others as "cranky." In these cases it seems to have an antiaggressive/antiimpulsive effect, although there is no strong body of literature to support this other than what has been reported anecdotally.

Another agent that psychologists need to be aware of is the anticonvulsant clonazepam (Klonopin) (Pollack, Tesar, Rosenbaum, et al., 1986). Although it is primarily used by neurologists for seizures, it has been used as an antipanic medication. Because it is fairly sedating, most physicians give it at bedtime, with smaller doses earlier in the day. As with all BZs, clonazepam is a CNS depressant and can induce depressive symptoms.

There were a few initial reports suggesting that some of the BZs may have antidepressant benefit, but few clinicians find this to be the case, and typically one would not expect an antidepressant response from a medication that has CNS depressant effects. Rarely, if ever, would a BZ be used to treat a clear depressive-affective syndrome. The only cases in which I see BZs being used at this point, tend to be situations of acute situational stress and anxiety disorders, but only at very low doses and frequently on a p.r.n. (as needed) basis. Another possible use might be to counteract the activating (insomnia, agitation, restlessness, and anxiety) that is temporarily induced by the use of the selective serotonin-reuptake inhibitor (SSRI) drugs. Still another use might be the rapid tranquilization effect that one might want to get in an inpatient psychiatric setting or emergency room to control agitation related to a manic/psychotic episode. For this, the benzodiazepine is used in conjunction with one of the neuroleptics (antipsychotic drugs) or one of the mood stabilizers like lithium or valproic acid (Depakote). When it is used in conjunction with one of the new SSRIs, one does need to be concerned about some of the pharmacokinetic interactions that might decrease the metabolism and increase the half-life of the medication. More simply stated, this combination could result in additive side effects and/or toxicity. In that case, the typical doses of the BZ might need to be reduced by no less than half of what might normally be considered.

In summary, I find a national trend of prescribers moving away from using these agents other than for very brief periods of time and at the lowest possible doses. Because the newer agents have a broad-spectrum efficacy in co-morbid conditions, more clinicians are moving to the use of the SSRIs, which appear to be able to "kill three birds with one stone." That is to say, they generally have very clear and obvious antidepressant efficacy but simultaneously have anxiolytic and antiobsessive (with the fourth possibility being anticompulsive) efficacy. In addition, because they are not habituating and not CNS depressants, they are generally the first-line treatment for chronic anxiety. This is a much safer strategy and, in addition, is much more effective in co-morbid conditions and avoids the potential for addiction issues altogether. For patients who specifically request BZs or who present with anxiety as a symptom, clinicians need to be aware of the possible use and abuse of these agents and the tendency on the part of some patients to manipulate physicians into prescribing these drugs.

Clinicians also need to be aware that many patients are far more comfortable at describing either the subjective symptom of anxiety or the somatic manifestations of anxiety, and one might be easily fooled into thinking that this represents a primary Axis I disorder, when in fact the anxiety and its accompanying cognitive, emotional, and physical symptoms are often harbingers of an oncoming major depressive episode (MDE). Therefore, it is often difficult in the early stages of diagnosis/assessment to determine whether one meets criteria for an anxiety or mood disorder. In these situations many patients are mistakenly given an anxiolytic for what appears to be an anxiety syndrome, when in fact the oncoming depression is totally nonresponsive or even exacerbated by the use of the anxiolytic. In these cases, one might do well to use a broad-spectrum efficacy antidepressant that would simultaneously have anxiolytic properties without all the complication related to the use of the BZ anxiolytics.

HYPNOTICS

The use of hypnotics at this point in psychopharmacology practice is moving toward being more limited in view of concerns of many prescribers about problems of dependency on these agents. As a result, even though newer agents are being developed, and over-the-counter (OTC) products are being promoted, in general the trend is to move away from the use of these agents and toward the use of other "hypnotic strategies." The most common example of this statement is a national trend to make use of the antidepressant trazodone (Desyrel) in nonantidepressant doses so as to take advantage of its sedative (but relatively nonanticholinergic) properties. In this way, an individual can get improvement in sleep without any CNS depressant effects or any risk of habituation.

Assuming the sleep disturbance is not due to a medical condition, it may be related to a specific situation in the person's life or may meet criteria for a primary sleep disorder. In one very common scenario, a patient will go to a family doctor describing problems with insomnia (either initial insomnia, middle insomnia, or terminal insomnia) and be prescribed one of the benzodiazepine (BZ) hypnotics, when in fact the insomnia problem is simply one of

a number of symptoms of an underlying clinical or major depression. The pharmacologic strategy employed may help with the symptom of sleep disturbance but does not address the underlying affective disorder. In fact, depending on the dose and duration of the BZ use, it may actually exacerbate the mood disturbance (Langtry & Benfield, 1990).

In another very common situation, a patient complains of sleep disturbance as part of a substance abuse disorder and as part of a withdrawal syndrome. Often, these patients are actively seeking to maintain their addiction by securing a benzodiazepine from one of several prescribers. For this group, any and all BZs (both antianxiety agents or hypnotics) should be actively avoided. Once the patient is sober, the clinician may carefully suggest the use of a non-BZ agent. On the U.S. market, zolpidem (Ambien) is the only non-BZ hypnotic currently available. Unlike the BZs, zolpidem has little in the way of antianxiety or anticonvulsant properties. The manufacturer of zolpidem, however, does advise that the agent not be used in conjunction with alcohol or other CNS depressants, and that caution be used when performing activities that require alertness and coordination because the drug may cause drowsiness. The chemical class to which zolpidem belongs is known as an imidazopyridine. At present the general trend among prescribers is to use hypnotics in insomnia only for brief periods (less than one week) or "as needed" (p.r.n.) in transient insomnia caused either by acute life stressors or major shifts in diurnal rhythm such as jet lag.

Currently, the primary classes of hypnotics include the benzodiazepines, of which there are five (see Table 12.5), the barbiturates, the barbiturate-like compounds, chloral derivatives, antihistamines, and the nonbenzodiazepine hypnotic mentioned earlier (zolpidem).

Although all BZs produce sedation or drowsiness, only those listed here have a formal (FDA) indication for insomnia. The other benzodiazepines have a formal indication only for the treatment of anxiety.

With the advent of the new, less sedating, more activating antidepressants (e.g., the SSRI's), a subset of patients experience insomnia as an activating side effect of these agents. This should not be con-

Table 12.5 Hypnotics

GENERIC NAME	TRADE NAME	DOSE RANGE (mg/d)	APPROXIMATE HALF-LIFE (h)	ACTIVE METABOLITES
Benzodiazepine				
Estazolam	ProSom	0.5–2.0	8–24	N
Flurazepam	Dalmane	15–30	0.5–1	Y
Quazepam	Doral	7.5–15	39	Y
Temazepam	Restoril	7.5–30	3.5–18.5	N
Triazolam	Halcion	0.125–0.5	1.5–5.5	N
Non-Benzodiazepine				
Zolpidem	Ambien	5–1 0	2.6	N

fused with an unexpected sleep disorder but, rather, seen as a (typically) brief side effect of the antidepressant, which generally levels off and/or disappears. If it does not level off or disappear, simply lowering the dose of the antidepressant, waiting it out if the sleep disturbance is not too severe, or adding a low dose of the sedating antidepressant trazodone are all common strategies. Because of the problems with contamination, the FDA withdrew the amino acid L tryptophan from the market so that this over-the-counter (OTC) agent is no longer available.

In my clinical practice, the use of BZ hypnotics is limited to extremely short-term, p.r.n. (as needed) use in situations where there is an acute situational stressor or where there is severe activation from the use of an SSRI. Often a very limited number and specific number of pills will be prescribed so as to actively avoid potential for addiction. In general, in treating sleep disturbances, all efforts must be made to make use of nonpharmacology strategies prior to the use of agents that have CNS depressant and/or habituating properties.

Any patient who presents on a barbiturate or requests a barbiturate is probably someone with an addiction problem who is seeking to have the prescriber or therapist enable him or her to continue the habit. In addition, one of the more popular over-the-counter (OTC) strategies is to use the sedative antihistamine diphenhydramine (Benadryl).

In general, the use of the BZ hypnotic changes the pattern of sleep architecture. Specifically, there is a decrease in alpha activity and a decrease in sleep latency. Stage 1 sleep is generally decreased. Time in Stage 2 sleep tends to increase, whereas Stages 3 and 4 sleep are reduced and Stage 4 sleep is often accompanied by a reduction in nightmares. REM sleep is often shortened, with the resultant effect being an overall increase in total sleep time. Patients who have been on BZ hypnotics for a long time should be advised to discontinue their use. Because of the rebound and withdrawal effects from tampering with these medications, however, patients should be tapered off these agents very slowly. Patients who have been using these agents for lengthy periods of time are very difficult to convince of the need to discontinue their use. Even when tapering is done very slowly, the instant they have any kind of withdrawal or rebound symptoms, they will unilaterally increase the dose without consulting their physician and frequently switch from one physician to another until they can find someone who will perpetuate their dependency on these agents.

MOOD STABILIZERS/ANTIMANICS

The term *mood stabilizer* first came into vogue with the realization that lithium salts were effective in treating both manic highs and depressive lows. Clearly, the drug of choice for a number of decades in the treatment of bipolar disorder (previously known as manic-depressive illness) has been lithium (Carlson & Goodwin, 1973). With the onset of use of some of the new anticonvulsants, one of which has recently been FDA-approved in the treatment of bipolar disorder, new options are available to clinicians. The three primary agents used in the treatment of bipolar disorder are lithium (in its various forms), valproic acid (VA; Depakene or the slow-release form called Depakote), and carbamazepine (Tegretol) (Ballenger & Post, 1980). Only the final agent is not formally approved in the treatment of bipolar disorder. Depakote was recently approved by the FDA for treatment of bipolar disorder following carefully controlled trials that clearly point to the effectiveness of VA in acute mania.

Overall, the diagnosis of bipolar disorder has gained increased acceptance in view of the fact that numerous famous people have written books or are touring the country addressing television audiences, discussing their bipolar disorder, and recommending pharmacologic treatments. In addition, the Lithium Information Center at the University of Wisconsin–Madison has some excellent materials that are available not only to bipolar patients but to families and clinicians of such patients as well.

Bipolar Type I is considered to be classically defined as episodes of mania and depression, whereas Bipolar Type II disorder is viewed as episodes of hypomania interspersed with classic episodes of major depression. Bipolar Type III disorder is viewed as related to cyclothymic personality or cyclothymia, and Bipolar Type IV disorder is an iatrogenic (precipitated by medication) hypomania or mania. An example of this is a patient who presents to the clinician with indications of depression and is put on an antidepressant. Shortly thereafter, the patient "flips up" into a "high," and the diagnosis is revised to a bipolar diagnosis. What manifestly appears to be a unipolar affective syndrome latently develops into a bipolar affective disorder. In these cases, the antidepressant is quickly withdrawn, and the mood stabilizer of choice is initiated (Weber, Saklad, & Kastenholz, 1992).

Studies are now under way comparing lithium, which has been the standard therapy for acute mania for more than two and half decades, to valproic acid. Some prescribers are finding that VA is not only equally efficacious but may be better tolerated as well as able to achieve rapid stabilization in acute manic episodes. If someone is having a second or third episode of mania that was previously responsive to lithium, most prescribers would continue

with that particular antimanic. In patients who may be "rapid cyclers," however, many prescribers are using VA as a first-line treatment both because of the ability to achieve therapeutic levels very quickly and because of its better side effect profile. One advantage cited for the use of VA is that therapeutic levels can be achieved a little more quickly than with lithium, often within a day. These newer agents and alternative agents are important in view of the fact that approximately 40% of patients placed on lithium suffer relapse over a one-year follow-up. Approximately two-thirds of patients suffer a breakthrough of a manic or depressive episode within two years of starting lithium, even though their lithium levels are in a therapeutic range.

Anticonvulsants such as VA and carbamazepine (Tegretol) have found an increase in use (Post, Ballenger, Uhde, & Bunney, 1984) especially since VA's formal approval from the FDA for bipolar disorder. The rationale for using some of these anticonvulsants in the treatment of bipolar disorder is a function of: (1) the fact that combining these medications may have beneficial effects in selected patients, and (2) possible improved efficacy for specific subtypes of bipolarity. Some of the studies that correlate with a lower response to lithium include co-morbidity (Axis II personality disorder), dysphoric or mixed mania, rapid cycling, and an episode sequence of depression–mania–euthymia.

A significant factor that affects compliance rates in using lithium is the side effect profile (Vestergaard, Amdisen, & Schow, 1980). The risk of many of the side effects increases in direct relation to the serum lithium levels (Gelenberg & Schoonover, 1991). Dosage reduction is always a treatment consideration, with changes being made very cautiously while observing for any signs of relapse. The various side effects of lithium can be classified as neurologic effects (e.g., tremor), hypothyroidism (which occurs in approximately 10% of patients), diarrhea, renal effects, and others (including a wide range of less frequent but not rare side effects, such as hair loss).

Because both lithium and VA have very clear therapeutic windows, blood levels are routinely used with both agents. This ensures that the patient maximizes the likelihood of efficacy by getting blood plasma levels into a "therapeutic window." With low blood levels, partial or no response is likely to occur, and above a ceiling figure, toxicity is likely to occur. In general, lithium has a relatively slow onset of action and may take as long as three weeks or longer to result in a therapeutic response (Jefferson & Greist, 1977). Too often, because patients are not educated about the latency of onset or action of lithium, they may discontinue the drug prematurely, claiming it was not helpful, when in fact they are simply slow responders. This same principle is often found to be the case in treating unipolar depression with antidepressants. An adequate trial of an agent is best defined by making sure there was an adequate dose for an adequate duration (Jefferson, Greist, Ackerman, et al., 1986). Many patients referred to me for so-called treatment-resistant depression or treatment-resistant bipolar disorder are simply referred back to the referral source with a recommendation to raise the dose closer to therapeutic levels.

For example, a patient was referred to me who had been diagnosed with clinical depression and who had been on fluoxetine (Prozac) 20 mg for the past year. The referral physician felt the patient was nonresponsive to Prozac because of how long the patient had been on the drug, and wondered what was the next antidepressant to try. Rather than seeing the patient as truly "treatment-refractory," I found that simply increasing the dose to 30 mg and ultimately to 40 mg resulted in complete symptom reduction.

Other experimental therapy in the treatment of bipolar disorder includes the use of the noradrenergic agent clonidine, the use of psychostimulants, atypical antipsychotics, and calcium channel blockers such as verapamil. Although these alternatives appear interesting, they are not routinely used and are not formally approved for use in bipolar disorder. Initial concerns about the blood disorder side effect of carbamazepine (CBZ) have led some clinicians to be wary of prescribing it. However, the incidence seems to be less than original estimates. A probable more significant concern with CBZ is its numerous drug–drug interactions. Because of the pharmacokinetics involved, CBZ can accelerate the metabolism of various drugs and therefore lower

neuroleptic plasma levels. Similarly, other agents can lower CBZ levels, thereby reducing efficacy and increasing the likelihood of a manic breakthrough set of symptoms.

A key to compliance with the mood stabilizers, and perhaps with all psychotropics, is the education given to patients prior to initiating drug therapy. This can significantly enhance compliance rates because side effects are not so unexpected, and patients can be informed about how the medications work. For example, the mood stabilizers are not addictive, and patients need to be instructed that there is a high recurrence rate if patients go off these drugs. Many patients end up needing a maintenance dose indefinitely or throughout their entire life span (Post, Weiss, & Chuang, 1992).

When the mood stabilizers, particularly lithium, are used in patients who do not have bipolar disorder, the primary reason usually is that the individual meets criteria for a treatment-resistant/treatment-refractory major depression or treatment-resistant obsessive-compulsive disorder (OCD). Very frequently, lithium is the augmenting or potentiating agent of choice to add to the primary medication for use in either depression or OCD. Table 12.6 lists some of the characteristics of the various mood stabilizers.

ANTIDEPRESSANTS

In this section we will focus on the major groupings of antidepressants. Ever since the onset of fluoxetine (Prozac), introduced in 1988, there has been a flurry of antidepressant activity that has resulted in eight new antidepressant compounds. One can distinguish the currently available antidepressants (approximately 20) between these eight new ones and the rest. The primary indication for the use of these agents is moderate to severe major depressive episodes (MDE). This is probably one of the most frequent conditions seen in clinical practice (Prien, Kupfer, Mansky, et al., 1984). Very commonly, these agents are used in conjunction with interpersonal, cognitive, or cognitive-behavioral therapies to create a synergistic effect for the patient, especially with MDE. In the 1990s more and more emphasis has been placed on specific neu-

Table 12.6 Mood Stabilizers

GENERIC NAME	TRADE NAME	USUAL ADULT DOSE (mg/d)	PLASMA LEVELS	HALF-LIFE (h)	INDICATION(S)
Approved					
Lithium carbonate	Lithium	600–1,800	0.6–1.2 mEq/L	24	Bipolar
Valproic acid	Depakote	750–4,200	50–100 mg/ml	16–16	Seizure/Bipolar
Experimental					
Carbamazepine	Tegretol	400–1,600	4–12 mg/ml	25–65	Seizure/Bipolar

rotransmitters and biologic etiologies of depression, in addition to the interpersonal and cognitive schools of thought. Much of the emphasis among the neurotransmitters has been on serotonin, as reflected in the development of four similar agents known as the selective serotonin-reuptake inhibitors (SSRIs).

Two of the groups of antidepressants, the tricyclic antidepressants (TCAs) and the monoamine oxidase inhibitors (MAOIs) were initially introduced for the treatment of depression in the late 1950s (Bielski & Friedel, 1976). Improved psychopharmacologic approaches to mood disorders have been a major advance and have become one of the cornerstones in treating this class of disorders. None of the antidepressants are addicting or habit-forming. Each of the antidepressants, as well as each of the classes of antidepressants, has equal efficacy, both intra- and interclass. Thus, at this point, no one agent can claim superiority over another agent in terms of ameliorating or alleviating symptoms of major depression (Stewart, Quitkin, & Klein, 1992). In addition, all of the antidepressants are felt to have an equal latency or onset of action. In other words, the length of time it takes for each of these agents to begin to work is equivalent and is roughly 3 to 6 weeks. This time frame may be different in special populations (geriatric) or special disorders (e.g., OCD), but generally most clinicians will alert patients who are beginning an antidepressant not to expect a significant benefit until they have been on it at least a month (Cole & Bodkin, 1990). Although there may be individual, idiosyncratic responses to specific agents, one generally does not expect this. Many patients who come for treatment, and who indicate that they have tried a

particular antidepressant before and that it did not work, in fact have not had an adequate trial. They have had either an inadequate dose or an inadequate duration of the antidepressant. Typically, the patient will not have had a good education about what side effects to expect, and discontinues the drug. Then the patient indicates that he or she tried that particular agent, when in fact had he or she taken it for a longer period of time or started on a lower dose, the patient might well have been able to stay with it and tolerate the antidepressant. The general pharmacologic rule of thumb among prescribers of antidepressants is "Start low, go slow, work high"—that is, start the dose low enough so as not to hit the person hard with side effects, but then begin to titrate the dose up to therapeutic levels where it can begin to do its work.

The first class of antidepressants that we will discuss are the tricyclic antidepressants, better known as the TCAs. As indicated, these agents were developed almost forty years ago and are only now beginning to fall out of favor. Among the TCAs, there are basically two groups, the tertiary amines and the secondary amines (Coccaro & Siever, 1985), differentiated by the number of methyl groups in each. The tertiary amines were developed first, but because of their side effects, the secondary amines were introduced. In general, the tertiary amines have been described as "dirty" medications because they are so difficult to tolerate, even at subtherapeutic levels. As seen in Figure 12.1, five medications are included in this group and, as can be seen in the fourth and fifth columns, their anticholinergic and sedative side effects (on a scale of 0–5) are generally very high. That is, even at subtherapeutic levels, patients often complain of such side effects as

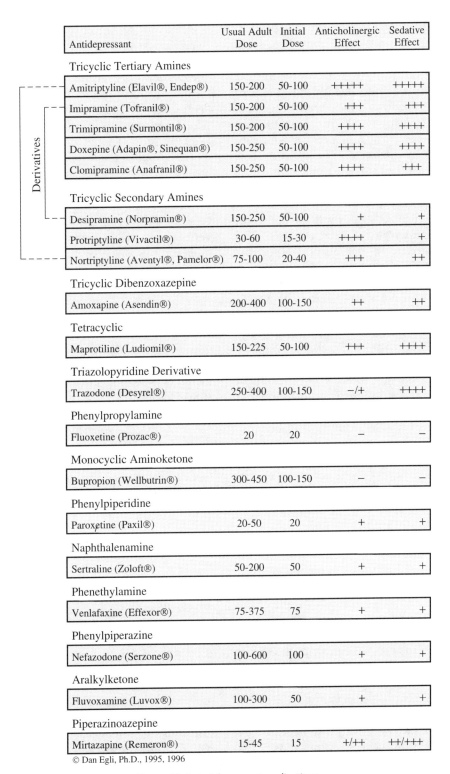

Antidepressant	Usual Adult Dose	Initial Dose	Anticholinergic Effect	Sedative Effect
Tricyclic Tertiary Amines				
Amitriptyline (Elavil®, Endep®)	150-200	50-100	+++++	+++++
Imipramine (Tofranil®)	150-200	50-100	+++	+++
Trimipramine (Surmontil®)	150-200	50-100	++++	++++
Doxepine (Adapin®, Sinequan®)	150-250	50-100	++++	++++
Clomipramine (Anafranil®)	150-250	50-100	++++	+++
Tricyclic Secondary Amines				
Desipramine (Norpramin®)	150-250	50-100	+	+
Protriptyline (Vivactil®)	30-60	15-30	++++	+
Nortriptyline (Aventyl®, Pamelor®)	75-100	20-40	+++	++
Tricyclic Dibenzoxazepine				
Amoxapine (Asendin®)	200-400	100-150	++	++
Tetracyclic				
Maprotiline (Ludiomil®)	150-225	50-100	+++	++++
Triazolopyridine Derivative				
Trazodone (Desyrel®)	250-400	100-150	−/+	++++
Phenylpropylamine				
Fluoxetine (Prozac®)	20	20	−	−
Monocyclic Aminoketone				
Bupropion (Wellbutrin®)	300-450	100-150	−	−
Phenylpiperidine				
Paroxetine (Paxil®)	20-50	20	+	+
Naphthalenamine				
Sertraline (Zoloft®)	50-200	50	+	+
Phenethylamine				
Venlafaxine (Effexor®)	75-375	75	+	+
Phenylpiperazine				
Nefazodone (Serzone®)	100-600	100	+	+
Aralkylketone				
Fluvoxamine (Luvox®)	100-300	50	+	+
Piperazinoazepine				
Mirtazapine (Remeron®)	15-45	15	+/++	++/+++

Derivatives

© Dan Egli, Ph.D., 1995, 1996

Figure 12.1. Antidepressant medications.

constipation, dry mouth, weight gain, and postural or orthostatic hypotension. In addition, because of the sedative properties, patients may complain of drowsiness or fatigue.

The five agents represented in this group of tertiary tricyclics do have some current usage both within and outside of psychiatry. Elavil is frequently prescribed by neurologists for pain syndromes. There was a time in recent years where Tofranil was in use as a panicolytic (antipanic) medication as a substitute for the habit-forming benzodiazepines, and Anafranil was the first agent approved in the United States for the treatment of obsessive-compulsive disorder (OCD).

A significant concern with all of the TCAs is their lethality in overdose as well as their cardiotoxicity. At this point, because of its side effect profile, Anafranil has fallen out of favor in the treatment of OCD. There are currently four additional agents, all SSRIs, formally approved for the treatment of OCD (Baxter et al., 1992). In order of U.S. approval, they are fluoxetine (Prozac), sertraline (Zoloft), fluvoxamine (Luvox), and paroxetine (Paxil). Although Figure 12.1 indicates the usual starting dose and typical therapeutic range for these medications, these figures may need to be lowered in pediatric, adolescent, geriatric, and certain side effect–sensitive adults.

The secondary tricyclics were developed next as a result of the side effect problems with tertiary amine tricyclics (DeVeaugh-Geiss, Landau, & Katz, 1989). As can be seen in Figure 12.1, this group of antidepressants comprises three agents. These are generally better tolerated and have far fewer anticholinergic and sedative properties. Even these three agents, however, have fallen out of favor and have generally been replaced by some of the newer, broad-spectrum-of-efficacy agents. If a patient's history indicates that a family member previously had a good response to a tricyclic, then it is possible that the prescriber would consider using the TCA, as there may be a genetic predisposition to having a preferential response to a specific agent. One potential benefit or advantage of the tricyclics in some situations would be their cost. Because they frequently come in generic formulations, the monthly costs may be significantly less than for the newer agents, and this may be one of the bases for selecting one of these as a first-line agent for some patients.

Heterocyclics or HCAs is a term given to some of the older antidepressants that are not tricyclic antidepressants but may be either bicyclic or tetracyclic. An example of the only tetracyclic currently available in the United States is maprotiline (Ludiomil). Another tetracyclic, which is not yet available in the United States, is mianserin. Maprotiline (Ludiomil) is sometimes argued not to be a tricyclic but, rather, a tricyclic with a bridge across one of the central tricyclic rings. Because of this, it parallels very closely many of the TCA side effects. Although it may have slightly fewer drying effects than some TCAs, it is lethal in overdose and may lower the seizure threshold, thereby increasing the risk of seizures.

Another atypical agent among the older ones is amoxapine (Asendin). It is unusual in that it not only has some antidepressant properties but also may have some dopamine-blocking properties and therefore is possibly effective in psychotic depressions. Because of its dopaminergic properties, however, one must be concerned about some of the usual side effects with neuroleptics, such as tardive dyskinesia (TD). At this point, with better developed antidepressants and newly developed neuroleptics that have been recently approved (e.g., clozaril and risperdal), as well as other neuroleptics that are at phase III level of development or beyond (meaning that they will soon be approved by the FDA), this agent has essentially fallen into disuse.

A final older agent that is somewhat atypical is trazodone (Desyrel). At present it has fallen into relative disuse as an antidepressant even though it has fewer anticholinergic side effects than others mentioned. Because it does have some sedating properties, it has become one of the most widely prescribed agents for symptoms of insomnia. Although it is not formally approved as a hypnotic by the FDA, many prescribers are using a very low dose of trazodone to take advantage of its sedating properties in order to help the patient get a good night's rest, without morning hangover, without risk of habituation, and without any CNS-depressant side effects. As can be seen in the chart, trazodone is neither a TCA or HCA but, rather, a triazolopyridine derivative. Some concern has been raised about the use of trazodone in therapeutic levels because of priapism (prolonged painful erection) in men. Though rare, this condition in isolated cases requires surgical intervention and may result in permanent impotence.

Another benefit of these older antidepressant agents is the fact that therapeutic drug monitoring (TDM) has been developed to allow clinicians to assess through blood plasma levels whether the amount of medication that the patient is taking has reached "therapeutic levels" (Goodwin, Prange, Post, Muscettola, & Lipton, 1982). For each of the agents that has a relatively well developed TDM literature base, clinicians can do a blood plasma level to assess whether the patient may be noncompliant with taking the medication or to head off potential toxicity. Such medications include imipramine, amitriptyline, desipramine, doxepin, and nortriptyline. Of these five compounds, the TDM that has been viewed as the most reliable and most specific is with nortriptyline. With newer agents, the manufacturers neither recommend doing TDM, nor have procedures been developed to a level that are either cost-efficient or as accurate as they need to be.

In summary, the older agents have generally fallen out of use and are rarely, if ever, used as first-line agents. They are equal in efficacy to the newer agents, have an equal latency of onset of action, are less costly, but are very lethal in overdose, are cardiotoxic, and generally have far more of a burdensome side effect profile.

SELECTIVE SEROTONIN-REUPTAKE INHIBITORS (SSRIs)

In the last few years there has been an increasing amount of evidence suggesting that serotonin neurotransmission is decreased during an episode of major depression (Richelson, 1988). Zimelidine was the first SSRI available for worldwide use, in 1982, but it was withdrawn because of problems associated with its use. Since that time, four SSRIs have been introduced to the U.S. market and, in order of introduction, include fluoxetine (Prozac),

sertraline (Zoloft), paroxetine (Paxil), and fluvoxamine (Luvox). Both Prozac and Zoloft are currently approved in the United States for both major depression and OCD (Rapoport, 1991). Paxil was initially approved for major depression only but in recent months received its additional approval for both OCD and panic disorder. Luvox was just approved by the FDA as a treatment for OCD in children.

These four agents tend to be more similar than they are different. As Figure 12.1 shows, these drugs have much less in the way of anticholinergic (e.g., blurred vision, dry mouth, constipation) and sedating effects than the older agents. In general, the most prominent side effects that occur with the SSRIs include mild nonmigrainous headaches, GI distress, and activation. The GI distress can come in the form of upset stomach, nausea, or diarrhea, and the activation tends to present as restlessness, agitation, anxiety, or insomnia. Typically, these agents are given in the morning as opposed to nighttime, so that patients are less likely to have any problem with sleep disturbance.

Another of the more common side effects of the SSRIs is sexual dysfunction, which can present as decreased libido, delayed orgasm, or anorgasmia (failure to achieve orgasm) for both men and women (Cooper, 1988). This is one of the more common side effects that can occur with this class of antidepressant. It may affect as many as 15% to 30% of patients. However, the biggest advantage of the SSRIs is the fact that their side effect profile, overall, is much more favorable than that of the older agents, and many patients report notable improvement without significant side effects. Often, the initial side effects that do occur level off and/or disappear completely within a short period of time. If the side effects are intolerable or do not level off, however, then switching to another SSRI can reduce the problem.

In contrast to the older agents, the SSRIs are extremely safe in overdose and are not cardiotoxic. The cost of these agents is much higher than that of the older agents, as they are currently not available generically. When one considers the overall efficacy and speed of improvement, however, some studies are beginning to suggest that even though the initial outlay of money for these medications may be greater, in the end they may actually lead to lower health costs when compared to the older agents.

Several of the differences between the SSRIs have to do with (1) teratogenicity (adverse fetal effects); (2) drug–drug interactions; and (3) half-life. The current teratogen rating system includes categories A (very low risk), B (mild), C (moderate), D (severe), and X (extreme and contraindicated). Of the SSRIs, the only Category B teratogen is fluoxetine, with the others having a less benign rating of Category C.

In terms of drug–drug interactions, there are a number of growing concerns and in some cases outright contraindications between the SSRIs and other classes of drugs that are metabolized by isoenzymes in the liver known as the P450 hepatic isoenzymes. There is a flurry of research in this area at this time, and it seems that each week the manufacturers of the respective SSRIs are adding new drug–drug interaction precautions or contraindications. As an example, the manufacturer of fluvoxamine (Luvox) now indicates as a contraindication drugs within the specific P450 isoenzyme subclass 3A4. These medications include a number of antihistamines (Seldane and Hismanal) as well as a medication frequently used by gastronenterologists (Propulsid), and the triazolo-benzodiazepine triazolam (Halcion). This means that if this particular SSRI is given in conjunction with any of these four medications, the pharmacokinetic interaction of these agents is likely to be seen in significant elevations in blood levels of the other drug, resulting in symptoms of drug toxicity or in other physical complications such as cardiac arrhythmias. Another SSRI drug, sertraline (Zoloft), also has some precautions noted in regard to the P450 3A4 isoenzyme, and fluoxetine (Prozac) has some precautions related to the P450 2D6 isoenzymes (Hirschfeld & Goodwin, 1988).

This is a fairly complicated issue, but it does raise important considerations about drug–drug interactions, and it is helping clinicians to become more astute and able to select a specific SSRI depending on what other medications the individual may be on

(Beasley & Dornseif, 1991). This issue has significant relevance to geriatric populations who are frequently on many other psychotropic and nonpsychotropic medications (often as many as ten).

The half-life of a drug is a measure of the time required for the serum level of the drug to decrease by 50%, assuming no further drug is being administered. The half-lives of sertraline (Zoloft) and paroxetine (Paxil) are approximately one day, whereas the half-life of fluvoxamine (Luvox) is much shorter, necessitating multiple dosing per day. The half-life of fluoxetine (Prozac) and its active (noninert) metabolite is very long (approximately 168 hours or longer). This is both an advantage and a disadvantage, as is a short half-life. A short half-life is an advantage when it comes to switching from one drug to another, whereas a long half-life is an advantage if the patient decides unilaterally not to take the medication on a particular day. With the long-life agent, blood levels are less likely to fluctuate, resulting in a lower likelihood of any change in mood or reemergence of mood symptoms. In contrast, the long half-life of fluoxetine and its metabolite (norfluoxetine) is problematic when one might be switching from an SSRI to a MAOI because the washout period (time on *no* drug at all) can be in the range of 5 to 6 weeks (Feighner, Herbstein, & Damlouji, 1985). When switching from a short-half-life SSRI to a MAOI, however, the washout period is generally considered much shorter, specifically two weeks. A disadvantage of a short half-life is that if patients unilaterally decide to skip or discontinue a dose, they often may experience a fairly rapid reemergence of depressive symptoms. In addition, tapering off the short-half-life medications is far more likely to induce a withdrawal-like syndrome if the titration decrements are too large or too fast.

At this point in time, the SSRIs are clearly the first-line agents of choice for the treatment of major depression. They are well tolerated by many people, are not lethal in overdose, are noncardiotoxic, and have a broad spectrum of efficacy. Specifically, their broad spectrum of efficacy includes at least three or four benefits. The three clear benefits for each of the SSRIs include the fact that they are effective antidepressants, good anxiolytics (antianxiety) agents, and excellent antiobsessional agents. A fourth possible benefit is that they may, in addition to their antiobsessional efficacy, have anticompulsive efficacy. That is why all four SSRIs (Prozac, Luvox, Zoloft, and Paxil) are currently formally approved for the treatment of OCD.

Before looking at the MAOIs, we will now review the other four new agents that are available in the United States in addition to the four SSRIs just reviewed. Those four agents, in order of introduction to the United States, include bupropion (Wellbutrin), venlafaxine (Effexor), nefazodone (Serzone), and mirtazapine (Remeron).

ATYPICAL ANTIDEPRESSANT: BUPROPION (WELLBUTRIN)

This newer agent is marketed primarily as an "atypical" antidepressant, so named because its mechanism of action is still unclear. Some investigators feel that it is a DNRI, a dopamine–norepinephrine reuptake inhibitor, because of some anecdotal reports of EPS-like side effects similar to those of neuroleptics. The primary way in which the maufacturer of this agent tends to market the drug is to emphasize the fact that it has very little likelihood of causing sexual dysfunction. In the clinical trials, the incidence of impotence and decreased libido was not statistically significantly different from placebo (Gardner, 1983).

The primary concern of the manufacturer and prescribers is the fact that it is slightly more epileptogenic (seizure-producing) than other antidepressants, specifically with an incidence of approximately 0.4% (4/1,000). On closer examination in the clinical trials, those who had seizures tended to be individuals whose dose was elevated above 450 mg per day and whose titration rate was greater than the recommended 150 mg per dose increase. Bupropion is contraindicated in three specific situations: (1) any history of prior seizure or head trauma, (2) CNS tumor, and (3) any concomitant medications or treatment regimens that lower the seizure threshold (e.g., antipsychotics, other antidepressants, or abrupt benzodiazepine discontinuation). In general, this medication is relatively

well tolerated by many patients and is an option to consider if sexual dysfunction is a concern. In the clinical trials, approximately 10% of the patients discontinue treatment because of side effects. Common side effects (those occurring with a greater than 20% incidence in the clinical trials) include tremor (21.1%), dizziness (22.3%), increased sweating (22.3%), nausea (22.9%), weight loss (23.2%), migraine/headache (25.7%), constipation (26.0%), dry mouth (27.6%), and agitation (31.9%). Another contraindication would be in someone who has a known allergy or hypersensitivity to the drug or who is in concomitant MAOI therapy.

VENLAFAXINE (EFFEXOR)

This newer antidepressant is generally viewed as a serotonin norepinephrine reuptake inhibitor (SNRI). As such, it has both the advantages and disadvantages of serotonin but without all the side effects of the earlier/older antidepressants. In the clinical trials, the main concern was a sustained increase in supine diastolic blood pressure (SDBP). However, this side effect is typically found to be dose-dependent with approximately 1% to 2% of patients experiencing it on doses between 100 and 150 mg, 3% to 4% on 200 to 300 mg, and approximately 6% of patients experiencing it on doses higher than 300 mg. The drug has a relatively low propensity to induce seizures, and ejaculatory inhibition was seen in approximately 10% of the cases in the clinical trials. A possible disadvantage of this agent, which would make it more likely to be a second-line than a first-line agent, is the fact that it requires a b.i.d. (twice a day) or t.i.d. (three times a day) dosing. If the medication is effective but at the same time produces an increase in blood pressure, often the patient can be kept on the therapeutic dose of the drug, along with standard antihypertensive treatment (ACE inhibitors, beta blockers, vasodilators, calcium-channel blockers, etc.).

Approximately 19% of those in the clinical trials discontinued treatment because of side effects. The most common of these include dry mouth (22%), somnolence (23%), headache (25%), and nausea (37%).

NEFAZODONE (SERZONE)

Nefazodone is an analog of trazodone. It is generally considered to be a serotonin-norepinephrine reuptake inhibitor presynaptically and a serotonin (5-HT) subreceptor-2 antagonist postsynaptically. Its mechanism of action is generally indicated by SNRI-5HT$_2$. It is viewed by many as a "mixed" reuptake inhibitor in that it has action on both sides of the synapse. Although this does make nefazodone unique, it does not suggest any greater efficacy or any decreased latency of onset of action. The main concern clinicians need to have is what its side effect profile is like compared to those of the other newer agents. The most significant side effects experienced in the clinical trials included nausea (22%), somnolence (25%), dry mouth (26%), and headache (36%). Its half-life is approximately 2 to 4 hours, so it needs to be given in multiple dosing per day. Like all of the newer antidepressants, it has a relatively low risk of lethality in overdose and is associated with a low incidence of drug-induced sexual dysfunction in both men and women. Other risks are still somewhat unknown because of the newness of the agent.

MIRTAZAPINE (REMERON)

Like nefazodone, mirtazapine is a "mixed" reuptake inhibitor in that it also exerts action on both sides of the synapse. It is an analog of another antidepressant available in Europe, known as Mianserin, and is actually a tetracyclic antidepressant. Its dual mechanism of action is that it is (presynaptically) an alpha 2 adrenergic autoreceptor blocker and a 5-HT (serotonin) 3 antagonist postsynaptically. The "bottom line" of this dual mechanism of action is that it also does not have a greater efficacy or a shorter latency of onset of action. In this case, the main clinical concern would be that of its side effect profile compared to those of the other newer agents. As of this writing, mirtazapine has been approved for a short period of time, so data are lacking as to its long-term effects and efficacy. More double-blind placebo-controlled studies are needed for further evaluation.

In general, the newer antidepressant agents are generally far better tolerated than the previous older agents. In my experience, the SSRIs tend to be chosen as first-line agents, with the other four newer medications being chosen as second-line agents. The older agents are being relegated to the "Smithsonian Institute of Psychopharmacology" except for rare occasions (e.g., treatment-refractory augmentation, family history of a specificity of response to an older agent, or having exhausted adequate clinical trials of all of the newer agents).

MONOAMINE OXIDASE INHIBITORS (MAOIs)

An early MAOI that was widely prescribed was known as iproniazid (Marsilid) (Quitkin, Rifkin, & Klein, 1979). When it was discovered that it could cause liver toxicity, it led to the development of the three currently available MAO inhibitors, which include the nonhydrazine MAOIs such as tranylcypomine (Parnate), the hydrazine MAOIs such as isocarboxazid (Marplan), and phenelzine (Nardil). Marplan, however, is generally not in use and at present there exists only a one- or two- year supply that is available only on a compassionate use basis.

In general, the MAOIs are not a first-line agent for depression because of the dietary restrictions and contraindications with other prescription and over-the-counter (OTC) medications (McGrath, Quitkin, Harrison, & Stewart, 1984). Once patients learn the diet, however, these drugs are far better tolerated than most people think they would be. Some research groups and clinicians believe that the MAOIs, as a class, may be the treatment of choice for so-called atypical major depression, which would include such symptoms as oversleeping (hypersomnia), overeating (hyperphagia) with weight gain, rejection sensitivity, panic-type anxiety, and reverse diurnal variation in mood (mood worsening as the day goes on, as opposed to improving or lifting). In addition, the MAOIs are typically reserved for cases of treatment-resistant major depression (Rabkin, Quitkin, McGrath, Harrison, & Tricamo, 1985). In cases where other antidepressants are being used, a "washout" period is needed before switching to the MAOI. For example, with three of the four new SSRIs (Zoloft, Paxil, and Luvox), a two-week washout is generally recommended, whereas with fluoxetine (Prozac) a five- to six- week washout is recommended because of the long half-life of norfluoxetine, a noninert metabolite of the parent compound (Lemberger, Bergstrom, Wolen, Farid, Enas, & Aronoff, 1985).

As indicated, the primary concern with this class of antidepressant is the restricted diet and avoidance of medications that contain sympathomimetic amines (Shulman, Walker, MacKenzie, & Knowles, 1989). Although toxic reactions to this class are uncommon, they do necessitate immediate discontinuation and treatment of the symptoms of hypertensive crises, which can pose a severe and potentially fatal situation. When MAOIs are taken with tyramine-containing foods or medications, symptoms need to be treated immediately and aggressively while the drug is quickly discontinued. Examples of foods with high tyramine content that should be avoided are sauerkraut, broad-bean pods, aged meats, pickled herring, and aged cheese. The main concern resulting from the use of these agents and tyramine-containing products and/or sympathomimetic drugs is a hypertensive crisis that in the worse-case scenario could result in a serious stroke. Hepatotoxicity occurs in rare cases with the currently available hydrozine MAOIs, and a central serotonin syndrome (marked by severe agitation) is also something that can occur with the MAOIs when they are combined with the newer SSRIs.

In general, the MAOIs are relegated to use in atypical depression that has been nonresponsive to other newer antidepressants and/or in treatment-refractory major depression. Because of the dietary restrictions and drug–drug contraindications, MAO inhibitors are not as widely used as the other non-MAO inhibitor antidepressants, but they still remain, with good patient education, an effective treatment of choice.

PSYCHOSTIMULANTS

This group of agents has been studied in the treatment of hyperactivity since the late 1930s. The three agents that are approved by the Food and Drug Administration (FDA) to treat ADHD in children and adolescents are dextroamphetamine (Dexedrine, Adderall), magnesium pemoline (Cylert), and methylphenidate (Ritalin). The term used to describe these medications, *psychostimulants*, is derived from their tendency to increase CNS activity in some regions of the brain (Chiarello & Cole, 1987). Though formally approved for use in narcolepsy as well, these three agents are used primarily for the treatment of ADD/ADHD in children and adolescents.

In recent years, with the growing awareness of ADD/ADHD, more adults have been diagnosed and treated with the same agents used in child and adolescent populations (Rickels, Gordon, Gansman, et al., 1970). In general, these three agents are used to target such cognitive and behavioral symptoms as inattention, difficulty with concentration, overall cognitive functioning, irritability, and impulsivity.

Some of the typical dosing strategies and various pharmacologic properties of these three agents are listed in Table 12.7. It should be noted that methylphenidate (MPH) also comes in a sustained-release (SR) formulation in light of the fact that it has a relatively short half-life of approximately 2 to 4 hours. Parents and teachers will often note a rebound-like effect at the end of the dosing period, when some of the ADD/ADHD symptoms begin to emerge (Wender, Reimherr, Wood, et al., 1985). Of the three agents available, MPH is probably the most widely used worldwide. One special concern related to the use of dextroamphetamine is the fact

Table 12.7 Psychostimulants

GENERIC NAME	TRADE NAME	DOSE RANGE	HALF-LIFE	SR FORMULATION	DURATION OF EFFECT
Dextroamphetamine	Dexedrine	5–60	6–8 h	N	3–5 h
Methylphenidate	Ritalin	5–80	2–4 h	Y	2–4 h
Pemoline	Cylert	18.75–112.5	8–12 h	N	5–8 h

that it is a Schedule II controlled substance. As such, it raises implications about issues of addiction/dependence and, for this reason, has been used less frequently than the other medications.

A less common use of the psychostimulants is in treatment-resistant/refractory major depressive episode, although this is an off-label indication for their use. This strategy is sometimes employed as an augmentation or potentiation strategy along with a concurrently administered antidepressant in major depression that is not responding or is only partially responding to typical agents.

Some of the more typically reported side effects from these agents include an activation syndrome, which includes nervousness and insomnia. Headaches can occur as well as upset stomach and loss of appetite, with related weight loss. These side effects often lessen or disappear after the initial few weeks of treatment. Other less common but more serious side effects that can occur with the use of psychostimulants include increased blood pressure, nightmares, rash, rapid heartbeat (tachycardia), and altered liver functioning (more likely with pemoline).

Some initial reports suggested that the use of these agents may stunt growth if they are used for extended periods of time, but investigations pursuant to these initial studies have mixed results. What seems to be developing as a literature and clinician consensus is that once psychostimulants are discontinued in adolescence, the growth spurt that frequently occurs at that same time may likely compensate for any stunting of growth that may have occurred earlier. The overall eventual height is not compromised.

One interesting factor to note in making use of these agents is that the clinician can expect to have a much quicker onset of action, often within a day or two of reaching therapeutic levels. This stands in contrast to some of the more traditional agents used in psychopharmacology, such as the antidepressants, which often have a latency of onset of action of approximately one month. The prescriber can get a fairly quick sense of whether the patient is going to be a responder or not.

Complicating the use of psychostimulants in ADD/ADHD is co-morbidity. For example, many children with ADD have co-morbid oppositional-defiant disorder (ODD) or conduct disorder. Other co-morbid conditions not infrequently occurring are mood and anxiety disorders, as well as learning disabilities. These examples of co-morbidity may affect both the pharmacologic and the psychosocial treatment interventions. It should also be noted that the use of these agents is rarely done outside the context of simultaneously employing psychoeducational and cognitive-behavioral strategies. Often, through the use of numerous parent-rating and teacher-rating ADD/ADHD scales, a pre- and post-test assessment of the effect of the medication can be done. This can provide invaluable assistance to the clinician in getting a sense of whether the psychostimulant is effective.

Approximately 5% to 20% of patients do not respond well to stimulant medications for one reason or another and end up trying another type of medication for its possible anti-ADD effects. Examples of some of these agents include several of the tricyclic antidepressants, clonidine, and buproprion. The use of some of the newer antidepressants in the treatment of ADD/ADHD is not well known, and studies are limited.

Overall, the risk of long-term side effects remains low and thus the overall benefit-to-risk ratio of this group of medications remains very good. Implementing drug holidays and making use of the various rating scales in a serial fashion will help the clinician know how to titrate the drug up to therapeutic levels as well as when to begin tapering and discontinuing the medication. It should also be noted that these agents are not approved for use in children under 6 years of age.

THE PSYCHOLOGIST AS A PRESCRIBER?

In recent years there has been an increasing interest on the part of certain psychologists, primarily clinicians, in obtaining prescription privileges. This has been a hotly debated subject within psychological circles. At the 1996 annual convention in Toronto, the Council of Representatives formally approved two documents that had to do with a model curriculum and model legislation developed by the APA Committee for the Advancement of

Professional Psychology (CAPP) Task Force on Prescription Privileges, which I chaired. This task force submitted their findings to CAPP, which then took the recommendations regarding model curriculum and model legislation to a tridirectorate group composed of the Board of Educational Affairs (BEA), the Board of Professional Affairs (BPA), and the Board of Scientific Affairs (BSA). The latter group reviewed the documents and made recommendations to the board of directors and council, and it was ultimately adopted at the aforementioned meeting in Toronto, Ontario, Canada. Thus, for the first time, a formal statement was made by APA to those within the organization that they were giving their "blessing" to proceed with developing these two areas for those who had an interest in the formal pursuit of prescription privileges.

Historically, there were some very early and interesting developments that related to prescription privileges. Within the Indian Health Service (IHS), there were a number of prescribing psychologists who typically prescribed from a limited formulary (a list of agents they were allowed to use) and in a dependent fashion. That is to say, they wrote the prescription and it was co-signed by a supervising physician. Obviously, these were psychologists who were placed in extremely rural settings, where psychiatric coverage for the prescribing of psychotropics was limited, if not nonexistent. It was not until recent years that the American Psychiatric Association (ApA) realized that this was occurring and, through legislative and political pressure, forced this practice to discontinue. This development, however, was more an offshoot of another attack that ApA was waging against the American Psychological Association (APA) in relation to another program within the military.

Another early development that was spawned in California was a degree in the 1970s called the Doctorate in Mental Health (DMH), in which there was an attempt to blend clinical psychology and psychiatry training. Those few trainees from that DMH program essentially took courses similar to a psychiatric residency and graduated with this unique degree, but never did end up formally prescribing. Ultimately the program went into nonexistence.

More recent developments in the early 1990s occurred when the Department of Defense, at the request of Senator Daniel Inouye (D-Hawaii) recommended a Psychopharmacology Demonstration Project (PDP), which is now in its fourth iteration. The first iteration of the PDP has graduates, two of whom are now prescribing within a military hospital setting from a limited formulary. Their prescriptions are co-signed by a supervising prescribing physician.

This program has been the object of intense scrutiny and opposition from the ApA, and the cost-effectiveness of the program will be evaluated by the National College of Neuropsychopharmacology. The initial iteration of the program was one that paralleled very closely a medical school training program, but more recent iterations/versions of the PDP have been pared down, primarily eliminating some of the more technical classwork and emphasizing more of the clinical practicum with supervision experience. The initial trainees from the program who are now prescribing felt that many of the courses they took prior to the practicum were totally irrelevant to their actual clinical prescription practice. New graduates from the third and fourth iterations of the program will soon be graduating, but the program continues to be a target for the American Psychiatric Association. They consistently target this program for funding cuts and ultimately discontinuation based on the premise that in their view, it is harmful to the consumer to have psychologists prescribing.

In the early 1990s, the Board of Professional Affairs (BPA), sponsored a fall retreat in which they began to focus on the feasibility of psychologists prescribing. Out of this fall retreat came a general consensus that it would be reasonable and feasible for individuals who get appropriate retraining to move toward prescription privileges. Their work was ultimately passed along to various factions within APA administration and governances, and the following year the APA Task Force on Prescription Privileges was created by the board of directors. On this task force were primarily academicians and one full-time clinician (myself). Out of this task force, which primarily addressed the feasibility and desirability of psychologists prescribing, came the now infamous Level I, Level II, and Level III differentiation. Level I simply had to do with exposure to psychopharmacology. Level II generally had to do with experiences leading to a more active collaboration with physicians in the prescribing of psychotropics. Level III was seen as representing unlimited, independent prescription privileges for psychologists. The recommendations from the APA Task Force on Prescription Privileges were forwarded to the board of directors, and various leaders within the APA's governance began to define what curriculum and legislative models would be needed to move toward the establishment of prescription privileges.

Shortly before the development of the aforementioned CAPP Task Force, a blue-ribbon panel was established in the state of California, which also, through group consensus, developed a model curriculum for psychologists that might be interested in developing this subspecialty. This blue-ribbon panel comprised both prescribers and nonprescribers, and the 30 or so members of the panel developed their set of curriculum recommendations. Shortly thereafter, the CAPP Task Force on Prescription Privileges was given the goal of developing their own model legislation and curriculum. As part of their work, they reviewed the model curriculum of the blue-ribbon panel and adopted many of their recommendations with a few revisions.

Along with the growing interest among clinicians in support of prescription privileges for psychologists, there are a number of competing forces within the profession that are actively opposed to this goal. Many articles critical of this movement have appeared in the monthly magazine for psychologists, the *APA Monitor,* and there are even one or two specific organizations that are marketing themselves as actively opposed to prescription privileges. For the most part, however, these organizations were formed and maintained by academic psychologists as opposed to full-time clinicians.

At the same time as this opposition group grew and began to mobilize itself, more and more divisions within the APA began to take a serious look at how to integrate psychopharmacology practice into clinical practice. As an example, Division 16 (School Psychology) developed a task force to look at the psychopharmacology issue. This was because many of their members are working in educational settings where a large percentage of children are diagnosed with ADD/ADHD and are taking psychostimulants. These psychologists often find themselves in the position of (informally) making recommendations about psychostimulants to general/family practitioners. In addition, Division 39 (Psychoanalysis) has also begun to become more receptive to ways they could integrate psychopharmacology with psychoanalysis. In Division 39's 1994 board decision, there was an affirmative vote in the direction of supporting those psychologists who are inclined to seek retraining that would ultimately lead to prescription privileges.

In addition to the various division activities, an increasing number of state and provincial psychological associations (SPPAs) are developing their own prescription privilege task forces within their respective state or province. At this point, a number of states have attempted to introduce legislation regarding prescription privileges bills. Most of the states that have done this are largely rural and have been met with tremendous opposition from the medical (specifically psychiatric) community. Two states that have been very aggressive in trying to get a bill into their legislatures are Hawaii and California. As of this writing, it is estimated that anywhere between five and ten states will shortly begin a coordinated effort (with legal and advisory input from the Practice Directorate) to introduce a prescription privileges bill into legislation. At this point, the model legislation and model curriculum developed by the CAPP Task Force on Prescription Privileges is generally seen as the basis on which most, if not all, of the state and provincial psychological associations will proceed.

Another development within the APA, as a function of the larger emphasis on psychopharmacology and subspecialization, is the possibility that the National College will offer credentialing as a formal subspecialty area. This would allow members who are looking to get retrained to market this subspecialty to the public. The National College has already developed an exam to test for competency in the area of addictions and substance abuse, and is contemplating developing a module in the area of psychopharmacology.

A further development that grew out of the earlier task force on psychopharmacology is that the Board of Educational Affairs (BEA) is working on specifying what Level I training would look like at both the undergraduate and graduate levels. This Level I Task Force is chaired by Dr. Marlyne Kilbey, an academician/researcher in Michigan. Their goal is to develop a model curriculum that would be consistent with Level I (exposure) training. In addition, more pharmaceutical companies seem to be in attendance at the annual APA meetings, setting up booths and distributing literature, while more CE (continuing education) firms are marketing psychopharmacology workshops, home study courses, and specialty certifications based on varying numbers of hours of training.

It appears that the majority of clinicians (approximately two-thirds) favor supporting prescription privileges, while the support of academicians/researchers is generally not as strong. More and more state and provincial psychological associations (SPPAs) are requesting psychopharmacology continuing education modules at their annual meetings. At their annual meeting, Division 12's (clinical) Post-Doctoral Institute (PDI) always has at least one program on psychopharmacology. As of this writing, the trend is clearly moving toward trying to provide support for those who have an interest in getting retrained in this subspecialty area. This will certainly be much easier if it is supported by the profession at large. The recent formal recognition of the model legislation and model curriculum pieces that were sent to the Council of Representatives and approved at the 1996 annual meeting in Toronto are a large step in this direction.

However, opposition to this subspecialty will continue. The primary reasons given by those opposed have to do with believing that it will dramatically increase malpractice insurance rates and that it will fundamentally change the identity of psychologists—for example, that pursuing prescription privileges will simply turn psychologists into "junior psychiatrists." Obviously, those in favor of the goal can offer many reasons that these arguments are not valid. At this point, it seems as though a number of rural states will probably develop legislation leading to a successful bill long before the political tug of war within the American Psychological Association is resolved. This will force a training module to be developed in any such state, and once this occurs, other states are likely to follow suit.

Psychology is also legitimately concerned with interfacing with both the Boards of Nursing and the Boards of Pharmacy in each of the respective states so that when psychologists obtain prescription privileges, those efforts can be coordinated by those who would fill the prescriptions and/or dispense the medication. Even if psychiatry is successful initially in "shooting down" the PDP through political means, it is likely that the momentum within psychology is large enough so that eventually one state will succeed. This is likely to follow the development within other fields such as optometry, nursing, pharmacy, and so on, where each of these groups has successfully developed legislation related to prescription privileges within their scope of practice. They have been able to convince legislators and the consumer that they can safely dispense medications related to their scope of practice and that being able to do so only broadens their ability to be effective. This idea is attractive to many consumers. At the same time, many consumers of psychological services would welcome the opportunity to have effective psychotherapy and pharmacotherapy occur in one setting, and by one provider.

FUTURE TRENDS

The field of psychopharmacology continues to change rapidly. Recently introduced medications are rapidly becoming "antiquated" with the advent of even newer agents with equal or greater efficacy, fewer and less serious side effects, and better drug–drug interaction profiles. The next major advances are likely to be in the area of finding antidepressants with a shorter latency of onset, and finding neuroleptic/antipsychotic drugs that do not have the serious long-term side effects of some of the current medications. Of course, the ultimate goal is to find a cure for one or more of the serious mental illnesses.

Another burgeoning field is that of brain mapping and neuroimaging techniques (e.g., PET, SPECT, fMRI). Much recent interest has focused on repetitive transcranial magnetic stimulation (rTMS) in order to help map and modify brain–behavior relationships. Through these new methods, researchers may be able to test long-standing models of the etiology of various disorders (e.g., OCD or major depression). As a result, clinicians in the future may be able to have much more specificity in drug treatment. That is, we will have access to technology and medications that help us know more quickly which part of the brain or which neurotransmitter system/subsystem is involved, and which treatment will be most efficient and efficacious.

Ultimately, psychologists will succeed in developing the curriculum and legislative models to begin prescribing. Like many other current professional groups (nurse practitioners, optometrists, etc.), they will be able to provide pharmacologic interventions consistent with the scope and practice of treating mental illness.

REFERENCES

Baldessarini, R. J. (1985). *Chemotherapy in psychiatry* (2nd ed.). Cambridge, MA: Harvard University Press.

Ballenger, J. C., Burrows, G. D., DuPont, R. L., Lesser, I. M., Noyes, R., Pecknold, J. C., Rifkin, A., & Swinson, R. P. (1988). Alprazolam in panic disorder and agoraphobia: Results from a multicenter trial: I. Efficacy in short-term treatment. *Archives of General Psychiatry, 45*, 413–422.

Ballenger, J. C., & Post, R. M. (1980). Carbamazepine (Tegretol) in manic-depressive illness: A new treatment. *American Journal of Psychiatry, 137*, 782–790.

Baxter, L. R., Schwartz, J. M., Bergman, K. S., Szuba, M. P., Guze, B. H., Marriota, J. C., Alazvaki, A., Selin, C. E., Feung, H. K., Munford, P., & Phelps, M. E. (1992). Caudate glucose metabolic rate changes with both drug and behavior therapy for obsessive-compulsive disorder. *Archives of General Psychiatry, 49*, 681–689.

Beardsley, R. S., Gardocki, G. J., Larsen, D. B., & Hidalgo, J. (1988). Prescribing of psychotropic medication by primary care physicians and psychiatrists. *Archives of General Psychiatry, 45*, 1117–1119.

Beasley, C. M., & Dornseif, B. E. (1991). Fluoxetine and suicide: A meta-analysis of controlled trials of treatment of depression. *British Medical Journal, 303*, 685–692

Benet, L. Z., Mitchell, J. R., & Sherner, L. B. (1990). Pharmacokinetics: The dynamics of drug absorption, distribution and elimination. In A. G. Gilman, T. W. Rall, A. S. Nies, & P. Taylor (Eds.), *Goodman & Gilman's: The pharmacological basis of therapeutics* (pp. 1–32). New York: Pergamon Press.

Bielski, R. J., Friedel, R. O. (1976). Prediction of tricyclic antidepressant response: A critical review. *Archives of General Psychiatry, 33*, 1479–1489.

Carlson, G. A., & Goodwin, F. K. (1973). The stages of mania. *Archives of General Psychiatry, 28*, 221–228.

Carpenter, W., Heinrichs, D. (1983). Early intervention, time-limited targeted pharmacotherapy of schizophrenia. *Schizophrenia Bulletin, 9*, 533–542.

Carpenter, W. T., Hanlon, T. E., Heinrichs, D. W., Summerfelt, A. T., Kirkpatrick, B., Levine, J., & Buchanan, R. W. (1990). Continuous versus targeted medication in schizophrenic out-patients: Outcome results. *American Journal of Psychiatry, 147*, 1138–1148.

Chiarello, R. J., & Cole, J. O. (1987). The use of psychostimulants in general psychiatry: A reconsideration. *Archives of General Psychiatry, 44*, 286–295.

Coccaro, E. F., & Siever, L. J. (1985). Second generation antidepressants: A comparative review. *Journal of Clinical Pharmacology, 25*, 241.

Cole, J. O., & Bodkin, J. A. (1990). Antidepressant drug side effects. *Journal of Clinical Psychiatry, 51*(Suppl. 1), 21–26.

Comaty, J. E., & Janicak, P. G. (1987). Depot neuroleptics. *Psychiatric Annals, 17*, 491–496.

Cooper, G. L. (1988). The safety of fluoxetine—an update. *British Journal of Psychiatry, 153*(Suppl. 3), 77–86.

Davis, K., Kahn, R., Ko, G., & Davidson, M. (1991). Dopamine in schizophrenia: A review and reconceptualization. *American Journal of Psychiatry, 148*, 1474–1484.

DeVeaugh-Geiss, J., Landau, P., & Katz, R. (1989). Preliminary results from a multicenter trial of clomipramine in obsessive-compulsive disorder. *Psychopharmacology Bulletin, 25*, 36–40.

Donaldson, S. R., Glenberg, A. J., & Baldessarini, R. J. (1983). The pharmacological treatment of schizophrenia: A progress report. *Schizophrenia Bulletin, 9*, 504–527.

Erickson, S. H., Bergman, J. J., Schneeweiss, R., & Smithson, E. (1980). The use of drugs for unlabeled indications. *Journal of the American Medical Association, 243*, 1543–1546.

Feighner, J.P., Herbstein J., Damlouji, N. (1985). Combined MAOI, TCA, and direct stimulant therapy of treatment-resistant depression. *Journal of Clinical Psychiatry, 46,* 206–209.

Gardner, E. (1983). Long-term preventive care in depression: The use of bupropion in patients intolerant of other antidepressants. *Journal of Clinical Psychopharmacology,* 44, 163–169.

Gelenberg, A. J., & Schoonover, S. C. (1991). Bipolar disorder. In A. J. Gelenberg, E. L. Bassuk, & S. C. Schoonover (Eds.), *The practitioner's guide to psychoactive drugs* (3rd ed., pp. 127–131). New York: Plenum Press.

Goodwin, F. K., Prange, A. J., Jr., Post, R. M., Muscettola, G., & Lipton, M. A. (1982). Potentiation of antidepressant effects by L-Tri-iodothyronine in tricyclic nonresponders. *American Journal of Psychiatry, 139,* 34–38 .

Greenblatt, D. J., Shader, R. I., & Abernethy, D. R. (1983). Current status of benzodiazepines. *New England Journal of Medicine. 309*, 354, 410.

Hansten, P. D., & Horn, J. R. (1990). Drug interaction mechanisms and clinical characteristics. In *Drug interactions and updates.* Vancouver, WA: Applied Therapeutics.

Hirschfeld, R. M., & Goodwin, F. K. (1988). Mood disorders. In J. A. Talbott, R. E. Hales, & S. C. Yudofsky (Eds.), *The American Psychiatric Press textbook of psychiatry* (pp. 38–49). Washington, DC: American Psychiatric Press.

Jefferson, J. W., & Greist, J. H. (1977). *Primer of lithium therapy.* Baltimore, MD: Williams & Williams.

Jefferson, J. W., Greist, J. H., & Ackerman, D. L. (1986). *Lithium encyclopedia for clinical practice* (2nd ed.). Washington, DC: American Psychiatric Press.

Kales, A. (1982). Benzodiazepines in the treatment of insomnia. In E. Usdin, P. Skolnick, & J. F. Tallman (Eds.), *Pharmacology of benzodiazepines* (pp. 199–217). New York: Macmillan.

Kales, A. (1990). Quazepam: Hypnotic efficacy and side effects. *Pharmacotherapy, 10*, 1–12.

Koch-Weser, J., & Frishman, W. H. (1981). Beta-adrenoceptor antagonists: New drugs and new indications. *New England Journal of Medicine, 305*, 500–506.

Langtry, H. O., & Benfield, P. (1990). Zolpidem: A review of its pharmacodynamic and pharmacokinetic properties and therapeutic potential. *Drug, 40*, 291–313.

Lemburger, L., Bergstrom, R. F., Woolen, R. L., Farid, N. A., Enas, C. G., & Aronoff, G. R. (1985). Fluoxetine: Clinical pharmacology and physiology disposition. *Journal of Clinical Psychiatry, 46*(3),14–19.

Levenson, J. (1985). Neuroleptic malignant syndrome. *American Journal of Psychiatry, 142*, 1137–1145.

Lieberman, J., Kane, J., & Johns, C. (1989). Clozapine guidelines for clinical management. *Journal of Clinical Psychopharmacology, 50*, 329–338.

Lieberman, J. (1996). Atypical antipsychotic drugs as a first-line treatment of schizophrenia: A rationale and hypothesis. *Journal of Clinical Psychiatry, 57*, 68–71.

McGrath, P. J., Quitkin, F. M., Harrison, W., & Stewart, J. W. (1984). Treatment of melancholia with tranylcypromine. *American Journal of Psychiatry, 141*, 288–289.

Pisciotta, A. V. (1969). Agranulocytosis induced by certain phenothiazine derivatives. *Journal of the American Medical Association, 208*,1862–1868.

Pollack, M. H., Tesar, G. E., & Rosenbaum, J. F. (1986). Clonazepam in the treatment of panic disorder and agoraphobia: A one-year follow-up. *Journal of Clinical Psychopharmacology, 6*, 302–304.

Post, R. M., Ballenger, J. C., Uhde, T. W., & Bunney, W. E. (1984). Efficacy of carbamazepine in manic-depressive illness: Implications for underlying mechanisms. In R. M. Post & J. D. Ballenger (Eds.), *Neurobiology of mood disorders.* Baltimore, MD: Williams & Wilkins.

Post, R. M., Weiss, S. R. B., & Chuang, O. (1992). Mechanisms of action of anticonvulsants in affective disorders: Comparisons with lithium. *Journal of Clinical Psychopharmacology, 12*, 23S–35S.

Prien, R. F., Kupfer, D. J., Mansky, P. A., & Eversole, D. (1984). Drug therapy in the prevention of recurrences in unipolar and bipolar affective disorders. *Archives of General Psychiatry, 41*, 1096–1104.

Quitkin, F. M., Rifkin, A., & Klein, D. F. (1979). Monoamine oxidase inhibitors. *Archives of General Psychiatry, 36*, 749–760.

Rabkin, J. G., Quitkin, F. M., McGrath, P., Harrison, W., & Tricamo, E. (1985). Adverse reactions to monoamine oxidase inhibitors: Part II: Treatment correlates and clinical management. *Journal of Clinical Psychopharmacology, 5*, 2–9.

Rapoport, J. L. (1991). Recent advances in obsessive-compulsive disorder. *Neuropsychopharmacology, 5*, 1–10.

Richelson, E. (1988). Synaptic pharmacology of antidepressants: An update. *McLean Hospital Journal, 13*, 67–88.

Rickels, K., Gordon, P., Gansman, D., & Spotts, T. (1970). Pemoline and methylphenidate in mildly depressed outpatients. *Clinical Pharmacotherapy, 11,* 698–710.

Shulman, K. I., Walker, S. E., MacKenzie, S., & Knowles, S. (1989). Dietary restriction, tyramine, and the use of monoamine oxidase inhibitors. *Journal of Clinical Psychopharmacology, 2,* 397–402.

Smith, D. E., & Wesson, D. R. (1983). Benzodiazepine dependency syndromes. *Journal of Psychoactive Drugs, 15,* 85–95.

Stewart, J. W., Quitkin, F. J., & Klein, D. F. (1992). The pharmacotherapy of minor depression. *American Journal of Psychotherapy, 46,* 23–36.

Ulenhuth, E. H., DeWit, H., Balter, M. B., Johanson, C. E., & Mellinger, G. D. (1988). Risks and benefits of long term benzodiazepine use. *Journal of Clinical Psychopharmacology, 8,* 161–167.

Vestergaard, P., Amdisen, A., & Schow, M. (1980). Clinically significant side effects of lithium treatment. *Acta Psychiatrica Scandinavica, 62,* 193–200.

Watsky, E. J., & Salzam, C. (1991). Psychotropic drug interactions. *Hospital and Community Psychiatry, 42,* 247–256.

Weber, S. S., Saklad, S. R., & Kastenholz, K.V. (1992). Bipolar affective disorders. In M. A. Koda-Kimble, L. Y. Young, W. A. Kradjan, & B. J. Guglielmo (Eds.), *Applied therapeutics: The clinical use of drugs* (5th ed., 201–233). Vancouver, WA: Applied Therapeutics.

Wender, P. H., Reimherr, F. W., Wood, D., & Ward, M. (1985). A controlled study of methylphenidate in the treatment of attention deficit disorder, residual type in adults. *American Journal of Psychiatry, 142,* 547–552.

Winter, M. E. (1988). *Basic clinical pharmacokinetics.* Vancouver, WA: Applied Therapeutics.

FOR FURTHER READING

For psychology students who are interested in learning more about psychopharmacology and would like beginner-level texts, J. Preston, J. H. O'Neal, and M. C. Talaga (1994) have a handbook that is specifically targeted "for therapists." It is called *Handbook of Clinical Pharmacology for Therapists.* It covers psychopharmacologic interventions both by diagnosis and drug class. An earlier brief manuscript by J. Preston and J. Johnson (1993) entitled *Clinical Psychopharmacology Made Ridiculously Simple* is just that and gives a good overview of the psychotropics based on the various clinical syndromes (depression, psychosis, etc.). Gelenberg and Schoonover's (1991) book is also targeted for the nonprescribing psychotherapist and provides an overview based on the major psychotropic drug classes (see reference list). J. S. Maxmen and N. G. Ward (1995) *Psychotropic Drugs: Fast Facts* was written for the lay public and provides a very user-friendly summary of psychopharmacology for the student based on nine medication categories most relevant to mental health practice.

Several new newsletters (e.g., *Child and Adolescent Psychopharmacology News,* published by Guilford Press) and journals (e.g., *CNS Spectrums,* published by MBL Communications) are excellent resources for students who want to keep abreast of the ever-changing field of psychopharmacology.

CHAPTER 13

BEHAVIORAL MEDICINE/HEALTH PSYCHOLOGY

Kathy Sexton-Radek

INTRODUCTION

Behavioral medicine and health psychology as areas of specialization came into existence in the late 1970s. The public health revolution during those years accentuated a focus on psychological factors contributing to illness and disease. Historically, psychological factors were considered to be immeasurable in physical illness and disease and thereby were inferred to be involved. Freud (1940) purported the term *neurosis* originally to describe such conditions. The famous case of Anna O. treated by Freud involved her conversion of her feelings of anxiety into the physical symptom of mutism, among other things. This historical early practice is in contrast to present-day work that has identified physical symptoms, usually measured by medical tests/instrumentation, and a clear understanding of possible physiological/biological links to the presenting complaint. Alexander (1950) was first to use the term *psychosomatic medicine* to refer to these conditions. With ensuing advances in medical science, early detection and diagnosis led to treatment classifications of physical illnesses. Initially, client complaints of physical symptoms or disease in the absence of physical pathology were designated *somatoform disorders* (e.g., conversion and hysterical disorders), whereas observable physical symptoms resulting from measurable disease process were classified as *psychophysiological disorders* and were listed on Axis III of the *Diagnostic and Statistical Manual* (DSM) taxonomy. The new DSM-IV (1994) considers such conditions in various places throughout its classification system.

Blanchard (1982) identified the emergence of behavioral medicine resulting from three sources: (1) application of behavior change technology to mental health problems, (2) development of the field of biofeedback, and (3) increased mortality in the 1960s caused by cardiovascular disease.

Given the premise of the interchange between psychological factors and disease process, a clear demarcation of the physical and psychological components of a disorder is not easily discerned. Bakal (1979) posited his psychosocial model to explain this interdependence of biological, psychological, and social factors in illness/disease process. This model identified the reciprocal, interdependent relationship among biological, psychological, and social factors (Meyers, 1991). Recent research investigations of individuals with the AIDS virus have identified the association between stress levels and environmental conditions in the exacerbation of this disease process. It is also known that other viral infections such as herpes simplex are worsened in stressful conditions.

BEHAVIORAL MEDICINE

Behavioral medicine is defined as the application of behavioral science to prevent, diagnose, and treat illness and disease. Schwartz and Weiss (1978) indicate behavioral medicine to be "the field concerned with the development of behavioral-science knowledge and techniques relevant to the understanding of physical health and illness and the application of this knowledge and these techniques to prevention, diagnosis, treatment, and rehabilitation." Psychosis, neurosis, and substance abuse are included only insofar as they contribute to physical disorders as an endpoint (Schwartz & Weiss, 1978). The presence of either symptom (physical or psychological) does not rule out the other. That is to say, physical change does not rule out the need to examine psychological variables. The field is interdisciplinary, with clinical psychologists working professionally with other medical professionals, such as physicians, nurses, physical therapists, and occupational therapists. The primary responsibilities of clinical psychologists in behavioral medicine are similar to those in other areas of specialization (Gentry, Street, Masur, & Asken, 1981). Diagnosis, assessment, and treatment practice serve to detect and facilitate the restoration of functioning. Miller (1983) identified the symbiosis between basic and applied science and in so doing carved out the scope of the field of behavioral medicine. He described the synergy between the laboratory findings and the field setting as essential to the enhancement of understanding illness behavior. The extension of the findings from experimental laboratory studies to practices in the field and the resultant reciprocity have led to well-researched techniques of intervention used in the field of behavioral medicine/health psychology (Miller, 1983).

Concepts of disease and sickness have been derived from applications of psychological models of stress. Hans Selye hypothesized from animal studies that organisms respond with stages of physiological states of alarm, resistance, and adaptation after toxin injection. Although each state refers to physiological changes, these concepts are commonly expanded to encompass a psychological dimension. It has been commonly hypothesized from Selye's work that physical symptoms can result from prolonged exposure to stress. Although Selye's stress was physical, it has been assumed that psychological reactions to stress (i.e., emotional and behavioral responses) are also sufficient to precipitate physical symptom complaint. Thus, psychological stress is part of the process and outcome of stress. Additionally, Sarason (1980) hypothesized that stress responses in conjunction with emotional or physical vulnerability levels tax the organism's ability to cope. It is assumed that maladaptive behavior results from a disproportionate amount of stress, vulnerability to stress, and inadequate coping (Sararon, 1980). Figure 13.1 illustrates the detail of this model about the interrelationships among stress, life events, and coping.

Correspondingly, illness behavior occurs when a disease process is present, although individuals may or may not manifest symptomatology (Mechanic & Volkart, 1961). Extreme symptomatic responses and pathological illness behavior are characteristics of hypochondriasis. If professionals in this field work in a medical setting, they may encounter individuals with this condition. Such individuals commonly go doctor shopping and obtain many treatments and prescriptions because they are not satisfied or are unable to accept that they are healthy and not in need of medical attention.

Medical professionals and clinical psychologists use the terms *acute* versus *chronic* to describe the intensity or severity of symptoms and *adaptation/maladaptation* to describe behaviors. Paramount to the clinician's understanding of an individual's response is an understanding of a client's state of mind when diagnosed with a disease or illness. Seligman (1975) proposed a model whereby the client's illness precipitates a perception of loss that integrates motivational, emotional, cognitive, and behavioral deficits. This behaviorally based model presumes that the individual's response

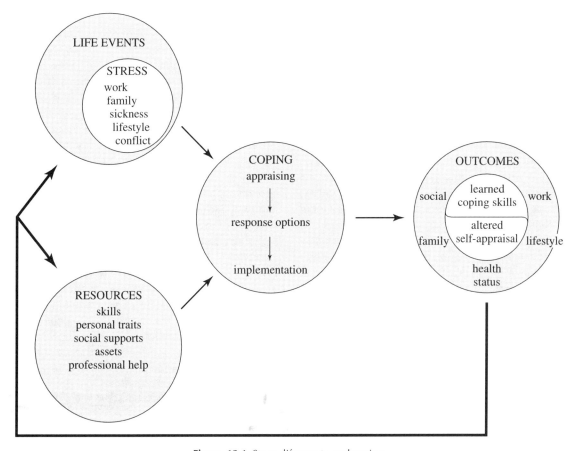

Figure 13.1. Stress, life events, and coping.

Source: From Eldon Tunks and Anthony Bellissimo, *Behavioral Medicine: Concepts and Procedures,* p. 6, Figure 1.1. Copyright © 1991 by Allyn and Bacon. Reprinted by permission.

generalizes across situations, thereby rendering a self-perception of illness as the person's identity. Actually, the reverse may occur: When my son split his head open, medical personnel referred to him as the "split head" for shorthand purposes. This comment is meant tongue in cheek to highlight personal identity and medical condition matching.

The generalization of a loss-of-control attitude is believed to propel the individual into symptomatic behavior. Tunks and Belissimo (1991) indicated the following to be indicative of this loss-of-control generalization:

- Physiological over-arousal giving rise to symptoms
- Interference with attentional capacities

- Overload of memory functioning and problems of retrieval of information
- Arousal of conflicts, symbolically or behaviorally
- Inappropriate use of information
- Helpless behavior that confirms the original loss-of-control attitude

The prevailing themes about the client's loss-of-control generalization and other illness features serve to guide the clinical psychologist. The role of the clinical psychologist is, in fact, to impart these important themes to the client. Restoration of health, reestablishment of self-control, development of self-efficacy, and development of goal-directed behavior are key to assisting the client (for an example, see Manning & Wright, 1983). Assessment methods and treatment techniques that are carefully chosen and skillfully enacted after an accurate diagnosis serve as the means for accomplishing this task. Assessment and treatment are typically behavioral or cognitive-behavioral in perspective. Clinical psychologists in this area strive for outcome measures such as symptom remission and reduction in severity or duration of symptoms. The characteristic method of education and/or demonstration that is used in these methods provides a means of altering beliefs and guiding the individual to gaining self-control. Several theorists have postulated this as an essential curative factor in the therapeutic process. The development of a sense of competence (Erickson, 1950), self-efficacy (Bandura, 1977), and instillation of a positive expectation or hope (Frank, 1973) are all involved in the therapeutic process. In fact, these factors are needed to impart change. Consonant to the behavioral focus, a faulty learning pattern also has been identified as a contributing factor to the occurrence of the illness or disease. For example, an individual may have tension headaches partly due to an inability to manage his or her schedule or interactions with people. The result is often an overcommitted, chaotic lifestyle with little time for relaxation. This may possibly result from the need to cope or sustain a defensive posture, which usually takes the form of sustained muscle tension. Soon this behavior pattern becomes ingrained.

In clinical practice, a diagnosis is determined from a psychological assessment, which usually includes sources of interview, observation, and psychological testing. In addition, a functional analysis (Haynes & Wilson, 1979), which is a behavioral/cognitive-behavioral assessment tool, can be used by the clinician to identify antecedent and consequential behaviors related to the presenting behaviors. The result of this assessment is a framework for treatment planning. This methodology utilizes the clinical methods of establishing a collaborative relationship with the client to set up treatment compliance. The request to record behaviors followed by the self-monitoring together provide rich information about baseline symptom intensity, duration, and severity that can be used for treatment goal planning. Figure 13.2 provides an algorithm for behavioral medicine and suggests that clients' pre-

senting complaints are the focal point of their illness behavior.

Clinicians use relaxation techniques to induce a slowing down of the autonomic nervous system, and, in turn, an increase in the sense of self-control and self-regulation. Benson (1975) initially proposed the use of relaxation techniques to effect behavior change. In the 1960s, progressive relaxation was held in high regard. Today, more cognitively oriented approaches involving the use of imagery or self-statements (Everly, 1989) have greater support in the scientific community. Modulation of the autonomic nervous system–sympathic division of the peripheral nervous system occurs by voluntary concentration on the alteration of arousal behavior. Classically, muscle tension is reduced, and breathing is slowed down. Relaxation training as developed by Jacobson was advanced by Bernstein and Borkovec (1973). The sequencing of muscle groups to relax, the criteria used to detect relaxation, and self-report before and after the relaxation are the keys to clinical effectiveness. Note that sample scripts of relaxation instructions can be found in the Further Reading section.

Biofeedback is the electronic monitoring and recording of physiological responses within the body—"reinserting into the system the results of past performance" (Norbert Weiner, mathematician). The goals of biofeedback are to increase awareness of internal events, to establish control over these events, and to generalize control from the laboratory into other areas of one's life (Budzynski, 1973). Treatment efficacy shows mixed results, largely due to the inability to measure whether control of physiological variables occurs (Budzynski, 1973). Jessup, Neufeld, and Merskey (1979) reported efficiency of biofeedback to be equivalent to that of relaxation techniques. Muscles commonly used for electromyograph (EMG) biofeedback are identified and matched to the presenting complaint. Thus, tension-type headache sufferers receive frontal or neck muscle biofeedback. Outcome studies of biofeedback with tension-type headaches report reductions in the number of headaches at two- and three-year follow-up points (Blanchard, 1987).

Meichenbaum (1976) theorized that the integration of a behavioral expansion of the cognitive ap-

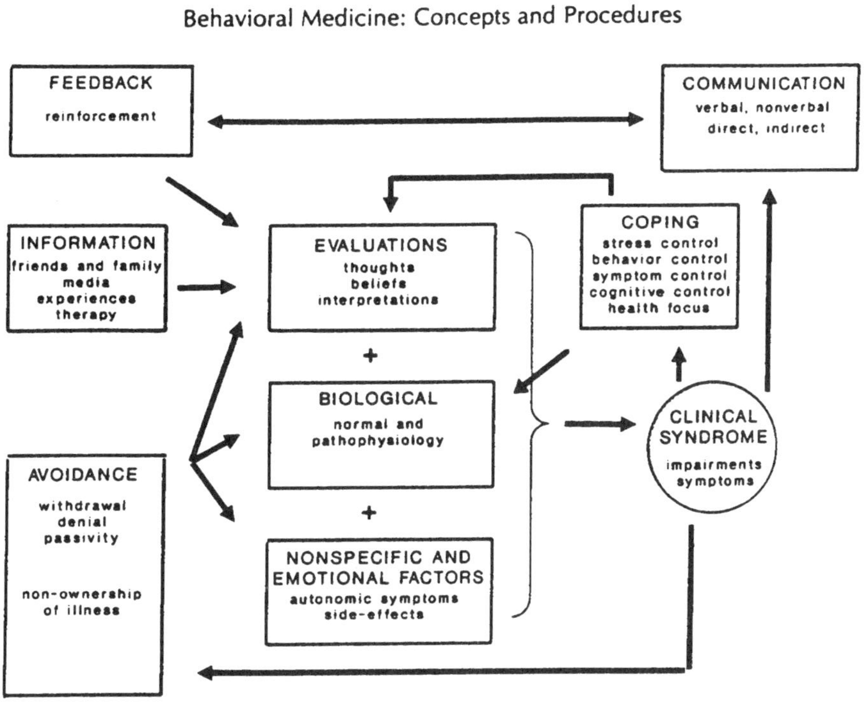

Behavioral Medicine: Concepts and Procedures

Figure 13.2. Algorithm for behavioral medicine.

Source: From Eldon Tunks and Anthony Bellissimo, *Behavioral Medicine: Concepts and Procedures,* p. 54, Figure A. Copyright © 1991 by Allyn and Bacon. Reprinted by permission.

proach of rational-emotive therapy may explain illness behavior. Specifically, the altering of one's internal dialogue in conjunction with relaxation will lead to behavior change. Meichenbaum described this use of "positive self-talk" dialogue as confirmatory to a person's coping goals. Stress inoculation techniques involve using a functional analysis to identify a target behavior and its corresponding antecedents and consequences. This modification of stress reactions breaks up the automatic thinking that is characteristic through the use of an educative phase in which triggers to the problematic behavior are identified and then a second phase in which behavior "practice" using new skills of reduction is done. The instruction and practice of relaxation teach the individual how to relax. Relaxation is a very effective treatment. Blanchard and Andrasik (1989) state that biofeedback is second to relaxation in the reduction of headaches. The specific physiologic response (e.g., frontalis muscle tension) that is altered in biofeedback is considered

to be the effective part of the process. That is, results from biofeedback studies by these authors conclude that there is reduction in headache activity as compared to no treatment and plausible factors. Relaxation has been demonstrated to be quite effective. Argas, Taylor, Kraemer, Allen, and Schneider (1980) report differences in both systolic and diastolic blood pressure measures in diagnosed hypertensives following relaxation training. Progressive muscle relaxation, deep breathing, and imaging a pleasant setting were used in combination for each relaxation training. Interestingly, the subjects were asked to stop practicing relaxation per the reversal design requirements, and lowered blood pressure measures were found. The authors concluded the subjects may have generalized the relaxation training.

Skill acquisition techniques used by clinical psychologists globally refer to the education of clients and their eventual skill development. Skills of assertion and self-control (e.g., weight control, exercise scheduling, relaxation, self-monitoring) and others represent various general skills taught to clients for therapeutic purposes. Clinical techniques for cognitive restructuring are also used frequently in behavior medicine to provide relief from a focus on symptoms. The diversion of attention away from oneself is accomplished with awareness of negative self-talk and practice of constructive statements (i.e., cognitive restructuring). In a recent study, behavioral medicine intervention practices of relaxation training and cognitive restructuring were found useful in reducing physical discomfort levels and psychological distress compared to pretreatment. Impressively, patients in the study reduced the number of service visits from 5.7 to 1.8 in six months (Bengen-Seltzer, 1997). Caudill, Schnable, Zuttermeister, Benson, and Friedman (1991) reported a 36% reduction in clinic visits at one-year follow-up of cognitive-behavioral treatment (i.e., education, relaxation training, logging, exercise, nutrition education). Preparation for possible reoccurrences of the behaviors are also planned through relapse prevention techniques (Brownell, Marlatt, Lichtenstein, & Wilson, 1986).

BEHAVIORAL MEDICINE RESEARCH PRACTICES

Behavioral medicine research typically uses the application of descriptive and inferential statistical analysis on data generated from controlled designs. Treatment outcome research conducted with repeated measures and, to some extent, meta-analytic procedures are common. Given the training of most clinical psychologists as scientist practitioners, systematic studies of intervention (via behavioral medicine or otherwise) are performed. Barlow, Hayes, and Nelson (1984) point out that traditional research methodology has made considerable contribution to behavior change in clinical research. These authors highlight the theme of clarifying the research question in order to select the most appropriate research design. Although it is difficult to conduct research in applied settings for the clinical psychologist, given role constraints, scheduling difficulties, and training (Haynes, Lemsky, & Sex-

ton-Radek, 1987), several alternatives exist for plausible designs such as single subject designs (Kazdin, 1996).

Alternative methods of design used in behavioral medicine research include quasi-experimental designs and applied research models (Campbell & Stanley, 1963; Monette, Sullivan, & DeJong, 1994). Methods such as observation, evaluation, survey research, and single-subject design are represented in the field of behavioral medicine. See Kazdin (1996) for a complete discussion of applied research methods in clinical psychology. Haynes and Wilson (1979) is a thorough resource on observation study methodology, and works by Barlow and Hersen (1984) and Kazdin (1982) discuss single-subject design.

Representative Studies in Behavioral Medicine

In the field of behavioral medicine, striking findings have been identified from investigations of relaxation with clients who have severe illnesses such as breast cancer. Spiegel and Bloom (1991) report findings from 86 women who had breast cancer that had metastasized already and who had a life expectancy of two years. The investigation was focused on helping these subjects cope with their poor prognosis. The findings indicated that subjects in the treatment group that included relaxation (in addition to self-hypnosis, which necessitates induction of relaxation that is sometimes taught in a group therapy format) outlived members of the control group that received medical treatment alone.

Lynch, Thomas, Mills, Malinow, and Katcher (1974) report empirical evidence of psychosocial factors affecting biological functioning. On the basis of case study/single-subject design data, a 72-year-old woman's irregular heart rhythm was reduced measurably during the time the nurse took her pulse—seemingly as a result of the nurse's focus of attention on her.

Lichtenstein (1982) identified cigarette smoking as a risk factor in the three leading causes of death: heart disease, malignant neoplasms, and stroke. As an observable behavior, smoking lends itself to being suitable for behavioral assessment and intervention. Behavioral analysis of smoking views cigarette smoking as complex but modifiable by contingency management techniques. These techniques are applicable throughout the phases of smoking (i.e., signals in the environment to smoke, immediate positive consequences). Research findings generated by Lichtenstein (1982) indicate the value of a variety of approaches that address the complex nature of smoking, such as aversion strategies, nicotine fading, use of nicotine chewing gum, and controlled smoking. Klesges, Benowitz, and Meyers (1991) examined the reinforcing qualities of cigarette smoking from both a behavioral and a biologic view. Changes in metabolic rate occur every time a person smokes; consequently, smoking cessation precipitates a weight gain from the energy increases experienced after smoking ceases. The combined behavioral (energy increase) and biological (metabolic rate) changes resulting from smoking cessation point to the need to combine behavioral therapy strategies with pharmacological treatment. Jason et al. (1995) innovatively studied various types of smoking cessation treatments. Self-help manuals, monetary incentives, and monthly booster support group meetings were used as treatment interventions. The findings from the treatment interventions, findings from previous studies, and the literature conclude that these interventions are effective. Quit-rates were highest for those individuals receiving all three treatments as compared to self-help manuals and support groups alone. (Importantly, support groups are to be conducted at the subjects' work site.)

Brownell (1982) suggests the pivotal strength of dieting to treating effectively the refractory disorder of obesity. With estimates that 30% of Americans meet criteria for obesity, treatment effectiveness is a key component of treatment essential for changing behavior. It has been reported that obesity is associated with hypertension, hyperlipidemia, diabetes mellitus, carbohydrate intolerance, surgical risk, risk with anesthesia, pulmonary and renal problems, and complications during pregnancy (Dawber, 1980). To treat the refractory disorder of obesity effectively, Brownell (1982) suggests that the fixed strength of dieting must be addressed. Attrition rates for traditional treatments run from 20%

to 80% (Stunkard, 1975), with weight loss programs weighing in at a 20% attrition range with behavior therapy. Attrition rates are higher for physical training/exercise groups.

Headache disorders are prevalent. In a survey of problems reported by a managed health care plan, headache was the third most common presenting complaint. Headaches are believed to be caused by changes in the cerebral vascular flow due to enhanced cognitive activity (e.g., worry) and sustained muscle tension (Haynes, et al., 1983). Dated studies identified headache sufferers with more stressful events. Behavioral treatments of relaxation and biofeedback are effective (Blanchard & Andrasik, 1982). Specifically, thermal biofeedback is effective with migraine headaches and EMG biofeedback with the more common tension-type headache (Budzynski, Stoyva, Adler, & Mullaney, 1973; Blanchard, Theobald, Williamson, Silver, & Brown, 1978).

Of the sleep disorders, insomnia is the most commonly reported. It is triggered by a number of events, including biological (e.g., medication reaction, psychiatric symptoms), psychological (e.g., worry, anxiety, and panic attacks), and social (e.g., work schedule, sleeplessness induced by caring for newborn; Haynes, Adams, & Franzen (1981). Relaxation and more specific treatments such as stimulus control (Borkovec, 1982) and sleep restriction (Sexton-Radek & Overton, 1996) provide a means of helping clients to consolidate their sleep and reduce presleep apprehensions. In studies conducted at sleep laboratories, individuals with insomnia secondary to chronic pain also benefited from sleep restriction (Morin, Kowatch, & Wade, 1989). Physiological arousal precipitated by cognitive activity (e.g., worries) and muscle tension was first identified in Monroe's (1967) seminal study of good and poor sleepers, where insomniacs displayed physiological activation levels significantly greater than those of good sleepers. The physiological activation levels stem from increased mentation (i.e., worry) and could be offset quite effectively by good health habits, collectively titled "sleep hygiene" (Lacks, 1987). Sexton-Radek, Carter, Netz, Heinz, and Adams (1997) report the use of sleep hygiene habits to enhance sleep quality by helping subjects become more "good sleepers" than "bad sleepers."

Rachman and Hodgson (1974) indicate that dyssynchronic patterns of behavior such as pain responses alert the body to activation which in turn maintains the pain response. Pain is a complex, multifaceted array of responses with psychological, social, and biological dimensions. Clinical psychologists working in the area of behavior medicine are likely to work with chronic pain patients, where the focus is on reducing the potency of stress-related perceptions (Caudill et al., 1991). Pain responses are limited largely to sensory information. Keefe (1982) advocates the use of a behavioral interview, the collection of objective data using questionnaires, and behavioral observation. Turk, Meichenbaum, and Genest (1983) categorize pain as follows: (1) acute pain such as dental pain; (2) periodic pain such as migraine headache; (3) chronic, intractable, benign pain such as low-back pain; (4) chronic progressive pain such as cancer pain; and (5) experimentally induced pain such as electric shock. Pain is considered to involve the individual's perception of the pain, the person's past history, ability to understand the nature of the pain, psychological factors, and the biological sensory information (Turk, Wack, & Kerns, 1985). Melzack and Wall (1988) additionally conclude that the sensory input is very much influenced by motivational and by affective and cognitive components of the individual, with neural mechanisms opening and closing off neural information. Barber (1984) was quoted as stating that distraction of attention is the "final common pathway" of all cognitive strategies. Although distraction techniques are helpful in pain reduction, it is also believed that cognitive coping strategies, which imply a more expanded mentation of distraction to a focused imagery, increase effectiveness. Further, the pairing of relaxation treatments with the cognitive approach enhances the utility of this treatment. Meichenbaum's (1983) technique of stress inoculation is also helpful in alleviating pain. Paramount to this area is Fordyce's operant conditioning of pain responses through the reinforcement of appropriate behavior contingencies (Fordyce, 1976).

Heart disease has been a leading cause of death. In 1974 Friedman and Rosenman identified the personality of a Type A individual as including patterned behaviors of time urgency, competitive stressing, and hostility that may be linked to cardiovascular deficiencies. Behavioral assessment that includes a standardized interview has been instrumental in identifying these patterns of behavior in individuals. Chesney and Rosenman (1985) later added hostility as a key clinical feature in the health consequences of Type A behavior. It was concluded that hostility represents suppressed anger and that the Type A behavior is an expression of this condition. Relaxation and counterconditioning are helpful in reducing anger. Nakano (1990) reports statistically significant decreases in speed and impatient behaviors of individuals diagnosed as Type A after behavioral treatment. Self-monitoring of daily activities identified the dependent variable of behavior (i.e., presence or absence of speed/impatience) instead of the more traditionally used measure of the Jenkins Activity Scale scores. The recording of speed/impatience behaviors along with thoughts and feelings was reported to have an impact on other displayed Type A behaviors, such as putting words into a speaker's mouth and being inattentive to lengthy comments (Nakano, 1990). A stress inoculation approach for anger/hostility regulation has been helpful in the treatment of Type A behavior as well.

Epstein and Masek (1978) have produced a number of studies underscoring the importance of compliance with treatment. Mean rates for long-term medication treatment are 54%; however, there is a dearth of literature in this area with a majority of studies at the descriptive/case study level. Self-report and measurement of therapeutic outcome have provided some promise as means of improving treatment adherence rate (Epstein & Wing, 1979; Martin & Dubbert, 1984).

Considerable speculation about the psychological and behavioral effects of exercise exist. Martin and Dubbert (1982) report health benefits of exercise for metabolic control, increased cardiac efficiency, and possible reduction in blood pressure. Stimuli control and reinforcement strategies have been suggested as means of increasing exercise adherence. Adherence behavior is likely to increase when instructions are specific and individuals understand the necessity for the change in behavior (Carmen Luciano & Herruzo, 1992).

Levy (1987) concludes that there are a number of reasons for treatment noncompliance. To avoid noncompliance, the clinician needs to address the following: insufficient skills or knowledge necessary to do the assignment, patient's beliefs not supportive of compliance, and patient's environment not supportive or interferes with complaint. Levy (1987) states that clinicians need to structure the therapy session to introduce, review, and provide the necessary skill training. Ultimately, it is the therapist's reinforcement of this training that leads to compliance in treatment. The cognitive-behavioral perspective is dominant in this type of approach, with increased self-efficiency, self-control, and empowerment as treatment goals. As in all experimental designs used by clinicians, good clinical decision making as to clinical realities and assumptions and the logical steps of the scientific procedure are needed (Hayes, 1981) (see Chapter 10 for further discussion of treatment adherence).

Belar (1988) describes graduate-level training of psychologists to work in the area of behavioral medicine/health psychology. It was recommended that core training in the social bases of health and disease as well as continued training in the scientist-practitioner model be required to practice as a clinical psychologist. Formal guidelines for the specialized and popular field of behavioral medicine/health psychology are anticipated (Belar, 1988; Boll et al., 1983; Sheridan et al., 1988).

HEALTH PSYCHOLOGY

Winett, King, and Altmann (1989) contend that health knowledge is positively correlated with health behaviors. Psychologists such as G. Stanley Hall and William James presented health issues in their writings. Schofield's (1969) classic article spawned the health psychology movement with its conclusions from a content analysis of psychology journals that psychologists were not studying physical health and illness. In 1979, Stone, Cohen, and Adler published one of the first books on health psychology and the journal *Health Psychology* was founded. Health psychology is consonant with Engel's (1977) work of integrating theory (literally laboratory findings) with field applications and the reciprocal feedback of field applications to theory (Feurstein, Labbé, & Kuczmierczyk, 1987). Matarazzo (1980) defined health psychology as the aggregate of the specific educational, scientific, and professional contributions of the discipline of psychology to the promotion and maintenance of health as well as the prevention and treatment of illness. Similar to behavioral medicine, health psychology is a multidisiplinary research and intervention field.

Health Psychology Research Practices

In addition to traditional and applied research methods, health psychologists employ epidemiological studies to investigate issues (Palinkas & Hoiberg, 1982; Singer, 1987). Congruent with Bandura's concept of building self-efficacy, health psychology interventions represent efforts to promote disease prevention and healthful behavior (Tulkin, 1987). Table 13.1 lists the types of incentives to consider when implementing a prevention strategy for both programs and individuals.

Representative Issues in Health Psychology

Anderson and Masur (1983) review the literature in terms of outcome studies that use therapeutic techniques to alleviate anxious responses. The responses were characterized by emotional distress, confusion, rapid breathing and/or hyperventilation, fidgeting, and vomiting prior to medical and dental procedures. This meta-analytic study indicated positive effects in general, although the heterogeneity of methods warned against definitive conclusions. The interventions in the review were broad in scope and ranged from dental restoration to burn debridement to renal analysis. The alleviation of fear included fear of pain and discomfort, the un-

Table 13.1 Types of Incentives

LEVEL OF DELIVERY (SOURCE)	DIRECT PAYMENT	PRICE REDUCTION	REDUCE RESPONSE COST	PRICE INCREASE	INCREASE RESPONSE COST
Individual	Self-contracting, e.g., for weight loss	Voluntary pre-payment, which reduces price, membership, insurance	Procure equipment, facilities; change schedule of work	Self-contracting, e.g., penalties and fines	Self-control strategies, e.g., stimulus control for smoking
Interpersonal	Family, group contracting, e.g., for weight loss	Group procurement and payment so that each member pays less	Reciprocal arrangements, e.g., buddy systems	Family, group contracting, e.g., penalties and fines	Mutually agreed-on restrictions, e.g., stimulus control for smoking
Organizational	Participation incentives; payment for changes	Subsidized participation; reduced fees for behavior	Procure facilities; flexible schedules; family/group participation	Fines, penalties for health/safety violations; open access	Restrict behaviors; restrict terms of employment
Institutional	Federal funds for enacting health and safety standards	Itemized deductions; deductible rates; decreased insurance rates for lower risk	Allow deductions for preventive services	Excise taxes; effluent taxes	DRG; no federal funds if no health and safety standards

Source: From Richard A. Winett, Abby C. King, and David G. Altman, *Health Psychology and Public Health: An Integrative Approach.* Copyright © 1989 by Allyn and Bacon. Reprinted by permission.

known, use of instruments, bleeding, destruction of body image, disruption of life plans, loss of control, and death. The early work of Janis (1958) identified that individuals with anticipatory fear at a moderate level were less vulnerable to postoperative emotional stress. Importantly, this work generated informative approaches to prepare individuals—a type of emotional inoculation. It was also determined that the viewing of such approaches (i.e., model receiving information) was successful in moderating stress (Anderson & Masur, 1983).

Booth-Kewley and Friedman (1987) broadened the view of type A characteristics. Their meta-analysis identifies for the first time the additional personality variables of negative emotions. These are added to the clinical picture of competitive/achievement striving, time urgency, and impatience. In health psychology, the preventive focus applied to the Type A personality issue takes the form of detection. Early detection of responses of individuals and groups provides health psychologists with intervention planning information

(Taylor, 1979, 1991). McMurray, Hardy, Roberts, Forsythe, and Mar (1989) reported a higher neuroendocrine response (greater levels of norepinephrine and beta-endorphin) by Type A than by Type B personality types. The measurement of "fitness" preceding exercise intervention is one example. However, these heightened levels may reflect a greater reactivity allowing for suppression of fatigue rather than increased activation (McMurray et al., 1989).

Flor, Turk, and Birbaumer (1985) conducted a psychophysiological assessment that measured muscle tension, heart rate, and skin resistance as subjects rested, described their pain, and rested again. Additionally, measures of depression and perceived control were done with standard measures in the field such as the Beck Depression Inventory and the State–Trait Anxiety Inventory. Pain responses as detected by heightened levels of muscular reactivity were predicted by the depression ratings. Support for the role of measuring and treating psychological factors comes from these results, highlighting the importance of evaluating stress-related responses. Moses, Steptoe, Mathews, and Edwards (1989) compared the effects of two aerobic training programs on mood and mental well-being as compared to placebo. Significant differences between the initial and final date of the two week exercise group on a commonly used measure called the Profile of Mood States (POMS) were found.

Physically fit individuals react to physical load and perhaps to stress with a smaller sympathetic response than do less fit subjects (van Doornen & deGeus, 1989). Doyne, Chambless, and Beutler (1983) report sustained positive gains in mood and cognitive function in four depressed women who underwent aerobic exercise. The four separate single-subject designs allowed for baseline, treatment, and posttreatment measurements that facilitated the tracking of the depression relief these individuals felt. An additional advantage of exercise has been reported to be alleviation of dysmenorrhea and possible relief of premenstrual syndrome (Gannon, 1988; Gannon, Luchetta, Pardie, & Rhodes, 1989). Adherence to exercise has been accomplished with the use of contracting. Wysocki, Hall, Iwata, and Riordan (1979) report increases in the number of aerobic points earned for each week in an exercise program by 7 of 8 participants using contract contingencies. See Martin and Dubbert (1984) and Dishman (1982) for comprehensive reviews of behavior change methods applied to exercise regimens to increase adherence. Exercise adherence could be enhanced with the identification of where an individual's thought and behavior patterns reside. Marcus, Rossi, Selby, Niaura, and Abrams (1992) report increased exercise adherence among individuals who are more committed to behavior change than "precontemplators."

With 50% to 90% of cancer patients experiencing pain, interventions that supplement medical treatment to reduce pain when it is expected are essential (Bonica, 1987). Such interventions aimed at alleviating pain typically involve relaxation, relaxation with mental imagery that entails cognitive focusing, or distraction training and biofeedback. Gil, Williams, Keefe, & Beckham (1990) investigated the self-report thought patterns of pain

patients during a pain flareup using test measures of thought patterns and coping strategies. A checklist of symptoms of psychological distress (e.g., depression, anxiety, anger) was also given. Findings indicate that subjects with more severe pain also had higher levels of psychological distress.

Keefe, Dunsmore, and Burnett (1992) identified the measurement of cognitive variables. From these, it is believed that cognitions influencing pain responses can be found and appropriate treatment matched to patient needs. Cognitive variables such as a person's belief to control an event are relevant to therapeutic gain. Negative self-image and depression are other cognitive variables that influence pain responses. Cognitive-behavioral treatment entails a combination of relaxation, exercise, activity pacing, and cognitive interventions (e.g., distraction). Although the mechanism and "potent" ingredients are not identified in this combination, outcome studies indicate the success of such approaches in reducing pain.

Several studies have linked stress with headache pain. Andrasik (1990) identified recurrent tension-type headache pain as associated with stress and being apprised of stressful events. Sexton-Radek (1994) concluded from an investigation of new and recurrent headache sufferers that the experience of being a headache sufferer was sufficient to induce a stress response and consequentially a headache. Psychosocial stressors precipitate headache pain as measured by cephalic blood flow in migraine and tension-type headaches (Haynes, Gannon, Bank, Shelton, & Goodwin, 1990; Haynes et al., 1983).

Biofeedback instrumentation also assists the clinician in identifying arousal symptoms characteristic of a stress response (i.e., sympathetic nervous system activation). Blanchard et al. (1983) designed a psychophysiological assessment of muscle tension, skin temperature, and heart rate that correctly predicted (31.5% to 70.2%) the variance in posttreatment headache activity. See a review by Haynes, Falkin, and Sexton-Radek (1988) for more information on psychophysiological assessment. Biofeedback successfully modulates the intensity and duration of headache pain in migraine headache sufferers (Price & Tursky, 1976). Blanchard and Andrasik (1989) have stated that biofeedback is second to relaxation in the reduction of headaches. The specific physiologic response (e.g., frontalis muscle tension) that is altered in biofeedback is considered to be the effective part of the process. In general, results from biofeedback studies by these authors conclude that a reduction in headache activity occurs with the use of biofeedback treatment. The confidence of these findings is highlighted by the fact that biofeedback treatments were compared to no-treatment and placebo conditions.

Baltimore and Wolff (1986) published a study identifying issues and concerns in the AIDS epidemic in the United States. This widely received work identifies the issue of "modes of transmission" and "accuracy of knowledge and groups at risk" as corresponding concerns. It was commented that public health models testing high-risk behaviors and screenings may address these issues as well as others related to the AIDS epidemic. Current health psychology efforts are aimed at preventive actions such as explicit education programs, availability of condoms, and voluntary testing. Self-control strategies such as self-monitoring are used for both educative and treatment adherence goals of such programs. With cases of AIDS in women on the rise, health psychology interventions to prevent disease spread are of paramount importance. Galavotti et al. (1995) report a shift to increased use of contraceptives in women at high risk for HIV contraction and transmission that corresponded with increased self-reported self-efficacy level. It is hypothesized that some individuals may present themselves in a certain fashion in order to achieve social goals. The presentation of self may include hazardous health behaviors, such as taking inadequate precaution against the spread of AIDS. With the largest group of sexually active but irregular condom-using individuals being college students, the importance of negotiating for this behavior is evident (Leary, Tchividjian, & Kraxberger, 1994). Some researchers have speculated that excessive embarrassment and worry in sexual encounters may stem from a perception that the behavior was planned. This perception of a lack of spontaneity in sexual encounters may contribute to the behavior of irregular condom use. Thus, health psychology interventions, while appropriately focused on in-

stilling condom use, need to expand into the realm of interpersonal relationships in order to succeed with their goal. Gartner, Gartner, and Ouellette Kabasa (1988) maintain that the broad scope and large volume of self-help materials and groups provides women with effective means of health promotion. It seems that a salient feature of the self-help movement is the variable of control. The insight and awareness achieved by self-help information that is broadly disseminated facilitates health and preventive approaches. An individual's experience with self-control is enhanced by self-help efforts that provide opportunities to become committed to one's health and oneself and challenge with additional perspectives (Maddi & Kabasa, 1984).

Research methods in the field of health psychology involve the use of traditional designs, quasi-experimental designs, and to some extent single-subject design. Applied methods entail the use of surveys and program evaluation assessments. Epidemiological studies and other broad-based census survey techniques are used to identify incidence and prevalence of a target behavior (Winett, King, & Altman, 1989). Belar (1988) has been instrumental in the design of graduate-level training programs in health psychology. Bresler (1988) described the expansion of predoctoral training in clinical psychology to include theory and practicum of health promotion in the community. The community focus to the training was thought to be more in line with the intentions of the National Institutes of Health's funding of cardiovascular disease prevention programs. In this manner, students were exposed to health promotion and community practice as alternatives to costly, office- or hospital-based interventions.

FUTURE DIRECTIONS

In today's market of health care budgets, the training and practice of clinicians to work in behavioral medicine and health psychology areas will change to more of a treatment-outcome focus. The maximization of clinical care with the current health care structure is one of the challenges for future clinicians interested in working in these areas (Friedman, Sobel, Myers, Caudill, & Benson, 1995;

Yates, 1995). Winett (1995) proposed future directions in health psychology that would better utilize epidemiological data, formulate better prevention programs that are closely linked to timing of client change, and focus on approaches to marketing such programs. Evidence exists of heightened risk behavior among certain ethnic minority groups—African Americans, Asian/Pacific Islanders, Latinos, and Native Americans (Myers, Kagawa-Singer, Kumanyika, Lex, & Markides, 1995). Cigarette smoking, excessive intake of dietary fat, limited exercise, being overweight, and alcohol consumption in minorities all point to a substantial need for behavioral medicine/health psychology treatment.

REFERENCES

Agras, W. S. (1982). Behavioral medicine in the 1980s: Nonrandom connections. *Journal of Consulting and Clinical Psychology, 50,* 797–803.

Alexander, F. (1950). *Psychosomatic medicine.* New York: Norton Press.

Anderson, K. O., & Masur, F. T. (1983). Psychological preparation for invasive medical and dental procedures. *Journal of Behavioral Medicine, 6*(1), 1–40.

Andrasik, F. (1990). Psychologic and behavioral aspects of chronic headache. *Neurologic Clinics, 3*(4), 961–975.

Agras, W. S., Taylor, C. B., Kraemer, H. C., Allen, R. A., & Schneider, J. A. (1980). Relaxation training. *Archives of General Psychiatry, 37,* 859–863.

Bakal, D. A. (1979). *Psychology and medicine psychobiological dimensions of health and illness.* New York: Springer.

Baltimore, D., & Wolff, S. M. (1986). *Confronting AIDS: Directions for public health, health care, and research.* Washington, DC: National Academy Press.

Bandura, A. (1977). Self-efficacy: Toward a unifying theory of behavioral change. *Psychological Review, 84,* 191–215.

Barber, T. X. (1984). Hypnosis, deep relaxation, and active relaxation: Data, theory, and clinical application. In R. L. Woolfolk & P. M. Lerner (Eds.), *Principles and practice of stress management* (pp. 1–23). New York: Guilford Press.

Barlow, D. H., Hayes, S. C., & Nelson, R. O. (1984). *The scientist practitioner: Research and accountability in clinical and educational settings.* New York: Pergamon Press.

Barlow, D. H., & Hersen, M. (1984). *Single case experi-* mental designs strategies for studying behavioral change (2nd ed.). New York: Pergamon Press.

Belar, C. (1988). Education in behavioral medicine: Perspectives from psychology. *Annals of Behavioral Medicine, 14,* 11–14.

Bengen-Seltzer, B. (1997). HMO case study demonstrates value of integrating behavioral health, primary care. *Behavioral Health Outcomes, 1*(12), 1–3.

Benson, H. (1975). *The relaxation response.* New York: William Morrow.

Bernstein, D. A., & Borkovec, T. D. (1973). *Progressive relaxation training: A manual for the helping professions.* Champaign, IL: Research Press.

Blanchard, E. B. (1982). Behavioral medicine: Past, present, and future. *Journal of Consulting and Clinical Psychology, 50*(6), 795–796.

Blanchard, E. B. (1987). Long-term effects of behavioral treatment of chronic headache. *Behavior Therapy, 18,* 375–385.

Blanchard, E. B., & Andrasik, F. (1982). Psychological assessment and treatment of headache: Recent developments and emerging issues. *Journal of Consulting and Clinical Psychology, 50*(6), 795–796.

Blanchard, E. B., & Andrasik, F. (1989). *Management of chronic headaches: A psychological approach.* New York: Pergamon Press.

Blanchard, E. B., Andrasik, F., Arena, J. G., Neff, D. F., Saunders, N. L., Jurish, S. E., Teders, S. J., & Rodichak, L. D. (1983). Psychophysiological responses as predictors of response to behavioral treatment of chronic headache. *Behavior Therapy, 14,* 357–374.

Blanchard, C. B., Theobald, D. E., Williamson, D. A., Silver, B. V., & Brown, D. A. (1978). Temperature biofeedback in the treatment of migraine headaches. *Archives of General Psychiatry, 35,* 581–588.

Blechman, E. A., & Brownell, K. A. (Eds.). (1988). *Handbook of behavioral medicine for women.* New York: Pergamon Press.

Boll, T. J., Thorensen, C., Adler, N., Hall, J., Millon, T., Moore, D., Olbrisch, M. E., Perry, N., Weiss, L., Woodring, J., & Wortman, C. (1983). Working group of predoctoral education/doctoral training. *Health Psychology, 2,* 122–130.

Bonica, J. J. (1987). A short course on the management of cancer pain. *Journal of Pain and Symptom Management, 2*(2), Suppl. 3.

Booth-Kewley, S., & Friedman, H. S. (1987). Psychological predictors of heart disease: A quantitative review. *Psychological Bulletin, 101*(3), 343–362.

Borkovec, T. D. (1982). Insomnia. *Journal of Consulting and Clinical Psychology, 50*(6), 880–895.

Bresler, C. (1988). Health promotion in the community: Development of a curriculum for predoctoral clinical psychologists. *Professional Psychology: Research and Practice, 19*(1), 87–92.

Brownell, K. D. (1982). Obesity: Understanding and treating a serious, prevalent, and refractory disorder. *Journal of Clinical and Consulting Psychology, 50*(6), 820–840.

Brownell, K. D., Marlatt, A., Lichtenstein, E., & Wilson, G. T. (1986). Understanding and preventing relapse. *American Psychologist, 41*, 765–782.

Budzynski, T. H. (1973). Biofeedback procedures in the clinic. In L. Birk (Ed.), *Biofeedback: Behavioral medicine* (pp. 484–496). New York: Grune & Stratton.

Budzynski, T. H., Stoyva, J. M., Adler, C. S., & Mullaney, D. G. (1973). EMG biofeedback and tension headache: A controlled outcome study. *Psychosomatic Medicine, 35*, 484–496.

Campbell, D. T., & Stanley, J. C. (1963). *Experimental and quasi-experimental designs for research*. Chicago: Rand McNally.

Carmen Luciano, M., & Herruzo, J. (1992). Some relevant components of adherence behavior. *Journal of Behavior Therapy and Experimental Psychiatry, 20*(2), 117–124.

Caudill, M., Schnable, R., Zuttermeister, P., Benson, H., & Friedman, R. (1991). Decreased clinic use by chronic pain patients: Response to behavioral medicine intervention. *Clinical Journal of Pain, 7*, 305–310.

Chesney, M. A., & Rosenman, R. H. (1985). *Anger and hostility in cardiovascular and behavioral disorders: The series in health psychology and behavioral medicine*. New York: Hemisphere.

Dawber, T. R. (1980). *The Framingham study: The epidemiology of atherosclerotic disease*. Cambridge, MA: Harvard University Press.

Dishman, R. K. (1982). Compliance/adherence in health-related exercise. *Health Psychology, 1*(3), 237–267.

Doyne, E. J., Chambless, D. L., & Beutler, L. E. (1983). Aerobic exercise as a treatment for depression in women. *Behavior Therapy, 14*, 434–440.

Engel, G. L. (1977). The need for a new medical model: A challenge for biomedicine. *Science, 196*, 129–136.

Epstein, L., & Wing, R. (1979). Behavioral contracting: Health behaviors. *Clinical Behavior Therapy Review, 1*, 1–15.

Epstein, L. H., & Masek, B. J. (1978). Behavioral control of medical compliance. *Journal of Applied Behavior Analysis, 11*, 1–9.

Epstein, L. H., & Wing, R. R. (1980). Aerobic exercise and weight. *Addictive Behaviors, 5*, 371–388.

Erickson, E. H. (1950). *Childhood and society*. New York: W.W. Norton.

Everly, G. S. (1989). *A clinical guide to the treatment of the human stress response*. New York: Plenum Press.

Feurstein, M., Labbé, E. E., & Kuczmierczyk, A. R. (1987). *Health psychology: A psychobiological perspective*. New York: Plenum Press.

Flor, H., Turk, D. C., & Birbaumer, N. (1985). Assessment of stress-related psychophysiological reactions in chronic back pain patients. *Journal of Consulting and Clinical Psychology, 53*(3), 354–364.

Fordyce, W. E. (1976). *Behavioral methods for chronic pain and illness*. St. Louis: C. V. Mosby.

Frank, J. (1973). *Persuasion and healing: A comparative study of psychotherapy*. Baltimore, MD: Johns Hopkins University Press.

Freud, S. (1940). The justification for detaching from neurasthenia a particular syndrome: The anxiety-neurosis. In *Collected papers* (Vol. 1). New York: Basic Books.

Friedman, M., & Rosenman, R. H. (1974). *Type A behavior and your heart*. New York: Knopf.

Friedman, R., Sobel, D., Myers, P., Caudill, M., & Benson, H. (1995). Behavioral medicine, clinical health psychology, and cost offset. *Health Psychology, 14*(6), 509–518.

Galavotti, C., Cabral, R. J., Lansky, A., Grimley, D. M., Riley, G. E., & Prochaska, J. O. (1995). Validation of measures of condom and other contraceptive use among women at high risk for HIV infection and unintended pregnancy. *Health Psychology, 14*(6), 570–578.

Gannon, L. (1985). *Menstrual disorders and menopause: Biological, psychological, and cultural research*. New York: Praeger.

Gannon, L. (1988). The potential role of exercise in the alleviation of menstrual disorders and menopausal symptoms: A theoretical synthesis of recent research. *Women and Health, 14*(2), 105–127.

Gannon, L., Luchetta, T., Pardie, L., & Rhodes, K. (1989). Perimenstrual symptoms: Relationships with chronic stress and selected lifestyle variables. *Behavioral Medicine, 3*, 149–159.

Gartner, A., Gartner, A.J., & Ouellete Kobasa, K. (1988). Self-help. In E. A. Blechman & K. D. Brownell (Eds.), *Handbook of behavioral medicine for women* (pp. 330–342). New York: Pergamon Press.

Gentry, W. D., Street, W. J., Masur, F. T., & Asken, M. J. (1981). Training in medical psychology: A survey of graduate and internship training programs. *Professional Psychology: Research and Practice, 12,* 224–228.

Gil, K. M., Williams, D. A., Keefe, F. J., & Beckham, J. C. (1990). The relationship of negative thoughts to pain and psychological distress. *Behavior Therapy, 21*(3), 349–362.

Hayes, S. C. (1981). Single case experimental design and empirical clinical practice. *Journal of Consulting and Clinical Psychology, 49*(2), 193–211.

Haynes, S. N., Adams, A., & Franzen, M. (1981). The effects of pre-sleep stress on sleep-onset insomnia. *Journal of Abnormal Psychology, 90*(6), 601–606.

Haynes, S. N., Falkin, S., & Sexton-Radek, K. (1988). Psychophysiological assessment in behavior therapy. In G. Turpin (Ed.), *Handbook of clinical psychophysiology* (pp. 175–214). New York: Wiley.

Haynes, S. N., Gannon, L. R., Bank, J., Shelton, B., & Goodwin, J. (1990). Cephalic blood flow correlates of induced headaches. *Journal of Behavioral Medicine, 13*(5), 467–480.

Haynes, S. N., Gannon, L. R., Cuevas, J., Heiser, P., Hamilton, J., & Katranides, M. (1983). The psychophysiological assessment of muscle-contraction headache subjects during headache and nonheadache conditions. *Psychophysiology, 20*(4), 393–399.

Haynes, S. N., Lemsky, C., & Sexton-Radek, K. (1987). The scientist-practitioner model in clinical psychology: Suggestions for implementing an alternative model. In J. R. McNamara and M. A. Appel (Eds.), *Critical issues, developments, and trends in professional psychology* (Vol. 3, pp. 1–26). New York: Praeger Press.

Haynes, S. N., & Wilson, C. (1979). *Behavioral assessment.* San Francisco: Jossey-Bass.

Janis, I. L. (1958). *Psychological stress.* New York: Wiley.

Jason, L. A., McMahon, S. D., Salina, D., Hedeker, D., Stockton, M., Dunson, K., & Kimball, P. (1995). Assessing a smoking cessation intervention involving groups, incentives, and self-help manual. *Behavior Therapy, 26*(3), 393–408.

Jessup, B. A., Neufeld, R. W., & Merskey, H. (1979). Biofeedback therapy for headache and other pains; an evaluative review. *Pain, 7,* 225–270.

Kazdin, A. E. (1982). *Single-case research designs: Methods for clinical and applied settings.* New York: Oxford University Press.

Kazdin, A. E. (Ed.). (1996). *Methodological issues and strategies in clinical research.* Washington, DC: American Psychological Association.

Keefe, F. J., Dunsmore, J., & Burnett, R. (1992). Behavioral and cognitive-behavioral approaches to chronic pain: Recent advances and future directions. *Journal of Consulting and Clinical Psychology, 60*(4), 528–536.

Keefe, F. J. (1982). Behavioral assessment and treatment of chronic pain: Current status and future directions. *Journal of Consulting and Clinical Psychology, 50*(6), 896–911.

Klesges, R. C., Benowitz, N. L., & Meyers, A. W. (1991). Behavioral and biobehavioral aspects of smoking and smoking cessation: The problem of postcessation weight gain. *Behavior Therapy, 22*(2), 179–200.

Lacks, P. (1987). *Behavioral treatment for persistent insomnia.* New York: Pergamon Press.

Leary, M. R., Tchividjian, L. R., & Kraxberger, B. E. (1994). Self-presentation can be hazardous to your health: Impression management and health risk. *Health Psychology, 13*(6), 461–470.

Levy, R. L. (1987). Compliance and clinical practice. In J. A. Blumenthal & D. C. McKee (Eds.), *Applications in behavioral medicine and health psychology: A clinician's handbook* (pp. 567–588). Sarasota, FL: Professional Resource Exchange.

Lichtenstein, E. (1982). The smoking problem: A behavioral perspective. *Journal of Clinical and Consulting Psychology, 50*(6), 804–819.

Lynch, J. J., Thomas, S. A., Mills, M. E., Malinow, K., & Katcher, A. H. (1974). The effects of human contact on cardiac arrhythmia in coronary care patients. *Journal of Nervous and Mental Disease, 158,* 88–99.

Maddi, S. R, & Kabasa, S. C. (1984). *The hardy executive: Health under stress.* Homewood, IL: Dow Jones-Irwin.

Manning, M. M., & Wright, T .L. (1983). Self-efficacy expectancies, outcome expectancies, and the persistence of pain control in childbirth. *Journal of Personality and Social Psychology, 45,* 421–431.

Marcus, B. H., Rossi, J. S., Selby, V. C., Niaura, R. S., & Abrams, D. B. (1992). The stages and processes of exercise adoption and maintenance in a worksite sample. *Health Psychology, 11*(6), 386–395.

Martin, J. E., & Dubbert, P. M. (1982). Exercise applications and promotion in behavioral medicine: Current status and future directions. *Journal of Clinical and Consulting Psychology, 50*(6), 1004–1017.

Martin, J. E., & Dubbert, P. M. (1984). Behavioral management strategies for improving health and fitness. *Journal of Cardiac Rehabilitation, 4,* 200–208.

Matarazzo, J. O. (1980). Behavioral health and behavioral medicine: Frontiers for a new health psychology. *American Psychologist, 35,* 807–817.

Matthews, K. (1982). Psychological perspectives on the Type A behavior pattern. *Psychological Bulletin, 91,* 293–323.

McMurray, R. G., Hardy, C. J., Roberts, S., Forsythe, Q. A., & Mar, M. H. (1989).Neuroendocrine responses of Type A individuals to exercise. *Behavioral Medicine,* 84–92.

Mechanic, D., & Volkart, E. H. (1961). Stress, illness behavior, and the sick role. *American Sociological Review, 26,* 51–58.

Meichenbaum, D. (1976). Toward a cognitive theory of self-control. In G. E. Schwartz & D. Shapiro (Eds.), *Consciousness and self-regulation—Advances in research* (Vol. 1). New York: Plenum Press.

Meichenbaum, D. (1983). Stress-inoculation therapy. In *Clinical Psychology Practitioners.* New York: Pergamon Press.

Melzack, R., & Wall, P. O. (1988). *The challenge of pain* (3rd ed.). London: Penguin Books.

Meyers, A. (1991). Biobehavioral interactions in behavioral medicine. *Behavior Therapy, 22,* 129–131.

Meyers, H. F., Kagawa-Singer, M., Kumanyika, S. K., Lex, B. W., & Markides, K. S. (1995). Behavioral risk factors related to chronic diseases in ethnic minorities. *Health Psychology, 14*(7), 613–621.

Miller, N. E. (1983). Behavioral medicine symbiosis between laboratory and clinic. *Annual Review of Psychology, 34,* 1–31.

Monette, D .R., Sullivan, T. J., & DeJong, C. R. (1994). *Applied social research tool for the human services* (3rd ed.). Chicago: Harcourt Brace.

Monroe, L. J. (1967). Psychological and physiological differences between good and poor sleepers. *Journal of Abnormal Psychology, 72*(3), 255–264.

Morin, C. M., Kowatch, R. A., & Wade, J. B. (1989). Behavioral management of sleep disturbances secondary to chronic pain. *Journal of Behavior Therapy and Experimental Psychiatry, 20*(4), 295–302.

Moses, J., Steptoe, A., Mathews, A., & Edwards, S. (1989). The effects of exercise training on mental well-being in the normal population: A controlled trial. *Journal of Psychosomatic Research, 33*(1), 47–61.

Nakano, K. (1990). Operant self-control procedure in modifying Type A behavior. *Journal of Behavior Therapy and Experimental Psychiatry, 2*(4), 249–256.

Palinkas, L. A., & Hoiberg, A. (1982). An epidemiology primer: Bridging the gap between epidemiology and psychology. *Health Psychology, 1*(3), 269–287.

Price, K. P., & Tursky, B. (1976). Migraineurs and non-migraineurs: A comparison of responses to self-control procedures. *Headache, 16,* 210–217.

Rachman, S., & Hodgson, R. I. (1974). Synchrony and desynchrony in fear and avoidance. *Behavior Research and Therapy, 12,* 311–318.

Sarason, I. G. (1980). Life stress, self-preoccupation, and social supports. In I. G. Sarason & C. D. Spielberger (Eds.), *Stress and anxiety* (pp. 73–94). New York: Hemisphere Publishing.

Schofield, W. (1969). The role of psychology in the delivery of health services. *American Psychologist, 24,* 568–584.

Schwartz, G. E., & Weiss, S. M. (1978). Yale conference on behavioral medicine: A proposed definition and statement of goals. *Journal of Behavioral Medicine, 1,* 3–12.

Seligman, M. E. P. (1975). *Helplessness: On depression, development, and death.* San Francisco: W. H. Freeman.

Sexton-Radek, K. (1994). The nature of recurrent tension-type headache and stress experiences. *Psychotherapy in Private Practice, 13*(3), 63–72.

Sexton-Radek, K., Carter, I., Netz, K., Heinz, E., & Adams, R. (1997). Sleep hygiene habits as an individualized treatment to enhance sleep. Poster presentation at the Society for Behavioral Medicine Conference, San Francisco, April 1997.

Sexton-Radek, K., & Overton, S. (1996). Practical treatment considerations: Compliance with sleep restriction treatment in a non-disordered sample of sleepers. *Psychotherapy in Private Practice, 15,* 1–12.

Sheridan, E. P., Matarazzo, J. D., Ball, T. J., Perry, N. W., Weiss, S. M., & Belar, C. D. (1988). Postdoctoral education and training for clinical service providers in health psychology. *Health Psychology, 7*(l), 1–17.

Singer, J. E. (1987). Training for applied research in health psychology. In G. C. Stone, F. Cohen, & N. E. Adler (Eds.), *Health psychology* (pp. 107–118). San Francisco: Jossey-Bass.

Spiegel, D., & Bloom, J. R. (1991). Group therapy and hypnosis reduce metastic breast carcinoma pain. *Psychosomatic Medicine.*

Stone, G. C., Cohen, F., & Adler, N. E. (1979). *Health psychology.* San Francisco: Jossey-Bass.

Stunkard, A. J. (1975). From explanation to action in psychosomatic medicine: The case of obesity. *Psychosomatic Medicine, 37,* 195–236.

Taylor, S. E. (1991). *Health psychology* (2nd ed.). New York: McGraw Hill.

Taylor, S. E., (1979). Hospital patient behavior: Reactance, helplessness, or control? *Journal of Social Issues, 35*, 156–184.

Tulkin, S. R. (1987). Health care services. In G .C. Stone, S. M. Weiss, J. D. Matarazzo, N. Miller, J. Rodin, C. D. Belar, M. J. Follick, & J. E. Singer (Eds.), *Health psychology: A discipline and a profession* (pp. 126–136). Chicago: University of Chicago Press.

Tunks, E., & Belissimo, A. (1991). *Behavioral medicine concepts and procedures.* New York: Pergamon Press.

Turk, D. C., Meichenbaum, D., & Genest, M. (1983). *Pain and behavioral medicine: A cognitive-behavioral perspective.* New York: Guilford Press.

Turk, D. C., Wack, J. T., & Kems, R. D. (1985). An empirical examination of the "pain behavior" construct. *Journal of Behavioral Medicine, 8*, 119–130.

Van Doornen, L. J., & deGeus, E. J. (1989). Aerobic fitness and the cardiovascular response to stress. *Psychophysiology, 26*(1), 17–28.

Winett, R. A. (1995). A framework for health promotion and disease prevention programs. *American Psychologist, 50*(5), 341–350.

Winett, R. A., King, A. C., & Altman, D. G. (1989). *Health psychology and public health: An integrative approach.* New York: Pergamon Press.

Wysocki, T., Hall, G., lwata, B., & Riordan, M. (1979). Behavioral management of exercise: Contracting for aerobic points. *Journal of Applied Behavior Analysis, 12*, 55–64.

Yates, B. T. (1995). Cost-effectiveness analysis, cost-benefit analysis and beyond: Evolving models for the scientist-manager-practitioner. *Clinical Psychology: Science and Practice, 2*(4), 385–398.

FOR FURTHER READING

Blumenthal, J. A., & McKee, D. C. (Eds.). (1987). *Applications in behavioral medicine and health psychology: A clinician's source book.* Sarasota, FL: Professional Resource Exchange. *This is a very helpful guide for someone starting to work in this field who wishes to get an overview of the translation of behavior therapy to behavioral medicine and health psychology practice.*

Hollandsworth, J. G. (1986). *Physiology and behavior therapy: Conceptual guidelines for the clinician.* New York: Plenum Press. *The material in this book is suitable to advanced psychology undergraduates as a preparation for graduate study in behavioral medicine. Conceptual themes of behavior therapy and clinical implications sections make this a very useful resource for the serious student.*

Schwartz, M. S. (1987). *Biofeedback: A practitioner's guide.* New York: The Guilford Press. *This is the definitive textbook on biofeedback. Material is appropriate to a broad readership. Topics such as the conceptual basis for biofeedback and listings of instrumentation manufacturers' addresses are presented.*

Taylor, S. E. (1991). *Health psychology* (2nd ed.). New York: McGraw-Hill.

Taylor, S. E. (1995). *Health psychology.* (3rd ed.). New York: McGraw-Hill. *This book is appropriate for an undergraduate-level or perhaps beginning graduate-level seminar that explains health psychology. The topics in the chapter are represented very expansively in the book, as are the secondary areas in the field.*

CHAPTER 14

COMMUNITY PSYCHOLOGY

Karen Grover Duffy

If the world already has clinical psychology, why does it need community psychology? The answer simply stated is that there are not enough psychologists for one-to-one intervention with all the individuals in the world who are disenfranchised and disaffected. The American Psychological Association (APA) has almost 80,000 members (APA, 1995), but this number is insufficient given that as many as one in three or four Americans may have a diagnosable disorder (Regier et al., 1993). Community psychologists, because they work on a large scale and because they emphasize prevention wherever possible, are quite different from clinical psychologists. At the same time, clinical and community psychologists can and do work together.

Various definitions of the field have been given since it was founded in Swampscott, Massachusetts, in 1965. The following definition incorporates most aspects that community psychologists agree are crucial to community psychology: ***Community psychology*** *focuses on social issues, social institutions, and other settings that influence groups and organizations as well as the individuals in them, with the primary goal being to optimize the well-being of communities and their citizens with innovative and alternative interventions* (Duffy & Wong, 1996).

This definition merits closer examination. The social issue crucial to the present book is mental disorder. Like clinical psychologists, community psychologists are extremely interested in this issue. Community psychologists also have a strong interest in other disaffected groups, such as the homeless, school dropouts, juvenile delinquents, and the elderly, because they, too, are community members. Community psychologists utilize many innovative interventions beyond psychotherapy and psychoactive medications. For example, a community psychologist would attempt to manage delinquency not just by counseling the youths but also by means of parent education. In fact, many of the methods and interventions that community psychologists enlist are not typically applied by clinical psychologists. By examining some of the goals of community psychology, the reasons that community psychologists apply alternative interventions will become clearer.

GOALS OF COMMUNITY PSYCHOLOGY

As mentioned in the definition, the primary goal of community psychology is to enhance the well-being of individuals, groups, organizations, and communities. Enhancing well-being is another goal of clinical psychology. Beyond that, however, clinical and community psychology part company. Other goals of community psychology include prevention rather than treatment of social problems; examination of extrapersonal (i.e., environmental and social) causes of disordered behavior; an emphasis on empowerment; choices among available interventions and treatments; and the development of a sense of community.

Prevention

As mentioned in the opening of this chapter, there simply are not enough psychologists and therapists for all individuals who may need them. When the United States was an agrarian and rural society, family members and neighbors used to look after one another. With urbanization and industrialization, however, society today seems colder and harsher. Individuals are less self-reliant and therefore turn to the government and a variety of professionals to meet their needs (Duffy & Wong, 1996). However, the logical implication is that not everyone with a mental disorder or other condition will be able to receive treatment from professionals, including clinical psychologists and psychiatrists. Similarly, mental disorders will probably never be totally eliminated with one-to-one therapy. Community psychologists, in large part because of the shortcomings of clinical psychology in managing the large numbers of individuals who require treatment, have determined that mass intervention may be a better vehicle for overcoming some mental disorders. The purpose of such mass or community intervention is typically to prevent mental disorder altogether wherever and whenever possible. Yes, it is true that some disorders are probably genetically and biochemically determined. However, other disorders might be completely preventable if we re-duce instigating stimuli such as stress. Community psychologists, then, rely on community-level interventions such as education and alteration of the environment to reduce the likelihood of mental disorder.

How can community psychologists accomplish the noble but enormous task of changing large numbers of people at once? One method for achieving this is *mental health education. In this type of education, people acquire knowledge, skills, and attitudes that directly contribute to their mental health and to their effect on the mental health of others.* The purpose of mental health education is to teach people *how* to think instead of just instructing them on *what* to think (Cowen, 1980). In this way, people learn to make reasonable choices and decisions and to feel a sense of responsibility for their own well-being. In other words, mental health education ensures the ability to think well, which paves the way for emotional relief, which in turn prevents dysfunction (Shure & Spivack, 1988).

Muñoz, Glish, Soo-Hoo, and Robertson (1992) designed a mental health education program to improve the knowledge and competency of citizens of San Francisco by broadcasting a series of televised segments about depression, self-control, and other aspects of mental health. One segment included information on the importance of relaxation and of finding time to relax. Another segment highlighted how to identify self-defeating thoughts and how to stop having such thoughts. Muñoz and associates utilized phone interviews of randomly selected individuals to collect data. For individuals who reported feeling depressed, Muñoz and associates demonstrated a decrease in depression from pre- to posttest. Participants also noted an increase in the use of the televised techniques as compared to the time period prior to the broadcasts.

The results of Muñoz's study demonstrated that depressed individuals experienced some relief from their depression via mental health education. *When a disorder such as depression or other problem already exists and is alleviated, secondary prevention* has occurred. In those viewers who were already mentally healthy and who used relaxation more frequently after the broadcasts, *primary prevention* occurred. ***Primary prevention*** *attempts to forestall a problem from occurring altogether*. Primary prevention refers to activities that can be undertaken with a healthy population to maintain or enhance its health, both physical and emotional (Bloom & Hodges, 1988).

The Ecological Perspective

Community psychologists are highly interested in the ***person–environment fit***—*the suitability of the person to the setting and the setting to the person*. To assure such fit, an *ecological perspective* is extremely important. *This perspective recognizes that there exists a transaction between people and settings. Individuals influence the settings in which they find themselves; settings influence the individuals in them* (Seidman, 1990). To find the best *person–environment fit, one needs to examine both entities as well as the relationship between them.* Establishing an optimal match between the individual and the environment is a goal of community psychology. In this way, community psychologists eschew labeling individuals who do not fit well into a particular setting as "misfits." Similarly, community psychologists typically avoid controlling the environment simply to control the individuals in it.

Again, a sample program may prove enlightening. Dropping out of school is common in the United States; the estimated national rate is 20%. Because the educational requirements of most jobs will increase in the future (Rumberger, 1987), dropping out of school needs to be reduced. Many factors have been posited as reasons that youths drop out of school. It may be easy to blame the youths themselves by noting that some of them have low self-esteem or school failure. However, the concept of ***alienation from school*** (Bronfenbrenner, 1986; Sarason, 1983), *which means lacking a sense of belonging to the school*, also accounts for a significant number of dropouts. The concept of alienation from school helps psychologists understand that often the school climate, not the youth, is responsible for the youth's dropping out of school. This ecological approach suggests that changing the youth's personality or study skills will

not prevent dropping out. Something in the school itself must be changed.

Felner, Ginter, and Primavera (1982) designed a school with an enhanced role for the homeroom teacher, who became a counselor and guide to the students. For example, the teacher helped first-year students to cope better with the transition from junior to senior high school. Likewise, the complexity of the school was reduced. Participants took classes in only one wing of the large school and shared classes with one another, so that they could perceive the school as friendlier and smaller. By merely restructuring the school in this fashion, Felner and his colleagues increased the students' attendance and grade point averages. The students also reported more stable self-concepts compared to nonparticipants.

Empowerment

Another assumption in community psychology is that individuals living in particular settings and circumstances best know the ramifications of life in those settings. The client, then, is as important as the professional, or more so.

Empowerment *is the process of enhancing the possibility that people can more actively control their own lives* (Rappaport, 1987). In other words, community psychologists hope to keep people from feeling powerless. Empowerment provides individuals with control and mastery over their own lives and democratic participation in their communities. Empowerment, then, means *doing* (Swift & Levin, 1987). However, the service to individuals is indirect. Rather, community psychologists provide the tools, environments, and information that engender collaboration so that affected individuals can do things for themselves. For example, community psychologists would not necessarily write grants for community mental health organizations. Instead, community psychologists would educate community agencies about *how* to write grants and *where* to look for grant money so that after the psychologists leave, the organizations can continue to seek their own funding.

Let us examine a program related to mental health that utilized empowerment. Perhaps the most classic and often cited program concerns lodge societies as developed by George Fairweather and his colleagues (Fairweather, Sanders, Maynard, & Cressler, 1969). Lodge societies are halfway houses or group homes for the mentally disordered that emphasize skill building and, of more importance to the present discussion, shared responsibility and decision making. In other words, the residents in the group homes decide their own work schedule, policies, and so forth. The residents are gradually empowered to have more control over their own lives, especially in comparison to their level of control in institutional settings. In institutions, the staff and administration generally exert much control over the residents. The lodge was designed to increase freedom and decrease the stigma attached to mental disorder.

The Fairweather group was able to document that, compared to control groups, the lodge participants were able to function longer in the community and to be more productive members of society, for example by holding jobs. Interestingly, the control participants reported that when they returned to the institution, it was because of pressure from a significant other. This reason was almost never cited by lodge participants. The lodge participants also were better able to tolerate one another's behavior. Fairweather and his colleagues' results therefore demonstrate the importance of ecology or of the social environment for those coping with mental disorder.

Choices among Alternative Interventions

Part of the philosophy of empowerment is that each individual is unique and therefore ought to have control over his or her life because the individual best knows his or her circumstances. The diversity of groups in the United States in terms of race, ethnicity, age, socioeconomic status, religion, and special needs speaks to the need to develop a variety of programs rather than a single program for everyone. Community psychologists, in fact most psychologists, respect diversity among people. As part of the recognition of uniqueness and diversity, community psychologists recognize that one intervention or one community service probably will not help all individuals equally well. Community psychologists consequently seek to establish a number of alternative services in various communities in recognition of the diversity in our communities. As part of this diversity of populations and services, community psychologists also concur that accessibility is of utmost importance. A service that is not readily available has no client base. Again, a model program can demonstrate this concept.

The United States has the highest teen pregnancy rate of any industrialized society (Lawson & Rhode, 1993). The relevance of teen pregnancy to clinical psychology is not necessarily evident. Suffice it to say here that young mothers represent one of the groups most at risk for child maltreatment (Patteson & Barnard, 1990). Although prevention programs (e.g., sex education) do exist, the teen pregnancy rate nonetheless remains high. Therefore, secondary prevention programs need to be in place. One such program allows pregnant teens to remain in school both during their pregnancies and after they give birth (Seitz, Apfel, & Rosenbaum, 1991). The program enables the teens to finish their education and provides day care for their children as well as counseling, health care, and parenting classes. This program recognizes that the needs of teen parents are sometimes quite different from those of other teens and from those of other parents. In other words, an alternative program to the traditional high school is offered to the pregnant teens. These teens appear to complete the program with good academic success and become better parents than they otherwise would have been.

A Sense of Community

Research has demonstrated that the subjective sense of well-being is often positively related to the sense of community or the sense of belonging in the community (Davidson & Cotter, 1989). *Sense of community is the feeling of the relationship an individual holds for his or her community* (Heller, Price, Reinharz, Riger, & Wandersman, 1984). *Specifically, sense of community includes a perception of similarity to others in the community, a willingness to maintain and acknowledge interdependence with others, and the feeling that one is part of a larger dependable and stable structure* (Sarason, 1974).

Community and sense of community relate to mental health in a number of ways, one of which can be detailed here. Alternative care for the mentally disordered typically involves settings in which a smaller number of clients are served compared to the large number served by a psychiatric hospital. One might conclude that such smaller settings result in a greater sense of community and/or a greater sense of self-efficacy. This is indeed the case; Kiesler (1982a, 1982b) examined 10 different alternative programs and found that individuals treated in the alternative settings improved more and were less likely to be rehospitalized than those who were treated in a hospital setting. This finding offers a vivid example of how the general public may be misinformed about and hold negative stereotypes of mental illness.

A second way in which sense of community relates to interventions with the mentally disordered is that some communities do not want alternative facilities in their neighborhoods (Miller, 1982). Community residents give many reasons for rejecting alternative services such as psychosocial clubs and group homes (to be described). Because residents generally have little information about mental illness and therefore stereotype and stigmatize the mentally ill as dangerous, some residents fear that the patients will commit crimes or will be inadequately supervised by the staff. Other residents feel that if they accept one such service, others will follow and thus property values will decrease (Arce, 1978; Johnson & Beditz, 1981).

Davidson (1981) conducted research on community-based treatment centers to determine how low-resistance neighborhoods differed from high-resistance neighborhoods. He found that often the low-resistance neighborhoods are typified by poverty. However, Davidson also documented that middle-class communities will accept low-stigma clients, such as maltreated children, in preference to mentally disordered adults who have formerly been hospitalized.

Other research suggests that communities of various sizes may or may not be appropriate for placement of the formerly hospitalized. For example, Kruzich (1985) found that small cities may be friendly and personalized, but they lack necessary services. On the other hand, cities of 10,000 to 100,000 residents have sufficient community resources for clients but still are not so large that residents feel lost or depersonalized in them. Although helping agencies may be plentiful, cities larger than 100,000 are so large that the mentally disordered find depersonalization to be a problem.

THE IMPORTANCE OF SOCIAL CHANGE

The foregoing discussion of acceptance of the mentally disordered in different types of communities provides a smooth transition to the next topic, social change. Social change is important to community psychologists because they see the cause of many disorders as lying in the environment and in society. If society causes distress, then society must change.

Social change gallops toward us every day. Much of it, unfortunately, is random. International wars, natural disasters, population swings, health epidemics, technological advances, and other major transformations are often uncontrollable and unpredictable, yet all influence each and every one of us. Community psychologists, however, revere planned social change because it can be shaped and managed in positive ways. ***Planned social change*** *is intentional; it is also planned in advance of any problems and so is quite different from random and unplanned change. Planned or induced social change is also distinguished from unplanned change in three ways. Planned social change is always meant to enhance well-being, is limited in scope to certain communities and/or affected groups, and provides a role for those influenced by the change (i.e., empowerment).*

METHODS OF PLANNED SOCIAL CHANGE

Education and Information Dissemination

Community psychologists often simultaneously engage a number of the following techniques in order to better society. Already mentioned is one extremely important change technique, mental health education and information dissemination. Let us discuss this in more detail.

Education is venerated in the United States. Educational strategies can be used to promote large-scale change, particularly given the advent of distance-learning technologies such as television, radio, the Internet, and satellite communications. The Muñoz and associates research that promoted adoption of strategies designed to optimize the mental health of the citizens of San Francisco was showcased earlier. Other than this sample program, how else can education and information dissemination create other planned and positive social changes? As mentioned previously, much research exists demonstrating that the general public is rejecting of people with mental disabilities (Duffy & Wong, 1996). Morrison (1980) claims that mental health education can be particularly valuable in "demythologizing" the public's perceptions of mental illness. Community members often view the mentally disordered as dangerous or as persons with a disease. Mental health education, according to Morrison, can alter this view. After public education about mental illness, community members come to see the mentally disordered individual as less dangerous and more in need of skills to cope with problems of living. This makes community members more likely to accept these individuals as neighbors.

Do education and information dissemination work? The answer is a resounding "yes." A marvelous book published by the American Psychological Association, *Fourteen Ounces of Prevention*, details program after program where education was used to reduce a social or personal problem. Only one program will be highlighted here, the Life Skills Training (LST) program designed for junior high school students as a substance abuse prevention program.

Experimentation with one psychoactive substance often precedes the use of other drugs in a relatively predictable and well-defined sequence. Individuals generally begin with tobacco and alcohol and progress to marijuana and then to other illicit substances. Some individuals ultimately progress to opiates and other addictive substances. Psychological factors such as low self-esteem, depression, and poor coping skills are significant for predicting subsequent progression to problematic forms of substance use (Botvin & Tortu, 1988). Experimentation generally commences during preadolescence or adolescence (Millman & Botvin, 1983).

In the LTS program, junior high school students were provided with the necessary skills via education to resist direct social pressures to smoke, drink alcohol, or use marijuana. To enable students to resist indirect social pressures to use various substances, they were helped to develop greater autonomy, self-esteem, self-mastery, and self-confidence. Students' knowledge of the immediate consequences of smoking and illicit substances was also enhanced by providing them with accurate information about the prevalence rates of use. In LTS, education was used to prevent experimentation and use of illicit and harmful substances. Results demonstrated that compared to control students, 75% fewer program students began smoking, 54% fewer program students reported drinking alcohol, and 79% fewer program participants reported getting drunk. On the basis of this sample program, we might tentatively conclude that educational programs designed to promote physical and mental health are effective.

Citizen Participation and Grass-Roots Efforts

Another planned change technique is citizen participation or grass-roots efforts. Citizen participation involves empowerment. Change then comes from the bottom of the community, from the citizens, rather than from the top or from the government. Citizens living in communities know better than psychologists what the problems of their community are and what methods to address the problems will be most accepted by other community members. Another advantage of citizen-planned change is that individuals who participate in change decisions are more motivated to abide by the decisions and to live comfortably with the changes.

One concrete example of citizen participation or of a grass-roots effort is the National Alliance for the Mentally Ill (NAMI). NAMI is a grass-roots, family and consumer self-help support and advocacy organization dedicated to improving the lives of people with severe mental illnesses. NAMI publishes its own newsletter, the *NAMI Advocate*; supports the need for continuing research; lobbies for improved legislation for the mentally ill; educates the public in part by providing a clearinghouse of information; and pursues other avenues that will enhance the life of the mentally disordered and their families and friends.

Do not forget one of the oldest forms of planned change and citizen participation—voting or electoral participation. Each citizen can use his or her vote to change public policy or to elect officials more friendly to various solutions to community problems. For example, families who have a mentally disordered member can vote for candidates who support mental health policy reform, increased funding for programs, or research on their family member's illness. A community citizen might run for the zoning board in a community that has thus far banned group homes for the mentally disordered so that the disabled family member must live farther away from his or her family.

Consultants and Professional Change Agents

Citizens sometimes do not know where to begin to change their communities, and they may call on community psychologists to act as consultants or professional change agents. In this capacity, community psychologists should always keep in mind the concept of empowerment. If community members become too dependent on the consulting psychologists, the change effort may collapse when the psychologist leaves. Consultants, then, should always include input from community residents in their decision making, suggested program designs, and so forth. The result should be that community members are empowered to continue with planned positive change long after the consultant exits the community.

Again, an example is appropriate. Suppose that at a medium-sized college campus in the southwestern United States there have been many budget and staff cuts—so many cuts, in fact, that the professors and clerical staff are feeling overworked. At the same time, because of the publicity about the cuts, admissions applications are dropping, so the remaining staff fear that they will eventually lose their jobs, too. Needless to say, stress levels are very high.

Consultants could be asked to develop stress management programs designed to help the campus community better cope with the distress. If the consultants do not take into consideration that they will have to leave the campus when the training is completed and that staff members need to continue to practice stress management, the consultants' visits are pointless. The stress management trainers need to fortify in participants' minds that they can continue the components of the stress management program without the presence of the consultant. For example, college members should continue to monitor their diets and to exercise even after the psychologists leave, because both practices have been demonstrated to enhance individuals' sense of well-being (Brown, 1991; Sime, 1984). Sime found that not only did exercise help diminish mild to moderate depression, but that avid exercisers, overall, frequently report an increased sense of accomplishment, worth, and well-being as well as feelings of relaxation, euphoria, and elation during and after exercising.

Community psychologists now understand that many stress management programs, such as exercise programs, are maintained after training *only if* there are social supports in place. ***Social support*** *is an exchange of resources between two individuals perceived by the provider or the recipient to be intended to enhance the well-being of the recipient* (Shumaker & Brownell, 1984). For example, if individuals who share the same problem come together to encourage one another and share coping strategies, this exemplifies social support. Consultants would try to build social support into stress management programs. In regard to stress management and exercise, researchers have discovered that if exercise is performed in groups (e.g., in groups of other faculty members or family members), exercise programs are more likely to be maintained (Bloom, 1988). Therefore, it is incumbent upon community psychologists to educate participants about *maintenance* of well-being after training. In this case, social support optimizes the likelihood that participants in stress management seminars will continue their stress management techniques when they feel a sense of community with others desiring the same outcome as well as a decrease in stress because of exercise and the other stress management techniques. Social support will be discussed in detail.

One caveat is needed here. Consultants usually become expert at program design and implementation. It is easy for them to transplant a program from one location to another. Programs, however, sometimes do not transplant well because of the idiosyncrasies of each community and each population. Although fidelity to the original design is often important, so, too, is consideration of the uniqueness of each setting (Blakely et al., 1987).

Networking of Community Agencies

Just as community members need to support one another so that a sense of community develops and so that they can encourage one another to live more satisfactory lives, so, too, must community organizations be networked or connected. *Networks are confederations of organizations with common interests that share resources and information with each other.* Networks ensure that member organizations remain strong through unity and that clients do not fall through service cracks. Already mentioned was the National Alliance for the Mentally Ill (NAMI). Another well-known networking or umbrella organization is United Way. United Way not only provides funding to member organizations; it also ensures that no two agencies will compete with each other for the same clients, that competition for resources such as money is reduced, and that member agencies know about and collaborate with one another. In this way, clients are better served and the health and longevity of each member organization is assured.

Policy Science and Public Policy

Two final, extremely important, and interrelated planned change techniques are policy science or

policy research and public policy. *Policy science is the science of making findings from science (including community psychology) available and relevant to governmental, community, and organizational (i.e., public) policy. Public policy*, of course, *refers to policy at the community or governmental levels that influences what resources are allocated where so that the quality of life is improved.* Community psychologists firmly believe that policy science or action research should drive public policy.

In fact, community psychologists hold this change technique in such high regard that some have studied ways to increase voter registration and electoral participation. Some of the most disenfranchised individuals in our society are least likely to participate in electoral actions. Many people of color find themselves in the lower socioeconomic classes and are also diagnosed with mental illness. It is these individuals who most need to express loudly and clearly which policies they believe will enhance their lives. Sadly, research demonstrates that these individuals are the ones least likely to be registered or to vote.

Fawcett, Seekins, and Silber (1988) wanted to encourage more voter registration among impoverished classes, so in true community psychology fashion they took the services to the people rather than making the people come to the services. The researchers instituted voter registration in locations that were frequented by such individuals. For example, when impoverished individuals came to collect their allocations of cheese and other food products, voter registration information was available and citizens were encouraged to register to vote. Fawcett and his co-workers found an amazing 100% increase in registrations and a 51% increase in actual voting.

Another example relates more to mental health. Psychologists as well as government leaders have long noted that the mentally disordered are sometimes institutionalized against their will, then heavily medicated, rebuffed, and sometimes maltreated by the mental health care system (e.g., Rosenhan, 1973). The return of individuals to their communities (deinstitutionalization) for both humanistic and economic reasons resulted from the passage of the Community Mental Health Centers

Act of 1963. This act established community mental health centers across the United States. The centers were to provide outpatient, emergency, and educational services, among others. Five essential services were required to qualify for federal funds. Local groups had to demonstrate that they could provide inpatient services, outpatient services, partial hospitalization services (e.g., patients receive treatment during the day and return home at night), a 24-hour emergency service, and consultation and education programs. Perhaps the most radical change provided by this act was the provision for 24-hour emergency service (Heller et al., 1984). This practice jolted the mental health professions because most psychotherapies were not prepared to deal with current crises and, in fact, believed that to do so would encourage neurotic "acting out" (Heller et al., 1984)

The use of all mental health services, including outpatient services, by all segments of the population initially increased as a result of this community mental health centers legislation (Veroff, Douvan, & Kulka, 1981). It is unknown, however, whether the increase was caused by the availability of the centers or by other intervening factors, such as the increase in number of depictions of psychotherapy and mental disorder on television which occurred at about the same point in time.

As desirable as they are, policy science and policy change are not always easy. One reason is that many individuals resist change of any type. Often the status quo is most comfortable, whereas the unknown is uncomfortable. Another reason that sweeping policy changes are resisted is because competing groups want different legislative outcomes, so lobbying occurs. **Lobbying** *means that certain collectives of individuals promote their own political causes.* Often these lobbying groups work at cross-purposes with one another. For example, while one group (the American Psychiatric Association) lobbies for increased funding for research on psychoactive drugs to assist the mentally disordered, another group (managed health care organizations) lobbies for legislation that would control or limit prescriptions to save money.

Another very important reason that public policy often fails to address real needs in meaningful ways is that policy change and community research are extremely difficult, often far more difficult than research that takes place in a laboratory. In community psychology, the community becomes the laboratory. Depending on the design, the number of subjects can soar; lack of control over research design and extraneous variables increases, and correlational methods where cause and effect are more difficult to ascertain prevail over experimental methods (Duffy & Wong, 1996; Speer et al., 1992).

We have now examined the purposes, goals, and history of community psychology. Although we could focus here on a variety of groups in our communities, such as maltreated children, the homeless, the elderly, juvenile delinquents, and the chemically dependent, we will instead turn our attention to the mentally disordered in our communities. The focus of this book is clinical psychology, and the population with whom clinical psychologists are most likely to work is this clinical population. Community psychologists are also interested in this population because they, too, are citizens of our communities. In a brief history we will first explore how the mentally disordered came from the asylums and hospitals of several decades ago to our modern communities .

THE MENTALLY DISORDERED IN OUR COMMUNITIES

In the 1960s, the prescription of psychoactive drugs became prevalent. Psychopharmacological medications include antidepressants, anxiolytics, mood stabilizers, neuroleptics (or antipsychotics), psychostimulants, and others, as described in Chapter 12. The use of these medications meant that some formerly institutionalized individuals could be returned to the community for treatment and care. The 1960s also saw the passage of the Community Mental Health Centers Act, meant to ensure that when patients returned to their communities, community mental health centers would be available to them that could address their daily and emergency needs. Thus, many patients moved from inpatient treatment in hospitals or institutions to outpatient status in our communities.

The process of moving the mentally disordered from institutions and hospitals to the community is called deinstitutionalization. Some authors, however, feel that because in reality the mentally disordered really move from one "single, lousy institution to multiple wretched ones " (Talbott, 1975, p. 530), a better term would be *transinstitutionalization*. **Transinstitutionalization** *refers to the notion that an individual spends his or her life moving from one institution to the next* (although not all of the institutions are hospitals). We will look shortly at where the deinstitutionalized mentally disordered do find themselves in U.S. communities.

Another reason for deinstitutionalization in many states has been a general economic downswing since the 1960s. Government budget cuts often translate into slashing of mental health budgets (Dumont, 1982). If insufficient funds exist to house the mentally disordered in hospitals, however, there is probably insufficient money to support them in the community. Couple this poor funding situation with the fact that the deinstitutionalized mentally disordered are unwelcome on the streets of many communities. The result is an unhappy state of affairs.

Furthermore, there is a strong causal link between mental disorder and poverty. Bruce, Takeuchi, and Leaf (1991) examined patterns of new disorders that developed over a 6-month period in an epidemiological study of various racial and ethnic groups. **Epidemiology** *examines the occurrence and distribution of health-related conditions in populations* (Duffy & Wong, 1996). The researchers found that a significant proportion of *new* episodes of mental disorder could be attributed to poverty. Therefore, just when the economy is at its worst and the institutions are shutting down, so, too, are citizens under duress and most in need of additional mental health services. Because of budget cuts, these services are not likely to be in place.

MEASURING SUCCESS OF COMMUNITY LIVING FOR THE MENTALLY DISORDERED

According to community psychologists, the ideal setting for the mentally disordered is one that enhances well-being and provides an optimal fit between the individual's competencies and the amount of support provided in the environment. If an individual lives successfully in a community, psychologists ought to be able to measure the individual's success.

Some clinicians and community psychologists have suggested that various scales might be employed to avoid prematurely placing into the community individuals who might have difficulty adjusting. One such scale is the Community Competence Scale developed by Searight, Oliver, and Grisso (1986). This scale has multiple subscales that measure an individual's problem-solving ability, appropriateness of social judgment, and other factors related to social competence. Searight and associates also found that the scale discriminates effectively between client groups requiring differing levels of guidance in the community.

When an individual is released to the community, what exactly is meant by success and how can it be measured? Typical measures of success in community living are social integration and recidivism. **Social integration** *is defined as people's involvement in a community's formal institutions (such as work organizations) as well as their participation in the community's informal social life.* **Recidivism** *means relapse or return to the institution or to some form of intensive care or treatment.* The first term is of immense interest to psychologists, especially community psychologists. Being socially integrated signifies that an individual is reliably connected to others in the community. Those others in the community, such as family and friends, can function as informal advisors and case managers to some extent for the mentally disordered individual who may not have the incentive or wherewithal to follow through on his or her own aftercare once out of the institution (Belcher, 1988). The latter term, *recidivism*, is primarily of interest to government officials who hope to keep hospitalization to a minimum because it is so expensive.

Some psychologists have examined recidivism. Maier, Morrow, and Miller (1989) developed a pre-release program for forensic mentally disordered individuals. (For more information on forensics, see Chapter 16 on forensic clinical psychology.) These individuals not only have a diagnosable mental disorder, they also have committed a crime—hence the term *forensic*. The release of these individuals into the community is problematic because they suffer from the dual stigma of being criminal and being emotionally disturbed. Morrow and Miller's program contained modules that reoriented the participants to the community and to social skills, but it also contained provisions for a buddy system, brief visits to the community before final release, and meetings with community leaders. The psychologists encouraged participants to take small steps, one at a time, before release, rather than just casting them out abruptly into society. Over a 24-month period, only one crime was committed even though the participants made over 11,000 excursions into the community.

Other measures of successful community living again vary according to who is asked to provide a definition. Staff of community services and family members of the mentally disordered often cite quality of life as an important criterion of successful community living. Quality of life is often described as having clean clothes, a clean place to live, useful tasks to occupy one's time, nutritious food, a sense of happiness, and so forth. Psychiatrists and some clinical psychologists might also cite lack of symptomatology as another desirable measure of efficacy of community living.

Clinical psychologists have also been queried about whether and why clients will be successful when placed in the community. Stack, Lannon, and Miley (1983) asked clinicians to judge whether they thought individuals would be readmitted to an institution within two years of release. The clinicians' judgments were biased with regard to the patients' ethnicity. That is, African Americans were judged more likely to be rehospitalized than were Whites. A second finding was that the clinicians were unduly influenced in their perceptions by the severity of the patients' disorder instead of other, more favorable factors such as lack of prior hospitalizations, youthfulness of the individual under consideration, and living circumstances in stable neighborhoods. Clinicians, then, need to attend to the whole client *and* his or her environment, not just to selected and perhaps biasing characteristics.

THE REALITIES OF COMMUNITY LIFE FOR THE MENTALLY DISORDERED

Homelessness

No one knows the exact number of homeless persons in the United States. Estimates range from 200,000 to over 3 million (National Coalition for the Homeless, 1988). Americans are somewhat desensitized to big numbers, but do not ignore this latter figure. Three million individuals is the population of a large city; in fact this figure surpasses the populations of Wyoming, Vermont, or Alaska (Kuhlman, 1994). No one is certain how many of these homeless persons are also mentally disordered. Many studies have found that the mentally disordered make up a sizable number of the homeless (e.g. Morse, Calsyn, & Burger, 1992; Mowbray, Bybee, & Cohen, 1993). Rossi (1989) administered a symptom scale to his homeless participants and found evidence of clinical depression or psychotic thinking in 20% to 30% of them. Rossi's homeless group proved to be significantly more impaired on these scales than was his control group of domiciled poor persons. Living on the streets without shelter or living sporadically in a homeless shelter is one unfortunate community option for the deinstitutionalized mentally disordered.

Jails and Prisons

Prisons and jails seem to be used all too often to house the mentally disordered. Diamond and Schnee (1990) tracked chronically mentally disordered men and found that they were high users of jails. Over a two-and-a-half-year period, the men used 11 different service systems. Criminal justice services were the most frequently used. Unfortunately, the same study demonstrated that the mental health care services the men received were often only short-term, crisis-care services. (Crisis intervention is addressed later.)

Most psychologists agree that jails and prisons are ill-equipped to provide therapeutic services for those with mental disorders (Freeman & Roesch, 1989). Prisons generally take a retributive approach to criminality rather than a rehabilitative approach. Further, most staff at correctional facilities are not trained in mental health, so the staff is concerned more with custodial matters. Perhaps if prisons do house some of the mentally disordered, justice system and mental health professionals need to take a more creative and integrative approach to their care (Pogrebin & Regoli, 1985).

Nursing Homes

It is ironic that most individuals deinstitutionalized from psychiatric hospitals still live in institutions. About 1.15 million former mental patients live in nursing homes (Bootzin, Shadish, & McSweeney, 1989). The nursing home industry is currently the largest system of long-term care for the severely and persistently mentally disordered (Bootzin et al., 1989). Perhaps because nursing homes benefit financially, these homes do not frequently return formerly institutionalized patients back to the hospitals or to the communities.

Board and Care Homes

These particular community-based shelters include group homes and family care homes. About 500,000 individuals with chronic mental disorders reside in these settings (U.S. Public Health Service, 1980). Although these homes may be smaller and more intimate than nursing homes, some of these shelters remain unregulated in various states.

Segal, Silverman, and Baumohl (1989) examined these facilities in California and described them. The family care home is typically small, has a family-like atmosphere, and is usually owner-occupied. These homes generally provide little in the way of therapy or medical supervision. These homes also are unlikely to conduct programming designed to make the residents more independent or to enhance the residents' well-being.

Group homes typically are somewhat larger than family care homes. These homes, according to the Segal group, serve an older population and do not typically control the residents as much as do the family homes. There are few rules, schedules, or curfews in most group homes. Some of the larger homes (more than 30 beds) do provide programming designed to enhance social skills. The larger homes also tend to exert more control over the residents than do the smaller group homes.

COMMUNITY INTERVENTIONS WITH THE MENTALLY DISORDERED

When community psychologists criticize other professionals for inadequate treatment of the mentally disordered, it is incumbent upon psychologists in the community to design and implement alternative interventions. Community psychologists have done just that. This section is dedicated to reviewing alternative community placements and interventions for this population. There are several alternative programs in place now; they include support groups, crisis intervention, psychosocial clubs, and assertive case management.

What features of community interventions and programs make such programs successful? Price, Cowen, Lorion, and Ramos-McKay (1988) give us some guidelines. First, the model programs are targeted; that is, they are focused at specific groups whose strengths and risks are well known to the program developers. Second, the programs are designed to alter the life trajectory of the people who participate in them. In other words, the programs are aimed at long-term rather than short-term change. Successful programs give the participants new skills to cope more effectively with life problems. The programs also provide social support so that individuals can make the transition from one life event to the next. Life transitions, such as the transition between junior and senior high school or between hospitalization and release to the community, are milestones or changes that produce stress and therefore can cause a person's trajectory to halt or to move downward (Duffy & Wong, 1996). In fact, model programs take advantage of natural supports (e.g., the family) that are already in place and strengthen those supports. Successful programs are constantly monitored and evaluated so that they can provide evidence of their success. Successful programs are transportable in whole or in part to other communities and other groups, so it is important that information about these programs be shared not only in psychological journals but with practitioners in the field.

Support Groups

Social support and support groups are not new ideas. Alcoholics Anonymous (AA) was one of the first support networks formed in the United States. Members of AA, or recovering alcoholics, come together as often as once or twice a day to give one another support and advice about coping with alcoholism. Members help one another to recognize that they are alcoholic, to recover from alcoholism, and to prevent relapse. From AA, other nationally recognized support groups have spun off. Another well-known group is Alanon, which provides support to families and friends of alcoholics. Still another is Narcotics Anonymous, which does the same for those recovering from addictions to other substances, such as heroin.

Such self-help groups provide social support. John Cassel (1974) and Gerald Caplan (1974) first identified and described social support. *Support groups*, otherwise known as *self-help groups* or *mutual help groups*, *include similar individuals who come together to provide assistance and emotional and other types of support for one another.* Contemporary researchers have recognized that social support need not take place in a formal support group; friends and family can also offer informal support, which is often as helpful as a formalized support group and sometimes as helpful as long-term psychotherapy with a clinical psychologist or psychiatrist. Like psychotherapy, social support is recognized as being transactional in nature. That is, the support is a two-way phenomenon in which provided support affects how well individuals function and how well they function influences how much support and attention they receive (Shumaker & Brownell, 1984).

Social support then is generally considered to enhance the well-being of involved individuals and to provide several benefits. Shumaker and Brownell (1984) review several of these benefits. First and most important to the present discussion, social support generally serves to enhance self-identity and self-esteem. Social support also serves to reduce stress, probably by broadening and clarifying the affected individual's understanding of the stressful events.

The concept of social support includes several subconcepts. *Social embeddedness is the number or quantity of connections an individual has to significant others who might offer assistance.* A well-embedded individual has many friends, family members, and other associates from whom he or she can probably draw support. *Enacted support is the availability of actual support. It refers to the concrete actions others perform when they render assistance.* Enacted support goes beyond merely having friends; it is more behavioral in that the friends actually provide support. *Perceived social support* is yet another related construct. *This is the most commonly researched concept in the literature and refers to one's appraisal of being reliably connected to others.* In other words, it is the perception of how available and how adequate social support is that makes it valuable (Duffy & Wong, 1996).

A second theme in the social support literature is *how or why* social support is effective, if at all. Brownell and Shumaker (1984) provide a good review of the modes by which social support might operate. Social support seems first to have direct effects. That is, it can have the effect of directly increasing healthier or better coping behaviors in the recipient. For example, when family members encourage a mentally disordered individual to stick to her medication regime because she will function better, these family members are providing direct social support.

Social support also can provide indirect effects. Social support can function to help recipients feel less stress or to perceive stressful events as less severe. For example, when a mentally disordered individual wants to see his psychologist but the psychologist is on vacation, a friend can remind the individual that during one other period when the psychologist was not available, the mentally disordered person managed to get through the experience unscathed.

Another effect of social support is its buffering or ameliorating effect. The support is buffering because a friend or family member points out that the distressed individual is coping as well as or better than other individuals in the same situation. For example, a person with a dual diagnosis (depression and alcoholism) might be reminded by friends in AA that many others have alcoholic relapses and that he is not a bad person because he had a moment of apparent weakness.

One last effect of social support is a boostering effect. Social support can sometimes make positive experiences more positive or more exhilarating. For example, when an individual who has been deinstitutionalized successfully makes it through her first month of independent living, friends can comment in positive ways and make this success even happier for the newly independent individual.

No studies have yet partialed out the exact effects of social support or self-help groups. In other words, psychologists do not yet know which, if any, of these effects is the single most important vehicle by which support works or whether all in combination are effective. While researchers continue to explore this very fertile and popular topic, for now it may be sufficient to recognize that the available studies all use different populations as well as different methodologies and statistics, thus rendering the studies incomparable. Tebes and Kraemer (1991) more fully explore this complexity of social support research for interested readers.

The concept of social support is not without controversy in the literature. Let us examine more of the topics related to social support and self-help groups. Another relevant issue is measurement of social support. Because there is some dispute about how to define social support, it is not surprising that there is disagreement about its measurement. A variety of measures have been developed, but the psychometric properties are still being examined (Fiore, Coppel, Becker, & Cox, 1986). *The Inventory of Socially Supportive Behaviors* or ISSB (Barrera, Sandler, & Ramsey, 1981) is a 40-item scale on which respondents report the frequency with which they were the recipients of supportive actions on a five-point scale. The authors report adequate test–retest reliability and internal consistency. Sample items include: "Was right there with you (physically) in a stressful situation" and "Assisted you in setting a goal for yourself."

A second scale is the *Social Support Behaviors Scale* (Vaux, Riedel, & Stewart, 1987). This 45-item scale taps five modes of support: emotional support, socializing, practical assistance, financial support, and advice. Respondents report separately on family and friends. The SS-B differs from the ISSB in that the ISSB asks about enacted or actual behavioral support, whereas the SS-B inquires about the likelihood of support or the availability of support.

Another issue related to social support is that it is not always helpful to the recipient. Research has demonstrated that when it is given at the wrong time or when it is perceived as threatening to self-esteem, it may have deleterious effects. Further, when the giver of support insinuates that the recipient must admit impairment, then social support is sometimes detrimental (Shinn, Lehmann, & Wong, 1984). Shinn and her co-workers also remind us that in the United States there exists a norm of reciprocity whereby, when help is given, there is an expectation that it will be repaid. This situation sometimes places the recipient in a lower status position until reciprocity can occur. Shinn and her co-workers suggest that under circumstances where reciprocity is impossible—for example, where a mentally disordered individual cannot for various reasons assist the supporter in return—professional help may serve the individual best (i.e., not threaten self-esteem), as no reciprocity is expected.

A final issue is that of the caregiver, family member, or friend. For them, giving intensive and continual social support can become distressing because of the demands of caring for a seriously mentally ill person and the social stigma attached to mental disorder. No recent study demonstrated this better than one by Rauktis, Koeske, and Tershko

(1995). These researchers investigated both positive and negative social interactions and their effects on the mental health of individuals caring for a seriously mentally ill family member. Although in general research supports the beneficial direct effects of social support, close relationships also can be a source of frustration and conflict. Research typically shows that caregivers have poorer physical health, poorer mental health, and a lower quality of life than the general population. The principal findings of Rauktis, Koeske, and Tershko are that negative social interactions significantly contribute to explaining caregivers' feelings of distress and depression, but positive social interactions make no significant contribution to feelings of mental health.

The results of this study have implications for both clinical and community psychologists. One clinical implication is that when working with family members who are caregivers to the mentally disordered, the clinician can prepare the family member for the possibility of negative social interactions, such as criticism by and distancing from friends. The preparation can help caregivers predict which individuals might be a source of positive rather than negative social interaction. Caregivers also can be taught how to request changes in others' behavior and how to indicate the need for empathetic listening.

At the community level, educating the caregivers' network of supports is important. Friends and family need to be informed about the symptoms, causes, and treatment of serious mental disorder. Such ongoing antistigma education is important in humanizing mental disorder, not just for the individual with the disorder but for the caregivers as well (Rauktis et al., 1995).

Psychosocial Clubs

Another form of community-based intervention for the mentally disordered is a club. *Psychosocial clubs* or *clubhouses* are community organizations designed to improve the quality of daily life for their members, who typically are the deinstitutionalized mentally disordered. This is accomplished by offering a protective, (usually) daytime, supportive environment and often by providing prevocational activities. Membership also gives these formerly hospitalized individuals a social support network of staff and other members, as well as structured activities which might include but are not limited to training in life management and interpersonal skills (Mastboom, 1992). The programs attempt to provide a community-based intervention for mentally disordered individuals to reintegrate them successfully into the community. Most clubs operate democratically, with members making many of the decisions. In this way, the programs meet some of the goals of community psychology.

Such organizations have witnessed phenomenal growth in the last two decades. No one knows how many exist, but in some locales there is an extensive network of clubhouses. For example, Massachusetts established an initial clubhouse program that included 18 different clubs around the state (Dudek & Stein, 1992). The Massachusetts clubhouses not only provide social support and training for the members, but also provide education about clubhouses for mental health professionals and family members of the mentally disordered. In fact, there are so many clubhouses available in the United States that there is a national organization, the National Clubhouse Expansion Program, and standards for establishment of clubhouses have been developed (Propst, 1992), which address membership eligibility, space, typical activities, employment, funding, and governance, among other issues. For example, with regard to policies, Glickman (1992) suggests that choice in the daily programs is essential because some members are so disabled by their illness that they are unable to participate actively in all clubhouse activities. Therefore, Glickman concludes, it is best not to make participation in activities mandatory.

Because these clubs have proliferated recently, some of them have been able to become more specialized or to offer specialized programs. Schartzer (1992) describes one psychosocial club that specialized in substance abuse among its members. Dual diagnosis is somewhat common among the mentally disordered. (Individuals with the dual diagnosis of mental disorder and chemical abuse are often labeled MICAs.) Schartzer describes a program called "Make Life Count," in which substance abuse is discussed openly and new members are questioned about such abuse in their initial assessments and screenings. Weekly drug screenings are set up for members who desire to remain drug-free. Contacts with other treatment programs, including Narcotics Anonymous and Alcoholics Anonymous, are also offered.

Other clubhouses specialize in job training (Vorspan, 1992). Often the training occurs in a work-ordered day, where a work schedule is set and prevocational training is offered. There is often some type of transitional employment situation consisting of part-time work with pay either within the club or external to it. Transitional employment helps members slowly regain entry into a sometimes rejecting society (Bilby, 1992). Such employment is not without controversy, for a variety of reasons. Some have argued that the transition to full-time employment is made more, not less, difficult by transitional employment (Bilby, 1992). Some clubs even emphasize college and posttechnical education in their programs (Dougherty, Hastie, Bernard, & Broadhurst, 1992).

Are such psychosocial clubs effective? One study examined the effects of clubhouse membership on participants from before their membership to after. The results showed that participants were hospitalized for psychiatric reasons five times as many days *before* their membership than they were *after* membership. The researcher (Wilkinson, 1992) suggests that this underscores the cost-effectiveness of clubhouse programs, as hospitalization is so expensive. Data from another study of clubs that provided educational opportunities demonstrated that after six months, 74% of the participants remained enrolled in the educational (college and posttechnical) programs, and 36.8% continued after 18 months with a mean grade point average of 3.0 (Doughtery et al., 1992). Corrigan and associates (1992) also found that in a club that emphasized job-finding skills, club members reported significantly improved job-interviewing skills and improved quality of life from before to after participation. Thus, from this initial evidence, psychosocial clubhouses appear to be quite effective.

Crisis Intervention

In many American communities, it is not the mental health professional but, rather, the police who are called when an individual is in a state of crisis (Baumann, Schultz, Brown, Paredes, & Hepeworth, 1987). Police often are not trained to cope with mental health and domestic situations; this also is not a good use of police time given that police are employed primarily to track crime. In an innovative program, Bauman and associates trained community volunteers on safety and crisis intervention techniques. When the police were called to a mental health or domestic crisis scene, an officer could call a trained team of volunteers to help with the crisis. The program generally resulted in less police time spent on each call. The results also indicated that trained lay people can be effective in intervening in a variety of crises. Olivero and Hanson (1994) suggest that the police should and can call mental health professionals and that collectively they need to develop linking agreements about how each will operate in different crisis situations.

The primary goal of psychological crisis intervention is to reach people in an acute state of distress and to provide them with enough support to prevent them from becoming chronically distressed (Slaikeu, 1984). This is consistent in part with one of the mandates of the Community Mental Health Centers Act, namely that 24-hour emergency care be made available to the mentally disordered. Because of the immediacy of the crisis and because responding to it requires flexibility and versatility, this type of intervention is quite different from traditional clinical interventions such as psychotherapy. The first crisis intervention programs were typically 24-hour phone services or "hotlines." Volunteers, who usually were trained in crisis intervention, staffed the phone lines at all hours. Many of these hotlines were established with the sole or primary purpose of suicide prevention.

Are these suicide prevention efforts effective? Caution is needed here because this research is difficult to do well. For example, it is difficult to find control groups for crisis intervention studies. Some studies utilize wait-listed clients; however, it would be unethical to wait-list suicidal individuals. These individuals simply cannot wait, because their crisis is often acute and very painful. One study used a pre–post design and a large number of participants to compensate for design problems. Leenaars and Lester (1995) conducted a large-scale study across Canada to determine whether the presence of crisis centers had changed Canada's suicide rates. Correlations were calculated between the presence of crisis services in 1985 and 1991 and changes in suicide rates over this period of time. The correlations indicated that the more crisis services were present in a region, the more likely it was that the suicide rate had decreased over the six years in question.

The system of telephone intervention also has been studied as to *how* and *when* it is effective. Echtering and Hartsough (1989) monitored 59 calls on a volunteer-staffed crisis intervention phone line. The volunteers' statements were recorded and coded to determine the sequence and usefulness of the steps in the process. There seemed to be three important phases of this type of short-term crisis intervention:

1. Assessment or evaluation of the nature and intensity of the crisis
2. Emotional integration (responding to the caller's emotions)
3. Problem solving or focusing on specific actions to be taken

These three steps, in this order, were most likely to end in success—that is, in alleviation of the caller's distress.

Crisis services have grown beyond this initial model. Not only do such services no longer take place exclusively by phone, but these services are designed to intervene in a variety of situations, not just for potential suicides. Much crisis work is now done face to face. One example of this is the mobile mental health team approach. These teams often go to the scene of a crisis for immediate intervention. In larger cities, some teams specialize in children and adolescent mental health services, some in alcohol and substance abuse or domestic violence, and so forth. A recent study has examined the effectiveness of round-the-clock mobile psychiatric crisis intervention. Reding and Raphelson (1995)

evaluated the effect of a 24-hour crisis intervention team on the number of psychiatric admissions to hospitals. Specifically, they examined whether adding a psychiatrist (who, for example, could provide medication) on the team was useful. The results indicated that the number of admissions to the hospitals during the program period (six months) was significantly lower than admissions during the same period for the previous two years. When the psychiatrist left the team, the number of admissions increased again.

A second study has also demonstrated that crisis intervention programs, although they can be expensive, really are cost-effective. Bengelsdorf, Church, Kaye, and Orlowski (1993) examined whether a professional mobile crisis intervention service was effective at diverting patients away from hospital admissions and into community-based treatments instead. Hospitalization is generally known to be more expensive than outpatient treatments. Fifty adults with mental disorders were tracked for six months. Although their crisis services cost over $54,000, hospital admissions would have cost at least another $43,000.

As mentioned previously, crisis services help people cope with more than suicidal tendencies. Various types of crisis intervention have helped individuals in communities cope with major school accidents (Weinberg, 1990), military disasters (McCaughey, 1987), international terrorism (Lanza, 1986), and air disasters (Kroon & Overdijk, 1993), to mention only a few crisis situations. Perhaps the other largest area of expansion is that of women's issues. Rape crisis intervention and temporary shelters for victims of domestic violence, which often provide on-the-spot counseling, also have proliferated since the early 1970s.

Assertive Case Management

Many community-based interventions for the seriously mentally disordered involve case management, whereby a case manager, for example a social worker, maintains contact with the client or consumer. These managers often act as advocates for the client, help broker other services in the community for the client, track medication regimes, teach daily living skills such as grocery shopping, and so on.

Recently, the literature has turned to **assertive case management**, known also as **intensive case management** or **assertive community treatment** (ACT), *where the caseload is small enough so that the case manager can provide intensive support to the client.* This case management technique is similar to other forms of case management, but it is more intense and the caseload typically is smaller—10 clients to one manager. The first assertive community treatment program was developed over twenty years ago in Madison, Wisconsin, by Stein and Test (1980). ACT has now emerged as one of the major treatment and rehabilitation approaches recognized for seriously mentally ill individuals (Bond, Witheridge, Dincin, & Wasmer, 1991; Mowbray, 1990). ACT is quite different from other interventions, especially in that the mental health professionals are "not only permitted but actually required to leave the comfortable surrounding of their hospitals and clinics, doing most of their work in their clients' own homes and neighborhoods" (Bond et al., 1991, p. 42). Most ACT programs also are willing to take on the most difficult clients.

Mowbray (1990) expressed surprise that ACT had not been more fully recognized by community psychologists because it upholds some of the major tenets of community psychology. For one, ACT utilizes outreach and in vivo treatment and thus adopts an ecological approach. Further, the low staff-to-client ratio ensures that each team member is well acquainted with every client and his or her unique circumstances. ACT guidelines also include capitalizing on client strengths rather than weaknesses. Although ACT obviously is not a primary prevention program, it was originally designed as an alternative to hospitalization. Because they work closely with clients, ACT staff members can detect early warning signs of clients' stress or of acute phases of disorders. Thus, the program provides secondary prevention. Because ACT emphasizes the integration of services for the client and because it takes a holistic approach to identifying client needs, ACT also parallels community psychology.

Preliminary research suggests that ACT is effective. Bond and associates (1990) found overall that

after one year, 76% of ACT clients remained involved with ACT, as compared to 7% of the clients who remained involved at a drop-in center. The ACT clients averaged significantly fewer hospitalizations and fewer days per hospital stay. The clients themselves reported greater satisfaction with the ACT program, fewer contacts with the police, and more stable housing situations than did the clients from the drop-in center.

Neale and Rosenbeck (1995), in a more recent study, found that a strong alliance between case managers and clients was associated with reduced symptom severity and improved global functioning as rated by independent assessors. Strong manager–client alliances also resulted in high client ratings of their community living skills. Essock and Kontos (1995) also found that ACT clients were hospitalized about half as often and were less likely to be without a permanent residence as compared to clients in standard services. Finally, Dvoskin and Steadman (1994) found that ACT clients spend fewer days in prison or jail than members of a comparison group. At first blush, then, ACT appears to be highly successful.

ACT, however, has not been without criticism. Toro (1990) criticized the way ACT research is conducted. He notes that longer follow-up periods are needed after ACT is implemented. In other words, we need to examine the long-term effects of various interventions, track rehospitalization as a measure of success or failure, and examine other outcome measures such as employment rates and stability of housing.

Other criticisms include those of Solomon and Draine (1995), who found that case managers may be serving some of the same functions traditionally served by the families of the mentally disordered and thus ACT may have an adverse or dampening effect on family relations. Botterbusch (1994), in a study where she obtained data from 107 ACT clients and 25 case managers, found that the ACT consumer still had little support from the larger community and remained socially isolated. She also found that the case managers interacted mostly with other professionals rather than with other community members. Mowbray (1990) also commented that ACT might not be empowering; that is,

ACT programs might not do enough to support independence and growth in clients. In fact, client dependency on hospitals might merely be replaced by dependency on the ACT case manager; if so, clients are not really empowered by ACT.

To correct the social isolation of persons with mental disorders, even with ACT, some mental health professionals have suggested combining ACT with psychosocial rehabilitation efforts such as clubhouses. In fact, Macias, Kinney, Farley, and Jackson (1994) found that case management integrated with psychosocial rehabilitation resulted in higher client functioning and less symptomatology than found in clients who received only psychosocial rehabilitation. Bond (1994) has called for more research on this suggestion. Corrigan and Kayton-Weinberg (1993) have also supported moving from aggressive or assertive case management to problem-focused case management for the severely mentally disordered in order to reduce dependency on mental health professionals. Problem-focused case management teaches clients how to identify and resolve community-based predicaments themselves so they become more independent of the mental health system.

In summary, assertive community treatment offers great hope for the deinstituionalized mentally ill, but program refinement needs to continue.

SPECIAL PROGRAMS FOR THE FUTURE OF COMMUNITIES: CHILDREN

Most of the programs discussed thus far are for adults. Yet children account for a large component of our community populations, and nearly everyone agrees that children hold the key to our future communities in their hands. We will briefly turn our attention to the role of community psychology in relation to children.

A Program for Parents

When children are aggressive, overactive, or fearful, and/or do not mind their parents, others respond to these children in repressive or dysfunctional ways. Thus, a vicious cycle of antisocial behavior and social rejection develops. The Houston Parent–Child Development Center houses a program to prevent this cycle from commencing (Johnson, 1988). The program, presented in the book mentioned earlier, *Fourteen Ounces of Prevention,* is truly a primary prevention program, as it starts with children at age one and with their parents. The Mexican American families who participated were considered to be at risk for the cycle of antisocial behavior in the children and for social rejection of the children by others. The risk factors were poverty and minority status.

An important feature of the program, and one that is consistent with community psychology, is that it was designed for this specific group of families. For example, the program was conducted primarily in Spanish. Second, a survey of these families revealed that the Mexican American women were very unlikely to leave their homes and that social interaction of the mother with people who were not her immediate relatives was considered undesirable. Another essential feature of the program is that transportation was provided for the mothers' trips to the center and for community health clinic visits. Still another feature is that program participants included more than just the mother and the infants; fathers and other family members were included as often as possible, even if this meant conducting some of the programming on weekends. The program was also very intensive. Parents had to participate for 550 hours, the equivalent of three semesters of college work.

The program took place in two stages. In the first stage, when the child was one year old, staff members visited the homes. The focus of these sessions was on the mother's and father's understanding of the infant's developmental progress and of the impact the parents would have on development. Parents were educated about such developmental aspects as language development, toys and games that are enriching, and physical growth. Interestingly, the staff members were not professionals but, rather, other women from the *barrio.*

In the second year of the program, families came to the center, where they interacted in groups. The 2-year-olds participated in a nursery school while their mothers attended classes on home management, consumer cooperatives, and so forth. The parents were educated about dealing with problem behaviors such as temper tantrums. Parents also were invited to suggest program modules.

Short- and long-term results are remarkable. First, the researchers videotaped mother–child interactions and found that the program mothers, compared to control mothers, were more affectionate, used more praise, used less criticism, were less rigidly controlling, and were more encouraging of their child's verbalizations. The homes of the program mothers also were more educationally enriching. The children were also assessed from grades 2 through 5. The program children were found to act out less, to be less impulsive and disruptive, and to be involved in fewer fights. Control children were more hostile, more dependent, and less considerate of others. Using a standardized measure of need to refer for clinical assistance, the researchers found that control children would have been more likely to be referred for assistance.

The Houston Parent–Child Development Center, designed to reduce children's behavior problems, did so through their parents. Are there programs that focus primarily on the child to prevent problem behaviors from developing? Of course.

A Program for Children

Various skills seem to distinguish children as early as age 4 as to who will show behavior problems and who will not. One skill is alternative-solution thinking: the ability to think of multiple means to solve an interpersonal problem, such as how two children can play with the same single toy. Children who cannot think of more than one or two ways to solve these problems are often impatient, overemotional, aggressive, withdrawn, or unconcerned about the feelings of others (Shure & Spivack, 1988). Such children often fail to weigh the effects of their actions on others. The fact of being stuck on one solution seems to be more crucial than the solution's content in determining whether the child's behavior is problematic. Shure and Spivack asked: Would enhancing these children's problem-solving skills reduce their impulsivity and other dysfunctional behaviors?

Shure and Spivack developed interpersonal cognitive problem-solving (ICPS) to focus children away from single solutions to a process of developing a number of solutions and weighing the pros and cons of each. ICPS is predicated on the premise that a person who is preoccupied with the end goal rather than how to attain it is likely to make impulsive mistakes, become frustrated, show aggressive behavior, or withdraw from the situation. ICPS also assumes that this more productive type of thinking facilitates interpersonal adjustment and psychological health.

Shure and Spivack found that 4 years of age was the earliest that language was sufficient to teach ICPS. Either teachers or mothers acted as trainers of the children. Specific program elements include first teaching negotiation, helping children understand some key words such as the difference between *some* and *all* and word strings such as *if . . . then*; identifying and then being sensitive to other's feelings; influencing others; and so forth. Children later master interpersonal problem-solving skills by being given stories and role-plays. The children's trainers also are trained to manage problem behaviors during the program, for example children who are disruptive or dominant.

Program results indicate that trained children as compared to a control group give more relevant solutions and potential consequences of the solutions to hypothetical problems. Prosocial behaviors are significantly enhanced in the program children, and problematic behaviors are significantly reduced. At one- and two-year follow-up, gains were maintained. For example, program children were still less likely to show problem behaviors. More important, the behaviors learned during ICPS seem to generalize from home to school and from school to home. Therefore, these positive results hold no matter who the trainer is, mother or teacher. This finding is particularly exciting to community psychologists because it means that the program probably can be transplanted to other communities.

These two programs highlight how by working with communities—parents and children—community psychologists can prevent long-range problem behaviors in children who need to be the mentally healthy adults of tomorrow.

WHAT CAN BE LEARNED FROM COMMUNITY PSYCHOLOGY

Various community interventions and programs have now been reviewed. Most incorporated a variety of the principles of community psychology, including but not limited to empowerment, prevention (rather than treatment), and large-scale rather than one-on-one intervention. All of the programs were effective in their own way, whether designed for children or adults and whether their efforts were aimed at primary or secondary prevention. What else can collectively be said of these programs?

First, programs implemented by community psychologists often are custom designed or tailored to the needs of their clients. The same is generally true of clinical interventions. The difference is that in clinical psychology the intervention is typically designed for one person, whereas in community psychology a group as large as a whole community is the target population. A second feature of community psychology interventions is that they recognize uniqueness or diversity in the population. In clinical psychology, the psychologist is often trained in one or two paradigms or one or two models of psychotherapy; thus, the clinical psychologist often assumes that many people can profit from the same intervention. The same assumption does not always hold for community psychology.

Another feature of community psychology programs is that they use a multifocused approach. A single method of intervention is often inadequate. Usually, several methods are employed together and are deemed more successful than one. For example, in interpersonal cognitive problem solving, children do not just learn to differentiate words such as *some* and *all* but, rather, learn a multitude of skills to help them cope with others. One limitation, however, is that combining treatment modalities in community psychology makes it difficult during program evaluation to tease out which component or components caused the efficacy. This is less likely to be the case in clinical psychology. Similarly, in community psychology a number of people, not just the individual at risk, typically participate in the program. For example, for pregnant teens, community psychologists hope to engage the teen's own parents as well as the father in any inter-

vention effort. Unless clinicians practice family, milieu, or group therapy, their interventions are usually aimed at the individual.

Another feature of community programs is that often the interventions are taken to the client's ecological setting. For example, programs for school dropouts are implemented in the schools, and programs for Hispanic mothers are implemented in their homes and neighborhoods. In clinical psychology, by contrast, the client typically has to meet the clinician on the clinician's turf.

Another important property of community programs is that they recognize the importance of assistance and support from nonprofessionals. No concept better illustrates this idea than the notion of *social support*. Social support can come from friends, family, and even other disaffected members of society. A professional, such as a clinical psychologist, is not always necessary. The concept of social support also insinuates that a professional does not always know best, a circumstance that takes aim at the intensive training and licensing required of clinical psychologists.

Most community psychology programs are also innovative and creative. This novelty sometimes can be problematic. George Fairweather and Bill Davidson (1986) remind their readers that individuals embarking on social change efforts need to be realists. Although the programs may be innovative and creative, the programmers might also experience much resistance, just as a clinician encounters resistance in a client who is undergoing change. In the case of community psychology, resistance sometimes comes from large groups of citizens. Often, the more novel the program, the more it changes the status quo. The more the status quo is changed, the more resistance is likely to occur (Duffy & Wong, 1996).

Probably the most important lesson from community psychology is that interventions and community services need to be coordinated. Too many clients fall through service cracks or receive only partial assistance. When agencies keep to themselves or are not networked, not only do the agencies encounter difficulties keeping themselves viable, so too do clients encounter difficulties by not receiving full sets of services, by receiving duplicate or unnecessary services, or by receiving no service. Community interventions, then, need to be fully integrated both into the community and with one another.

COMMUNITY PSYCHOLOGY: TOWARD THE FUTURE

Community psychology appears to be an energetic and promising field. We have seen where it has been, but where is it going? Glimpses of changes in the field's research methodology, employment opportunities, and educational opportunities might prove revealing.

Research Methodology

Both Lounsbury and associates (Lounsbury, Leader, Meares, & Cook, 1980) and Speer and his fellow researchers (1992) examined the topics, populations, and specific measures and research methodologies used in community psychology over two different decades. They discovered that the number of experiments in which variables were actively manipulated had decreased over the years, while the number of field studies actually increased. In field studies there is generally no manipulation of variables. Thus, over the years there was also a decline in the use of control groups and an increase in correlational analyses. In fact, some very sophisticated and nonexperimental analyses are currently capturing the field's attention. These include *meta-analysis, a statistical review of the literature to determine the robustness of trends in the literature.* For readers seeking more information, meta-analysis is described in more detail in the chapter on research.

Second, the same authors note that there exist today fewer studies of the mentally disordered in the community psychology literature. This change signals a trend toward working with more diverse populations, such as juvenile delinquents, pregnant teens, and parents who maltreat their children. Community psychology is indeed outgrowing its mental health roots.

Community psychologists also espouse inclusion of a wide diversity of groups in their research. Loo, Fong, and Iwamasca (1988) reviewed the top community psychology journals and found that before 1988 only about 11% of the articles pertained to ethnic minorities. My own quick analysis of articles from the 1990s indicates that over 35% of articles include people of color and other diverse groups (Duffy & Wong, 1996). There appears to be an increase in the kinds of individuals being studied in community psychology, such that the field is practicing what it preaches. We might conclude, then, that research in community psychology continues to evolve in interesting ways that are often divergent from the rest of the field of psychology.

Educational Opportunities

Most concentrated or specialized training in community psychology occurs at the graduate level. There are only a few stand-alone community psychology graduate programs at the master's and doctoral levels. Many graduate programs combine community psychology with clinical psychology. However, a chapter in an undergraduate text like this one is a good start. Several undergraduate colleges offer a course in community psychology, community internships or volunteer work, and perhaps one or two courses.

It is at the graduate level that specialization in community psychology takes place. At this level, most universities utilize the scientist–practitioner model (the Boulder model) consistent with training in clinical psychology. Students are trained to conduct research and to practice the discipline on the basis of scientific foundations. Some community psychology programs are freestanding, but many are combined clinical–community psychology programs. In the 1970s there were very few community psychology graduate programs. The number grew in the 1980s and has held steady in the 1990s.

Employment Opportunities

Walfish, Polifka, and Stenmark (1986) surveyed graduates with community psychology training and found that of the doctoral students surveyed, 83% reported obtaining a job at their first-choice placement. The major employment settings were community mental health centers, medical schools, consulting firms, universities, and health care facilities. Hoffnung, Morris, and Jex (1986) conducted a similar survey of master's-level graduates and found equally favorable results. The respondents also reported high employment rates (90%), with most individuals employed in human or social services. These same researchers also included measures of job satisfaction and found them to be moderately high.

The Future of the Field

Most community psychologists would gladly be put out of business. That is, most individuals in the field would be very happy if there were few or no social problems and no disaffected groups. But this will probably never be a reality, because when one social problem has been eradicated, a new one seems to arise to take its place. Witness our major health epidemics, for example. Smallpox was erased in time for us to have a more recent, disastrous encounter with AIDS.

No one can predict for sure where societies are headed or what the future holds for a particular discipline. Given that communities are likely to continue to diversify and that citizens probably will always want to better their communities and to need a guiding hand when doing so, community psychology will continue to flourish. What might change this picture, however, is continual changes in funding and therefore availability of various community programs. Some authors argue that there is a shifting of responsibility from federal governments to state governments (Linney, 1990), which makes the future of communities and community psychology murkier and less certain. However, it is community psychologists, not clinical psychologists, who best know how to interface with legislators and others who influence public policy. Given this trend, the health of community psychology appears certain.

REFERENCES

American Psychological Association. (1995). *APA membership directory*. Washington, DC: Author.

Arce, A. A. (1978). Approaches to establishing community services for the mentally disabled. *Psychiatric Quarterly, 50,* 264–268.

Barrera, M., Sandler, I. N., & Ramsey, T. B. (1981). Preliminary development of a scale of social support: Studies on college students. *American Journal of Community Psychology, 9,* 435–448.

Baumann, D. J., Schultz, D. F., Brown, C., Paredes, R., & Hepeworth, J. (1987). Citizen participation in police crisis intervention activities. *American Journal of Community Psychology, 15,* 459–472.

Belcher, J. R. (1988). Are jails replacing the mental health care system for the homeless mentally ill? *Community Mental Health Journal, 24,* 185–195.

Bengelsdorf, J., Church, J. O., Kaye, R. A., & Orlowski, B. (1993). The cost effectiveness of crisis intervention: Admission diversion savings can offset the high cost of service. *Journal of Nervous and Mental Disease, 181,* 757–762.

Bilby, R. (1992). A response to the criticisms of transitional employment. *Psychosocial Rehabilitation Journal, 16,* 69–82.

Blakely, C. P., Mayer, J. P., Gottschalk, R. G., Schmidt, N., Davidson, W. S., Roitman, D. B., & Emshoff, J. G. (1987). The fidelity–adaptation debate: Implications of the implementation of public sector social programs. *American Journal of Community Psychology, 15,* 253–268.

Bloom, B. L. (1988). *Health psychology: A psychosocial perspective*. Englewood Cliffs, NJ: Prentice-Hall.

Bloom, B. L., & Hodges, W. F. (1988). The Colorado Separation and Divorce program: A preventive intervention program for newly separated persons. In R. Price, E. W. Cowen, R. P. Lorion, & J. Ramos-McKay (Eds.), *Fourteen ounces of prevention* (pp. 153–164). Washington, DC: American Psychological Association.

Bond, G. R. (1994). Case management and psychosocial rehabilitation. Can they be synergistic? *Community Mental Health Journal, 30,* 341–346.

Bond, G. R., Witheridge, T. F., Dincin, J., & Wasmer, D. (1991). Assertive community treatment: Correcting some misconceptions. *American Journal of Community Psychology, 19,* 41–51.

Bond, G. R., Witheridge, T. F., Dincin, J., Wasmer, D., Webb, J., & DeGraaf-Kaser, R. (1990). Assertive community treatment for frequent users of psychiatric hospitals in a large city: A controlled study. *American Journal of Community Psychology, 18,* 865–891.

Bootzin, R. R., Shadish, W. R., & McSweeney, A. J. (1989). Longitudinal outcomes of nursing home care for severely mentally ill patients. *Journal of Social Issues, 45,* 31–48.

Botterbusch, K. F. (1994). Summary of: Community support networks for persons with psychiatric disabilities. *Vocational Evaluation and Work Adjustment Bulletin, 27*, 57–61.

Botvin, G. J., & Tortu, S. (1988). Preventing adolescent substance abuse through life skills training. In R. H. Price, E. L. Cowen, R. P. Lorion, & J. Ramos-McKay (Eds.). *Fourteen ounces of prevention* (pp. 98–110). Washington, DC: American Psychological Association.

Bronfenbrenner, U. (1986, February). Alienation and the four worlds of childhood. *Phi Delta Kappan*, 430–436.

Brown, J. D. (1991). Staying fit and staying well: Physical fitness as a moderator of life stress. *Journal of Personality and Social Psychology, 60*, 555–561.

Brownell, A., & Shumaker, S. A. (1984). Social support: An introduction to a complex phenomenon. *Journal of Social Issues, 40*, 1–9.

Bruce, M. L., Takeuchi, D. T., & Leaf, P. J. (1991). Poverty and psychiatric status: Longitudinal evidence from the New Haven Epidemiologic Catchment Area Study. *Archives of General Psychiatry, 48*, 470–474.

Caplan, G. (1974). *Support systems and community mental health*. New York: Behavioral Publications.

Cassel, J. (1974). Psychosocial processes and "stress": Theoretical formulations. *International Journal of Health Services, 4*, 471–482.

Corrigan, P., & Kayton-Weinberg, D. (1993). Aggressive and problem-focused models of case management for the severely mentally ill. *Community Mental Health Journal, 29*, 449–458.

Corrigan, P. W., Reedy, P., Thadani, D., & Ganet, M. (1995). Correlates of participation and completion in a job club for clients with psychiatric disability. *Rehabilitation Counseling, 39*, 42–53.

Cowen. E. L. (1980). The wooing of primary prevention. *American Journal of Community Psychology, 8*, 258–284.

Davidson, J. L. (1981, June). Location of community-based treatment centers. *Social Science Review*, 221–241.

Davidson, W. B., & Cotter, P. R. (1989). Sense of community and political participation. *Journal of Community Psychology, 17*, 119–125.

Diamond, P. M., & Schnee, S. B. (1990). *Tracking the costs of chronicity: Towards a redirection of resources*. Presented to the Annual Meeting of the American Psychological Association, Boston.

Dougherty, S., Hastie, C., Bernard, J., & Broadhurst, S. (1992). Supported education: A clubhouse experience. *Psychosocial Rehabilitation Journal, 16,* 91–104.

Dudek, K. J., & Stein, R. (1992). Organizing for clubhouses: The Massachusetts success story. *Psychosocial Rehabilitation Journal, 16*, 141–146.

Duffy, K. G., & Wong, F. Y. (1996). *Community psychology*. Boston: Allyn and Bacon.

Dumont, M. P. (1982). Review of "Private Lives/Public Spaces," by E. Baxter & K. Hopper, and "Shopping Bag Ladies," by A. M. Rousseau. *American Journal of Orthopsychiatry, 52*, 367–369.

Dvoskin, J. A., & Steadman, H. J. (1994). Using intensive case management to reduce violence by mentally ill persons in the community. Special Issue: Violent behavior and mental illness. *Hospital and Community Psychiatry, 45*, 679–684.

Echtering, L. G., & Hartsough, D. M. (1989). Phases of helping in successful crisis telephone calls. *Journal of Community Psychology, 17*, 249–257.

Essock, S. M., & Kontos, N. (1995). Implementing assertive community treatment teams. Special Section: Assertive community treatment. *Psychiatric Services, 46*, 679–683.

Fairweather, G. W., & Davidson, W. S. (1986). *An introduction to community experimentation: Theory, method, & practice*. New York: McGraw-Hill.

Fairweather, G. W., Sanders, D. H., Maynard, H., & Cressler, D. L. (1969). *Community life for the mentally ill*. Chicago: Aldine.

Fawcett, S. B., Seekins, T., & Silber, L. (1988). Low-income voter registration: A small-scale evaluation of an agency-based registration strategy. *American Journal of Community Psychology, 16*, 751–758.

Felner, R. D., Ginter, M., & Primavera, J. (1982). Primary prevention during school transitions: Social support and environmental structure. *American Journal of Community Psychology, 10*, 277–290.

Fiore, J., Coppel, D. B., Becker, J., & Cox, G. B. (1986). Social support as a multifaceted concept: Examination of important dimensions for adjustment. *American Journal of Community Psychology, 14*, 93–111.

Freeman, R. J., & Roesch, R. (1989). Mental disorder and the criminal justice system. *International Journal of Law and Psychiatry, 12*, 105–115.

Glickman, M. (1992). The voluntary nature of the clubhouse. *Psychosocial Rehabilitation Journal, 16*, 39–40.

Heller, K., Price, R. H., Reinharz, S., Riger, S., & Wandersman, A. (1984). *Psychology and community change*. Homewood, IL: Dorsey.

Hoffnung, R. J., Morris, M., & Jex, S. (1986). Training community psychologists at the master's level: A case study of outcomes. *American Journal of Community Psychology, 14,* 339–349.

Johnson, D. L. (1988). Primary prevention of behavior problems in young children: The Houston Parent–Child Development Center. In R. H. Price, E. L. Cowen, R. P. Lorion, & J. Ramos-McKay (Eds.), *Fourteen ounces of prevention* (pp. 98–110). Washington, DC: American Psychological Association.

Johnson, P. J., & Beditz, J. (1981). Community support systems: Scaling community acceptance. *Community Mental Health Journal, 17,* 153–160.

Kiesler, C. A. (1980). Mental health policy as a field of inquiry for psychology. *American Psychologist, 35,* 1066–1080.

Kiesler, C. A. (1982a). Mental hospitals and alternative care: Noninstitutionalization as potential public policy for mental patients. *American Psychologist, 37,* 349–360.

Kiesler, C. A. (1982b). Public and professional myths about mental hospitalization: An empirical reassessment of policy-related beliefs. *American Psychologist, 37,* 1323–1339.

Kroon, M. B., & Overdijk, W. I. (1993). Psychosocial care and shelter following the Biljmermeer air disaster. *Crisis, 17,* 117–125.

Kruzich, J. M. (1985). Community integration of the mentally ill in residential facilities. *American Journal of Community Psychology, 13,* 553–564.

Kuhlman, T. L. (1994). *Psychology on the streets: Mental health practice with homeless persons.* New York: Wiley.

Lanza, M. L. (1986). Victims of international terrorism. *Issues in Mental Health Nursing, 8,* 95–107.

Lawson, A., & Rhode, D. L. (1993). *The politics of pregnancy: Adolescent sexuality and public policy.* New Haven, CT: Yale University Press.

Leenaars, A. A., & Lester, D. (1995). Impact of suicide prevention centers on suicide in Canada. *Crisis, 16,* 39.

Linney, J. A. (1990). Community psychology into the 1990s: Capitalizing opportunity and promoting innovation. *American Journal of Community Psychology, 18,* 1–17.

Loo, C., Fong, K. T., & Iwamasca, G. (1988). Ethnicity and cultural diversity: An analysis of work published in community psychology journals, 1965–1985. *Journal of Community Psychology, 16,* 332–349.

Lounsbury, J. W., Leader, D. S., Meares, E. P., & Cook, M. P. (1980). An analytic review of research in community psychology. *American Journal of Community Psychology, 18,* 917–921.

Macias, C., Kinney, R., Farley, O. W., & Jackson, R. (1994). The role of case management within a community support system: Partnership with psychosocial rehabilitation. *Community Mental Health Journal, 30,* 323–339.

Maier, G. J., Morrow, B. R., & Miller, R. (1989). Security safeguards in community rehabilitation of forensic patients. *Hospital and Community Psychiatry, 40,* 529–531.

Mastboom, J. (1992). Forty clubhouses: Models and practices. *Psychosocial Rehabilitation Journal, 16,* 9–24.

McCaughey, B. G. (1987). U.S. Navy special psychiatric rapid and intervention team (SPRINT). *Military Medicine, 152,* 133–135.

Miller, R. (1982). The least restrictive alternative: Hidden meanings and agendas. *Community Mental Health Journal, 18,* 46–55.

Millman, R. B., & Botvin, G. J. (1983). Substance use, abuse, and dependence. In M. D. Levine, W. B. Carey, A. C. Crocker, & R. T Gross (Eds.), *Developmental behavioral pediatrics* (pp. 683–708). Philadelphia: W. B. Saunders.

Morrison, J. K. (1980). The public's current beliefs about mental illness: Serious obstacle to effective community psychology. *American Journal of Community Psychology, 8,* 697–707.

Morse, G. H., Calsyn, R. J., & Burger, G. K. (1992). Development and cross-validation of a system for classifying homeless persons. *Journal of Community Psychology, 20,* 228–242.

Mowbray, C. T. (1990). Community treatment for the seriously mentally ill: Is this community psychology? *American Journal of Community Psychology, 18,* 893–902.

Mowbray, C. T., Bybee, D., & Cohen, E. (1993). Describing the homeless mentally ill: Cluster analysis results. *American Journal of Community Psychology, 21,* 67–94.

Muñoz, R. F., Glish, M., Soo-Hoo, T., & Robertson, J. (1982). The San Francisco Mood Survey project: Preliminary work toward the prevention of depression. *American Journal of Community Psychology, 10,* 317–329.

National Coalition for the Homeless. (1988). *Precious resources: Government owned housing and the needs of the homeless.* New York: Author.

Neale, M., & Rosenheck, R. A. (1995). Therapeutic alliance and outcome in a VA intensive case management program. Special Section: Assertive community treatment. *Psychiatric Services, 46,* 719–723.

Olivero, J. M., & Hanson, R. (1994). Linkage agreements

between mental health and law enforcement agencies. *Administration and Policy in Mental Health, 21,* 217–225.

Patteson, D. M., & Barnard, K. E. (1990). Parenting of low birth weight infants: A review of issues and interventions. *Infant Mental Health Journal, 11,* 37–56.

Pogrebin, M. R., & Regoli, R. M. (1985). Editorial. Mentally disordered persons in jail. *Journal of Community Psychology, 13,* 409–412.

Price, R. H., Cowen, E. L., Lorion, R. P., & Ramos-McKay, J. (1988). Introduction. In R. H. Price, E. L. Cowen, R. P. Lorion, & J. Ramos-McKay (Eds.), *Fourteen ounces of prevention* (pp. 98–110). Washington, DC: American Psychological Association.

Propst, R. N. (1992). Standards for clubhouse programs: Why and how they were developed. *Psychosocial Rehabilitation Journal, 16,* 25–34.

Rappaport, J. (1987). Terms of empowerment/Exemplars of prevention: Toward a theory for community psychology. *American Journal of Community Psychology, 15,* 121–148.

Rauktis, M. E., Koeske, G., & Tershko, O. (1995). Negative social interactions, distress, and depression among those caring for a seriously and persistently mentally ill relative. *American Journal of Community Psychology, 23,* 279–299.

Reding, G. R., & Raphelson, M. (1995). Around-the-clock mobile psychiatric intervention: Another effective alternative to psychiatric hospitalization. *Community Mental Health Journal, 31,* 179–187.

Regier, D. A., Narrow, W. E., Rae, D. S., Manderscheid, R. W., Locke, B. Z., & Goodwin, F. K. (1993). The de facto U.S. mental and addictive disorders service system. *Archives of General Psychiatry, 41,* 971–978.

Rosenhan, D. L. (1973). On being sane in insane places. *Science, 179,* 250–258.

Rossi, P. H. (1989). *Down and out in America: The origins of homelessness.* Chicago: University of Chicago Press.

Rumberger, R. W. (1987). High school dropouts: A review of issues and evidence. *Review of Educational Research, 57,* 101–121.

Sarason, S. B. (1974). *The psychological sense of community: Prospects for a community psychology.* San Francisco: Jossey-Bass.

Sarason, S. B. (1983). *Schooling in America: Scapegoat and salvation.* New York: Free Press.

Schartzer, J. E. (1992). Dealing with substance abuse behavior in the clubhouse. *Psychosocial Rehabilitation Journal, 16,* 107–110.

Scott, R. R., Balch, P., & Flynn, T. C. (1983). A comparison of community attitudes toward CMHC services and clients with those of mental hospitals. *American Journal of Community Psychology, 11,* 741–749.

Searight, H. R., Oliver, J. M., & Grisso, J. T. (1986). The community competence scale in the placement of the deinstitutionalized mentally ill. *American Journal of Community Psychology, 14,* 291–301.

Segal, S. P., Silverman, C., & Baumohl, J. (1989). Seeking person–environmental fit in community care placement. *Journal of Social Issues, 45,* 49–64.

Seidman, E. (1990). Pursuing meaning and utility of social regularities for community psychology. In P. Tolan, C. Keys, F. Chertak, & L. Jason (Eds.), *Researching community psychology: Issues of theory and methods* (pp. 91–100). Washington, DC: American Psychological Association.

Seitz, V., Apfel, N. H., & Rosenbaum, L. K. (1991). Effects of an intervention program for pregnant adolescents: Educational outcomes at two years postpartum. *American Journal of Community Psychology, 19,* 911–930.

Shinn, M., Lehmann, S., & Wong, N. W. (1984). Social interaction and social support. *American Journal of Community Psychology, 40,* 55–76.

Shumaker, S. A., & Brownell, A. (1984). Toward a theory of social support: Closing conceptual gaps. *Journal of Social Issues, 40,* 11–36.

Shure, M. B., & Spivack, G. (1988). Interpersonal cognitive problem solving. In R. H. Price, E. L. Cowen, R. P. Lorion, & J. Ramos-McKay (Eds.), *Fourteen ounces of prevention: A casebook for practitioners* (pp. 69–82). Washington, DC: American Psychological Association.

Sime, W. E. (1984). Psychological benefits of exercise training in the healthy individual. In J. D. Matarazzo, S. M. Weiss, J. A. Herd, N. E. Miller, & S. M. Weiss (Eds.), *Behavioral health: A handbook for health enhancement and disease prevention.* New York: Wiley.

Slaikeu, K. A. (1984). *Crisis intervention: A handbook for practice and research.* Boston: Allyn and Bacon.

Solomon, P., & Draine, J. (1995). Consumer case management and attitudes concerning family relations among persons with mental illness. *Psychiatric Quarterly, 66,* 249–261.

Speer, P., Dey, A., Griggs, P., Gibson, C., Lubin, B., & Hughey, J. (1992). In search of community: An analysis of community psychology research from 1984–1988. *American Journal of Community Psychology, 20,* 195–209.

Stack, L. C., Lannon, P. B., & Miley, A. D. (1983). Accuracy of clinicians' expectancies for psychiatric rehospitalization. *American Journal of Community Psychology, 11,* 99–113.

Stein, L. I., & Test, M. A. (1980). An alternative to mental hospital treatment: Conceptual model, treatment program, and clinical evaluation. *Archives of General Psychiatry, 37,* 392–397.

Swift, C., & Levin, G. (1987). Empowerment: An emerging mental health technology. *Journal of Primary Prevention, 8,* 71–94.

Talbott, J. A. (1975). Current clichés and platitudes in vogue in psychiatric vocabularies. *Hospital and Community Psychiatry, 26,* 530.

Tebes, J. K., & Kraemer, D. T. (1991). Quantitative and qualitative knowing in mutual support research: Some lessons from the recent history of scientific psychology. *American Journal of Community Psychology, 19,* 739–756.

Toro, P. A. (1990). Evaluating professionally operated and self-help programs for the seriously mentally ill. *American Journal of Community Psychology, 18,* 903–907.

U.S. Public Health Service. (1980). *Toward a national plan for the chronic mentally ill.* Washington, DC: U.S. Department of Health and Human Services.

Vaux, A., Riedel, S., & Stewart, D. (1987). Modes of social support: The Social Support Behaviors (SS-B) Scale. *American Journal of Community Psychology, 15,* 209–237.

Veroff, J., Douvan, E., & Kulka, R. A. (1981). *The inner Americans: A self-portrait from 1957 to 1976.* New York: Basic Books.

Vorspan, R. (1992). Why work works: Sixth plenary session of the fifth international seminar on the clubhouse model. *Psychosocial Rehabilitation Journal, 16,* 49–54.

Walfish, S., Polifka, J. A., & Stenmark, D. E. (1986). The job search in community psychology: A survey of recent graduates. *American Journal of Community Psychology, 14,* 237–240.

Weinberg, R. B. (1990). Serving large numbers of adolescent victim-survivors: Group interventions following a trauma at school. *Professional Psychology Research and Practice, 21,* 271–278.

Wilkinson, W. H. (1992). New Day, Inc., of Spartanburg: Hospitalization study. *Psychosocial Rehabilitation Journal, 16,* 163–168.

FOR FURTHER READING

For students who are interested in reading more about community psychology, several textbooks are available. Two recent and leading books in the field are Duffy and Wong (1996) and Levine and Perkins (1997). Orford's (1992) book on theory and practice in community psychology offers the British perspective on the same topic.

Tolan, Key, Chertok, and Jason's (1990) edited volume on research in community psychology offers insights into the keys concepts, hypotheses, levels of analysis, and research methodologies utilized by community psychologists.

The casebook *Fourteen Ounces of Prevention* (Price, Cowen, Lorion, & Ramos-McKay, 1988) offers readers summaries of actual community problems that were resolved or treated with community psychology interventions. These programs were selected from among thousands across the United States by a blue-ribbon panel of experts.

CHAPTER 15

TRANSCULTURAL PSYCHOLOGY AND THE DELIVERY OF CLINICAL PSYCHOLOGICAL SERVICES

Juris G. Draguns

INTRODUCTION: CULTURE IN CLINICAL SERVICES

Clinical services in psychology are invariably delivered in a social context. In interactions between a clinical psychologist and a client, culture is always an implicit and silent participant (Draguns, 1975). In culturally diverse societies like those of the contemporary United States and Canada, clinical contact often takes place across a cultural divide or barrier. To put it differently, the clinician and his or her client bring to this transaction subtly or starkly different expectations based on their respective lifetimes of social learning and experience. Moreover, these differences in expectations may produce misunderstandings that can, to varying degrees, interfere with or complicate the desired beneficial effects of such contacts. For these reasons, it is essential to discuss the role of culture in the implementation of clinical services.

In this chapter, I will tackle four major tasks. First, I will introduce and explain the concept of culture and describe the available approaches to its scientific, empirical investigation. Second, I will present some of the findings on the role of culture in producing abnormal behavior. Third, I will survey the impact of cultural characteristics for the entire range of clinical psychological services, from initiation through termination to follow-up. Fourth and finally, I will try to sketch the ideal state of training for, and implementation of, culturally sensitive and effective services in clinical psychology.

Culture: A Concept Hard to Define

Culture is one of the concepts in social science that is implicitly and approximately understood by a great many people. Yet difficulties arise when attempts are made to squeeze the multiple and complex features of this concept into a succinct definition. This difficulty does not afflict only novices, students, and lay persons. Experts have sought in vain to arrive at a universally acceptable and comprehensive definition of culture. The failure of their quest is attested by Kroeber and Kluckhohn (1952), who devoted an entire monograph to the listing and scholarly analysis of the definitions of culture then extant—over 100 of them! This number has no doubt increased in the meantime.

Instead of adding to this complexity and the frustration it would inevitably generate, let us limit ourselves to the pithy statement by Herskovits (1948, p.

17), who defined *culture* as the human-made part of the environment. This definition encompasses, first of all, the myriad artifacts created by human beings—from the simplest tools to the most complex computers, from makeshift huts to high-rise buildings, from slings to ballistic missiles. At the same time, Herskovits emphatically intended to include the socially shared products of human minds: the languages spoken around the world; the ideas expressed and understood; the rules, values, and beliefs people live by; and the cumulative experience of human groups accumulated over centuries and millennia. One of the distinctive features of the human species is that human beings create, use, and take seriously symbols, socially agreed-on signs that have a potentially profound impact on experience and behavior.

Triandis (1972) introduced the concept of *subjective culture*, which refers to the way in which, within a specific human group, events are categorized and labeled through language and by means of which these categories, norms, roles, and values are interrelated and grouped. It is very important to note that subjective culture includes specifications on how the various concepts enumerated above are linked to behavior.

Another feature of culture that must be emphasized is that culture constitutes a bridge across time. Culture is not created anew by each generation. Instead, of necessity, it is continuous and cumulative. Culture can be equated with the accumulated experience of a group over time and, perhaps, with that group's shared wisdom.

Along similar lines, Stewart (1995) has distinguished surface, deep, and procedural cultures. *Surface culture* is expressed through observable behavior, in speech, gestures, and action as well as in artifacts such as food, dress, buildings, and tools. *Deep culture* refers to thoughts, feelings, and self-experience in time and space. *Procedural culture* is manifested in performance and communication, by pursuit of goals through action, formulating and implementing decisions, experiencing and resolving conflicts among people, and a host of meaningful and/or social activities.

Culture, then, is especially relevant to social behavior. All human groups feature—and regulate—interaction among their members. The specific patterns of social behavior are prescribed by culture and are transmitted through socialization.

From Culture to Cultures

In defining *culture*, social scientists refer to it in the singular. In describing specific tribes or other groupings, however, they inevitably come to grips with a multitude of human *cultures*. It is the variety of cultures that is of paramount concern in designing and implementing clinical psychology services. Cultures, to be sure, differ across distances and geographical and social barriers; no one would assert that the cultures of the contemporary United States, Japan, and Ethiopia are identical. Yet, as a result of population shifts and migrations of the last four centuries, and especially those of the last few decades, persons from a variety of cultures of origin find themselves thrown together in the same location and in the same habitat. This is especially the case in the United States and Canada, which were conceived as nations of immigrants and continue to experience an influx of newcomers from all or most regions of the world. Not only the migrants but also their descendants, sometimes for many generations, continue to harbor traits of surface, deep, and procedural cultures brought from their countries of origin.

Nor should it be forgotten that the locations in which the new settlers arrived were inhabited by peoples which possessed their own distinctive cultures. Centuries later, the descendants of these indigenous inhabitants cling to certain parts of their ancestral cultures or, in some cases, are in the process of reviving and reasserting them. Culture, then, is a concept that is helpful for understanding people in remote and exotic locations, but it is as relevant around the block as it is around the globe. Mental health professionals in particular, in North America and elsewhere, are inescapably confronted with cultural diversity among their clientele. The American Psychological Association has made it an official requirement for clinical psychologists to know the cultural characteristics of their clientele and to take these into account in rendering their services (Korman, 1974). The assumption on which this requirement rests is that clinical services must be culturally sensitive and appropriate in order to be effective and beneficial to their recipients.

Emic and Etic: Two Contrasting Views in Conceptualization and Investigations

Regardless of the topic of their study, social scientists tend to proceed to the study of culture from one of the two contrasting points of view. The *emic* position is often articulated by theoreticians and investigators who concentrate on the study of social phenomena, including those of psychological disturbance, within its specific cultural context of occurrence. What preceded this event, what accompanied it, and what followed it are sought within the context of the culture in which the phenomenon occurred. In the case of an extreme fear reaction, for example, the observer would note when and how this pattern of behavior occurred, what meaning was attributed to it, how it was counteracted and treated, and what consequences it entailed over time—all within the setting of the specific culture. An emic investigator would not be interested in fright reactions across cultures, nor would such an investigator be inclined to generalize observations at a specific time and place to some or all other cultures.

Contrast this orientation with the mode of operation of a researcher who proceeds from the assumption that a fear response observed at a specific time and place is but the local variant of a universal phenomenon. Such an investigator would be quick to apply quantitative ratings and to compare them across cultures. This mode of operation is designated *etic*. An etically oriented scientist would not neglect or overlook the culturally distinctive features of a pattern of behavior. In an etic context, however, such local characteristics would be subordinated to cross-culturally comparable features. In general, etic investigators assume cultural differences to be quantitative. Emic researchers are impressed with the futility of counting and comparing that which can only be described on its own terms. Historically, cultural anthropologists typically espoused an emic position, whereas psychiatrists often gravitated toward the etic view. A pure, classical expression of emic orientation was provided by the

eminent anthropologist Ruth Benedict (1934), who was impressed with the plasticity of psychological disorders across cultures. The characteristics that, in one culture, would be ascribed to madness would, in another, be prized as marks of leadership, creativity, or healing powers. Every culture, then, would create its own unique and recognized categories of psychological disturbance.

The most outspoken expressions of the etic perspective are more difficult to pinpoint. Eric Berne (1956, 1959), a prominent psychiatrist and originator of transactional analysis, asserted that serious mental disorder, such as schizophrenia, is basically alike wherever it may occur. Culture, in this view, provides no more than external trappings and minor nuances or accents to this disorder and presumably many others.

Contemporary investigators are rarely engaged in the defense of, or assault on, either of these extreme positions. Rather, they would be likely to shift from emic to etic modes of operation, empirically and theoretically, and to be aware of the possibility of combining and integrating these points of view.

THE CURRENT STATE OF KNOWLEDGE

Historical Origins

Kraepelin (1904), often considered the founder of scientific psychiatry, pursued as an avocation the observation of psychiatric patients of remote and exotic lands. He traveled to Algeria and Java (now in Indonesia) and concluded that depression, for example, was differently expressed and experienced in these two countries than in his native Germany. His observations, though duly noted by his colleagues and contemporaries, did not lead to the development of a systematic, continuous, and expanding program of investigations until many years later, in the 1960s and 1970s. By now, study of abnormal behavior across and within cultures is being rigorously pursued, and the scope of such investigations is spreading while their pace is accelerating. It is now possible to offer a limited number of conclusions based on systematic research and consonant with several recent reviews of literature (Al-

Issa, 1995; Draguns, 1995; Pfeiffer, 1994; Tanaka-Matsumi & Draguns, 1997):

1. The two most serious mental disorders, schizophrenia and major depression, have been encountered and described over a wide range of cultures, in all regions of the world. It may be rash and premature at this time to say that schizophrenia and/or serious, disabling depression is found in each and every culture of the world. Such an assertion would be subject to disproof by just one negative instance. As yet, there is no description extant of a culture in which, on the basis of an exhaustive epidemiological, census-type study, cases of schizophrenia and/or depression have been found to be absent. However, the possibility—though not the probability—remains that such a culture will be identified at some time and place. In the meantime, absolute statements are premature.

Investigators have gone further and have pinpointed a limited number of symptoms that for schizophrenia appear to be cross-culturally constant. On the basis of World Health Organization (WHO) comparison of 10 nations widely different in economic, historical, and political characteristics from all major regions of the world, the following symptoms were found to be minimally variable across cultures (WHO, 1973, 1979; Jablensky et al., 1992):

Restricted affect
Poor insight
Thinking aloud
Poor rapport
Incoherent speech
Unrealistic information
Bizarre/nihilistic delusions

For depression, an analogous list of symptoms was identified on the basis of a four-country comparison by the World Health Organization (WHO, 1983; Jablensky, Sartorius, Gulbinat, & Ernberg, 1981):

Sad affect
Loss of enjoyment
Inability to concentrate
Ideas of insufficiency

Ideas of inadequacy
Ideas of worthlessness

The expectation is justified—even though as yet there is no proof—that other major categories of human distress and disability would also yield similar sets of symptoms tending toward universality. However, such studies, in the case of anxiety or impulse control for example, remain to be undertaken (Tanaka-Matsumi & Draguns, 1997).

2. The foregoing findings allow wide scope for cultural variation in symptoms and other variables across cultures. On the basis of WHO studies, schizophrenia, for example, exhibits a more benign course in developing than in developed countries. The ramifications of this result are far from being explored, but one possible explanation (Cooper & Sartorius, 1985) posits that the slower pace of life in rural, tradition-bound, low-technology environments is conducive to at least a passive acceptance of seriously disturbed individuals. By contrast, in modern, dynamic, technologically advanced, and economically developed settings, life is regulated by the car, the clock, and the computer—and the margin of tolerance is extremely narrow for escape from reality and for wishful or magical thinking divorced from facts and logic.

In the case of depression, cultural variations pertain to the experience of guilt (Marsella, Sartorius, Jablensky, & Fenton, 1985). It is now known that self-condemnation or self-mortification on a moral basis is not a fundamental feature of depression in a variety of cultures (WHO, 1983). At the same time, research results have demonstrated that the vegetative symptoms of depression are more constant across cultures than are the guilt-related, psychological ones (Murphy, Wittkower, & Chance, 1967). Hasty assertions of early observers (e.g., Carothers, 1953) that depression is virtually unknown in Africa have been refuted by more systematic and conclusive research (Prince, 1968). However, rates of depression vary to a much greater extent across cultures and, possibly, ethnic groups than do those of schizophrenia.

Conclusive international or cross-cultural comparisons of incidence of depression are stymied by the difficulties of case identification. In the absence of inside knowledge of a culture, the subtle, unobtrusive, and culturally specific signs of depression are easily missed by an outside observer (DeHoyos & DeHoyos, 1965; López, 1989; Tanaka-Matsumi, 1992). It has also been hypothesized (Draguns, 1996c) but not yet demonstrated that empathy may facilitate, and stereotyping and social distance may impede, the recognition of depression. If this expectation is upheld, it may explain why diagnosticians may underdiagnose depression across cultures, as they may lack empathy for, feel more distant from, and be likely to stereotype individuals in and from another culture.

3. There is solid evidence that experience and report of bodily distress is a prominent avenue of communicating negative psychological experiences (Kirmayer, 1984). Moreover, epidemiological and comparative data suggest that such a tendency to somatize is variable across time and cultures. Historically, it increases in prevalence and intensity in times of political and social uncertainty (Starcevic, 1991), as a result of traumatic and humiliating status loss (Kleinman & Kleinman, 1995), or in periods of disillusionment and hopelessness (Skultans, 1995) as an expression of a sense of personal apathy and despair. In reference to culture, the experience of bodily discomfort, ache, and pain has been investigated intensively in several Chinese milieus: on the mainland (Kleinman, 1982), in Hong Kong (Cheung, 1986), on Taiwan (Cheng, 1995), and by Chinese Americans (Sue & Morishima, 1982). Moreover, somatization is a prominent channel of experiencing personal distress in various Hispanic (Koss, 1990), African (Peltzer, 1995), and other groups. These cultural data alert clinical psychologists to the importance of physical discomfort in a variety of personally and/or socially stressful situations. These observations argue powerfully against the misguided practice of some North American clinicians of dismissing these complaints as psychologically trivial or explaining them away as signs of resistance against genuine self-understanding or insight. Instead, somatic complaints should be taken seriously and responded to sensitively. They may be culturally sanctioned calls for help. Even more specifically, a culturally specific code may operate. In

traditional Chinese medicine, the liver was linked to anger, the heart to anxiety, and the spleen to depression. Remarkably, some of these connections were discernible in the reports of bodily symptoms and the experience of modes of psychological distress of contemporary Chinese patients (Ots, 1990). The lesson for a contemporary clinician is that such symptoms should not be dismissed as indicative of lack of psychological sophistication or sensitivity. This caution applies especially to the communication of distress of culturally distinctive clients.

4. Over the hundred years after Durkheim's (1951/1897) classical sociological study of suicide, a great deal has been learned about lifetime stress, personal despair, and social disintegration as determinants of self-destructive acts. Paris (1991) has concluded that social disintegration is a powerful predictor of suicide across nations, cultures, and ethnic groups. The alternative hypothesis, rooted in psychoanalysis, that suicide is primarily self-directed anger has received much less support. The challenge remains to integrate social alienation, breakdown of personal relationships, and loneliness with other important influences in a cross-culturally valid and practical predictive model of suicide.

5. Early reports from the field were focused on the description of exotic patterns of disturbance at geographically remote locations and in culturally different milieus. By this time, such terms as *amok* (a destructive, but time-limited, state of frenzy observed in Southeast Asia), *susto* (a combination of physiological overarousal, loss of appetite and sexual motivation, and generalized fear response encountered in Central and South America), and *latah* (automatic and uncontrollable imitation of gestures, movements, and actions in states of anxiety and insecurity, in Malaysia) have entered the modern psychiatric vocabulary. In fact, a list of such culture-bound syndromes has been incorporated into an appendix to the current official *Diagnostic and Statistical Manual of Mental Disorders* (DSM-IV) (American Psychiatric Association, 1994). A practicing clinical psychologist in Canada or the mainland United States is not likely to

encounter most of these disorders in his or her practice, although exceptions may occur with recently arrived immigrants or sojourners experiencing extreme threat or stress. One culture-bound disorder somewhat more frequently seen in the continental United States is *ataque de nervios*, sometimes referred to as the "Puerto Rican syndrome," a trancelike state accompanied by psychophysiological overarousal, seizurelike episodes, and hallucinations. It usually occurs in the wake of the loss or termination of an important human relationship (Lewis-Fernandez, 1994). When faced with the symptoms of this disorder, the challenge for the working clinician is to respond with clinical realism, personal sensitivity, and cultural sophistication. The pitfalls to be avoided are to overestimate the degree of disturbance, to institute inappropriately restrictive treatment, and thereby to start the patient on the road to chronicity. Equally ominous, however, is the tendency to attribute the entire sequence of responses to culture and to assume that it is benign and self-corrective. In clinical settings where such syndromes have been seen before, it behooves the clinician to be informed in advance of their symptoms and to initiate workable, sensitive, and appropriate interventions.

6. The foregoing conclusions validate neither of the extreme theoretical positions that were introduced earlier in this chapter. Instead, a middle-of-the-road view is proposed: Psychological disturbance is cross-culturally variable, yet comparable. It is just not true that in each culture or society abnormal behavior is cut of different cloth, the relatively few culture-bound syndromes to the contrary notwithstanding. At the same time, the notion that psychological disturbance is essentially identical at all points of the globe and in all social groups has received no support.

Of course, it should not be assumed that all the findings extant have been covered under the preceding six headings. However, these six points have received relatively solid substantiation. Three or four decades ago, there were simply no confirmed or established cross-cultural findings in psychopa-

thology. Now there are, and the preceding section has provided a selective sampling of them.

What Do We Not Know?

As noted, cultural investigation of mental disorders has a number of achievements to its credit. Yet many important questions remain unanswered. Here is a sampling of them:

1. Are psychological disorders distributed differently across cultures and ethnic groups? The resolution of this issue would require the conduct of comparative epidemiological investigations across cultures. This is an extremely challenging task that entails consistent use of rules of diagnosis in several settings different in customs, language, and limits of socially acceptable behavior. Such studies have only recently begun to be implemented, for example, by Compton et al. (1991) in Taiwan and the United States, and it is premature to draw any definitive conclusions. Even in the multiethnic settings of Canada and the United States, "head counting" as psychiatric census research of mental disorders has rarely taken ethnicity or culture into account. The few studies that have done so (e.g., Srole, Langner, Michael, Opler, & Rennie, 1962) are not sufficient to permit us to make generalizations beyond their respective sites in space and in time.

2. In what manner does culture exercise its influence on mental disorder? How are culturally mediated experiences transformed into personal distress and disability? Of necessity, the answer to this question is complex. It is much easier to describe and compare the manifestations of disorder in various cultures than it is to observe the process of their emergence.

3. What are the specific cultural influences that are responsible for characteristic symptoms? To attempt to answer this question, it would be necessary to break down culture into its crucial or active components. As yet, this task has not even been attempted, let alone accomplished. Yet it is an essential step for future investigations to take, lest

we continue to invoke the concept of culture as an amorphous entity that makes this happen.

4. How do cultural and biological factors interact in producing specific mental disorder? The field of cultural study of mental disturbance is confronted with a paradox. On the one hand, the last few decades have been marked by spectacular advances in the understanding of the neurophysiology, neuropsychology, and biochemistry of mental illness, especially in the case of schizophrenia, major depression, bipolar mood disorder, and panic disorder. On the other hand, at the same time, increased awareness has been developing of the prominence of cultural and social influences in the development of abnormal patterns of behavior. Can these two trends be reconciled or, better yet, integrated, and if so, how? Perhaps future study of somatic distress, experienced within the body but shaped by culture, may provide the prospect of such integration.

5. So far, the focus has been on the role of culture in *shaping* the experience of disturbance and distress, rather than more fundamentally contributing toward its causation. Virtually nothing is as yet known about this potentially important and complex, and also controversial and possibly explosive topic.

CENTRAL CONCEPTS AND ISSUES

The Self as a Pivotal Concept at the Interface of Culture and Abnormal Psychology

To paraphrase William James (1952/1891), the *self* refers to everything a person would call his or her own—one's body, but also one's personal characteristics, social stimulus values, creative products, relationships, associations, and possessions. Several formulations (Chang, 1988; Kimura, 1972, 1995; Landrine, 1992; Markus & Kitayama, 1991; Triandis, 1989) have converged in suggesting that self-experience is subtly yet profoundly shaped by culture. In individual-centered cultures like those of northwestern Europe and North America, the self is experienced as an autonomous, indeed "Godlike"

(Landrine, 1992) structure. It constitutes an aggregate of fundamental personal traits that remain constant across space and time. Quite differently, in the cultures of East and South Asia, those of Latin America, and around the Mediterranean, a sociocentric orientation prevails that promotes a greater flexibility and permeability of self-experience. A sociocentric self is prominently composed of relationships with other people and of social roles in interacting with them. There is less emphasis on an immutable personal core of traits. As Chang (1988) put it, the sociocentric self of China and Japan primarily unites and joins a person to other people; the individualistic self prevalent in Europe and North America principally distinguishes and separates an individual from other persons. We should not, however, fall into the error of thinking that all sociocentric selves are alike or that there are no quantitative or qualitative distinctions among individualistic self-concepts or in individualistic self-experience. Roland (1988) uncovered subtle but significant distinctions between the self-experience of Japanese and Indian clients as observed by him in the course of psychoanalysis, even though both the Japanese and the Indians generally shared a sociocentric outlook. Among individualistic cultures, McClelland, Sturr, Knapp, and Wendt (1958) were able to identify a complex difference in the nature and balance of obligations to self and society between their German and American subjects, even though in both countries a self-contained and articulate sense of self prevailed. Moreover, sociocentric versus individualistic selves vary on a continuum. Such variation is encountered in clinical contact within the culturally diverse North American population of clients, although the measurement and determination of these two self-orientations is still in its infancy. Still, students of clinical psychology should be alerted to the potential importance of these aspects of self-experience in both assessment and intervention.

Social and Personal Dimensions Relevant to Self-Experience

Hofstede (1980, 1991) undertook research on work-related attitudes in 53 countries and 3 regions, with a total participation of over 100,000 persons. On the basis of the factor analysis of this mammoth collection of data, four dimensions were identified by means of which samples across cultures could be compared: individualism–collectivism, power distance, uncertainty avoidance, and masculinity–femininity. Hofstede (1980, 1986, 1991) has described the defining properties of these factors and specified their manifestations in the process of socialization, schooling, and interaction at the workplace. The importance of individualism–collectivism for self-experience has been especially noted by many authors (e.g., Triandis, 1989, 1994), but the other three dimensions are potentially relevant. Tables 15.1 and 15.2, taken from Draguns (1996f), summarize this information and bring it to bear on the concerns of clinical psychology assessment and intervention. The limits of their practical utility in the clinical setting remain to be established by research, from case studies to systematic multidimensional investigations.

Unconfounding Disturbance and Deviance

A major pitfall of practicing clinical psychology in a multicultural environment is equating social deviance with psychological disturbance. In its

Table 15.1 Hofstede's Dimensions and Related Personality Constructs

HOFSTEDE'S DIMENSIONS	RELATED CONSTRUCTS
Individualism–Collectivism	
"Individualism pertains to societies in which the ties between individuals are loose: everyone is expected to look after himself or herself and his or her immediate family. Collectivism pertains to societies in which people from birth onward are integrated into strong, cohesive ingroups, which throughout people's lifetime continue to protect them in exchange for unquestioning loyalty." (Hofstede, 1992, p. 51)	Allocentrism vs. idiocentrism Field dependence vs. field independence
Power Distance	
"the extent to which the less powerful members of institutions and organizations within a country expect and accept that power is distributed unequally." (Hofstede, 1992, p. 28)	Authoritarianism vs. egalitarianism
Uncertainty Avoidance	
"the extent to which people within a culture are made nervous by situations which they perceive as unstructured, unclear, or unpredictable, situations which they therefore try to avoid by maintaining strict codes of behavior and a belief in absolute truths." (Hofstede, 1986, p. 308).	Intolerance of ambiguity vs. tolerance of ambiguity Rigidity vs. flexibility Cognitive complexity
Masculinity–Femininity	
"Masculine pertains to societies in which social gender roles are clearly distinct (i.e., men are supposed to be assertive, tough, and focused on material success whereas women are supposed to be modest, tender, and concerned with the quality of life); femininity pertains to societies in which social gender roles overlap (i.e., both men and women are supposed to be modest, tender, and concerned with the quality of life)." (Hofstede, 1991, pp. 82–83)	Tough-mindedness vs. tender-mindedness

Table 15.2 Hofstede's Four Dimensions in Relation to Self and Others

INDIVIDUALISM–COLLECTIVISM		
	INDIVIDUALISM	COLLECTIVISM
Self:	Autonomous	Contextual
	Private, differentiated	Public, vague, "fuzzy boundaries" between self and others
	Immutable, permanent	Changeable
Socialization:	Intense, few relationships	Less intense, multiple relationships
Relationships:	Lifelong, few	Many, some changes with circumstance and situation

POWER DISTANCE		
	HIGH	LOW
Self:	Encapsulated	Permeable
	Status and wealth important	Friendship important
Socialization:	Harsh	Lenient
Relationships:	Hierarchical	Egalitarian

UNCERTAINTY AVOIDANCE		
	HIGH	LOW
Self:	Articulate, consistant	Partially unverbalized, somewhat inconsistent
Socialization:	Purposeful preparation for school, work, and life	Opportunity for exploration and fantasy
Relationships:	Tightly categorized, ritualized, formal	Spontaneous and unstructured, little ritual or formality

MASCULINITY–FEMININITY		
	MASCULINITY	FEMININITY
Self:	Pragmatic	Altruistic
Socialization:	Demanding	Relaxed
Relationships:	Instrumental	Expressive

most blatant form, this error occurs when a normal person from a different culture is assigned a psychiatric diagnosis on the basis of his or her seemingly bizarre and inappropriate behavior. Alas, such grievous misdiagnoses have occurred, and the interested reader is referred to the documented accounts by Jewell (1952) and Sue (1996). One would hope that such tragic incidents will never occur again, given the improved objectivity and cultural sophistication of the present diagnostic system, as embodied in the DSM-IV (American Psychiatric Association, 1994).

In a more subtle manner, however, confounding deviance with disturbance may be manifested through the clinician's inclination to diagnose a more severe degree of deviance outside of his or her familiar cultural group. An example of this trend was documented among the Amish of southeastern Pennsylvania.[1] Local mental health professionals—none of whom were Amish by affiliation or

---

[1] The Amish are a fundamentalist Protestant Christian group who reject modern lifestyles and espouse pacifism. They fled religious persecution in Switzerland and Germany and have formed communities in Ohio, Pennsylvania, Virginia, and elsewhere. For information on their behavior patterns, customs, values, and history, see Hostetler (1980).

background—typically assigned the diagnosis of schizophrenia to hyperactive and acutely disturbed Amish patients. These diagnoses were found to be erroneous in three-fourths of the cases in light of rule-based and objective diagnostic procedures. By means of the same diagnostic practices, manic phase of bipolar mood disorder was established as the valid and correct diagnosis in these cases (Egeland, Hofsteter, & Eshleman, 1983). Similar diagnostic misattributions have occurred with members of other culturally distinctive groups (López, 1989). Typically, a more serious, chronic, or less reversible disorder was diagnosed. However, there is at least one documented finding of diagnosticians imbued with cultural relativism mistakenly "excusing" the presence of genuine disorder and assigning diagnoses of lesser disruption and disturbance to members of minority groups, despite the seriousness of their symptoms (López & Hernandez, 1992). This instance, then, represents the opposite trend to that often observed: Instead of mistaking deviance for disturbance, disturbance was dismissed as deviance.

Empathy, Stereotyping, and Social Distance

Empathy, by definition, enhances the clinician's sensitivity to the client by acknowledging, with feeling, "There but for the grace of God go I." Empathy has two distinct aspects: *cognitive*, by means of which clinicians can experience reality from the client's point of view, and *affective*, which enables them to tune in to, and to share, the client's emotional state. Ridley and Lingle (1996) have recognized the difficulty involved in empathizing with a culturally different client. Subtle clues in such a client's communication and demeanor may be misunderstood, misperceived, or simply not noticed. Moreover, across cultural boundaries, the clinician may see the client as though from afar; subtle personal reactions may be overlooked, and only readily visible actions may be noted. Under these circumstances, conspicuous behavioral disturbance is likely to crowd out signs of more subjective and personal distress, such as that of depression.

Unfamiliarity or lack of experience with the client's culture may promote stereotypes and obliterate perception of the personal and unique aspects of experience. In the process, the client may run the risk of being deindividualized and seen as a "typical" member of his or her group. Empathy thus may be negatively related to stereotyping, whereas a positive correlation is expected between social distance and stereotyping. The less the clinician knows about the client's cultural group, the more he or she would be inclined to fill the gaps in his or her knowledge through stereotyping.

Beware of Stereotypes, But Do Not Overlook Cultural Differences

On the basis of the points advanced here, a clinical psychologist would be well advised to steer clear of stereotyping. Reliance on stereotypes in social interaction or clinical activity powerfully interferes with a person's cognitive operations in assessing another individual in his or her uniqueness and individuality. Moreover, the stereotypical labels affixed to another individual have a "sticky" quality. As social psychologists have amply demonstrated, such labels are easy to apply but difficult to remove, even in the face of massive invalidating evidence. And stereotypes, again as shown in both clinical and social-psychological laboratory studies, color and distort the perception, recollection, and interpretation of a great many acts and events. Once a stereotype has been applied, it serves as a filter through which incoming information is processed. Therefore, a virtual obligation for a clinician, especially if he or she is operating in a culturally diverse setting, is becoming aware of stereotypes, recognizing their limitations, and reducing their role, especially as automatic triggers of feelings, attitudes, and expectations.

However, let us not succumb to the opposite extreme. Some people, in their eagerness to counteract stereotypes, deny *any* cultural differences in psychological characteristics. The result is "culture-blind" delivery of services. Such an approach overlooks the social reality of cultural influences on all aspects of behavior, including the experiences of distress and disability that constitute the major criteria of psychological abnormality. In all clinical operations, then, it is advisable to be informed of the substantiated research-based cultural characteristics and experiences. This awareness should be coupled with the realization that trends, correlations, and significant differences between samples are not predictive of a specific group member's performance, score, or diagnosis. Integrative reviews of pertinent findings are available, for example, for China (Draguns, 1996a; Lin, Tseng, & Yeh, 1995) and Japan (Caudill, 1973; Lebra, 1976). Useful information has accumulated about the characteristic patterns of disturbance on the major officially recognized minority groups in the United States: Adebimpe (1981) for African Americans, Casas and Vasquez (1996) for Hispanics, Sue and Morishima (1982) for Asian Americans, and Trimble, Fleming, Beauvais, and Jumper-Thurman (1996) for Native Americans. Literature is sparse and/or scattered about the various ethnic groups of European descent in North America. A difficult and complex task was faced in surveying the accumulated findings on the mental disorders of the Jews, given the variety of available information and the heterogeneity of groups subsumed in this inclusive cultural category. Yet, Sanua (1992, p. 228) was able to conclude that:

> A number of findings appear to be consistent. There is a higher percentage of Jews who undergo psychotherapy, primarily of a psychoanalytic nature. Jews do seem to suffer more from depression and psychoneuroses, and they tend to have lower rates of schizophrenia (except for two studies conducted in Europe—and these rates may be consequent to the German occupation). Jews seem to have less paranoid symptomatology perhaps because they tend to internalize their aggression. This is somewhat surprising, in view of the Jews' minority status and experiences of discrimination. In spite of this internalization of aggression, the rate of suicide is low among Jews. Studies have revealed that alcohol and drugs are used minimally. There is some evidence that strong family attachment, ethnic identity and religiosity have a positive effect on the mental health of Jews. With the weakening of the relatedness to the group, both alcohol and drug use are now on the increase. Jewish alcoholics, drug users and criminals may be more likely than those from other ethnic groups to be suffering from psychiatric problems.

These conclusions are reproduced here in their entirety because they represent a commendable blend of realism and caution. The knowledge of these findings is relevant and applicable to the operations of the clinician on the case level, provided caution is exercised and the leap from trend to type is avoided.

CULTURE AND CLINICAL PSYCHOLOGISTS' ACTIVITIES I. ASSESSMENT

Introduction

Clinical psychologists spend a substantial share of their professional time in interviewing, observing, and testing their clients. The general purpose of these activities is to obtain information that is needed for determining appropriate treatments and interventions. In the process, understanding the client within the context of his or her lifetime experience may be fostered and the diagnosis of the client's disorder if any may be accomplished. All of these operations are affected by the client's and the clinician's cultural backgrounds and by any discrepancy between them.

A Comprehensive Scheme for Cultural Assessment

Kleinman (1992) (as cited by Castillo, 1996) has proposed an elaborate model for cultural assessment that apparently incorporates all aspects of the client's cultural experience. The steps involved in this procedure are as follows:

1. The client's cultural identity must be ascertained. How does the patient describe himself or herself in cultural terms? What is the client's self-designation or label? Is there one such self-designation, or are there several? If the client's identities are multiple, what are their relationships? What are the client's feelings about his or her ethnic identity? How does it affect his or her behavior, self-concept, and interaction with in-group and out-group members?

2. At this point, the clinician is encouraged to learn more about the group with which the client identifies on the basis of available references and resource persons.

3. What is the cultural meaning of the client's key complaints, the expression of his or her dis-

tress, and the culturally shaped pattern of disturbance?

4. How do the client and/or his or her family explain the experience of illness and impose meaning on it?

5. What is the emotional effect of the client's family, work, and community on the experience of patient's illness?

6. What is the social response to the client's illness, including any socially significant forms of stigma?

7. Are there any ethnocentric biases on the part of the clinician, and what is their potential effect on treatment?

8. Finally, a treatment plan must be developed, negotiated, and agreed on by the client, his or her family, and the clinician.

It is unlikely that all of these steps would need to be traversed in every encounter between the culturally distinctive client and the clinician. However, the various components of this sequence may be kept in mind and examined for their applicability, especially in cases of cultural contrast between the patient and the clinician.

Interview

Like all the other assessment operations, an interview needs to make sense to the client and must relate to the goals of the clinical contact. To that end, information and structure may need to be provided, and the expectations and the outlook of the client may need to be accommodated. The greater the culture gulf, the greater the need for modification and improvisations. Clinicians working with migrants and sojourners from Africa (e.g., Nathan, 1994) have found it necessary to resort to metaphoric, indirect, and symbolic communications in order to make the interview a more meaningful experience for their clients. In general, contact across culture lines is obstructed by ambiguity and by the lack of direction and structure. Under such conditions, an increase in anxiety is likely to occur, and spontaneity and openness of communication may be impaired. Is it better for the interviewer to ask closed (e.g., yes/no) questions or to encourage self-exploration by open-ended questions (e.g., "Tell me about your marriage")? No unequivocal answer can be provided at this point. Often, however, the urgency of the client's need for help should be recognized (e.g., "Help me first, ask me questions later"). The client's idiom of distress—the words and concepts used in couching his or her suffering—must be respected, and hasty interpretations should be avoided (e.g., "When you are telling me of your wounded heart, you are telling me how sad and hurt you feel"), although the clinician's empathy may need to be communicated, perhaps nonverbally and unobtrusively.

It is difficult to provide generic suggestions for cross-cultural interviewing lest they become stereotypical. The client's and/or his or her culture's stylistic preferences and aversions may need to be ascertained and incorporated into the interviewer's technique. Two cultural sources of variation come to mind in this connection. In some cultures, the acquiescent response style is a mark of politeness and deference, especially with a professional person of a perceived prominent status. If such a possibility is hypothesized, it may be advisable to vary the format of the questions (e.g., "Here is a list of several symptoms you might or might not have. Please pick the ones you have experienced within the last two weeks, if any."). Cultures may also vary in the amount of intrusiveness they are prepared to tolerate. If the limits of such tolerance are in danger of being tapped, the interviewer may weigh the advantages and the disadvantages of pursuing particularly sensitive topics. The question may be asked if the explanation of such topics is indispensable in the client's specific situation. Another aspect of the same problem pertains to the readiness to self-disclose as a cultural variable. It has been suggested (Partridge, 1987) that self-disclosure just comes more easily in those cultures where the self is experienced as self-contained and autonomous. Conversely, where the boundaries of the self are less well delineated and where the self is more subject to fluctuation across both situations and time, genuine difficulties may be experienced when the interviewee is asked to describe what he or she is like. If needed, additional time should be allocated so that a relationship can develop and trust and confidence are built up. Finally, flexibility and accommodation are important ingredients for helping overcome cultural misunderstandings. Technique in any case should be subordinated to the objective of obtaining the information needed in a realistic way.

The interviewer's tools to that end are primarily attitudinal. A receptive, flexible, and spontaneous stance is helpful and appropriate in most situations. Two of the points from Kleinman's list provided in the preceding section are worth keeping in mind. First, the available resources—scholarly, personal, and social—should be used to overcome any impasse that may develop. Second, the possibility should be entertained (but not assumed!) that the interviewer's attitudes toward the client's ethnicity and/or his or her own may bias the resulting judgment. Limitations of the interviewer's own outlook, if any, should then be recognized, and steps should be taken to overcome them.

Standardized Personality Tests 1: Paper-and-Pencil Inventories, with Emphasis on the MMPI

The Minnesota Multiphasic Personality Inventory (MMPI) has emerged as the most widely used personality test in the direct self-report format. Its original validation in Minneapolis was undertaken without any reference to the ethnic or racial composition of the several normal and clinical validation samples. Decades later it was discovered (Gynther, 1972) that, compared with Whites, African Americans were more likely to be psychiatrically diagnosed. Specifically, Scales F, 8, and 9 were elevated in African Americans by comparison with their White counterparts, both normal and psychiatrically diagnosed. A more recent, comprehensive review of all MMPI studies on the four major U.S. minority groups (African Americans, Hispanics, Native Americans, and Asian Americans) by Greene (1987) failed to substantiate a consistent pattern of differences between any two ethnic groups involved in the comparison. Greene therefore argued against developing separate norms for specific ethnic groups. Meanwhile, the original MMPI has been replaced by the revalidated MMPI-2 (Butcher, Dahlstrom, Graham, Tellegen, &

Kaemmer, 1989). In contrast to the original validation, proportionate numbers of African Americans, Hispanics, Native Americans, and Asian Americans were included in the large and representative revalidation groups. These developments suggest that the ethnic disparities on the MMPI-2 are likely to have decreased rather than increased by comparison with the original MMPI. Still, there are new reports of ethnic differences in psychopathology indicators, this time between Asian Americans and Whites, and especially so for relatively unacculturated immigrants within that group (Sue, 1996). Thus, the risk of confounding social deviance with personal disturbance, which was discussed in an earlier section, has not disappeared even from the new and substantially improved version of the MMPI. Elsewhere (Draguns, 1996b, p. 69) it was concluded that "the MMPI is a usable, but imperfect, tool of appraisal within the multicultural American setting." Still, a number of precautions should be observed. In the case of a culturally distinctive client, automatic—and mindless—use of cutoff scores for diagnostic and treatment purposes is to be avoided. The scores and profiles are to be noted but interpreted more tentatively, with a bigger proverbial grain of salt, than in the cases of more typical, majority-group clients. Impersonal—computerized and/or blind—interpretation of the MMPI scores should never serve as the basis for real-life decisions involving the client's life and welfare—and especially so if the client is culturally atypical.

Unstructured Personality Tests 2: Projective Measures

In contrast to the MMPI, no systematic and cumulative body of findings pertaining to ethnic differences in scores and responses has emerged on the Rorschach Inkblot Test, even though the first culturally oriented studies with this instrument go back to the 1940s (e.g., DuBois, 1944). For a couple of decades the Rorschach was the measure of choice in the anthropological culture and personality research, until Lindzey (1961) demonstrated the inherent inconclusiveness of this effort. This, however, does not imply either the uselessness of the

Rorschach with minority members or the absence of cultural problems with its application across ethnic lines. Although the inkblots may be culturally neutral, the context of testing rarely is (Dana, 1993; Ritzler, 1996). At the very least, the expectations and interpretations of the situation and rationale of testing by the tester and testee almost invariably differ (Fulkerson, 1965), and this difference is likely to be augmented across ethnic lines. The situation here is similar to that in the diagnostic interview, except that both stimulus and situational ambiguity are essential parts of the procedure of projective testing (Draguns, 1996a; Fulkerson, 1965). Under these circumstances, distrust, anxiety, and insecurity cannot help but distort and interfere with the production of meaningful and spontaneous responses to the inkblots. Again, realistic recognition of these obstacles and sensitive rapport building would appear to be the most likely measures for counteracting or preventing such disruption.

In the case of thematic tests, prominently exemplified by the TAT, the ethnic-cultural issue has revolved around the unmistakably Caucasian features of all the human figures depicted on the original TAT cards. For African American testees, Thompson (1949) devised a set of virtually identical pictures with African facial features. Since its introduction, this test has seen little research and not much clinical use. More potentially viable is another set of thematic pictures specifically devised to reflect the emic concerns of African American individuals within contemporary U.S. culture, *Themes Concerning Blacks* (Williams, 1972). This test is designed to supplement, rather than replace, the TAT and other general thematic tests.

The future appears to portend the development of more specific thematic tests, with stimuli custom made for specific segments of the U.S. population, including ethnic groups. TEMAS, introduced and described by Costantino and Malgady (1996), is a harbinger of this trend. It consists of ethnically relevant contemporary stimuli depicting a variety of interpersonal situations and features persons with Caucasian, Hispanic, and African characteristics. Validation of TEMAS has been systematically pursued, and the results of this effort appear promising.

Thus, clinical psychologists may be faced with more rather than fewer choices among projective tests, some of which incorporate cultural awareness and design even into their test stimuli. In using projective techniques, the culturally sensitive psychologist must keep in mind the relevance of cultural factors in all phases of assessment. As Dana (1993) has emphasized, constructing culturally appropriate norms and devising culturally fitting stimuli is necessary but not sufficient. Cultural considerations impinge upon all stages of this transaction, from the social context in which testing is embedded to the interpretation and communication of the findings into which the intertwining of cultural and personal characteristics must be incorporated.

Intelligence Testing: An Unending Controversy

The use of intelligence tests with educationally and economically disadvantaged cultural minorities involves intractable problems, and no generally satisfactory solution to this dilemma is as yet in sight. At the dawn of the twentieth century, when the first usable intelligence tests were introduced, Alfred Binet, William Stern, Lewis Terman, and other pioneers of intelligence test construction were aware of the makeshift nature of their instruments. They knew that they had succeeded in developing tests of cognitive ability that were useful and, to an imperfect degree, valid at a specific point in space and time rather than universal instruments applicable and valid everywhere and for all times. These pioneers, however, were hopeful that a culture-free test of intelligence would eventually be constructed. With the benefit of hindsight, contemporary psychologists know that this hope is unrealizable. In the meantime, the linear descendants of the early intelligence tests continue to be used in the multicultural society of the United States, even though it is widely recognized that disparities in economic, political, educational, and social opportunity place a number of minority group members at a distinct disadvantage. The situation is patently unfair. Yet there are those who assert that persons of all cultural backgrounds and all walks of life must be tested—not for the purpose of establishing their "true" or "real" intelligence level, but for realistic prediction of appropriate educational steps to be taken in the near future. Also, what the testee can do at this point is a valid diagnostic and clinical concern. Thus, there is a delicate balance to be established whereby intelligence tests are used helpfully and flexibly for practical, specific purposes rather than being proscribed altogether (as, incidentally, was done in the dogmatically egalitarian Soviet Union in 1935) because of their widely known imperfections.

Against this background, the following guidelines are offered for future clinical psychologists at the brink of the new millennium:

1. Abide by all the administrative regulations and legal requirements of your institution, jurisdiction, and state. In some states, it is illegal to use intelligence tests with persons within a specific age range and/or minority status. In other places, specific rules exist on when, where, how, and to whom test-based information about a person's intelligence may or may not be released.

2. Proceed from the recognition that IQ is just one quantitative indicator derived from a person's intelligence test performance. Segments of the general public stand in awe of the IQ; informed psychologists do not. They are aware both of the legitimate uses of this score and of its multiple limitations.

3. Therefore, regard the results of the intelligence test as a complex, qualitative sample of a person's cognitive and problem-solving performance, which must be described, reported, and interpreted in their entirety.

4. Consider the respective advisability of excluding the IQ from the actual report or including this score. If the client's IQ is reported, it is the psychologist's responsibility to make sure that this datum is interpreted realistically and fairly.

5. Steer clear of any automatic use of cutoff scores and never allow a real-life decision concerning the client to be made entirely or primarily on the basis of his or her IQ (or any other single score).

6. Look beyond the test and gather observations about the client's problem-solving skills in a variety of real-life, practical situations, especially within the client's accustomed milieu and habitat.

7. Acquire thorough knowledge about the complex issue of the interrelationship of intelligence test scores, social or cultural disadvantage, and cultural characteristics, and apply this expertise in interpreting specific test findings. A recent article by Neisser et al. (1996) represents current experts' reasoned consensus on the controversies related to intelligence.

Two future trends may be anticipated. First, intelligence test findings will increasingly be supplemented—though probably not replaced—by non-test-based systematic information about the testee's social competence—his or her actual coping in relevant practical situations. To this end, Mercer (1979) has developed the System of Multicultural Pluralistic Assessment (SOMPA). This procedure incorporates scores from standardized intelligence tests, but goes beyond them in taking into consideration four additional kinds of data, on socioeconomic status, acculturation to the contemporary mainstream U.S. milieu, family structure, and family size. All of this information is assigned weights and then pooled in order to arrive at a more comprehensive and culturally sensitive appraisal of a person's intelligence. SOMPA then takes into account test performance, cultural background, and the characteristics of the setting in which the person is currently functioning.

Second, the study of emic definitions of intelligence for various specific sociocultural groups is as yet in its infancy, but is likely to gain momentum and eventually be incorporated into a multifaceted culturally sensitive assessment of intelligence. In the A-chewa culture in Zambia, in South Central Africa, Serpell (1989) investigated the implicit local concepts of intelligence. Three interrelated, yet distinct notions were identified. They corresponded roughly to cleverness, resourcefulness, and socially sensitive helpfulness. Whereas the first two components closely correspond to the features of intelligence as the term is understood in modern Euro-American culture, the third characteristic comes as something of a surprise. Similarly, locally distinctive facets of intelligence may be uncovered in future research with various cultural and ethnic groups within the North American population. Two approaches may be useful in pursuit of this goal. Sociometric techniques of ascertaining who is intelligent/smart/clever may be employed by asking local informants to identify such individuals in their communities. Critical incidents may then be scrutinized in which that trait was exemplified. In this manner, the stranglehold of the IQ may eventually be loosened in order to give way to a more flexible and differentiated conception of intelligence.

Neuropsychological Tests: A New Area of Cultural Concern

Neuropsychological measures are designed to identify the presence and nature of psychological deficits and dysfunctions that are traceable to brain damage. For the most part, they consist of perceptual and cognitive procedures that typically are completed successfully by persons with unimpaired central nervous systems over a wide range of intelligence, but pose problems for the neuropsychologically impaired. Seemingly, this is an area of inquiry in which the impact of cultural differences should be minimal. However, perceptive neuropsychologists (e.g., Lezak, 1983) have recognized that this is not so. On the basis of largely clinical observations, Ardila, Rosselli, and Puente (1994) have offered practical suggestions for overcoming cultural barriers in neuropsychological assessment of Hispanic patients. Echemendia, Harris, Congett, Diaz, and Puente (1997) have reported the results of a survey of clinical neuropsychologists' experience with Hispanic populations. The participants have indicated that, although they conduct neuropsychological assessments with substantial numbers of Hispanic clients, few of them received training and supervision for working with this minority population. Such training is needed, the participants in this survey asserted, because of the intertwining of cultural factors and cognitive perceptual deficits that affect neuropsychological performance. Some of the items on neuropsychological tests tap overlearned and automatized responses for the majority group. Yet these items may be less familiar for cul-

turally distinctive individuals with a different educational background. Even such a mundane task as repeating digits may be subject to cultural influence. Spanish speakers may have more experience in grouping numbers (e.g., "389") rather than repeating them discretely ("3-8-9") (Echemendia et al., 1997). Above all, speakers of English as a second language should not be expected to perform comparably on language-mediated test items and tasks. Differences in their scores in such areas of performance should not be interpreted on a neuropsychological basis in the absence of strong supportive independent evidence. The results by Echemendia et al. pertain to one minority; they introduce a note of caution and indicate a need for research with other culturally atypical populations in North America.

A New Frontier: The Interface between Person and Culture

There has been a gradually increasing awareness of the importance of cultural factors in influencing all aspects of clinically relevant behavior. Pedersen (1990, 1991) has proposed that culturally oriented intervention in counseling and clinical psychology constitutes the "fourth force," coequal with psychodynamic, humanistic, and behavioral theories. If this stand has merit, it calls for the development of new methods of assessment for disentangling the threads of cultural influence in crucial domains of behavior and experience. With this new orientation in mind, the following promising potential developments are delineated:

1. In an earlier section of this chapter, the contrast between the sociocentric and individualistic selves was introduced. The origins of this distinction are traceable to clinical and social observations in contrasting cultures, supplemented by a mosaic of findings about culturally characteristic responses from a wide range of controlled experiments, statistical data, and naturalistic observation. As yet, however, no clinically useful measure of autonomous versus socially permeated self has been developed. The challenge for the field of clinical

psychology is to develop and validate a culturally sensitive and individually applicable instrument whereby a person's self-experience could be objectively and reliably assessed, on the individual-centered versus sociocentric axis and on other potentially relevant culturally variable dimensions.

2. Related to the foregoing objective, a need exists for personal and cultural identity scales. A lot of research has been conducted on the several empirically established types of African American identity (e.g., Carter, 1996; Cross & Fhagen-Smith, 1996), but clinicians have been slow to incorporate the resulting measures into their assessment procedures. Of special clinical interest is the way a person's cultural identity is interlaced and interpenetrated with his or her personal identity and self-concept.

3. Where does a person stand in relation to his or her culture of origin and current culture of residence? Acculturation scales have been developed and used extensively in research, both for specific cultural groups and for the generic population of immigrants and newcomers (e.g., Sodowsky & Plake, 1991). However, the next step remains to be taken—that is, the incorporation of data on acculturation into the assessment of individuals by clinicians. It would be of interest to ascertain not only the degree of acculturation quantitatively but also its variety qualitatively. To that end, scales incorporating, for example, Berry's (1990) fourfold scheme of assimilation, isolation, marginalization, and integration would be a welcome addition to the clinical psychologists' assessment armamentarium.

4. Research by Hofstede (1980, 1986, 1991), Triandis (1994, 1995), and others has brought to the fore the potential relevance for clinical exploration of a number of dimensions or traits that were discovered through cross-cultural research. Prominent in this respect is individualism–collectivism. Culturally sophisticated practitioners of clinical assessment would welcome the construction of self-report measures of this variable, perhaps supplemented by social ratings and even self-expressive and

semiprojective stimuli for this construct. However, individualism–collectivism is not the only measure with a potential for incorporation into person-centered assessment operation. Confucian dynamism, first investigated with Chinese populations in Hong Kong and elsewhere (Chinese Culture Connection, 1987; Cheng, 1990), also has been found to be applicable and meaningful in other cultures and to be relevant to clinical concerns and interventions (Hofstede, 1991).

5. Persons' world views are both culturally variable and pertinent to the objectives of understanding the mainsprings of their conduct and predicting their actions. Ibrahim and Kahn (1987) have developed such an instrument. By now, its factor-analytic composition has been ascertained (Ibrahim & Owen, 1994), and it has been proved useful in career assessment (Ibrahim, Ohnishi, & Wilson, 1994). The next step is to introduce it into the clinical context. Of special interest is this measure's overlap with personal identity.

INTERVENTION

Psychotherapy

Verbal psychotherapy involves human interaction that is crucially dependent on a trusting relationship, spontaneous communication, and mutual understanding. All of these essential components of psychotherapy are at risk and under strain when a cultural barrier exists between the client and the therapist. Pfeiffer (1996) has described five frequently encountered clashes of expectations:

1. The client expects the therapist to tell him or her what to do; the therapist insists on helping the client resolve his or her problem on the basis of available personal experience and resources.
2. The client seeks support by and participation of family, community, and friends; the therapist emphasizes individual and personal decision making and action.
3. The client seeks a solution on the basis of power distribution in a traditional patriarchal

family; the therapist encourages an egalitarian, task-oriented approach to the problem.

4. To the client, the problem is outside of the person, in the social environment; the therapist tries to increase greater self-awareness and, implicitly, places the problem within the individual.

5. The client's suffering is expressed in bodily terms; the therapist is more interested in the client's thoughts and feelings.

Pfeiffer identified these five contrasts on the basis of his experience in doing psychotherapy with Turkish guest workers in Germany. His formulation is applicable as well to many other cross-cultural encounters in psychotherapy.

In this country, it is well known that early termination rates of minority clients in psychotherapy are disproportionately high. Often, such clients seek therapy at a more painful and acute stage of the disorder than is typically true of clients closer to the cultural mainstream. What they need and expect is early and immediate relief; seeing no prospect of obtaining it, they quit in disappointment. These aborted therapy relationships often end on a note of mutual misunderstanding. The help seeker is frustrated and bewildered; the professional helper may sometimes attribute the failure of psychotherapy to a lack of motivation or of psychological-mindedness on the part of the client.

Over the last few decades, some progress has been achieved in correcting this situation. Specifically, steps have been taken to bridge the gap between the professional community of psychotherapists and their clients from all segments of the population. Although the great variety of these changes cannot be summarized adequately under headings, the following developments are especially worth articulating. Minority and other culturally distinctive clients are no longer expected to accommodate to preexisting and presumably immutable therapeutic services. In the optimal case, the culture accommodation model developed by Higginbotham, West, and Forsythe (1988) is applied whereby programs are initiated and shaped on the basis of matching community needs with professional resources. This approach can be imple-

mented on a systematic basis for a whole community, region, country, or even the entire world (Desjarlais, Eisenberg, Good & Kleinman, 1995), or it may be applied on an individual basis, for example by a single pioneering clinical psychologist attempting to set up therapeutic services in a number of African countries (Peltzer, 1995). It is also exemplified by the operations of a psychotherapist trying to meet the challenge of providing both meaningful and effective therapeutic services to newcomers with a very different background and outlook (Nathan, 1994). A similar situation is encountered by a clinical psychologist who finds himself in a culturally different setting and is trying to work out the appropriate combination of interventions that will be effective with his help-seeking clients (Fish, 1996). In all of these cases, the therapists succeeded in their objectives by taking seriously their clients' beliefs, values, outlooks, and attitudes. To put it differently, the psychotherapist's legitimate mandate is to relieve distress and to reduce suffering. It would only distract him or her from the attainment of these goals if the therapist undertook the difficult task of changing his or her clients' subjective culture. Instead, therapists' interventions must be adapted and accommodated to their clients' culturally based expectations.

Another possibility is to modify the format and the technique of psychotherapy. For Hispanic clients, for example, new, imaginative kinds of therapy have been pioneered. Costantino, Malgady, and Rogler (1988) have devised therapy approaches for adolescents based on stories (*cuentos*) of popular Hispanic sports figures and other folk heroes who would constitute attractive and glamorous models of prosocial and adaptive behavior. Zuniga has proposed the incorporation of well-known popular sayings (*dichos*) as aids for overcoming resistance in Hispanic clients. Javier (1990) raised the question of the potential relevance and effectiveness of insight-oriented psychotherapy for Hispanic and other minority clients who have been socialized in a culture of poverty. The triad of material deprivation, resignation or fatalism, and impaired object relations suggests that conventional approaches geared to self-exploration are not sufficient and may be only marginal in their utility for such populations. When and where services remain rigid and unmodified, an increasing gap between the need for services and their low rate of utilization results. In such cases, informal nonprofessional resources, such as those of a trusted confidant (*persona de confianza*) (Rosado & Elias, 1993), may be utilized. Much is written about traditional healers (Adler & Mukherji, 1995), but their availability and acceptability in the contemporary urbanized environment is limited, and, with worldwide trends toward modernization intensifying, their share of providing mental health services is expected to shrink (Claver, 1976; Scharfetter, 1985). Where such interventions are practiced, however, they should be taken seriously and incorporated as components into the total culturally oriented delivery system. In British Columbia, for example, Jilek (1988) has cooperated productively with Salish Indian shamanistic spirit dance rituals in counteracting depression, anxiety, somatic complaints, and alcohol and drug abuse.

A special problem is posed by the language in which psychotherapy is conducted. With many Asian, Hispanic, European immigrant, and other clients, psychotherapists communicate of necessity in English, even when the client's command of that language is imperfect. More subtly, even when the client is a competent and fluent English speaker, his or her subjective experience may be couched in another language. This writer remembers a case of a German-born man whose command of English was flawless. Nonetheless, he spontaneously shifted into German when topics pertaining to his childhood came up. Few therapists are bilingual or multilingual, and none of them can accommodate the tremendous variety of their clients' language backgrounds. There may be some merit in inviting the client to say a key word or phrase in his or her first language, even if the language is unfamiliar to the therapist—for example, to name an important feeling in that language so as to capture its full emotional impact. There is some systematic support for the notion that recollections in the person's first language have greater vividness and intensity, at least for Spanish–English bilinguals (Javier, Barroso, & Muñoz, 1993). Perhaps, at a minimum, even a monolingual therapist can enhance his or her effec-

tiveness by awareness of and attention to the issues of language, affect, experience, and communication in psychotherapy.

Therapy services also must be adapted to the needs and expectations of newcomers to Canada and the United States. Adaptation to a different culture is stressful and challenging even for voluntary immigrants and sojourners. In increasing numbers, however, refugees from wars, oppression, discrimination, and other social stress have been arriving in North America. Of necessity, their traumatic experiences in their countries of origin, as well as during and after their flight, have left emotional scars and have spawned in some cases cumulative and mushrooming problems. Increasingly, psychotherapists are called upon to participate in devising and implementing culturally appropriate services for survivors of torture, persecution, and other stressful or traumatic experience.

Therapy is often employed to cushion the effect of *culture shock*. Oberg (1958) coined this term to describe a mixture of cognitive disorientation, personal helplessness, and emotional distress that some people experience upon immersing themselves into a new and different cultural environment. Culture shock affects immigrants, sojourners, and refugees. A combination of orientation to the new culture through information, practice, and role playing and recognition of response to the client's emotional needs has produced positive results in cushioning against and overcoming its effects (Bemak, Chung, & Bornemann, 1996).

Acculturation stress is related to culture shock but is more protracted in its effects (Westermeyer, 1987). It refers to the pressures and stresses experienced by the newcomers in coming to grips with the demands for accommodation to the new environment. Appropriate approaches for mitigating this experience, especially in its more distressing aspects, are threefold: at policy, orientation, and therapy levels. First, the enlightened public of the host countries for immigrants has come to recognize that providing options and decreasing pressure toward conformity are humane policies that, moreover, reduce the direct and indirect costs of adaptation. The metaphor of a melting pot, with its connotation of a thorough and inevitable transformation, has been discarded in modern conceptualizations and practice in most countries that receive large numbers of immigrants. At the same time, there is a consensus on the urgent need to provide practically oriented guidance for the persons arriving in the country. Finally, there is a distinct place for therapeutic services to deal with the likely experiences of frustration, insecurity, and helplessness that the need for rapid change in adapting to a new environment entails. Such interventions should be focused on the present social reality and should be geared toward a prompt alleviation of depression, anxiety, sense of a personal inadequacy, and other related conditions. These interventions may also facilitate the migrant's choice of his or her own style and pace of acculturation, with their respective emphases on integrating the old and the new cultures, assimilating into the host culture, or preserving as much of the old culture as possible (Berry, 1990).

In the case of refugees and expellees, whose numbers have so tragically increased in recent decades, adaptation to the new setting is greatly complicated by the traumatic events experienced or witnessed before, during, and after their flight. By this time, a substantial literature exists on therapeutic intervention in response to these traumata (Arpin, Comba, & Fleury 1988; Marsella, Bornemann, Ekblad, & Orley, 1994; van der Veer, 1992). These authors are in agreement in proposing prompt and direct response to the distress experienced. Attention should be focused on the here and now. This objective should be accomplished in a manner that is culturally meaningful to the client, aiming to produce symptom reduction and relief from distress early in therapy, and confronting the prominent issue of painful personal losses as early in treatment as possible (cf. Draguns, 1996d). At the same time, such issues as the extent and nature of verbal interaction between the therapist and the client, and of their respective roles (Draguns, 1996d) are expected to vary across cultures, as is the nature of the cultural explanation of the disasters endured. In this new and prominent field of intervention, improvisation has of necessity prevailed. Still, there is a lot to be learned from the experience of clinicians who have had to intervene, often on a moment's notice and with little preparation (Marsella et al.,

1995). Future developments should include a more complete documentation of the results obtained. At some point, the various results obtained may be pooled and integrated. This will provide a more panoramic view of what kinds of interventions have generally worked and, more ambitiously, would yield data on the interaction of culture and approach to therapy in producing optimal results.

Emphasis in this section has been on attitude rather than technique. Specific techniques may well be found useful for particular populations, although there is no prospect of self-contained therapies uniquely devised for a given culture. The important thing to maintain is a maximal adaptability to needs and circumstances in the service of delivering the most effective interventions possible to a maximal diversity of populations.

Behavior and Cognitive Therapies

Cultural factors also matter in the design and delivery of behavior and cognitive therapy services. Tanaka-Matsumi and Higginbotham (1996) have addressed this issue. The objective of behavioral and cognitive interventions is to change specific overt or covert responses and to replace them with more adaptive and rewarding kinds of behavior. Although this goal appears to be specific and acultural, cultural characteristics are relevant to all stages of therapy planning, implementation, evaluation, and follow-up. The greater flexibility in the design of such services compared to traditional verbal psychotherapy allows for incorporation of cultural considerations of all of its phases. The culture accommodation model (Higginbotham, West, & Forsyth, 1988), already introduced in an earlier section of this chapter, can easily be applied to the planning and execution of behaviorally and cognitively oriented programs. To this end, the goals and techniques of intervention are not unilaterally imposed but are negotiated with the clients, their agents or guardians, and the community in which intervention occurs. Consensus among the participants in this transaction is sought concerning the goals of therapy. What responses should be targeted for the application of behavioral and/or cognitive principles? What is the prospective client's culturally rooted and personally held conception of the nature of his or her problematic behavior? What kinds of objectives does the client hope will be attained upon completion of intervention, if it is successful? What kinds of conditions might enhance the meaningfulness of planned interventions, and what expectations will increase the chances of their successful application? Should the program be implemented by members of the clients' ethnic group, or can it be carried out effectively by extraneous professional and trained personnel? Finally, what kinds of reinforcers would be optimally effective with a specific population and in reference to a specified target behavior (in those problem areas where these considerations are applicable)?

Although the framework for incorporating culture into these interventions is in place, Tanaka-Matsumi and Higginbotham (1996) have been able to find relatively few instances of its actual application with minority clients or members of other populations. What needs to be counteracted and overcome is a great many practitioners' "tunnel vision" of the target symptoms, which causes them to overlook or disregard the context in which an excess or deficit has occurred. Perceptive proponents of behavioral and cognitive intervention recognize the importance of the influences of the milieu, the lifetime experience, and the past formative and present active social interactions and relationships. All of these strands of experience are mediated by culture.

The behavioral and cognitive approaches have the further advantage of being focused on the client's complaints and of aiming at the direct and speedy change of problematic behavior. These features go a long way toward resolving one of the major sources of dissatisfaction by help-seekers of distinctive cultural backgrounds. In the case of verbal psychotherapy, a covert tug of war often results between the therapist and the client. The therapist is steering in a different direction from the one where the client wants to go; the client may feel that his or her suffering is not being taken seriously and remains unrelieved. In the course of a behavioral and cognitive therapy program, this problem does not arise. Thus, with appropriate cultural provisions incorporated for sensitive implementation, behavioral and cognitive approaches hold the promise of

being prominent components of culturally oriented therapeutic intervention.

Before and After Therapy: Its Planning and Evaluation

With the increasing emphasis on accountability and cost-effectiveness in providing psychological services, practicing clinical psychologists in the future increasingly will be called upon to justify their interventions. This anticipation dictates the need for detailed and rational plans in delivering services, for monitoring their effects, and for comparing them with other available but perhaps less innovative interventions. In all of these operations, cultural factors may have to be included, especially if the services in question are geared to a specific group and its problems. So far, therapy outcome research has rarely taken ethnic factors into account (Sue & Sundberg, 1996). The challenge is to demonstrate that ethnicity is a relevant factor in the evaluation of the effectiveness of intervention and that heeding it, rather than disregarding it, results in improved, and perhaps even more cost-effective, services.

Over and above these considerations, clinical psychologists of the next decades will have to bridge the gulf between service delivery and research data collection in their daily operation. Construing each case as a research project with an N of one, carefully monitoring interventions and their effects, and keeping a continuing record of these data may help establish a solid database and obliterate the distinction between clinical intervention and research, a goal that the founders of American clinical psychology in Boulder, Colorado, had prophetically envisioned.

TOWARD A CULTURALLY SENSITIVE CLINICAL PSYCHOLOGY

Future Trends

Not so long ago, cultural influences were on the periphery of clinical psychologists' concern. Self-assertion by American ethnic minorities; a greater influx of immigrants, refugees, and sojourners; and the increased flow of communication in a world in which distances have shrunk—all of these developments have pushed cultural issues to the foreground. Thus the admonition of the Vail conference (Korman, 1974) to pay heed to the needs of culturally diverse clients and to be sensitive to their concerns has become a general imperative in the professional lives of a great many clinical psychologists. To be knowledgeable and perceptive about cultural threads of experience has become a clinical and social reality. These trends are expected to intensify and accelerate in the next century. Clinical psychologists, then, must learn to operate in a variety of social environments, to appreciate the differences in their client's subjective culture, and to strive to reach out to persons seeking their services who come with distinctive expectations and different agendas.

Characteristics of Culturally Competent Clinical Psychologists

How do personal experiences, academic and professional training, and personality traits interact to facilitate optimal delivery of clinical services across cultural lines? As yet, we have only glimmers of an answer to this important question. Certainly, a culturally effective clinical psychologist should possess such attributes as flexibility, openness to experience, tolerance of complexity and ambiguity, and acceptance of self and others (Dinges & Duffy, 1979). This list, however, taken from the set of characteristics posited for an interculturally competent person, is general and somewhat vague. More to the point, recent research has attempted to pinpoint the traits of cross-cultural counselors that, by implication, would be applicable to culturally active clinical psychologists. This enterprise is in progress. On the basis of the results obtained so far, effective multicultural counselors possess a workable level of multicultural techniques and skills, are aware of their own cultural assumptions and beliefs, and are perceptive of other persons' psychological states and backgrounds; further, they bring to their professional multicultural contacts a high degree of self-confidence and social perceptiveness (Sodowsky, 1996). Thus, the desirable qualities represent a mixture of components that are general

and specific, personal and social, and skill-oriented and attitudinal.

CONCLUSIONS

In the multicultural environment in which many clinical psychologists will probably operate in the next few decades, their effectiveness will be significantly enhanced by their knowledge of the impact of cultural factors on the experience of distress and disability. However, information by itself is not enough. Its effective application will be promoted by the affective components that come into play in cross-cultural transaction: being open to new social encounters instead of anticipating them in a state of insecurity and worry, feeling self-confident rather than experiencing unresolved doubts, and actively seeking intercultural experience rather than avoiding and shrinking from such contacts. To be sure, skill building and practice are also needed. The product of such preparation is a flexible and competent clinical practitioner who is not beholden to a static rule-following model. Such a person, moreover, knows the limitations of stereotypes. Cautiously, he or she may be guided by some of them as hypotheses without ever confounding them with facts. The culturally sensitive clinician, moreover, does not crystallize his or her cultural knowledge and sophistication into immutable categories. Above all, culture—whether the psychologist's or the client's—does not obscure his or her view of the individual—a person whose suffering and its alleviation are the clinician's paramount concerns. The ideal or optimal outcome is the ability to feel with one's client, even if his or her subjective experience is couched in a manner that at first glance appears baffling or incomprehensible. The skilled and sensitive clinician also should be able to find words or other means to communicate empathy and concern across cultural lines. And the competent clinician is well aware that deviance from his or her cultural perspective should not be equated with disturbance and that other explanations must be sought and considered on their merits before the diagnosis of mental disorder is legitimately applied to a person of a distinctive cultural background. If current trends continue, the competent clinician will cross cultural frontiers in his or her daily rounds, easily and confidently, though never mindlessly or automatically.

We do not know all there is to know, but we know that multicultural skills can be learned and perfected, even though they rest on the foundation of an individual's personal experience. Thus, helping people from a diverse set of backgrounds to cope with the vicissitudes of life is a never-ending challenge, admitting of improvement, yet never attaining perfection.

REFERENCES

Adebimpe, V. R. (1981). Overview: White norms and psychiatric diagnosis of Black patients. *American Journal of Psychiatry, 138,* 279–285.

Adler, L. L., & Mukherji, R. R. (Eds.). (1995). *Spirit versus scalpel.* Westport, CT: Bergin & Garvey.

Al-Issa, I. (Ed.). (1995). *Handbook of culture and mental illness: An international perspective.* Madison, CT: International Universities Press.

American Psychiatric Association. (1994). *Diagnostic and statistical manual of mental disorders* (4th ed.). Washington, DC: Author.

Ardila, A., Rosselli, M., & Puente, A. (1994). *Neuropsychological evaluation of the Spanish speaker.* New York: Plenum Press.

Arpin, J., Comba, L., & Fleury, F. (Eds.). (1988). Migrazione e salute mentale in Europa. *Antropologia Medica, 4,* 3–107.

Benedict, R. (1934). Culture and the abnormal. *Journal of General Psychology, 10,* 59–82.

Bemak, F., Chung, R. C. Y., & Bornemann, T. H. (1996). Counseling and psychotherapy with refugees. In P. B. Pedersen, J. G. Draguns, W. J. Lonner, & J. E. Trimble (Eds.), *Counseling across cultures* (4th ed.) (pp. 243–265). Thousand Oaks, CA: Sage Publications.

Berne, E. (1956). Comparative psychiatry and tropical psychiatry. *American Journal of Psychiatry, 113,* 193–200.

Berne, E. (1959). Difficulties of comparative psychiatry. *American Journal of Psychiatry, 113,* 193–200.

Berry, J. W. (1990). Psychology of acculturation. In J. J. Berman (Ed.), *Nebraska Symposium on Motivation 1989* (pp. 201–234). Lincoln: University of Nebraska Press.

Brislin, R. W. (1993). *Understanding culture's influence on behavior.* Fort Worth, TX: Harcourt, Brace, Jovanovich.

Butcher, J. N., Dahlstrom, W. G., Graham, J. R., Tellegen, A., & Kaemmer, B. (1989). *Minnesota Multiphasic Personality Inventory—2 (MMPI-2) manual for administration and scoring.* Minneapolis: University of Minnesota Press.

Carothers, J. C. (1953). *The African mind in health and disease.* Geneva: World Health Organization.

Carter, R. T. (1996). Exploring the complexity of racial identity attitude measures. In G. R. Sodowsky & J. T. Impara (Eds.), *Multicultural assessment in counseling and clinical psychology* (pp. 193–224). Lincoln, NE: Buros Institute of Mental Measurement.

Casas, J. M., & Vasquez, M. J. T. (1996). Counseling the Hispanic: A guiding framework for a diverse population. In P. B. Pedersen, J. G. Draguns, W. J. Lonner, & J. E. Trimble (Eds.), *Counseling across cultures* (4th ed.) (pp. 146–176). Thousand Oaks, CA: Sage Publications.

Castillo, R. J. (1996). *Culture and mental illness: A client-centered approach.* Pacific Grove, CA: Brooks-Cole.

Caudill, W. (1973). The influence of social structure and culture on human behavior in Japan. *Journal of Nervous and Mental Diseases, 157,* 249–258.

Chang, S. C. (1988). The nature of self: A transcultural view: Part I. Theoretical aspects. *Transcultural Psychiatric Research Review, 25*(3), 169–204.

Cheng, S. K. (1990). Understanding the culture and behavior of East Asians: A Confucian perspective. *Australian and New Zealand Journal of Psychiatry, 24,* 510–515.

Cheng, T. A. (1995). Neuroses in Taiwan: Findings from a community study. In T. Y. Lin, W. S. Tseng, & E. K. Yeh (Eds.), *Chinese societies and mental health* (pp. 156–166). Hong Kong: Oxford University Press.

Cheung, F. M. C. (1986). Psychopathology among Chinese people. In M. H. Bond (Ed.), *The psychology of the Chinese people* (pp. 171–213). Hong Kong: Oxford University Press.

Chinese Culture Connection. (1987). Chinese values and the search for culture-free dimensions of culture. *Journal of Cross-Cultural Psychology, 18,* 143–164.

Claver, B. G. (1976). Problèmes de guerissage en Côte d'Ivoire. *Annales Médico-Psychologiques, 134,* 23–30.

Compton, W. M., Helzer, J. E., Hwu, H. G., Yeh, E. K., McEvoy, L., Topp, J. E., & Spitznagel, E. L. (1991). New methods in cross-cultural psychiatry in Taiwan and the United States. *American Journal of Psychiatry, 148,* 1697–1704.

Cooper, J. E., & Sartorius, N. (1977). Cultural and temporal variation in schizophrenia: A speculation on the importance of industrialization. *British Journal of Psychiatry, 26,* 493–503.

Costantino, G., & Malgady, R. (1996). Development of TEMAS: A multicultural thematic apperception test: Psychometric properties and clinical utility. In G. R. Sodowsky & J. C. Impara (Eds.), *Multicultural assessment in counseling and clinical psychology* (pp. 85–136). Lincoln, NE: Buros Institute of Mental Measurement.

Costantino, G., Malgady, R. G., & Rogler, L. H. (1988). Folk hero modeling therapy for Puerto Rican adolescents. *Journal of Adolescence, 11,* 155–165.

Cross, W. E., & Fhagen-Smith, P. (1996). Nigrescence and ego identity development: Accounting for differential Black identity patterns. In P. B. Pedersen, J. G. Draguns, W. J. Lonner, & J. E. Trimble (Eds.), *Counseling across cultures* (4th ed.) (pp. 108–123). Thousand Oaks, CA: Sage Publications.

Dana, R. H. (1993). *Multicultural assessment perspectives for professional psychology.* Boston: Allyn and Bacon.

DeHoyos, A., & DeHoyos, G. (1965). Symptomatology differentials between Negro and White schizophrenics. *International Journal of Social Psychiatry, 11,* 245–255.

Desjarlais, R., Eisenberg, L., Good, B., & Kleinman, A. (1995). *World mental health: Problems and priorities in low-income countries.* New York: Oxford University Press.

Dinges, N., & Duffy, L. (1979). Culture and competence. In A. J. Marsella, R. G. Tharp, & T. J. Ciborowski (Eds.), *Perspectives on cross-cultural psychology* (pp. 209–231). New York: Academic Press.

Draguns, J. G. (1975). Resocialization into culture: The complexities of taking a worldwide view of psychotherapy. In R. W. Brislin, S. Bochner, & W. J. Lonner (Eds.), *Cross-cultural perspectives on learning* (pp. 273–289). Beverly Hills, CA: Sage Publications.

Draguns, J. G. (1995). Cultural influences upon psychopathology: Clinical and practical implications. In R. A. Javier, W. G. Herron, & A. Bergman (Eds.), Special issue: Multicultural perspectives on mental illness. *Journal of Social Distress and the Homeless, 4,* 79–103.

Draguns, J. G. (1996a). Abnormal behavior in Chinese societies: Clinical, epidemiological, and comparative studies. In M. H. Bond (Ed.), *Handbook of psychology of the Chinese people* (pp. 412–428). Hong Kong: Oxford University Press.

Draguns, J. G. (1996b). Ethnocultural considerations in the treatment of post-traumatic stress disorder: Ther-

apy and service delivery. In A. J. Marsella, M. J. Friedman, E. T. Gerrity, & R. M. Scurfield (Eds.), *Ethnocultural aspects of post-traumatic disorder: Issues, research, and clinical applications* (pp. 459–482). Washington, DC: American Psychological Association.

Draguns, J. G. (1996c). Humanly universal and culturally distinctive: Charting the course of cultural counseling. In P. B. Pedersen, J. G. Draguns, W. J. Lonner, & J. E. Trimble (Eds.), *Counseling across cultures* (4th ed.) (pp. 1–20). Thousand Oaks, CA: Sage Publications.

Draguns, J. G. (1996d). Multicultural and cross-cultural assessment of psychological disorder: Dilemmas and decisions. In G. R. Sodowsky & J. Impara (Eds.), *Multicultural assessment in counseling and clinical psychology (Buros-Nebraska Symposium on Measurement and Testing)* (Vol. 9, pp. 37–76). Lincoln, NE: Buros Institute of Mental Measurement.

Draguns, J. G. (1996e). Projective techniques. In A. Kuper & J. Kuper (Eds.), *The social science encyclopedia* (2nd ed.) (pp. 679–681). London: Routledge.

Draguns, J. G. (1996f). Toward a more sensitive and realistic assessment in multicultural settings. In R. T. Carter (Ed.), *What is multiculturalism? 1995 Columbia University Teachers College Cross-Cultural Roundtable Proceedings* (pp. 23–29). New York: Columbia University Teachers College Press.

Draguns, J. G. (1997). Abnormal behavior patterns across cultures: Implications for counseling and psychotherapy. *International Journal of Intercultural Relations, 21,* 213–248.

DuBois, C. (1944). *The people of Alor.* Minneapolis: University of Minnesota Press.

Durkheim, E. (1951/1897). *Suicide: A study in sociology* (J. A. Spaulding & G. Simpson, Trans.). Glencoe, IL: Free Press (originally published in 1897).

Echemendia, R. J., Congett, S., Harris, J., Diaz, L., & Puente, A. (1997). Neuropsychological training and practices with Hispanics: A national survey. *The Clinical Neuropsychologist, 11*(3), 229–243.

Egeland, J. A., Hofsteter, A. M., & Eshleman, S. K. (1983). Amish study: The impact of cultural factors on diagnosis of bipolar illness. *American Journal of Psychiatry, 140,* 67–71.

Fish, J. (1996). *Culture and therapy: An integrative approach.* Northvale, NJ: Jason Aronson.

Fulkerson, S. C. (1965). Some implications of the new cognitive theory for projective tests. *Journal of Consulting Psychology, 29.*

Greene, R. L. (1987). Ethnicity and MMPI performance:

A review. *Journal of Consulting and Clinical Psychology, 55,* 497–512.

Gynther, M. (1972). White norms and black MMPIs: A prescription for discrimination? *Psychological Bulletin, 78,* 386–402.

Herskovits, M. (1948). *Man and his works.* New York: Knopf.

Higginbotham, H. N., West, S., & Forsyth, D. (1988). *Psychotherapy and behavior change: Social, cultural and methodological perspectives.* New York: Pergamon Press.

Hofstede, G. (1980). *Culture's consequences: International differences in work related values.* Beverly Hills, CA: Sage Publications.

Hofstede, G. (1986). Cultural differences in teaching and learning. *International Journal of Intercultural Relations, 10,* 301–320.

Hofstede, G. (1991). *Cultures and organizations: Software of the mind.* London: McGraw-Hill.

Holtzman, W. H., Diaz-Guerrero, R., & Swartz, J. D. (1975). *Personality development in two cultures.* Austin: University of Texas Press.

Hostetler, J. A. (1980). *The Amish society* (3rd ed.). Baltimore, MD: Johns Hopkins University Press.

Hsu, J., & Tseng, W. S. (1991). *Culture and family: Problems and therapy.* New York: Haworth Press.

Ibrahim, F. A., & Kahn, H. (1987). Assessment of world views. *Psychological Reports, 60,* 163–176.

Ibrahim, F. A., Ohnishi, H., & Wilson, R. P. (1994). Career assessment in a culturally diverse society. *Journal of Career Assessement, 2,* 276–288.

Ibrahim, F. A., & Owen, S. V. (1994). Factor analytic structure of the Scale to Assess World View. *Current Psychology: Development, Learning, Personality, Social, 13,* 201–209.

Jablensky, A., Sartorius, N., Ernberg, A. M., Anker, Korten, A., Cooper, J. E., Day, R., & Bertelson, A. (1992). *Schizophrenia: Manifestation, incidence, and cause in different cultures: A World Health Organization ten-country study.* Cambridge: Cambridge University Press.

Jablensky, A., Sartorius, N., Gulbinat, W., & Ernberg, G. (1981). Characteristics of depressive patients contacting psychiatric services in four cultures. *Acta Psychiatrica Scandinavica, 63,* 367–383.

James, W. (1952/1891). *The principles of psychology.* Chicago: Encyclopedia Brittanica.

Javier, R. A. (1990). The suitability of insight-oriented therapy for Hispanic poor. *American Journal of Psychoanalysis, 50,* 305–318.

Javier, R. A., Barroso, F., & Muñoz, M. A. (1993). Autobiographical memory in bilinguals. *Journal of Psycholinguistic Research, 22,* 319–338.

Jewell, D. P. (1952). A case of a psychotic Navaho Indian male. *Human Organization, 11,* 32–36.

Jilek, W. (1988). *Indian healing: Shamanistic ceremonialism in the Pacific Northwest.* Vancouver, BC: Hancock House.

Kimura, B. (1972). Mitmenschlichkeit in der Psychiatrie. *Zeitschrift für Klinische Psychologie, 20,* 3–13.

Kimura, B. (1995). *Zwischen Mensch und Mensch—Strukturen japanischer Subjektivität* (Egon Weinmayr, Ed. & Trans.). Darnstadt, Germany: Wissenschaftliche Buchgesellschaft.

Kirmayer, L. (1984). Culture, affect, and somatization: Parts 1 and 2. *Transcultural Psychiatric Research Review, 21,* 159–188, 237–262.

Kleinman, A. (1982). Neurasthenia and depression: A study of somatization and culture in China. *Culture, Medicine and Psychiatry, 6,* 117–190.

Kleinman, A. (1986). *Social origins of distress and disease.* New Haven: Yale University Press.

Kleinman, A. (1988). *Rethinking psychiatry: From cultural category to personal experience.* New York: Free Press.

Kleinman, A. (1992). How culture is important for DSM-IV. In J. E. Mezzich, A. Kleinman, H. Fabrega, B. Good, G. Johnson-Powell, K. M. Lin, S. Manson, & D. Parron (Eds.), *Cultural proposals for DSM-IV* (pp. 7–28). Pittsburgh: University of Pittsburgh (cited by Castillo, 1996).

Kleinman, A., & Kleinman, J. (1995). Remembering the Cultural Revolution: Alienating pains and the pain of alienation/transformation. In T. Y. Lin, W. S. Tseng, & E. K. Yeh (Eds.), *Chinese societies and mental health* (pp. 141–155). Hong Kong: Oxford University Press.

Korman, M. (1974). National conference on levels and patterns of professional training in psychology: Major themes. *American Psychologist, 29,* 441–449.

Koss, J. D. (1990). Somatization and somatic complaint syndromes among Hispanics: Overview and ethnopsychological perspectives. *Transcultural Psychiatric Research Review, 27,* 5–29.

Kraepelin, E. (1904). Vergleichende Psychiatrie. *Zentralblatt für Nervenheilkunde und Psychiatrie, 27,* 433–437.

Kroeber, A. I., & Kluckhohn, C. (1952). *Culture: A critical review of concepts and definitions.* Cambridge, MA: Peabody Museum.

Landrine, H. (1992). Clinical implications of cultural differences: The referential versus the indexical self. *Clinical Psychology Review, 12,* 401–415.

Lebra, T. S. (1976). *Japanese patterns of behavior.* Honolulu: University Press of Hawaii.

Lewis-Fernandez, R. (1994). Culture and dissociation. A comparison of *ataque de nervios* among Puerto Ricans and possession syndrome in India. In D. Spiegel (Ed.), *Dissociation: Culture, mind, and body* (pp. 123–167). Washington, DC: American Psychiatric Press.

Lewis-Fernandez, R., & Kleinman, A. (1994). Culture, personality, and psychopathology. *Journal of Abnormal Psychology, 103,* 67–71.

Lezak, M. (1983). *Neuropsychological assessment* (2nd ed.). New York: Oxford University Press.

Lin, T., Tseng, W. S., & Yeh, E. K. (Eds.). (1995). *Chinese societies and mental health.* Hong Kong: Oxford University Press.

Lindzey, G. (1961). *Projective techniques and cross cultural research.* New York: Appleton-Century-Crofts.

López, S. R. (1989). Patient variable biases in clinical judgment: Conceptual overview and methodological considerations. *Psychological Bulletin, 106,* 184–203.

López, S. R., & Hernandez, P. (1992). How culture is considered in evaluation of psychopathology. *Journal of Nervous and Mental Disease, 176,* 598–606.

Markus, H. R., & Katayama, S. (1991). Culture and the self: Implications for cognition, emotion, and motivation. *Psychological Review, 98*(2), 224–253.

Marsella, A. J., Sartorius, N., Jablensky, A., & Fenton, F. R. (1985). Cross-cultural studies of depressive disorders. In A. Kleinman & B. Good (Eds.), *Culture and depression* (pp. 299–324). Berkeley: University of California Press.

Marsella, A. J., Bornemann, T., Ekblad, S., & Orley, J. (Eds.). (1994). *Amidst peril and pain: The mental health and well-being of the world's refugees.* Washington, DC: American Psychological Association.

Marsella, A. J., Friedman, M. J., Gerrity, E., & Scurfield, R. M. (Eds.). (1996). *Ethnocultural aspects of post-traumatic stress disorder: Issues, research, and clinical applications.* Washington, DC: American Psychological Association.

McClelland, D. C., Sturr, J. F., Knapp, R. H., & Wendt, H. W. (1958). Obligations to self and society in the United States and Germany. *Journal of Abnormal and Social Psychology, 56,* 245–255.

Mercer, J. R. (1979). *Technical manual: System of Multicultural Pluralistic Assessment (SOMPA).* New York: Psychological Corporation.

Moghaddam, F. M., Taylor, D. M., & Wright, S. C. (1993). *Social psychology in cross-cultural perspective.* New York: W. H. Freeman.

Murphy, H. B. M., Wittkower, E. D., & Chance, N. A. (1967). Cross-cultural inquiry into the symptomatology of depression: A preliminary report. *International Journal of Psychiatry, 3,* 6–15.

Nathan, T. (1994). *L'influence qui quérit.* Paris: Odile Jacob.

Neisser, U., Boodoo, G., Bouchard, T. J., Boykin, A. W., Brody, N., Ceci, S. J., Halpern, D. F., Loehlin, J. C., Perloff, R., Sternberg, R. J., & Urbina, S. (1996). Intelligence: Knowns and unknowns. *American Psychologist, 51,* 77–101.

Oberg, K. (1958). *Culture shock and the problem of adjustment to new cultural environments.* Washington, DC: Foreign Service Institute.

Ots, T. (1990). The angry liver, the anxious heart, and the melancholy spleen: The phenomenology of perceptions in Chinese culture. *Culture, Medicine, and Psychiatry, 14,* 21–58.

Paris, J. (1991). Personality disorders, parasuicide, and culture. *Transcultural Psychiatric Research Review, 28,* 25–39.

Partridge, K. (1987). How to become Japanese: A guide for North Americans. *Kyoto Journal, 1*(4), 12–15.

Pedersen, P. B. (1990). The multicultural perspective as a fourth force in psychology. *Journal of Mental Health Counseling, 12,* 93–95.

Pedersen, P. B. (1991). Multiculturalism as a generic approach to counseling. *Journal of Counseling and Development, 70,* 3–14.

Pedersen, P. B., Draguns, J. G., Lonner, W. J., & Trimble, J. E. (Eds.). (1996). *Counseling across cultures* (4th ed.). Thousand Oaks, CA: Sage Publications.

Peltzer, K. (1995). *Psychology and health in African cultures: Examples of ethnopsychotherapeutic practice.* Frankfurt/Main: IKO-Verlag für interkulturelle Kommunikation.

Pfeiffer, W. M. (1994). *Transkulturelle Psychiatrie* (2nd ed.). Stuttgart: Thieme.

Pfeiffer, W. M. (1996). Kulturpsychiatrische Aspekte der Migration. In E. Koch, M. Özek, & W. M. Pfeiffer (Eds.), *Psychologie und Pathologie der Migration* (pp. 17–30). Freiburg/Breisgau: Lambertus.

Ponterotto, J. G., et al. (1995). *Handbook of multicultural counseling.* Thousand Oaks, CA: Sage Publications.

Prince, R. (1968). The changing picture of depression syndromes in Africa: Is it a fact or diagnostic fashion? *Canadian Journal of African Studies, 1,* 177–192.

Ridley, C. R. (1989). Racism in counseling as an aversive behavioral process. In P. B. Pedersen, J. G. Draguns,

W. J. Lonner, & J. E. Trimble (Eds.), *Counseling across cultures* (3rd ed.) (pp. 55–77). Honolulu: University of Hawaii Press.

Ridley, C. R., & Lingle, D. W. (1996). Cultural empathy in multicultural counseling: A multidimensional process model. In P. B. Pedersen, J. G. Draguns, W. J. Lonner, & J. E. Trimble (Eds.), *Counseling across cultures* (4th ed.) (pp. 21–46). Thousand Oaks, CA: Sage Publications.

Ritzler, B. A. (1996). Projective methods for multicultural personality assessment: Rorschach, TEMAS, and the Early Memories Procedure. In L. A. Suzuki, P. J. Meller, & J. G. Ponterotto (Eds.), *Handbook of multicultural assessment: Clinical, psychological and educational applications.* San Francisco: Jossey-Bass.

Roland, A. (1988). *In search of self in India and Japan.* Princeton, NJ: Princeton University Press.

Rosado, J. W., & Elias, M. J. (1993). Ecological and psychocultural mediators in delivery of services for urban, culturally diverse Hispanic clients. *Professional Psychology: Research and Practice, 24,* 450–459.

Sanua, V. D. (1992). Mental illness and other forms of psychiatric deviance among contemporary Jewry. *Transcultural Psychiatric Research Review, 29,* 197–233.

Sartorius, N., Jablensky, A., Korten, A., & Ernberg, G. (1986). Early manifestation and first contact incidence of schizophrenia. *Psychological Medicine, 16,* 909–928.

Scharfetter, C. (1985). Der Schamane-Zeuge einer alten Kultur wieder belebbar? *Schweizer Archiv für Neurologie und Psychiatrie, 136,* 81–95.

Serpell, R. (1989). Dimensions endogènes de l'intelligence chez les A-chewa et autres peuples africains. In J. Retschnitzky, M. Bossell-Lagos, & P. Dasen (Eds.), *La recherche interculturelle* (Vol. 2, pp. 164–182). Paris: L'Harmattan.

Skultans, V. (1995). Neurasthenia and political resistance in Latvia. *Anthropology Today, 11,* 14–17.

Sodowsky, G. R. (1996). The Multicultural Counseling Inventory: Validity and applications in multicultural training. In G. R. Sodowsky & J. C. Impara (Eds.), *Multicultural assessment in counseling and clinical psychology* (pp. 241–246). Lincoln, NE: Buros Institute of Mental Measurement.

Sodowsky, G. R., & Impara, J. C. (Eds.). (1996). *Multicultural assessment in counseling and clinical psychology.* Lincoln, NE: Buros Institute of Mental Measurement.

Sodowsky, G. R., & Plake, B. (1991). Psychometric properties of the American International Relations

Scale. *Educational and Psychological Measurement, 51,* 207–216.

Strole, L., Langner, T., Michael, S. T., Opler, M. K., & Rennie, T. A. (1962). *Mental health in the metropolis: The midtown Manhattan study.* New York: McGraw-Hill.

Starcevic, V. (1991). Neurasthenia: A paradigm of social psychopathology in a transitional society. *American Journal of Psychotherapy, 45,* 544–553.

Stewart, E. C. (1995). The feeling edge of culture. *Journal of Social Distress and the Homeless, 4,* 163–202.

Sue, S. (1996). Multicultural assessment in counseling and clinical psychology. In G. R. Sodowsky & J. C. Impara (Eds.), *Multicultural assessment in counseling and clinical psychology* (pp. 37–84). Lincoln, NE: Buros Institute of Mental Measurement.

Sue, S., & Morishima, J. (1982). *The mental health of Asian Americans.* San Francisco: Jossey-Bass.

Sue, D., & Sundberg, W. D. (1996). Research and research hypotheses about effectiveness in intercultural counseling. In P. B. Pedersen, J. G. Draguns, W. J. Lomer, & J. E. Trimble (Eds.), *Counseling across cultures* (4th ed.) (pp. 323–352). Thousand Oaks, CA: Sage Publications.

Suzuki, L. A., Meller, P. J., & Ponterotto, J. G. (Eds.). (1996). *Handbook of multicultural assessment.* San Francisco: Jossey-Bass.

Tanaka-Matsumi, J. (1992). *Cultural and social factors in depression.* Unpublished paper.

Tanaka-Matsumi, J., & Draguns, J. G. (1997). Culture and psychopathology. In J. W. Berry, M. H. Segall, & C. Kagitcibasi (Eds.), *Handbook of cross cultural psychology: Vol. 3. Social behavior and applications* (2nd ed.) (pp. 449–491). Boston: Allyn and Bacon.

Tanaka-Matsumi, J., & Higginbotham, H. N. (1996). Behavioral approaches to counseling across culture. In P. B. Pedersen, J. G. Draguns, W. J. Lonner, & J. E. Trimble (Eds.), *Counseling across cultures* (4th ed.) (pp. 266–292). Thousand Oaks, CA: Sage Publications.

Thompson, C. E. (1949). The Thompson modification of the Thematic Apperception Test. *Rorschach Research Exchange, 13,* 469–478.

Triandis, H. C. (1972). *The analysis of cognitive culture.* New York: Wiley.

Triandis, H. C. (1989). The self and social behavior in differing cultural contexts. *Psychological Review, 96,* 506–520.

Triandis, H. C. (1994). *Culture and social behavior.* New York: McGraw-Hill.

Triandis, H. C. (1995). *Individualism and collectivism.* Boulder, CO: Westview Press.

Trimble, J. E., Fleming, C. M., Beauvais, F., & Jumper-Thurman, P. (1996). Essential cultural and social strategies for counseling Native American Indians. In P. B. Pedersen, J. G. Draguns, W. J. Lonner, & J. E. Trimble (Eds.), *Counseling across cultures* (4th ed.) (pp. 177–209). Thousand Oaks, CA: Sage Publications.

van der Veer, G. (1992). *Counselling and therapy with refugees: Psychological problems of victims of war, torture, and repression.* Chichester, England: Wiley.

Weidman, H. H., & Sussex, J. H. (1971). Culture values and ego functioning in relation to the atypical culture-bound reactive syndrome. *Journal of Social Psychiatry, 17,* 83–100.

Westermeyer, J. (1987). Cultural factors in clinical assessment. *Journal of Consulting and Clinical Psychology, 55,* 471–478.

Williams, R. L. (1972). *Themes concerning Blacks.* St. Louis: Robert L. Williams and Associates.

World Health Organization. (1973). *Report of the International Pilot Study of Schizophrenia.* Geneva: Author.

World Health Organization. (1979). *Schizophrenia: An international follow-up study.* Geneva: Author.

World Health Organization. (1983). *Depressive disorders in different cultures: Report of WHO collaborative study of standardized assessment of depressive disorders.* Geneva: Author.

Zuniga, M. E. (1991). "Dichos" as metaphorical tools for resistant Latino clients. *Psychotherapy, 28,* 480–483.

FOR FURTHER READING

The field of culture and mental health is growing at a fast pace and is experiencing rapid, almost kaleidoscopic transformation. Writers in the field typically address other specialists. Consequently, students' needs may be neglected. With these considerations in mind, the following selection of recent and relatively readable writings is offered.

On cross-cultural psychology, with emphasis on social behavior in the experimental laboratory and in real-life settings, Brislin (1993), Moghaddam et al. (1993), and Triandis (1994) effectively communicate the major current concerns and the principal recent findings in the field. They also do much to bridge the gap between the artificiality of the experiments and the "messiness" of social interaction, especially as it is regulated in several cultures.

In reference to abnormal behavior, the most comprehensive overview of cultural data (Pfeiffer, 1994) has not yet been translated into English. On a somewhat more limited range of topics, however, Al-Issa (1995) and Desjarlais et al. (1995) provide excellent and authoritative coverage. Reviews of research findings on the interface of mental disorder and cultural factors by Draguns (1995, 1997), Lewis-Fernandez and Kleinman (1994), and Tanaka-Matsumi and Draguns (1997) are also available. On the problems of assessment and testing, the interested reader may turn to Sodowsky and Impara (1996) and Suzuki, Meller, and Ponterotto (1996). On counseling and psychotherapy, there is the edited volume by Pedersen, Draguns, Lonner, & Trimble (1996), a comprehensive handbook by Ponterotto et al. (1995), and a book on a more specialized topic, the interface of culture, family, and disturbance, by Hsu and Tseng (1991). Three more experiential and personal volumes also have appeared recently: by Fish (1996) on the experience of an American psychologist trying to respond to the therapy needs of Brazilian clients, by Nathan (1994) on developing innovative therapy methods for reaching traditional African clients in Paris, and by Peltzer (1995) on designing and implementing clinical services for a wide-ranging clientele in a variety of African settings.

CHAPTER 16

FORENSIC PSYCHOLOGY

Gerald Cooke

DEFINITION AND SCOPE

Forensic psychology includes all areas where law and psychology interface. While many people think of evaluations of criminals when they think of forensic psychology, it is, in fact, a much broader area that encompasses both clinical and nonclinical topics. Among the other clinical areas of forensic psychology are evaluations in cases involving personal injury, child custody, child sexual abuse, and psychological malpractice. Personal injury includes not only reactions to physical injury but also cases involving harassment and/or discrimination. Clinical forensic psychologists also evaluate applicants for positions of police and correctional officers. An area that has recently gained a great deal of media, as well as professional, attention involves evaluations of potential for violence in the workplace after someone has made comments or threats that raise such a concern (see Table 16.1).

Clinical forensic psychologists provide psychotherapeutic treatment as well as conducting evaluations. Treatment of criminal populations may take place within prisons or in the community. Treatment of offenders within the community often is a condition of the offender's probation or parole.

Treatment of offenders involves special issues, considerations, and techniques, that differ from therapy with nonoffender populations (Milan & Evans, 1987). Clinical forensic psychologists also may provide treatment for individuals who have had personal injury lawsuits and suffer from depression, anxiety, or other problems secondary to the trauma or injuries. Those forensic psychologists who do custody and child sexual abuse evaluations also may provide treatment for children and families. Whenever treatment takes place within a legal context, there are special issues that do not exist for nonlegal cases.

Most clinical forensic psychologists have doctoral (Ph.D. or Psy.D) degrees in clinical psychology. Nonclinical forensic psychologists more often have their degrees in experimental, social, or other areas of psychology. Rather than focusing on the evaluation of a single individual, the nonclinical forensic psychologist is more likely to deal with issues that can be subjected to scientific experimental study. These include such areas as factors affecting eyewitness identification (Wells & Seelau, 1995), and evaluation of bias in criminal lineups and photo displays, jury selection, and jury dynamics (Coo-

Table 16.1 What Forensic Psychologists Do

Criminal Cases	**Administrative Law Cases**
Waivers between juvenile and adult status	Worker's compensation
Competency to understand and/or waive Miranda rights	State disability insurance
	Social Security disability
Competency to stand trial	**Other**
Not guilty by reason of insanity	Malingering
Guilty but mentally ill	Potential for dangerous behavior
Diminished capacity	Eyewitness identification
Mitigating psychological factors in death penalty cases	Jury selection
	Product liability
Disposition and treatment recommendations	Victim/witness evaluation
Predatory sex offender evaluations	Evaluation/training of police officers
Civil Cases	**Treatment**
Child custody	Incarcerated offenders
Child sexual abuse (may also be criminal)	Offenders on parole/probation
Psychological/neuropsychological damages in personal injury cases	Children and families in custody litigation
	Victims of crime
Termination of parental rights	Psychic trauma due to personal injury
Civil competency	
Involuntary commitment	

per, Bennett, & Sukel, 1996). Another major area of nonclinical forensic psychology, human factors engineering, addresses issues such as the characteristics and placement of warnings, adapting machinery/computers and the workplace itself to human physical and psychological needs, and the adequacy of guards and other safety features on dangerous machinery such as power saws. Each of these areas of forensic psychology will be discussed later in this chapter.

HISTORY AND LEGAL BACKGROUND

Medical doctors and psychiatrists have long been involved in the legal system, but the acceptance of psychologists as expert witnesses is of relatively recent origin. Although there was occasional testimony by psychologists as far back as the 1920s, the case that established psychologists as having expert status was *Jenkins v. United States* (1962). In this case, Jenkins raised an insanity defense. The trial judge instructed the jury to disregard the testimony of three defense psychologists because they were not competent to give a "medical opinion" regarding "mental disease." The court of appeals for the District of Columbia ruled, however, that a judge could not automatically disqualify a witness for lack of a medical degree but, rather, had to look at the specific credentials of a proposed expert before ruling on expert status.

In the years following the Jenkins case, psychologists became involved in an ever-increasing range of legal issues. This involvement varied by state and still does. For example, in some states a psychologist may testify in a proceeding for the involuntary commitment of a patient, whereas in other states that type of testimony is restricted to psychiatrists. But the overriding influence on psychologists' involvement has been based on an evolving standard of what constitutes an expert witness. The Frye standard was first formulated in the case of *Frye v. United States* (1923). Although this case involved the use of a precursor of the polygraph (lie detector), the standard was applied to psychology as well. It stated that novel scientific evidence "must be sufficiently established to have gained general scientific acceptance in that . . . field." This became known as the "general scientific acceptance test."

The formulation of the Federal Rules of Evidence in 1975 broadened the scope of testimony. Rule 702 states: "If scientific, technical, or specialized knowledge will assist the Trier of Fact to understand the evidence or to determine a fact in issue, a witness qualified as an expert by knowledge, skill, experience, training, or education may testify thereto in the form of an opinion or otherwise." The "Trier of Fact" is in some cases a jury and in other cases a judge without a jury. In either case the emphasis is on the expert's ability to "assist," which is a very broad standard. Because the standard is so broad, when an attorney objects to a witness being qualified as an expert, the judge will rarely sustain the objection. Rather, the judge will state that the judge or jury should take the credentials into account in determining the weight to be given to the testimony.

A recent case, *Daubert v. Merrell Dow Pharmaceuticals* (1993), though reinforcing Rule 702, has again modified the definition of expert testimony, although this case also had nothing to do with psychology. It states that to be admissible, expert testimony must be based on scientific methodology that does not "diverge significantly from the procedures accepted by recognized authorities in the field. If it does so diverge it cannot be shown to be generally accepted as a reliable technique" (p. 1128). *Daubert* is too recent a case to determine what its long-term effects will be on admissibility of testimony. It certainly seems broader than the Frye test but may be more conservative than Rule 702. For example, methodology in controversial emerging areas, such as the prediction of violent behavior and the distinction between false and accurate reports of child sexual abuse, may find it difficult to meet this standard.

It seems clear that psychologists have gained expert status in the courtroom, which in most cases equals or exceeds the weight given to psychiatric testimony. Many courts give more weight to psychological testimony because the use of psychological tests is viewed as providing additional data supportive of expert opinion.

TRAINING AND EDUCATION IN FORENSIC PSYCHOLOGY

To become an independently practicing forensic psychologist, one must obtain a Ph.D. or its equivalent. Prior to the 1970s there were no specialty doctoral programs in forensic psychology. The most that was available was an occasional graduate course in "correctional psychology" and the opportunity to serve a clinical internship within a prison or a correctional mental health facility.

The first Ph.D. forensic specialty program was instituted at the University of Nebraska in the 1970s. Since that time, several alternative models have been developed for specialty in forensic psychology at various educational institutions across the country (Metton, 1987). In the specialty program the student usually takes courses in various areas of the law (e.g., criminal, family) and a course in forensic assessment in addition to traditional psychology graduate courses.

Supervised Research, Seminars, and Practica Focused on Forensic Areas

Several universities have developed joint degree programs in which the student earns a combined J.D.–Ph.D., typically after six years of study. Although such a degree obviously provides the student with knowledge and sophistication in the areas of both psychology and the law, the employment advantage of the joint degree is controversial.

Another option open to the person who has traditional psychological training and wishes to become more involved in forensic psychology is to enroll in a post-doctoral program, usually lasting one to two years. These programs assume that students are already well grounded in psychology and focus on psycholegal issues. Classes, seminars, and practica are usually scheduled so that students can maintain their established practices.

Licensing

Most states have psychologist licensing statutes. To qualify to take the licensing examination, the psychologist must document a certain amount of supervised professional experience beyond the doctoral degree. One cannot practice as a psychologist without supervision, unless one has passed the licensing examination. The examination and license is either in psychology or clinical psychology, and not specific to forensic psychology.

There is, however, a practice called "boarding" in forensic psychology. After five years of experience in a forensic area, one may apply to the American Board of Forensic Psychology (now part of the American Board of Professional Psychology) for "diplomate" status. The applicant submits a written work sample, which is reviewed by three persons who already have diplomate status. If the work sample passes, there is then an oral examination of the applicant, typically lasting about three hours, by three other diplomates. Obtaining diplomate status (being "boarded") is a way of ensuring the consumer that the diplomate has demonstrated competency in a range of forensic areas, and special competency in those forensic areas in which expertise is claimed.

EVALUATION IN CRIMINAL CASES

Sources of Referral

Forensic psychologists typically get referrals for criminal evaluations from one of five sources: court appointments, prosecutors' offices, public defenders' offices, private defense attorneys, or forensic psychiatrists. The rules governing the evaluation and sometimes even the procedures employed depend in part on the source of the referral.

When the psychologist is directly appointed by the court (i.e., the judge), the person evaluated must be told that the evaluation is not privileged or confidential and that the evaluator will be reporting back to the court. The situation is essentially the same when the evaluation is conducted at the request of the prosecutor's office. The request for evaluation by the prosecutor's office usually arises after the defense, utilizing their own forensic mental health professional, has raised one of the mental health issues to be discussed next.

The situation is different when the referral comes from a public defender or private defense attorney. Here the evaluator is acting as an agent of the attorney, and therefore the communications and test results from the client are protected by attorney–client privilege. The psychologist communicates the findings back to the attorney. If the attorney and client believe that the findings will be helpful in the criminal case, then the report and/or testimony will be presented in court. If the findings are not helpful and/or are potentially damaging to the client, however, then the attorney will not use the information

in court. Because the findings are protected by attorney–client privilege, the prosecutor's office cannot obtain the psychologist's test results, notes, or report.

At times a defense attorney may retain one forensic mental health professional after another until the attorney finds one whose opinion is helpful to the case. Certainly psychologists have an ethical responsibility to be honest in providing their opinions, although some forensic psychologists, like some people in every profession, undoubtedly "sell" their opinions. There are also instances of genuine and valid disagreement among equally qualified forensic psychologists. The media often criticize this kind of "doctor shopping" by defense attorneys as unethical, but this is not so. To the contrary, the attorney's ethical responsibility is to provide the best representation and defense possible for the client. This may require, if possible, finding a psychologist whose opinion aids the defense.

Up until recent years it was usually the forensic psychiatrist who was appointed or retained. The psychiatrist would do a preliminary evaluation and, if the psychiatrist felt that psychological testing would be helpful, would then request that a psychologist be retained or appointed as well. Although the same privilege issues apply as were discussed above, the procedures may differ depending on the professional relationship between the psychiatrist and psychologist. There is a certain amount of overlap in psychiatric and psychological evaluations, as both involve taking a history and conducting a clinical interview. In some cases both professionals do this; in other cases the psychologist's role may be limited to administration and interpretation of psychological tests. Also, when the psychologist is retained separately, the report goes back to the referral source and, if testimony is needed, the psychologist would be called to testify. Where the referral is from the psychiatrist, the psychologist's report may go to both the attorney and the psychiatrist, or it may go only to the psychiatrist, in which case it is then either integrated into or attached to the psychiatric report. If testimony is needed, both professionals may be called to testify or only the psychiatrist, who will then rely in part on the information received from the psychologist. The kinds of tests used and the nature of the information they provide are discussed elsewhere in this text.

The Criminal Court System

Criminal cases may arise in state courts or in federal courts, depending on the crime charged and, in some cases, on whether a crime involved actions only within one state or across state lines. Federal judges are appointed for life. Federal juries are drawn from a wider geographical area than are state court juries.

State courts are administered by the individual counties in the state. The characteristics of these county courts may vary widely. In some states and counties judges are appointed, while in others they are elected. The terms they serve also vary. In some counties a particular judge or group of judges will hear a particular type of case throughout their terms. In other counties judges rotate every one to three years, so that a judge who has been hearing family court cases may be rotated to criminal cases. When there is rotation it is inevitable that judges will hear cases that were never part of their law practice. For example, an ex–district attorney who has become a judge may be hearing custody cases, and a former custody attorney may be hearing criminal cases. Judges develop a reputation for how they handle certain kinds of cases and for their attitudes toward mental health professionals. Some judges are known to rely heavily on input from mental health professionals; others are known to have little regard for mental health professionals and to be likely to ignore their input. Juries also vary from county to county on the basis of whether they are primarily urban, suburban, or rural, and also along ethnic and racial lines. Counties often develop reputations for having liberal or conservative juries. Attorneys often plan legal strategies based on the reputation of the judges and/or the probable makeup of the jury. The strategy may include whether and at what stage of the trial to call a psychologist to testify.

Legal Issues in Criminal Cases

Many legal issues arise in the course of a criminal case, but only a handful of these involve mental health professionals. The law specifies the issues on which testimony from mental health professionals

may be used, and testimony is allowed only on those issues. The attorney may be required to make an "offer of proof" to the court regarding an expert's testimony. This means explaining to the court how the testimony will be used and demonstrating that it is admissible under the law. For example, expert testimony *cannot* be introduced during the guilt phase of the trial (as opposed to the penalty phase) simply to explain the reason for the defendant's behavior or to indicate that the individual has personality characteristics that may or may not be associated with the type of offense charged. Only if the expert can offer an opinion on an issue in the language of the law is the opinion admissible.

Competency to Stand Trial

Although the exact language varies by jurisdiction, both state and federal law require that an individual be competent to proceed legally at every stage of the legal process. Criminal competency involves the capacity of the defendant to understand the nature and object of the proceedings and to aid the attorney in the preparation of the defense (Grisso & Siegel, 1986). The concept was originally based on physical illness. For example, an individual in intensive care for a heart attack certainly could not proceed. This concept was extended to mental illness and first defined in *Dusky v. United States* (1960). Competency is totally distinct from mental state at the time of the offense (responsibility).

As in all areas where law and psychology interface, in competency evaluations it is necessary to translate the legal standard into psychological terms in order for an opinion to be formulated. Understanding the nature and object of the proceedings generally means that defendants have to know, or have the capacity to learn, that they are the person charged, that there are possible plea alternatives, and that there are possible outcomes in which the penalties vary according to the seriousness of the charge. The defendant also must have at least a basic understanding of the roles of the judge, jury, prosecutor, and defense attorney. Further, the defendant must be able to relate to the attorney and must be able to provide pertinent facts to the attorney in order to assist in the preparation of the defense. The defendant has to have the capacity to testify in a relevant fashion and to help challenge prosecution witnesses. Finally, the defendant has to be capable of appropriate courtroom behavior and of being motivated to help in the legal process rather than engaging in self-defeating behavior. Both interview and psychological testing are helpful in evaluating these issues (Grisso, 1986) (see Table 16.2).

Making such a determination can be a complex and difficult task for the mental health professional. First, incapacity in any of the areas noted must be the result of a diagnosable mental illness or defect (e.g., retardation). The distinction is made between the *inability* to cooperate with the legal process and the *unwillingness* to do so. For example, some individuals, because of political or other attitudes, may feel that the legal system is unfair and may choose not to cooperate. Whether or not one agrees with their belief, if it is a function of a rationally derived attitude and not a function of mental illness, then the individual would be considered to be competent.

An individual's denial of the offense and the resulting plea of "not guilty," even if the evidence against the defendant is overwhelming, also does not constitute incompetency unless it is a function of mental illness. A defendant has the right to make the prosecution prove its case "beyond a reasonable doubt" and therefore may want to take the case to trial no matter what the strength of the evidence against the defendant. An example in which a defendant's denial of guilt would probably lead to a judgment of incompetency is one in which the individual is psychotic, has the delusion of being Christ, and has hallucinations in which God's voice is heard saying that, as Christ, the defendant can do no wrong and is above the laws of man.

Another issue has to do with real or feigned amnesia. Many individuals who commit crimes are under the influence of alcohol and/or drugs and may have partial or complete amnesia for their actions. Others are in a state of psychological distress or illness that also may produce a partial or complete amnesia. Many other individuals simply say they do not remember committing the act, even where intoxication or illness was absent. Claimed amnesia in and of itself is not a basis for incompetency as long as the defendant understands what he or she is being charged with and can relate some details before and/or after the act. Where the basis for amnesia was drug or alcohol intoxication, the amnesia is due to a failure of registration and the memory is likely never to be recovered. As a result, rarely is amnesia due to intoxication accepted as a basis for incompetency. Amnesia is sometimes accepted by the court as a basis for incompetency when it is the result of a psychotic episode at the time of the act and where the memory is likely to be recovered and the individual returned to competency through treatment with medication and therapy.

Mental retardation may be the basis for incompetency, although individuals with an IQ above 60 usually are capable of meeting the criteria unless there are other accompanying mental illnesses. On the other hand, even an extremely intelligent person may be incompetent if mental illness precludes assisting in the defense. For example, consider a case of a man with an IQ of 146 who suffered from paranoid schizophrenia and believed that the government had implanted a tiny radio transmitter in his tooth and therefore could listen to his conversations with his attorney. On the basis of this delusion, along with his belief that his own attorney was part of the plot against him, he refused to consult with

---

Table 16.2 Competency to Stand Trial

Areas for Evaluation
1. Appraisal of available legal defenses
2. Unmanageable behavior
3. Quality of relating to attorney
4. Planning of legal strategy, including guilty plea to lesser charges
5. Appraisal of role of:
   a. Defense counsel
   b. Prosecuting attorney
   c. Judge
   d. Jury
   e. Defendant
   f. Witnesses
6. Understanding of court procedure
7. Appreciation of charges
8. Appreciation of range and nature of possible penalties
9. Appraisal of likely outcome
10. Capacity to disclose to attorney available pertinent facts surrounding the offense
11. Capacity to realistically challenge prosecution witness
12. Capacity to testify relevantly
13. Self-defeating vs. self-serving motivation (legal sense)

the attorney and was found incompetent to proceed. After treatment brought his psychosis under control, he became competent and proceeded to trial.

The case of *Jackson v. Indiana* (1972) was the first to address what would become of an individual whose competency could not be restored through treatment. Prior to Jackson, defendants could be found incompetent, even on minor charges, and if they remained mentally ill could be kept in a mental hospital for the rest of their lives, often far beyond the statutory penalty if they had been found guilty. For example, there was a case of a man who, with a co-conspirator, attempted to rob a store. The co-conspirator was found guilty and served three years in prison. The other man was found incompetent and, twenty years later, remained a patient in the state's maximum-security forensic mental hospital. Following Jackson, states were required to pass laws to prevent such abuses. Typically these laws require that an individual can be held as criminally incompetent for the lesser of two periods of time: either the maximum sentence the defendant could have received on the charge, or a specified time period such as 5 years or 10 years (Winick, 1995). At the end of that time, the charges would have to be dropped and persons would be committable only if they met civil commitment criteria. Persons who were not civilly committable would have to be released. In some states, charges of homicide are an exception in that the charge is not dropped and can be reinstated at a later date should the person become competent.

A subcategory of competency involves the individual's ability to waive the Miranda rights (*Miranda v. Arizona*, 1973) and give a statement. If the individual suffers from mental illness that precludes a voluntary, knowing, or intelligent waiver, then the individual is not competent to waive the rights and the court may preclude the statement from being used as evidence.

Certification/Decertification

State law has distinguished juvenile criminal offenders from adult offenders, with different possible legal outcomes. Although it varies by jurisdiction, typically the law provides that all persons under a certain age, usually under 14, will be treated as juveniles, regardless of the charges, and cannot be tried in adult criminal courts or sentenced to adult criminal facilities. All defendants age 18 or older are handled by the adult criminal courts. Those in the 14- to 17-year-old age range may be placed in either the juvenile or the adult system depending on various criteria. Typically, if the charge is homicide, the defendant will be tried in adult court unless the defense is able to get the defendant decertified to juvenile court. If the charge is anything except homicide, the charge will be tried in juvenile court unless the prosecution is able to get the defendant certified through adult court. This most often occurs when it is a serious violent crime such as assault, rape, or armed robbery.

Laws and changes in laws often reflect the current political climate. Because of increased concern in recent years over juvenile crime, some states are modifying these laws so that all felonies originate in adult court.

Whether the process is certification or decertification (in some states referred to as a "waiver"), the criteria the mental health professional must address are essentially the same: The defendant must be amenable to treatment, supervision, and rehabilitation within the time allotted by the statute, usually by age 19 or 21, and within existing juvenile treatment facilities. The law specifies other criteria as well, but these are demographic, such as the age of the defendant and whether there is a prior criminal record, and are not issues to be addressed by the mental health professional. The forensic psychologist addresses this issue by evaluating the defendant through interview and psychological testing. It is also important to review records, such as school records, as these may be relevant to the ability of the juvenile to be supervised. Offering an opinion on rehabilitation may be difficult, as this is essentially a prediction of further aggressive and/or criminal behavior. Such predictions are problematic, as will be discussed elsewhere in this chapter. Legal outcomes are also related to the political climate: With the growing incidence of violent juvenile crime, courts are increasingly inclined to try juveniles in adult court and to place them in adult criminal facilities. The reason is that in most states a juvenile must be released by age 21 or shortly thereafter, no matter what the crime. Thus, a 16-year-old who commits murder but is adjudicated a juvenile may have to be released in five years, whereas the same juvenile, if certified to adult court, could potentially receive a life sentence.

Mental State at the Time of the Offense

Most states and the federal government have insanity statutes that deal with the individual's responsibility or culpability at the time of the offense. Some states also have additional statutes regarding mental state at the time of the offense, which fall under the concepts of "diminished capacity" and "guilty but mentally ill." The definition of *insanity* under the law and the procedures for its application have changed over time, again often as a result of the political climate and attitudes toward offenders. There was a liberalizing trend in the statutes throughout the 1960s and 1970s so that more individuals met the criteria for "not guilty by reason of insanity" (NGRI) and received treatment rather than incarceration. Then, in 1982, John Hinckley was acquitted "by reason of insanity" for the attempted assassination of President Reagan. In reaction, both federal and state laws became much more conservative. Currently, most states utilize the M'Naghten rule, based on a case in England in 1843. The actual wording varies by jurisdiction but essentially is that at the time of committing the act the accused suffered from a mental disease or defect that prevented the accused from knowing the nature and quality of the act or, if the accused did know it, from knowing that what was done was wrong. Some jurisdictions use a broader criterion developed by the American Law Institute (ALI): The defendant can be found NGRI if the defendant did not appreciate the criminality or wrongfulness of the act or was substantially unable to conform the behavior to the requirements of law.

Media attention notwithstanding, the insanity defense is rarely raised and, when raised, is rarely successful. Packer (1987) reports that in Michigan only 0.09% of the adults arrested for serious crimes and only 1.7% of adults arrested for homicide were found NGRI. Most defendants are aware of the nature and quality of their acts, as this is usually

defined very concretely in terms such as knowing that they had a gun that fired bullets that could harm or kill another person. An NGRI finding is more likely to result when, because of mental illness, the defendant did not know that what was done was wrong. This most often arises when the defendant's actions are based on psychotic delusions and/or hallucinations, so that defendants believe that what they were doing was right and justified. A typical case is one in which a man had several years of mental health treatment and was diagnosed as paranoid schizophrenic. He came to believe that his 13-year-old daughter was possessed by the Devil and that, through her, the Devil was going to destroy the world. Auditory hallucinations of God's voice instructed him to kill the Devil and thus save the world. Laboring under this belief, he stabbed his daughter to death and was screaming, "I have saved the world!" as family members and a neighbor pulled him off his daughter. Mental health experts often look at the defendant's behavior following the act to reach an opinion regarding whether the individual recognized that what he or she was doing was wrong. Attempts at flight or concealment are tantamount to demonstrating that the defendant knew that what was done was wrong.

A defendant found NGRI is committed to a forensic mental hospital. The law requires periodic reevaluation for recommitment, typically once a year. Technically persons can be released at one of these hearings if it is determined that they are no longer dangerous as a result of their mental illness. However, the final decision is up to the court, which is not required to accept the opinions of the hospital staff or other mental health professionals. Typically, persons found NGRI are recommitted for many years. However, NGRI is an acquittal. Thus, the person can never be placed in prison, and a significant number do eventually return to the community, particularly those who have been found NGRI on less serious charges.

Diminished capacity generally applies only to attempted homicide and homicide and refers to the fact that the prosecution must prove all elements of the crime. One of the elements of first-degree murder is that the defendant had to have formed a "specific intent to kill." Where, because of mental illness or defect, the defendant lacked the capacity to form a specific intent, this is known as *diminished capacity,* and the defendant must, if the judge or jury accepts the testimony, be convicted of something less than first-degree murder. The lesser degree of murder also, of course, carries a shorter sentence. Consistent with the trend in insanity statutes, the diminished capacity statutes have gradually narrowed the definition so that today defendants rarely meet the criteria.

"Guilty but mentally ill" (GBMI) statutes exist in a number of states. The defendant is found guilty and receives the same sentence for the act as would an individual who was not deemed mentally ill. With GBMI, the court has determined that the defendant is responsible for the actions and did not meet the insanity criterion, but was also mentally ill. Often, the ALI insanity standard is used for findings of GBMI. The statutes provide for the defendant to be placed first in a mental hospital and treated. Once the mental illness is controlled, however, the person is then transferred to prison to serve the remainder of the sentence.

Some critics see the GBMI statute as an unfortunate compromise that deprives defendants of legitimate NGRI determinations. However, this statute also allows for presentation of testimony that would not be admissible under the stricter NGRI standard and may influence the degree of guilt found by the judge or jury. For example, a jury hearing of the defendant's mental illness may find the defendant guilty of second- or third-degree murder rather than first-degree murder even though the facts could have justified a first-degree conviction.

Sentencing and Disposition

Though receiving less media attention than issues of competency and insanity, it is in the penalty phase that mental health professionals are most often called on to provide input. Courts frequently turn to mental health professionals for recommendations on whether an individual requires mental health treatment and whether such treatment should involve hospitalization or outpatient treatment. Mental health professionals also may recommend treatment as a condition of probation or parole. Opinions are also elicited from the court regarding potential for suicidal and aggressive behavior and whether the defendant can withstand the stress of incarceration.

Death Penalty Mitigation

When a defendant is convicted of first-degree murder, the judge and/or jury must, in those states that have death penalty statutes, determine whether the sentence is imprisonment or the death penalty. Death penalty statutes contain lists of aggravating and mitigating circumstances that the jury must consider in determining the sentence (see Table 16.3). Mitigating circumstances include several mental state factors that the expert may address, such as whether the defendant was suffering from mental illness at the time of the offense. There is also an "other" category in which testimony may be presented on such issues as a history of learning disability or history of being physically or sexually abused as a child. There is a substantial literature indicating that the death penalty is applied in an arbitrary and discriminatory manner (Bohm, 1991).

EVALUATION IN PERSONAL INJURY AND OTHER CIVIL LAW CASES

Introduction

Personal injury lawsuits, in which an individual attempts to get monetary compensation for injuries, may arise from a number of sources. The most common are from automobile accidents and slip-and-fall accidents. Additional sources include any other kind of accident, such as bus, train, or plane. Another significant group involves suits by individuals or their family claiming injury or death from improper or negligent medical practices. In all these kinds of cases, evaluation of the physical injury is outside the expertise of the forensic psychologist and is the province of other experts. The psychologist can, however, evaluate the individual's response to the physical injuries and the resulting disabilities.

Psychological Damages

Most individuals who sustain a physical injury do not suffer a significant or diagnosable psychological reaction. No one likes to be sick or injured,

Table 16.3 Mitigating and Aggravating Factors in the Jury's Consideration of the Death Penalty

Mitigating

1. The defendant has no significant prior criminal convictions.
2. The defendant was under the influence of extreme mental/emotional disturbance.
3. The defendant has substantially impaired capacity to appreciate the criminality/wrongfulness of conduct or to conform conduct to requirements of law.
4. Age
5. The defendant acted under extreme duress or substantial domination of another person.
6. The victim was a participant in the defendant's homicidal conduct or consented to the homicidal acts.
7. The defendant's participation in homicidal acts was relatively minor.
8. Other (e.g., The defendant had a history of abuse as a child, or of substance abuse).

Aggravating

1. The victim was a firefighter, police officer, or public servant killed in performance of duties.
2. The defendant paid or was paid by another person in conspiring to kill the victim.
3. The victim was held by the defendant for ransom or as a shield or hostage.
4. Death occurred while the defendant was flying an aircraft.
5. The victim was a prosecution witness against the defendant.
6. The killing was committed in the course of the perpetration of another felony.
7. The defendant knowingly placed another person in grave risk of death in addition to the victim.
8. The offense was committed by means of torture.
9. The defendant has a history of felony convictions involving the use or threat of violence.
10. The defendant has been convicted of another offense for which a life sentence or death was imposed, or committed the offense while serving a life sentence.

but a normal or expected reaction to injury is not considered compensable. Rather, the person must sustain a reaction that is beyond the expected and of a degree of severity that causes significant impairment in social, occupational/academic, or other areas of functioning. Diagnostic judgments are made on the basis of criteria listed in the *Diagnostic and Statistical Manual of Mental Disorders,* fourth edition (DSM-IV)(1994).

The most common psychological diagnosis due to an injury is an Adjustment Disorder, defined as the development of emotional or behavioral symptoms in response to an identifiable stressor occurring within three months of the onset of the stressor. The symptoms may include depression, anxiety, a disturbance of conduct, or any combination of these. To some extent, the psychological reaction is related to the course of recovery from the physical injuries and disabilities. If the individual recovers physically and is able to resume all or most of the previous activities, then the psychological reaction usually disappears. In some cases, physical recovery is not complete, but the individual adjusts to the new partially disabled level of functioning and, again, the psychological reaction disappears.

Some people, however, experience symptoms that either do not fall into the Adjustment Disorder category or that persist either because the physical disabilities themselves persist or because something in the individual's psychological makeup causes the psychological symptoms to persist even when the physical symptoms have largely disappeared. For example, following an automobile accident some individuals develop a phobia for automobiles. Two important aspects of phobias are anxiety and avoidance, and either or both may be present. In such cases the individual is afraid to get back into a car or experiences marked anxiety when in a car. The result may be months or years of inability to travel by car, which, of course, can significantly impair social and occupational functioning. Others show an increase in generalized anxiety rather than a specific phobia. One category that is sometimes found is referred to as Post-Traumatic Stress Disorder (PTSD). Anxiety disorders may include panic attacks. When individuals experience increased anxiety, they often show associated difficulties with attention, concentration, and memory, which can interfere with life functions.

Another frequent reaction to physical injury is depression, which usually occurs if the individual does not experience the expected course of recovery. Frustration and anger also often accompany the depression. People who are severely depressed often have difficulty initiating and sustaining activities necessary to daily living, as well as social or occupational activities.

Any of these reactions also can lead to a loss of pleasure of life (Andrews, Meyer, & Berla, 1996).

Neuropsychological Damages

Individuals who are involved in accidents sometimes sustain damage to the brain. This most commonly occurs when the person strikes his or her head, for example against the car windshield. Although the severity of the traumatic brain injury may be correlated with the length of loss of consciousness, this is not necessarily the case. In fact, an individual may sustain brain injury without a loss of consciousness. Further, one does not even have to strike one's head to sustain brain injury: The whiplash effect that occurs in some accidents may cause the brain to hit the inside of the skull, causing injury to brain cells.

Forensic psychologists with specialized training in neuropsychology can assess the deficits due to traumatic brain injury. The normal course of recovery for what is called a closed-head injury (when damage to the brain results without skull fracture and without penetrating wounds of the brain) is 18 to 24 months. However, many people recover much more quickly. Whatever deficits remain after about 24 months are likely to be permanent and irreversible. Deficits from brain injury can affect memory, thinking, language, perception, orientation, and/or emotional control (Reitan & Wolfson, 1986).

Worker's Compensation/SSI

States have worker compensation laws that compensate for illnesses and injuries, including mental illnesses, suffered in the course of employment. However, applicants must prove that the work situation was responsible for the injury and/or the psychological reaction, although the process and criteria vary from state to state.

The Social Security Act awards benefits to those whose disability is based on psychiatric impairment as well as to those with physical impairments. Many people are not eligible for disability insurance because they have not earned sufficient coverage

from their tax payments based on employment. There is, therefore, a program known as Supplemental Security Income (SSI) available to those whose income falls below a certain level. To receive such benefits, applicants must provide a mental health evaluation indicating that they are disabled by virtue of a mental illness and therefore unable to work. The government often will require an independent examination to confirm or dispute the claim. Forensic psychologists are frequently called on to perform evaluations for both workers' compensation and SSI benefits.

Harassment/Discrimination

When an individual experiences harassment or discrimination in the workplace due to gender, race, age, ethnic background, or a special condition or disability (such as HIV), that person may develop a psychological reaction (McDonalds & Kulik, 1994). As with other "injuries," this most often takes the form of depression or anxiety. However, harassment and discrimination also often affect self-esteem, confidence, and the ability to trust others. Here, as in other forensic evaluations, it is important to assess the individual's functioning prior to the harassment and discrimination because the individual may have had psychological difficulties before that had nothing to do with the harassment/discrimination. However, it is also necessary to evaluate whether the harassment/discrimination caused preexisting problems to worsen and/or caused new problems that never would have existed except for the harassment/discrimination (Cooke, 1996). This kind of case is, however, different from one in which there is a clearly documented physical injury. In harassment/discrimination cases, there is usually no objective evidence that the alleged acts took place. Thus, the forensic psychologist, whether retained by the plaintiff (the person claiming the injury) or by the defendant (the business or its insurance company against whom the claim is directed) must not assume that the harassment/discrimination actually did or did not take place. That is up to a jury or a judge to decide, and the psychologist must frame opinions in terms of the individual's perception of harassment/discrimination.

Psychiatric/Psychological Malpractice

Mental health professionals have both ethical and legal responsibilities to the patients they treat. Psychiatric/psychological malpractice generally arises in three contexts: (1) The therapist becomes sexually involved with the patient, (2) the patient commits suicide and the family claims the therapist was negligent and/or failed to meet the "standard of care" for treatment, or (3) the patient harms or kills someone else and the same negligence/standard of care issues are raised.

No therapist should become sexually involved with any patient. It has long been recognized that many patients become sexually attracted to their therapist, but it is the responsibility of the therapist to deal with this attraction in a therapeutic manner (Williams, 1992). When a patient claims that the therapist has become sexually involved, there is rarely objective evidence. If the therapist denies the charge, the situation is similar to the harassment/discrimination situation discussed earlier, and the forensic psychologist must approach it in a similar manner. In these cases, however, because the patient has some type of mental or emotional difficulty or would not have been seeing a mental health professional in the first place, the issue of the patient's prior mental difficulties also is usually raised.

When a patient commits suicide, the family may bring what is called a wrongful-death suit. It is impossible to predict or prevent every suicide, but a therapist has a responsibility to monitor patients appropriately and to be aware of the signs of a potential suicide so as to take appropriate action. A therapist who fails to do this may be found to have failed to meet the standard of care. Wrongful-death suits also may arise from homicide or medical malpractice.

The patient who harms or kills another person raises the same issues as well as an additional one. Most states have statutes that define patient–therapist privilege. That is, the therapist is precluded from releasing any information about the patient to a third party without the patient's consent. But both a famous case on this issue, *Tarasoff v. Regents of the University of California* (1976), and many of the state statutes provide for a "dangerous patient exception" to the privilege, so that a therapist has a duty to warn and protect a specific third party who is in danger from the patient if the therapist has reason to reach that conclusion. For example, the therapist may have to contact the party who is in danger or even contact the local police department. The issue is then whether the therapist followed the standard of care in determining whether the third party needed to be warned or protected.

Malingering

Some individuals who are injured in an accident or otherwise may not really have significant resulting physical or psychological problems but, motivated by the possibility of compensatory monetary damages, may try to fake or exaggerate resulting problems. This is known as *malingering*. Forensic psychologists are always attuned to the possibility of malingering in any type of forensic case. For example, an accused murderer claiming insanity may be malingering. On the other hand, parents in a custody case often malinger in the opposite direction by denying or minimizing problems and trying to present themselves as perfectly well-adjusted individuals and wonderful parents.

The forensic psychologist approaches the possibility of malingering in a number of ways (Hall & Pritchard, 1996). First, mental illness, like physical illness, usually has a cluster of symptoms that go together and follows a certain course of development. When an individual reports symptoms that are not expected as part of that cluster or reports a course of the illness that is not what is expected, then the psychologist becomes suspicious of malingering. For example, anyone can say that he hears voices—that is, that he has auditory hallucinations—but psychologists are familiar with the kinds of conditions that can lead to auditory hallucinations and what forms such hallucinations usually take.

Another approach to evaluating malingering is through psychological testing. This is discussed in more detail in another section of this chapter and is also discussed elsewhere in this book. Some of the objective personality tests have certain scales that will show whether an individual is exaggerating or minimizing problems. Other tests, such as the Rorschach Inkblot Technique, are much more difficult to fake and may produce findings inconsistent with what the individual is claiming.

Civil Competency

Whenever an individual enters into a relationship with another individual or with society that implies a "contract," that individual must be competent to do so. Civil competency is different from criminal competency (Slovenko, 1987) as defined earlier in this chapter, although an aspect of civil competency, competency as witness in a trial, may apply to either civil or criminal proceedings. Every witness is presumed competent but may not be if mental illness has impaired his or her memory, ability to communicate, or understanding of the oath to tell the truth. Special concerns are raised with child witnesses and are particularly important when allegations of child sexual abuse are raised.

Another type of competency involves the competency of professionals, including psychologists, psychiatrists, other medical doctors, and attorneys, because of the implied or actual contract when the professional provides services. An individual also must be competent to enter into an actual contract, such as buying a house or making other purchases, and more generally must be competent to handle his or her own funds. Competency may come into question regarding individuals' ability to make decisions regarding their own medical or psychiatric/psychological care. For example, whether or not a patient has the right to refuse psychiatric medication depends, in part, on whether that individual is competent to make such decisions. If not, a guardian or court may make what is called a "substituted judgment." Finally, a person executing a will may lack "testamentary capacity" because of mental illness, progressive brain damage, or other causes.

EVALUATION IN CHILD CUSTODY CASES

The laws regarding the criteria under which legal and physical custody of children are decided have changed markedly over the years. Today, most states have some wording that incorporates what is in the "best interest of the child." Here, as elsewhere, translating the legal jargon into the behavioral and psychological factors is difficult and controversial. The American Psychological Association (1994) has formulated guidelines for custody evaluations, which include assessing the child's characteristics and needs and the capacities of each parent in order to determine which is the "best fit."

In almost all cases where custody is contested, each parent will end up having some time with the child. Only in cases of physical abuse, sexual abuse, or extreme emotional abuse is the court likely to preclude any visitation or partial custody. Even in these cases, the court has the option of supervised visitation for that parent, with the reasoning that the combination of contact and protection may be more in the child's best interest than no contact at all. *Legal custody* is distinguished from *physical custody*. Legal custody has to do with decision making in three major areas: education, medical care, and religious training. It is totally independent of the physical custody arrangement, and the court will almost always grant shared legal custody.

Physical custody has to do with the time the child spends with each parent. It can vary from only a few hours once a week for one parent to equally divided time. The "standard" arrangement in the past, whereby one parent, usually the mother, had primary custody and the father saw the child on alternate weekends and for a few hours one evening per week is no longer standard, although it still occurs. The courts have rejected the "tender years" doctrine, which held that a young child was better off with the mother, and courts now frequently award primary custody to fathers as well. Also, in a growing number of cases both parents must work, and the custodial arrangement is often fashioned around each parent's availability to the child. If the parents live in geographically separated areas, one parent often has the child during the school year and the other for the greater part of school vacations and most of the summer.

Equally shared, or joint, custody gained widespread acceptance in the late 1970s and 1980s. Under such an arrangement, time is split equally—for example, alternating weeks with each parent. This arrangement presumes that it is in the child's best interest to have as much time as possible with each parent. Research has suggested that this is the best arrangement when the parents are cooperative and the agreement is voluntary, but it may not be the best for the children where the parents are hostile and uncooperative and the arrangement is forced by the court. Each case must be evaluated on the basis of its specific characteristics. However, an overriding factor in considering what is best for the child involves an understanding that the best predictor of a child's future adjustment is the level of conflict between the parents.

The specific features vary widely from case to case. In some cases parents may suffer from mental illness or substance abuse problems. In some cases there are allegations of sexual or physical abuse, which may or may not be true. Some cases involve what has been called the Parent Alienation Syndrome, in which one parent deliberately and methodically turns the children against the other parent (Gardner, 1987). Children with certain problems, such as Attention Deficit Disorder with Hyperactivity, or with special medical needs, may have their needs best met by a parent who has certain personality characteristics and parenting attitudes and practices. Forensic psychologists may utilize not only general assessment procedures but also special measures of parenting knowledge, attitudes, and practices. Observation of parent–child interaction, either in a home visit or in the office, is also crucial.

EVALUATION IN CHILD SEX ABUSE CASES

Allegations of child sexual abuse are sometimes brought as part of the custody suit. Although every such allegation must be considered important and investigated thoroughly, it has been found that the greatest number of false allegations occur in the context of child custody cases (Cooke & Cooke, 1991). Allegations also occur in a variety of other contexts. Contrary to the concept of a weird-looking stranger, the person who sexually molests a child usually is known to the child. It may be a par-

ent, a stepparent, a grandparent, another relative, an older sibling or stepsibling, or a neighbor. There also have been cases, some of which have gained great media attention, in which one or more school or preschool teachers have been accused of sexually molesting a number of children in their care.

The short- and long-term effects on individuals who are sexually abused as children vary widely, with some showing little or no effect and others developing serious reactions at the time and longer term personality problems or mental illnesses (Briere, 1992). Thus, it is extremely important to identify cases of abuse, to protect children from abusers, and to treat and/or incarcerate the abusers. But there are multiple problems in addressing these issues. First, even outside the custody context, false accusations are brought. Second, although some child molesters fit certain psychological profiles, many show no clear psychological signs that they have such proclivities. Also, unless there is actual penetration, there is rarely conclusive medical evidence of abuse, so authorities must rely on psychological evaluation, including interviewing. But here, too, there are serious problems. Children's psychological reactions to abuse overlap with their psychological reactions to other stresses in their lives, such as parental divorce, separation from one parent, beginning school, and the like. An even greater problem is that young children are very prone to influence when interviewed. Usually the first interview of a child is by a parent, who may, understandably, be quite emotional and upset. Also, one would not expect a parent to follow the guidelines for interviewing a child in a nonleading fashion. The problem is often compounded when the first official interview is by a police officer, an assistant prosecutor, or a case worker for child protective services. Often, these people are not adequately trained. They tend to assume that the abuse occurred and conduct an interview to validate that assumption. In doing so, they may influence the child to report abuse that has not actually occurred.

Why is it important to sort out false from accurate reports of sexual abuse? First, the process of repeated evaluation of the child and possible appearance in court is often as traumatic as the abuse itself. Second, where the accused is an important person in the child's life, such as a parent, separation from that parent may be traumatic. Third, social service agencies have limited budgets, and it is important to direct resources where they are needed rather than squandering them on false cases. Finally, accused persons may lose their jobs, be forced to undergo treatment, or even go to prison. There is currently a controversy raging over whether, when released from prison, convicted child molesters should be placed in a special status requiring notification of police departments, schools, and neighbors in the communities to which they return to live.

Recently, a new type of situation has emerged in which adults claim to recall instances of child abuse that occurred many years before and of which they previously had no memory (Pezdek & Banks, 1996). It is well documented that a single traumatic incident may be repressed and therefore not remembered until something happens to trigger that memory years later. However, there is considerable controversy whether a person can repress repeated instances over many years, as is often claimed in these cases. In addition, frequently the memory has been encouraged by a therapist who believes that the patient's problems in adult life were due to child sexual abuse. The term False Memory Syndrome has emerged to describe these cases in which evaluators believe that the "remembered" abuse never actually occurred. Often the individuals who make such claims are bringing civil suit against a parent or other person, and it is important to sort out accurate from false memories. The damage done to the relationship between the adult child and the parents is also considerable, and repair of that relationship can begin only if the child comes to understand that the memory was false.

WORKING WITH POLICE

Forensic psychologists may consult with police departments in a number of roles (Reiser & Klyver, 1987). One such role is the psychological evaluation of applicants for the position of police officer and, in some departments, as part of the screening procedure for promotion to higher ranks. The psychological screening is usually one of the last steps in the selection process and is performed only for those who have already been otherwise accepted. Although there is some controversy over how the psychological evaluation is to be utilized, it is generally accepted that the role of the psychologist is *not* to decide who would make a good police officer. Rather, the role is to screen out those with psychological problems or personality characteristics that would interfere with the special job duties and functions of a police officer. Interviews and general batteries of psychological tests are often used, and there are also special tests that have been developed for use with police. The importance of evaluation of police officers arises because police officers have a great deal of power and carry weapons; if one abuses that power, the consequences to others can be harmful and even fatal.

Forensic psychologists also do training with police officers. Police officers are often the first "therapists" on the scene in an emergency. Many of the situations police officers deal with cannot be handled physically, and the officer must rely on what has been learned about the psychology of people and how to deal with them verbally. For example, police officers need to learn how to talk to a person threatening suicide. Training is also offered in dealing with potentially dangerous individuals, particularly in hostage negotiation situations. Police officers also are often called on to deal with domestic conflict situations. Despite the fact that statistically these are the most dangerous situations for police officers, the initial interaction is usually verbal and requires the police officer to be sensitive to the dynamics and the emotionality of the domestic conflict in order to best resolve it.

Police work is very stressful, not only because of the potential danger but also because rotating shifts can disrupt family life, and for other reasons as well. Police officers who are called on to use their weapons, particularly if a death results, may experience guilt and doubt. Thus, providing counseling for police officers is part of the role of forensic psychologists who have special training and/or experience in police work.

COMMITMENT OF MENTALLY ILL PERSONS

All jurisdictions have laws for the voluntary and involuntary commitment of mentally ill persons. Although the wording varies according to jurisdiction, the basic concept is that for a person to be commited involuntarily, he or she has to demonstrate that within a recent period of time, usually the last 30 days, he has been a danger to himself or to others or is unable to care for himself because of mental illness. The initial commitment is on an emergency basis for a limited period of time, usually 72 to 120 hours. Before that period expires, a hearing is conducted to determine whether the danger or inability to care for oneself continues. Only if that is the case is the next level of commitment certified. This is usually for another 20 to 30 days, at which time another hearing is held to extend the commitment further.

These hearings provide "due process" legal protection for the person being committed. Although the commitment is in theory for the person's "own good," it does involve a deprivation of freedom and civil liberties. In the past there have been abuses of commitment. A series of cases beginning in the 1960s defined the limits of a person's right to treatment and right to refuse treatment. One of the important principles that has developed is that the person should be treated in "the least restrictive alternative." For example, if possible, the person should be in an open ward rather than a locked ward, or in outpatient rather than inpatient treatment.

Depending on the jurisdiction, forensic psychologists may be called on to testify regarding the mental illness, the need for treatment, and the types of treatment recommended.

TREATMENT

In Prisons

Living in a prison setting has its own unique stresses (Mobley, 1987). Some individuals develop apathy, a loss of initiative and individuality, and a sense of social isolation. Others adopt the counter-cultural attitudes and values often associated with prison inmates. Both of these trends have implications for therapy in the prison setting. Forensic psychologists not only have to deal with the realities of prison structure, discipline, and stress, but also with these specific problems. In therapy, for example, the therapist generally encourages the patient to trust others and express feelings openly to them. But such trust and openness can be counterproductive in the prison setting. The goals of therapy also differ depending on the inmate's sentence. For an inmate serving a life sentence, the goal is to facilitate the best possible adjustment within the prison setting. For the "short-timer" who will soon be returning to the community, the focus is on reinstating and maintaining adaptive social relationships and avoiding situations or individuals that are likely to lead to recidivism.

In Forensic Psychiatric Units

The states and federal government have special forensic mental health facilities for treatment of both pretrial and convicted prisoners. Individuals charged with a crime who require evaluation of their competency to stand trial and/or treatment to return them to competency are usually housed in one area. Those who are committed from prison and/or those commited after a finding of "guilty but mentally ill" are usually housed in a separate area. Those found "not guilty by reason of insanity" may be housed in another separate area if the size of the facility allows.

Treatment of each of these groups has a different goal. Most of those who are being evaluated and treated for incompetency are suicidal or psychotic. They require medication and therapy. They also require special therapy focusing on teaching them about the legal system, pleas, and other matters specifically targeted to return them to competency. The goal of treatment for convicted prisoners and GBMIs is, if they still have a long sentence to serve, to return them to a level of functioning at which they are capable of being transferred to the prison, even if that is done while retaining them on medication. A major difficulty is that whereas mental health facilities can go through procedures to medicate patients involuntarily, prisons usually cannot or will not. Patients who lack insight into their illness and need for medication may discontinue the medication after return to prison, decompensate, and need to be rehospitalized. For those whose remaining sentences are short, the focus of treatment would be return to the community. The goal for NGRIs is initially to bring the illness and the potential danger into remission so that these patients can be transferred from the forensic facility to a civil facility and gradually be given more privileges and responsibilities as they improve. The eventual goal is return to the community, although this may take many years to accomplish.

Treatment on Probation and Parole

Treatment of ex-offenders in the community is sometimes essential to the prevention of recidivism, and is often made a condition of parole and probation. Unfortunately, most ex-offenders cannot afford private treatment, but go to the same community mental health centers that provide care for nonoffender populations. These therapists often are not experienced in working with offender populations or trained in their special needs. Also, ex-offenders may be manipulative, hostile, or poorly motivated for treatment. When they begin to miss appointments, the therapist may not actively try to get them back into treatment, which may result in a violation of parole or probation and/or in recidivism. Many ex-offenders have substance abuse problems and are required as a condition of parole or probation to go first to an inpatient drug and alcohol program and subsequently to an outpatient program instead of or in addition to other treatment.

Treatment of Involuntarily Committed Persons

The initial phase of treatment for these individuals usually takes place in an emergency mental health facility. If they are returned to the community after the brief emergency commitment, arrangements are made for appropriate outpatient treatment. For those who are recommitted or who voluntarily agree to remain hospitalized, some will go into state facilities and others will be transferred to private hospitals. The type of medication and/or therapy will depend on the nature of the problem.

Personal Injury and Other Civil Cases

The types of disorders that result from physical and emotional injuries were discussed earlier in this chapter. Treatment may be afforded to the individual by private health insurance or from the defendant's insurance company. Most often the treatment is provided by private practitioners or clinics. Although the treatment will vary depending on the type of problem, cognitive and behavioral therapies are often used in conjunction with techniques such as biofeedback to deal with depression, anxiety, and pain. These therapies, unlike traditional talking therapies, usually do not involve investigation of childhood or other past feelings or experiences, but focus on the current symptoms and ways of modifying them.

Custody and Child Sexual Abuse Cases

A therapist working with a child in such cases must strike a delicate balance between protecting the privilege and the trust in the relationship with the child and the need to work with the other members of the family. With very young children, the primary intervention involves aiding the parents in their parenting practices. Special play therapy techniques, along with other therapy and behavioral techniques, are used with children. In some of these cases, the focus of therapy is reuniting a child with a parent from whom the child has been separated or alienated.

TESTING AND ASSESSMENT

Information on psychological tests is presented in other chapters and will be discussed only briefly here. Depending on the nature of the case, the forensic psychologist may utilize intelligence and memory tests, neuropsychological batteries for the evaluation of brain dysfunction, and objective and/or projective personality tests. Some tests such as the

Minnesota Multiphasic Personality Inventory—2 (MMPI-2)(1989) are particularly valuable in forensic cases because they have *validity scales* that reflect whether the individual is presenting emotional difficulties in a candid manner, is exaggerating or falsifying pathology, or is being guarded and defensive and minimizing even common faults and problems.

There are also specialized forensic tests (Grisso, 1986), which usually consist of checklists derived from the psychological and behavioral criteria for the particular legal issue. Items on the checklist are given weight, and cutoff scores are defined beyond which the individual is considered to meet the standard for that legal issue. Such measures exist for criminal competency and criminal responsibility (insanity). For use in custody cases, there are also specialized tests for "parental competency" and for children's perceptions of parents. The utility of these specialized tests is controversial because of methodological problems in the construction of the tests and problems in assessing their validity.

PREDICTION OF FUTURE AGGRESSIVE AND SEXUAL BEHAVIOR

Either directly or indirectly, forensic psychologists are regularly called on to predict future dangerous behavior. Questions about whether an individual needs to be hospitalized or can be placed on probation involve predicting dangerous behavior. Clinical research has questioned the ability of mental health professionals to make such predictions with adequate accuracy. Both the American Psychological Association and the American Psychiatric Association have expressed concern about mental health professionals engaging in such prediction. Yet courts, including the United States Supreme Court, have continued to rely on mental health professionals to aid them in making decisions that involve prediction.

In recent years the methodology for prediction has improved considerably (Menzies, Webster, McMain, Staley, & Scaglione, 1994). This methodology distinguishes the motivation for the offense and offender, the presence and recency of a history of violence, and the presence or absence of current verbalized intentions to commit violent acts. This methodology helps to define categories of individuals for whom predictions can be made more reliably and validly, but much more research and clinical work is needed. The growing frequency of violence in the workplace in recent years has prompted emphasis on special methodology for its assessment. This often involves protocols that include not only the standard test and historical predictors of aggressive behavior, but also focus on the individual's history, relationships, and attitude within the particular company or workplace.

Prediction of future sexual behavior has become even more important in the context of recent changes in sexual offender laws. Such laws attempt to define who are high-risk offenders and attempt either to have them kept for treatment beyond the statutory sentence for their crime, or to have notification of police, schools, and neighbors upon release (Schopp & Sturgis, 1995). Although the constitutionality of such laws has yet to be resolved, the other important issue is the ability of mental health professionals, courts, and correctional personnel to make such predictions about risk.

NONCLINICAL FORENSIC PSYCHOLOGY

There are several major areas of research within nonclinical forensic psychology. One of these is the study of eyewitness testimony. Our judicial system relies heavily on eyewitness testimony. However, many studies of the factors affecting human memory, face recognition, cross-racial identification, and the like have demonstrated that eyewitness testimony is quite fallible (Wells & Loftus, 1984).

Another area of study involves jury selection, dynamics, and decision-making processes. Scientific jury selection may involve extensive surveys to find the characteristics of jurors favorable to the defense or prosecution in a criminal case, or to the plaintiff or defendant in a civil case. Knowledge of jury dynamics is grounded in social psychology and the study of interpersonal influence.

Human factors engineering deals with adapting machinery and the work environment to human physical and psychological needs. For example, an individual injured by a piece of machinery may sue the maker of the machinery claiming that the warnings and safeguards were inadequate. Nonclinical forensic psychologists specializing in human factors engineering would be called on to conduct experiments and/or offer opinions on these issues.

THE FORENSIC PSYCHOLOGIST AS CONSULTANT TO ATTORNEYS AND AS EXPERT WITNESS

When a forensic psychologist is retained by an attorney, the role often involves not only a review of records and evaluation of the client, but also consultation with the attorney on a variety of issues. The forensic psychologist may be asked, for example, whether trial by judge or jury would be preferable, whether the client should testify, and how to prepare and present the psychologist's testimony. The forensic psychologist's initial commitment to the attorney is to conduct an evaluation. After that is done, the psychologist communicates the findings, and the attorney and client decide whether testimony would be helpful to the case. If so, then the psychologist will be called as an expert witness.

Testimony is often traumatic for the expert who is new to the courtroom. The psychologist must prepare individually and also with the attorney. This preparation (unless the psychologist is an independent court-appointed evaluator, as is often the case in custody litigation) is perfectly ethical. The psychologist needs to know what questions the attorney will ask, and the attorney needs to know what the psychologist's answers will be.

The purpose of cross-examination of the expert by the opposing attorney is to weaken the credibility and the basis for the opinion in the eyes of the judge or jury. The forensic psychologist should recognize this and not view the cross-examination as a personal attack. Although the psychologist is usually retained by one side in litigation, once the psychol-

ogist is testifying, the role should be that of an educator of the judge or jury, not of an advocate.

LEGAL/ETHICAL ISSUES

Privilege/Confidentiality

As described earlier in this chapter, whether privilege applies in an evaluation depends on the type of case and on who has retained the psychologist. Privilege also applies to treatment unless it is court-ordered and part of the order requires reporting back to the court. The privilege in therapy belongs to the client, not to the therapist. That is, the decision whether or not to release information to a third party lies with the patient. The therapist can neither release information nor refuse to release information if it is counter to the wishes of the patient. In most cases the patient must provide the therapist with a release of information in writing before the therapist will release information. However, the therapist may breech the privilege under special conditions, such as the dangerous patient exception discussed earlier in this chapter. If the client calls the therapist to testify in a trial, that also constitutes a waiver of the privilege.

Definition of the Client

In criminal and personal injury cases, the client is the attorney who retains the psychologist, although the psychologist always has an ethical and legal responsibility for the welfare of the person being evaluated, no matter which side retained the psychologist. In custody cases, however, if all parties participate, it does not matter which side retains the psychologist or which side paid for the evaluation. The child is always the client, and therefore information is released about what is in the best interest of the child whether or not the opinion favors the parent who retained the psychologist.

Ethical Guidelines

The American Psychological Association publishes ethical guidelines for psychologists and specialty guidelines for forensic psychology (1991).

The guidelines specify that psychologists must not enter into conflicting or multiple roles, must not practice outside the areas of their knowledge, and must not abuse the power they hold as evaluators and/or therapists. The guidelines also describe and define privilege and other duties to clients.

FUTURE TRENDS IN FORENSIC PSYCHOLOGY

Throughout this chapter situations have been described in which it was noted that further research is needed. These areas are likely where future trends will focus. The issue of prediction of future aggressive and sexual behavior, including violence in the workplace (Feldman & Johnson, 1996), is of primary importance. Further work on distinguishing false from true accounts of child sexual abuse is needed. As technology, particularly computers, expands into every aspect of our lives, new issues of damage and confidentiality will arise.

Future trends will also involve the development of new treatment techniques. Crime, particularly violent crime, is a major societal problem. Evaluative and therapeutic interventions need to be developed not only for those already charged with crimes, but also to identify and treat, within legal constraints, those who are potential offenders. New techniques need to be developed to treat the psychological problems underlying child sexual abuse, as the rates of recidivism in this area are quite high.

REFERENCES

American Psychiatric Association. (1994). *Diagnostic and statistical manual of mental disorders* (4th ed.) (DSM-IV). Washington, DC: Author.

American Psychological Association. (1991.) Specialty guidelines for forensic psychologists. *Law and Human Behavior, 15*, 655–685.

American Psychological Association. (1992). Ethical principles of psychologists and code of conduct. *American Psychologist, 47*, 1597–1611.

American Psychological Association. (1994). Guidelines for child custody evaluations in divorce proceedings. *American Psychologist, 49*, 677–680.

Andrews, P., Meyer, R. G., & Berla, E. P. (1996.) Development of the Lost Pleasure of Life Scale. *Law and Human Behavior, 21*, 99–111.

Bohm, R. M (Ed.). (1991). *The death penalty in America: Current research*. Cincinnati: Anderson.

Briere, J. (1992). *Child abuse trauma: Theory and treatment of the lasting effects*. Newbury Park, CA: Sage.

Cooke, G. (1996). The role of the mental health professional in harassment/discrimination cases: A moderate perspective. *American Journal of Forensic Psychology, 14*, 37–48.

Cooke, G., & Cooke, M. (1991). Dealing with sexual abuse allegations in the context of custody evaluations. *American Journal of Forensic Psychology, 9*, 55–67.

Cooper, J., Bennett, E. A., & Sukel, H. L. (1996). Complex scientific testimony: How do jurors make decisions? *Law and Human Behavior, 20*, 379–394.

Daubert v. Merrell Dow Pharaceuticals, Inc., 113 S.Ct. 2786 (1993).

Dusky v. U.S., 362 U.S. 402 (1960).

Feldman, T. B., & Johnson, P. W. (1996). Workplace violence: A new form of lethal aggression. In H. V. Hall (Ed.), *Lethal violence 2000* (pp. 311–338). Kamuela, HI: Pacific Institute for the Study of Conflict and Aggression.

Frye v. U.S., 293 F. 1013 (D.C. Cir. 1923).

Gardner, R. A. (1987). *The parent alienation syndrome and the differentiation between fabricated and genuine child sex abuse*. Cresskill, NJ: Creative Therapeutics.

Grisso, T. (1986). Competency to stand trial. In T. Grisso, *Evaluating competencies* (pp. 62–112). New York: Plenum Press.

Grisso, T., & Siegel, B. A. (1986). Assessment of competency to stand criminal trial. In W. J. Curan, A. L. McGarry, & S. A. Shah (Eds.), *Forensic psychiatry and psychology* (pp. 145–166). Philadelphia: Davis.

Hall, H. V., & Pritchard, D. A. (1996). *Detecting malingering and deception*. Delray Beach FL: St. Lucie.

Jackson v. Indiana, 406 U.S. 715 (1972).

Jenkins v. U.S., 307 F.2d 637 (D.C. Cir. 1962).

McDonald, J. J., & Kulick, F. B. (Eds.). (1994). *Mental and emotional injuries in employment litigation*. Washington, DC: Bureau of National Affairs.

Menzies, R., Webster, C. D., McMain, S., Staley, S., & Scaglione, R. (1994). The dimensions of dangerousness revisted: Assessing forensic predictions about violence. *Law and Human Behavior, 18*, 1–28.

Metton, O. (1987). Training in psychology and law. In I. B. Weiner & A. K. Hess (Eds.), *Handbook of forensic psychology* (pp. 681–698). New York: Wiley.

Milan, A. M., & Evans, J. H. (1987). Intervention with incarcerated offenders. In I. B. Weiner & A. K. Hess

(Eds.), *Handbook of forensic psychology* (pp. 557–601). New York: Wiley.

Minnesota Multiphasic Personality Inventory—2. (1989). Minneapolis: University of Minnesota Press.

Miranda v. Arizona, 384 U.S. 218 (1973).

Mobley, M. J. (1987). Psychotherapy with criminal offenders. In I. B. Weiner & A. K. Hess (Eds.), *Handbook of forensic psychology* (pp. 602–629). New York: Wiley.

Packer, I. K. (1987). Homicide and the insanity defense: A comparison of sane and insane murderers. *Behavioral Sciences and the Law, 5,* 25–35.

Pezdek, K., & Banks, W. P. (1996). *The recovered memory/false memory debate.* San Diego, CA: Academic Press.

Reiser, M., & Klyver, N. (1987). Consulting with police. In I. B. Weiner & A. K. Hess (Eds.), *Handbook of forensic psychology* (pp. 437–459). New York: Wiley.

Reitan, R., & Wolfson, D. (1986). *Traumatic brain injury.* Tucson: Neuropsychology Press.

Schopp, R. F., & Sturgis, B. J. (1995). Sexual predators and legal mental illness for civil commitment. *Behavioral Sciences and the Law, 13,* 437–458.

Slovenko, R. (1987). Civil competency. In E. B. Weiner & A. K. Hess (Eds.), *Handbook of forensic psychology* (pp. 188–201). New York: Wiley.

Tarasoff v. Regents of the University of California, 17 Cal. 3d 425, S. Ct. Cal., 1976.

Wells, G. L., & Loftus, E. F. (Eds.). (1984). *Eyewitness testimony.* Cambridge: Cambridge University Press.

Wells, G. L., & Seelau, E. P. (1995). Eyewitness identification: Psychological research and legal policy on lineups. *Psychology, Public Policy and Law, 1,* 765–791.

Williams, M. H. (1992). Exploitation and inference: Mapping the damage from therapist–patient sexual involvement. *American Psychologist, 47,* 412–421.

Winick, B. J. (1995). The side effects of incompetency labeling and implications for mental health law. *Psychology, Public Policy and Law, 1,* 6–42.

FOR FURTHER READING

Brodsky, S. L. (1991). *Testifying in court: Guidelines and maxims for the expert witness.* Washington, DC: American Psychological Association.

Ceci S. J., & Bruck, M. (1995). *Jeopardy in the courtroom: A scientific analysis of children's testimony.* Washington, DC: American Psychological Association.

Hill, H. V., & Pritchard, P. A. (1996). *Detecting malingering and deception.* Delray Beach, FL: St. Lucie Press.

Weiner, I. B., & Hess, A. K. (Eds.). (1987). *Handbook of forensic psychology.* New York: Wiley.

GLOSSARY

A-B-A design: See *Reversal design*.

Abreaction: The expression of emotions that, if harbored, lead to neurotic symptoms.

Acculturation: The process whereby a person socialized in another culture adapts to and learns to cope with a culture that is new and different to him or her.

Achievement test: A test designed to measure the degree of past learning in a subject matter.

Action potential: The chain reaction of events that involves the temporary loss or reversal of polarization at a segment of the axon for a micromoment and initiates the same repeating sequence of events in the immediately adjacent portion of the axon, ultimately resulting in neurotransmitter release from the nerve terminal.

Actuarial judgment: The kind of judgment in which an empirically derived formula is used to diagnose or predict behavior.

Adaptive behavior: The personal independence and social responsibility exhibited by an individual relative to the norm of their appropriate age group.

Adenosine triphosphate (ATP): A vital cellular energy molecule that powers many biochemical reactions within cells.

Age-equivalent scores: Scores representing the average performance of a child at a particular age in the normative sample.

Akathisia: A medication-induced (typically by neuroleptics) objective or subjective feeling of motor restlessness or anxiety.

Akinesia: A medication-induced (typically by neuroleptics) decrease in motor movements, rigidity, or apathy.

Alpha: The probability of committing a Type I error.

Alienation from school: A student's lack of a sense of belonging to the school.

Alternate-form reliability: The degree to which two different forms of the same test obtain similar results.

American Psychological Association (APA): The largest professional organization for psychologists in the United States.

Amnesia: Lack of memory for a period surrounding an event. It may be caused by mental illness, substance intoxication, or head injury.

Aptitude test: A test designed to measure specific abilities or general ability (intelligence).

Assertive case management: Also know as intensive case management or assertive community treatment (ACT): Case management where the caseload is small enough that the case manager can provide intensive support to the clients.

Assessment: Appraisal of a person's characteristics, strengths, and weaknesses as a basis for informed decision making.

Attorney–client privilege: A rule of law indicating that what a client says to his or her attorney is privileged/confidential and does not have to be revealed.

Attrition: Loss of subjects from a study, either during the active phase of the study or during follow-up.

Autonomy: The ethical standard stating that individuals have the right to decide what will happen to them. It is based on the Nuremberg Code and the Declaration of Helsinki. Autonomy implies free consent and informed consent, and requires the respect of people's ability and right to choose freely their own courses of action.

Autotroph: Organism that is able to synthesize all the organic molecules it needs for survival from inorganic substances and some form of energy such as sunlight.

Axon and terminal: The transmitting neurofilaments of neurons. Electrochemical impulses called action potentials travel down the axon, resulting in the release of neurotransmitters from the terminal area, where it is stored in discrete packages called vesicles. The axon terminals are small knoblike swellings sometimes referred to as *boutons,* from the French for "button." The terminal is synonymous with the presynaptic membrane.

Before–after trial: A quasi-experimental design in which people are evaluated before and after an intervention. Also called a one-group pretest/posttest study.

Behavioral assessment: A variety of approaches to assessment that focus on behavior itself rather than on inferred traits or causes of behavior.

Behavioral medicine: The application of behavioral science to prevent, diagnose, and treat illness and disease.

Behavioral rating scale: A scale that is used to rate behavior directly (e.g., present vs. absent) or along a dimension (e.g., never, occasionally, fairly often, all the time).

Behavior therapy: A model of psychotherapy based on concepts and methods derived from social learning theory, operant conditioning, and classical conditioning. Individuals are taught to modify pathological behavior in direct ways.

Beneficence: The ethical principle that requires the prevention of harm, the removal of harm, and the provision of benefit.

Best interest of the child: The current standard by which the court determines a child custody arrangement.

Beta: The probability of committing a Type II error .

Bias: Any factor, other than the intervention, which could affect the results of a study by acting more on one group than on the other—for example, if more disturbed patients are assigned to the treatment group than to the placebo group.

Biomolecules: Molecules that make up living matter. These are mostly proteins, carbohydrates, lipids, and nucleic acids.

Blended family: A family unit containing children with different biological parents living together as step-siblings with one parent married to an adult not related to all the children.

Boundaries: The parameters, or limits, of a professional relationship. The concept of boundaries helps define the behaviors that are or are not appropriate in a given relationship.

Boundary crossings: Behaviors that are not characteristics of a professional relationship.

Boundary violations: Harmful boundary crossings.

Brief dynamic therapy: Therapies generally distinguished by the selection of motivated, functional patients; the use of transference and countertransference; the confrontation and interpretation of focal, intrapsychic conflict; and emphasis on the psychological importance of termination.

Brief therapy: Therapy characterized by the planned use of specific concepts and principles in a focused, purposeful way. It emphasizes efficiency as well as efficacy. Underlying its variety of approaches, BT shares a set of clinical features and a value orientation.

Centrosomes: Organelles that play an important role in distributing chromosomes during cell division.

Cerebrospinal fluid (CSF): A fluid that circulates through and around the brain and spinal cord.

Certification/decertification (waiver): A process of moving a criminal defendant under the age of 18 from adult to juvenile court or vice versa.

Child abuse: The physical or sexual abuse or neglect of a child under the age of 18 by the parent or other person responsible for the welfare of the child.

Chorea: A movement disorder characterized by irregular and dancelike involuntary movements of various muscle groups.

Civil commitment: Procedures under civil law by which an individual may voluntarily or involuntarily be hospitalized. Involuntary hospitalization requires that the person be suffering from mental illness, a danger to self or others, or unable to care for self.

Civil competency: The capacity to manage one's own person and/or property.

Classical conditioning: Learning by association in which the probability of a response to a conditioned stimulus is increased as a result of pairings of that stimulus with an unconditioned stimulus.

Client–centered therapy: Also known as person-centered or nondirective therapy, this approach was developed by Carl Rogers, Ph.D. It emphasizes the reflection by the therapist of the client's feelings and experiences, in order to help the client grow beyond present psychological limitations.

Clinical diagnosis: Assessment of an individual in terms of the categories and concepts of the *Diagnostic and Statistical Manual of Mental Disorders, Fourth Edition* (DSM-IV).

Clinical judgment: The kind of judgment in which the clinician processes information in his or her head to diagnose or predict behavior.

Clinical psychology: The field that integrates science, theory, and practice to understand, predict, and alleviate maladjustment, disability, and discomfort as well as to promote human adaptation, adjustment, and personal development. Clinical psychology focuses on the intellectual, emotional, biological, psychological, social, and behavioral aspects of human functioning across the life span, in varying cultures and at all socioeconomic levels.

Coefficient alpha: An index of reliability based on internal consistency of scale items.

Cognitive-behavioral therapy: An approach to psychotherapy that integrates cognitive and behavioral techniques (see separate definitions).

Cognitive therapy: Largely developed by Aaron Beck, M.D., and Albert Ellis, Ph.D., this is an approach to psychotherapy that emphasizes the identification and correction of inaccurate and irrational ways of thinking.

Cohort study: See *Nonequivalent control study.*

Collaboration: The process of establishing treatment goals and outcomes that are satisfactory to patients. The therapist is in charge of the collaboration.

[a]**Collectivism:** "[P]ertains to societies in which people from birth onward are integrated into

[a]See references for Chapter 15.

strong, cohesive in groups which throughout people's lifetime continue to protect them in exchange for unquestioning loyalty" (Hofstede, 1991, p. 51).

Common (therapeutic) factors: The universal variables that have been linked to change in most systems of psychotherapy.

Community psychology: Branch of psychology that focuses on social issues, social institutions, and other settings that influence groups and organizations as well as the individuals in them. The primary goal of community psychology is to optimize the well-being of communities and their citizens with innovative and alternative interventions .

Compliance: Following the treatment recommendations of the therapist and maintaining the mutually agreed on commitments of therapy. This term is often used interchangeably with *adherence* and includes (among others) attending therapy, taking prescribed medication, and completing homework assignments.

Concurrent validity: A type of criterion-related validity in which the criterion measures are obtained at about the same time as the test scores.

Conditioned response: The response to a conditioned stimulus caused by pairing of the conditioned stimulus with an unconditioned stimulus.

Conditioned stimulus: A stimulus that elicits a response when paired with an unconditioned stimulus.

Confidentiality: The ethical rule of keeping disclosures private.

Confucian dynamism: A cultural characteristic based on adherence to precepts of the Chinese philosopher Confucius. It emphasizes acceptance of parental and other legitimate authority; promotes perseverance, effort, and thrift; and affirms the family-like character of the economic, social, and political organizations. Though explicitly based on Chinese values, Confucian dynamism has been found to be applicable in and comparable across other cultures.

Conjoint therapy: Two or more family members seen together in a psychotherapy session.

Construct validity: A type of validity that refers to the appropriateness of test-based inferences about the construct presumably measured by a test.

Content validity: A type of validity that refers to

the test items being representative of the behaviors that the test was designed to sample.

Countertransference: The unfolding of various thoughts, feelings, attitudes, and emotions toward the client by the therapist.

Criminal competency: A determination of whether a defendant understands the nature and object of the proceedings against him or her and can aid the attorney in the defense.

Criterion-referenced test: A test in which the objective is to determine where an examinee stands with respect to clearly defined educational objectives.

Criterion-related validity: A type of validity that is demonstrated when a test is shown to be effective in estimating an examinee's performance on an appropriate outcome measure.

[a]**Culture:** In addition to Herskovits's (1949) definition given in Chapter 15, culture is represented "first, as a combination of both social and material products of humankind; second, as already being there when the individual arrives in the world; and third, as more than all that is in the minds of individuals " (Moghaddam et al., 1993, p. 2).

Culture accommodations: A series of procedures whereby the preferences, needs, expectations, and conceptions pertaining to mental disorder and psychological problems are taken into account in designing and implementing mental health services in a culture in which they were not available.

Culture-bound syndromes: Patterns or groups of psychiatric symptoms that have been found to occur exclusively or predominantly within a cultural or ethnic group, in a delimited geographic area, or in a specific region of the world.

Culture shock: A psychological reaction compounded of distress and helplessness that has been found to occur among migrants, sojourners, and visitors upon their contact with or immersion into a new and different culture.

Cytoplasm: All of a cell's protoplasm except its nucleus; the living matter within a cell between its outer membrane and its nucleus.

Cytoskeleton: Microscopically thin protein threads, fibers, and tubules that function to help the cell keep its shape, anchor its organelles,

direct the flow of internal chemical traffic, and in some cases aid in motility.

Deception: Purposely lying to research subjects about the nature of or reason for a study.

Declaration of Helsinki: A series of ethical standards, following the Nuremberg Code, detailing the rights of subjects in human experiments.

Defendant: In civil law, the individual or group against whom the plaintiff makes a claim; in criminal law, an individual charged with a crime.

Deinstitutionalization: The process of moving the mentally disordered from institutions and hospitals to the community.

Dendrites: The receptive neurofilaments of neurons, containing receptors where neurotransmitters bind; also referred to as the *postsynaptic membrane*.

***Diagnostic and Statistical Manual of Mental Disorders, Fourth Edition* (DSM-IV):** A manual, prepared by the American Psychiatric Association in conjunction with other groups, which lists the criteria for different mental illnesses.

Diathesis–stress model of illness: A *diathesis* is a genetically based, constitutional predisposition toward a particular disease or disorder. *Stress*, in this context, refers to any environmental factor or circumstance that may have a negative impact on one's body and thus trigger the disease.

Diminished capacity: In state law, applies to psychological states that can reduce the level of homicide. In federal law, a psychological state that contributed to the crime and can be the basis for the judge in sentencing the defendant to less than the federal sentencing guidelines.

Diplomate: One who has passed written and/or oral tests of a specialty board. This informs the public of a level of competence in the specialty.

Disengagement: Occurs when inflexible family boundaries give too much independence and not enough support.

Due process: A process generated by the Constitution ensuring that every individual has certain rights under the law and access to the procedures to obtain those rights.

Dystonia: A medication-induced contraction of muscles (typically head, neck, jaws, or limbs), which may be brief or prolonged.

Ecological perspective: The perspective that recognizes that there exists a transaction between people and settings. Individuals influence the

[a]See references for Chapter 15.

settings in which they find themselves; settings influence the individuals in them.

Effectiveness: Whether an intervention will work with the types of patients and procedures encountered in actual practice. See *Efficacy*.

Effect size: The magnitude of the difference in outcome between the experimental and control groups, expressed in standard deviation units.

Efficacy: Whether an intervention can work under ideal circumstances. See *Effectiveness*.

Electroencephalography (EEG): A method utilizing electrodes placed on the scalp to measure the gross electrical activity of the brain. The actual instrument is the electroencephalograph and the brain graphic tracings it produces is the electroencephalogram.

Emic: An approach that emphasizes the unique character of each culture's phenomena and characteristics and promotes their study within the culture, on the basis of that culture's concepts.

Empathy: The process whereby a person's thoughts, feelings, and emotions are understood from that person's point of view, are so experienced on the affective plane, and are then communicated to the person.

Empowerment: The process of enhancing the possibility that people can more actively control their own lives.

Enacted support: The availability of actual support and the concrete actions others perform when they render assistance.

Endoplasmic reticulum: A network of interconnecting flattened sacs, tubes, and channels within a cell's cytoplasm, involved in the synthesis of various biomolecules and some detoxification processes.

Enmeshment: Occurs when family boundaries are diffuse or unclear, often restricting autonomy.

Epidemiology: Technique that examines the occurrence and distribution of health-related conditions in populations.

Ethical dilemma: A situation in which two or more courses of action can be justified by ethical principles.

Ethical guidelines: Guidelines set down by a professional organization regarding what constitute proper and appropriate arrangements and procedures.

Ethical imperialism: The imposition of Western ethical standards on cultures or groups that have different mores and beliefs.

Ethics of care: An orientation to professional ethics that is based on the internal characteristics of professional relationships, rather than on the imposition of external, abstract principles.

Etic: An orientation that emphasizes the universality of psychological and social phenomena and encourages their investigation and comparison across two or more cultures.

Eugenics: The selective breeding of human beings to improve the species.

Eukaryote: A cell having a membrane-bound nucleus and membrane-bound organelles.

Excitatory postsynaptic potential (EPSP) A depolarizing stimulus that increases the likelihood that the receiving neuron will "fire" or initiate an action potential.

Existential therapy: An approach to psychotherapy that incorporates attention to limitations to existence (death, separation, fate) that all persons face.

Experiential psychotherapy: A system that focuses on the patient's immediate emotional and physical state as the critical ingredients in change.

Expert witness: One who by training or experience can provide information to the court that would not normally be known to the lay person, and can provide the court with assistance in addressing certain issues.

Exposure: The gradual engagement with feared stimuli and events that leads to change. A process that is crucial in most therapies.

External validity: The degree to which a causal relationship seen in a study can be generalized to other settings, persons, times, and outcome measures.

Extrapyramidal side effects (EPS): Side effects most common after initiation of neuroleptic therapy. Examples include dystonia, akathisia, and pseudo-Parkinsonism.

Factor analysis: A group of statistical procedures used to summarize relationships and identify underlying factors that account for the interrelationships among several variables.

False memory syndrome: The term applied to the "remembering" of events that actually never happened. Usually applies to "recovered memories" of child sexual abuse.

Family of origin: The family in which one was raised.

Fidelity: The ethical rule of promise keeping.

Fiduciary relationship: A relationship characterized by trust; the client needs to trust the professional on the basis of the professional's expert knowledge.

File drawer problem: Because there is a bias toward publishing only studies which show statistical significance, many studies with null results may be buried in files, which could affect the results of any meta-analyses.

Forensic: Having to do with legal matters.

Free consent: The ethical standard that people should not be coerced, either overtly or covertly, into participating in a study. See also *Informed consent*.

Functional analysis: A behavioral assessment tool that suggests that the clinician identify antecedent and consequential behaviors relating to the presenting behaviors.

Gestalt therapy: A model of therapy that uses imagery, role playing, and other techniques to help the patient encounter deeply buried feelings and bodily states. Introduced by Fritz Perls, M.D.

Golgi bodies: Small groups of flattened membrane-bound sacs stacked loosely on one another that modify, package, and distribute cells' secretory products as well as distribute and recycle their membranes.

Grade equivalent scores: Represent the average performance of a child at particular grade level in the reference group.

Group therapy: Psychotherapy in which several people participate together in the treatment process at the same time with the therapist, and are helped by both the therapist and one another.

Half-life: The time taken for the concentration of a compound in a tissue to decrease by 50%.

Hawthorne effect: The change in performance or behavior of subjects in a study due simply to the fact that they know they are in a study, and not caused by the intervention itself.

Health psychology: The area of psychology that studies how psychological factors influence health, illness, and health-related behaviors. An emphasis is placed on prevention of behaviors that exacerbate and/or contribute to poor health.

Heterotroph: Organisms that cannot synthesize all their needed organic compounds and so must feed on organic materials found in the external environment.

Historical controls: A control group consisting of people who were diagnosed or treated at some time in the past.

Homework: Assignments designed to facilitate progress between sessions. Broadly considered, it develops skills or disturbs the system in which clients function and in which they are presumably "stuck."

Humanistic psychotherapy: A collective term that describes those therapies (experiential, existential, Gestalt, and client-centered) that emphasize as goals the enhancement of the person's full potential.

Hysteria: Derived from the Greek word for womb, hysteria was originally thought to be a woman's complaint. Especially in the late nineteenth century, physicians were intrigued with the myriad of symptoms thought to constitute hysteria, including seizures and paralysis. Other symptoms range from specific physical distress, such as headaches and feelings of numbness, to more generalized distress such as depression and extreme fatigue. Freud's earliest major work was entitled *Studies in Hysteria*.

Illusory validation: A phenomenon in projective testing in which the examiners ignore disconfirming instances and cling to their preexisting stereotypes.

[a]**Individualism:** "[P]ertains to societies in which the ties between individuals are loose; everyone is expected to look after himself or herself and his or her immediate family" (Hofstede, 1991, p. 51).

Individualistic self: Also referred to as referential self; the self prevalent in Western culture that is conceived as "the center of awareness, emotion, judgment and action" (Landrine, 1992, p. 403).

Informed consent: 1. An ethical doctrine that includes clients' rights to accept or refuse professional services, and the professionals' obligations to provide adequate and relevant information to clients in order for them to exercise their

[a]See references for Chapter 15.

rights. 2. The principle by which clients are fully and openly informed of the nature and purposes of a clinical interview and then give approval (usually in writing) to proceed. 3. The ethical standard that people must be told of the exact nature of a study and what will be required of them before they can be asked to participate in research. See also *Free consent.*

Inhibitory postsynaptic potential (IPSP): A stimulus that decreases the likelihood that the receiving neuron will fire, usually by hyperpolarizing the cell.

Insanity: The criteria vary by jurisdiction. A defendant, if found insane, is not held criminally responsible for the crime and is placed in a mental hospital rather than in the prison system.

Internal validity: The confidence with which statements about causality can be made on the basis of a study. Depends on (among other factors) the strength of the research design, the power of the statistical tests, and the reliability of the measurements.

Interpersonal therapy: Explicitly treats problems, especially depression, as being maintained by problematic relationships.

Interrupted time series: A quasi-experimental design in which there are numerous measures of the dependent variable over time, both before and after an intervention.

Interview: A face-to-face verbal exchange in which the interviewer attempts to elicit information or expressions of opinion as part of an assessment of a client.

Intrapsychic: The interaction of forces (often conflicting) within the mind or person.

Justice: The ethical principle of fairness, including treating equals equally.

Learning disability: A disorder in one or more of the basic psychological processes involved in understanding or using spoken or written language, resulting in an impaired ability to listen, think, read, write, spell, or to do mathematical calculations.

Legal custody: A determination resulting from custody litigation of whether one or both parents has decision-making powers regarding education, religion, and medical care.

Lysosomes: Membranous bags of destructive enzymes that break down large molecules into smaller ones.

Magnetic resonance imaging (MRI): A method of obtaining highly resolved and detailed images of all organs, especially the brain, which employs powerful magnetic pulses that are analyzed by a computer to produce the final image.

Malingering: Faking or falsifying, usually of mental illness when there is none, but also may apply to denying problems that in fact exist.

Managed care: An orientation to health care designed to contain the costs of treatment.

Manualized psychotherapies: An empirically driven approach to psychotherapy in which the therapist is directed specifically by predetermined and tested methods and concepts.

Mental health education: In this type of education, people acquire knowledge, skills, and attitudes that directly contribute to their mental health and to their effect on the mental health of others.

Mental retardation: Significantly subaverage general intelligence (IQ below 70 to 75) in combination with deficits in adaptive behavior and onset before age 18.

Mental status examination: A semistructured interview designed to assess the patient's current intellectual and emotional functioning.

Meta-analysis: A systematic way of combining the results of many studies to arrive at an overall estimate of the effectiveness of an intervention.

Mitochondria: Organelles that are the principle site of ATP production and thus can be thought of as the cell's power plants.

Multiple-baseline study: A quasi-experimental design in which a number of different behaviors are measured and the treatment is aimed at only one of them.

Myelin: A fatty substance that surrounds the axons of many neurons, thereby insulating them and allowing them to transmit impulses faster than nonmyelinated fibers.

Natural history: The most usual course of a disorder, in the absence of any intervention, from its onset to either remission or death.

Negative punishment: The withdrawal of a stimulus after the occurrence of a behavior that results in the decreased future probability of that behavior (e.g., time-out).

Negative reinforcement: The occurrence of a behavior associated with the removal of a stimulus, as in escape and avoidance learning.

Networks: Confederations of organizations with common interests that share resources and information with each other.

Neurofilaments: Fine threadlike structures that are special features of neurons that enable them to receive and transmit chemical messengers, viz. dendrites and axons.

Neuroglia: Literally, "nerve glue." Neural cells that support transmitting neurons both physically and nutritionally. There are two main types: (1) astrocytes, which are relatively large, star-shaped cells that connect neurons with the brain's blood supply and also anchor them in place, and (2) oligodendrogia, which function principally to encase axons in insulating sheaths called *myelin,* which increases the rate at which they can conduct impulses.

Neuroleptic: Refers to the effects of psychoactive drugs on the nervous system. Often refers to antipsychotic drugs that produce side effects resembling neurological disorders.

Neuroleptic malignant syndrome (NMS): An acute disorder of thermoregulation and neuromotor control associated with neuroleptic therapy. Frequent symptoms include fever, muscle rigidity, autonomic changes, and altered consciousness.

Neuron: A nerve cell that receives, integrates, and transmits electrochemical signals. The functional units of the nervous system.

Neuropeptide: A small protein neurotransmitter, such as beta-endorphin.

Neuropsychology: The study of relationships between brain function and behavior.

Neurotransmitter: A chemical messenger released by a neuron to excite or inhibit adjacent neurons.

Nondirective therapy: Empathic reflection of the patient's thoughts and feelings, rather than providing instruction or interpretation by the therapist.

Nonequivalent control study: A quasi-experimental design in which the control group may differ from the experimental group on one or more key variables. *Example*: Patients in therapy are compared to people with a similar disorder but who did not seek therapy. Also called a *cohort study*.

Nonmaleficence: The ethical principle that prohibits the infliction of harm.

Nonverbal behavior: The subtle forms of human communication expressed in gesture, body language, tone of voice, and facial expression.

Norm-referenced test: A test in which the performance of each examinee is interpreted in reference to a relevant standardization sample.

Nucleoli: Small spherical organelles found within the cell's nucleus that synthesize ribosomal RNA and assemble ribosome subunits.

Nucleus: A cytoplasmic organelle that usually occupies the central portion of the cell. The nucleus stores, duplicates, transfers, and transcribes genetic information.

Nuremberg Code: The first code of ethics governing the way human subjects in experiments should be treated, emphasizing the autonomy of the individual. This was followed by the Declaration of Helsinki.

Offer of proof: The rule requiring that the attorney notify the court what legal issue the expert witness will be addressing.

One-group pretest/posttest study: See *Before–after trial*.

Organelle: A discrete, formed body in the cytoplasm of a cell; literally, "little organ."

Organic compounds: Molecules that contain carbon atoms.

Pain response: An unpleasant sensation, physical discomfort, and/or suffering that occurs in varying degrees of intensity.

Paternalism: The overriding of a person's autonomy for beneficent reasons.

Patient advocate: A person appointed by the government who can give consent in lieu of the subject or patient. See *Surrogate*.

Patient–therapist privilege: Information from a patient to a therapist may not be released by the therapist without the patient's permission. There are some exceptions to the privilege defined by law.

Pediatric psychology: A field of research and practice concerned with a wide variety of topics in the relationship between the psychological and physical well-being of children.

Perceived social support: Social support concept in which an individual feels reliably connected to others.

Percentile rankings: The percentage of the comparison sample that the child's performance has surpassed.

Person–environment fit: The suitability of the person to the setting and the setting to the person.

Personal injury: A general term covering cases in which a plaintiff claims physical and/or psychological damages.

Pharmacokinetics: The body's effect on a drug. Four basic pharmacokinetics factors include absorption, distribution, transformation, and excretion.

Pharmacodynamics: The drug's effect on the body (both desirable and undesirable).

Physical custody: The specific arrangement, resulting from custody litigation, of time spent with each parent.

Placebo: An intervention that is not supposed to have any therapeutic effect.

Plaintiff: An individual who makes a claim or petitions the court.

Planned social change: Intentional or induced social change planned in advance of any problems.

Polarization: The state of having opposite qualities or powers. The difference in electrochemical charge that develops between the outside and inside of the neural membrane such that the interior is negatively charged relative to the exterior.

Policy science: The science of making findings from science available and relevant to governmental, community, and organizational (i.e., public) policy.

Positive punishment: The addition of a stimulus or consequence after the occurrence of a behavior that decreases the likelihood of the behavior (i.e., scolding).

Positive reinforcement: The occurrence of a behavior is followed by a stimulus that results in the increased probability of the future occurrence of that behavior (i.e., praising a child for being good).

Positron emission tomography (PET): A method that uses radioactively labeled glucose-sensitive detectors and powerful computers to indicate metabolic activity in regions of the brain.

Potentiation: The addition of a second drug to augment or enhance the effects of the original drug (e.g., adding lithium to potentiate the antidepressant effects of a selective serotonin-reuptake inhibitor [SSRI]).

Power: The ability of a statistical test to detect a significant difference between groups or relationship between variables, when in fact they exist. Defined as (1– beta).

Predictive validity: A type of criterion-related validity in which current test scores (e.g., SAT scores in high school) are effective at predicting a future criterion (e.g., college grades).

Primary prevention: Prevention that attempts to forestall a problem from occurring altogether. Primary prevention essentially refers to activities that can be undertaken with a healthy population to maintain or enhance its health.

Professional ethics: Standards of correct professional behavior.

Professional practice standard: A standard of informed consent that requires professionals to provide the level of information to clients that other professionals in the community provide.

Projective method: An assessment method in which the examinee encounters vague, ambiguous stimuli and is asked to provide a response.

Prokaryote: A cell lacking a membrane-bound nucleus or membrane-bound organelles.

Protoplasm: A richly complex mixture of water and organic substances within a cell that performs the countless, yet finely coordinated and integrated, biochemical reactions that give rise to and maintain life.

Pseudo-parkinsonism: A medication-induced muscle rigidity, decrease or lack of facial expression, or slowness of voluntary movements.

Psychoanalysis: A theoretical and therapeutic system that builds on the foundation and work of Sigmund Freud, M.D. Therapy in this framework focuses on the understanding and acceptance of the patient's unconscious motivations, fears, and conflicts.

Psychodrama: A group therapy technique in which participants role-play parts of their own lives or the lives of others to achieve new levels of self-understanding.

Psychodynamics: The theory of interplay between forces within an individual as the basis for understanding that person's motivation.

Psychological malpractice: Practices that fail to meet ethical guidelines and/or standards of reasonable care in the profession.

Psychosocial clubs or clubhouses: Community organizations designed to improve the quality of daily life for their members, who typically are the deinstitutionalized mentally ill.

Psychotherapy: The art and science of treating psychological, behavioral, and emotional problems by a trained and objective professional.

Psychotherapy integration: A relatively new approach to psychotherapy that is concerned with crossing the boundaries of the separate therapeutic systems in order to combine the most effective ingredients of each into a more powerful therapy.

Psychotropic drug: A drug acting on the brain to cause a change in mood or behavior.

Public policy: Policy at the community or government level that influences what resources are allocated where so that the quality of life is improved.

Quasi-experiment: Studies that do not use randomization to assign subjects to groups.

Randomization: A method of assigning subjects to groups in such a way that the chances of being allocated to a specific group are the same for all people.

Randomized controlled trial: See *True experiment*.

Reasonable-person standard: A standard of informed consent that requires professionals to provide the level of information to clients that a reasonable client, in similar circumstances, would want to know.

Receptor: A molecule, usually a protein, that is present on the surface of or within a cell and is the initial site of action of a biologically active agent.

Recidivism: 1. Relapse or need to return to an institution or to some form of intensive care or treatment for a particular disorder. 2. The frequency of repetition of a behavior (often applies to criminal behavior).

Reframing: A universal therapeutic technique, crucial to brief therapy. Generally, a therapist-induced change in perspective, which often leads clients to corresponding changes in attitude and behavior. Looks especially for positive intentions behind problematic behavior, the positive function of symptoms, or their positive unintended consequences.

Relationship: The mutual influence between two or more persons. In psychotherapy, the therapeutic relationship is often thought to be the driving force behind progress.

Relaxation techniques: Treatment methods involving breath regulation, muscle relaxation, and mental imagery to slow down the autonomic nervous system and, in turn, increase a sense of self-control/self-regulation.

Reliability: Consistency in measurement.

Reversal design: Studies in which the treatment is alternately given and withheld from the patient to determine its effect on some behavior. Also called an A-B-A design.

Ribosomes: Organelles in which amino acids are assembled into proteins.

Scientist/practitioner: A model of education and training for clinical psychologists established at the Boulder Conference in 1949. Participants recommended that clinical psychologists receive Ph.D.'s after being trained in general psychology as well as in clinical activities with a predoctoral internship. Graduate students in psychology were to learn to be scientists, able to conduct independent research, as well as practitioners skilled in assessment and psychosocial treatments. This model is still followed in most university-based clinical graduate programs within colleges of arts and sciences, in contrast to professional programs that offer Psy.D.'s and emphasize training for practice.

Secondary prevention: When a disorder such as depression or other problem already exists and is alleviated as early as possible.

Selective serotonin-reuptake inhibitor (SSRI): Antidepressants such as fluoxetine (Prozac) or sertraline (Zoloft) that show specificity in inhibiting the uptake of 5-hydroxytryptamine into platelets or brain tissue.

Sense of community: Feeling about the relationship an individual holds for his or her community Specifically includes a perception of similarity to others in the community, a willingness to maintain and acknowledge interdependence with others, and the feeling that one is part of a larger dependable and stable whole.

Single-subject design: An applied research design that determines the sources of variability in the individual.

Social desirability: The tendency of examinees to respond to test items in a socially desirable manner or to respond to a questionnaire or interview in such a way as to present themselves in the best possible light.

Social distance: The degree to which a person is reluctant to establish social contact and to interact with another person, often of a different social or ethnic background, in an egalitarian, mutual, intensive, and affective manner.

Social embeddedness: The number or quality of connections an individual has to significant others who might offer assistance.

Social integration: People's involvement in a community's formal institutions (such as work organizations), as well as their participation in the community's informal social life.

Social support: An exchange of resources between two individuals perceived by the provider or the recipient to be intended to enhance the well-being of the recipient.

[a]**Sociocentric self:** Also referred to as *indexical self.* The self that is prevalent in collective cultures. Such a self "includes other people and portions of the natural and supernatural world" (Landrine, 1992, p. 407), "is not a separate entity that can be referred to or reflected in isolation" (Landrine, 1992, p. 406), and "is principally manifested in a pattern of social roles" (Draguns, 1995, p. 93).

Solution-focused brief therapy: A particularly economical derivative of systemic therapy. It emphasizes the therapeutic use of questions, building on exceptions to problems, and rapid transitions to solutions intrinsic to a problem or client.

Soma: The cell body containing the nucleus and many other cytoplasmic organelles and the point of origin of the neurofilaments, dendrites, and axons.

Standard error of measurement: Refers to the component of measurement error found in the child's obtained score. Reflected by using a confidence interval around the obtained score in order to estimate the range of scores in which the child's true score really falls.

Standardization sample: A large group of subjects representative of the population for whom a test is intended.

Standard of care: A consensus among professionals regarding ethical and procedural practices in the specialty.

Steady state: Desired blood drug level that is reached when the total concentration of a drug in the blood plasma remains unchanged.

[a]**Stereotype:** A set of beliefs about a group of people that gives insufficient attention to individual differences among the members of that group (Brislin, 1993).

Strategic therapy: Generally refers to specific therapist-initiated interventions designed for specific problems. Sees problems as often maintained by efforts to change them. Symptoms are often treated as having a function. Change is effected primarily through treating a specific symptom. Implicitly systemic and interpersonal.

Structural therapy: Seeks to create change in immediate problems through altering transactional processes in a family system.

Structured interview: An interviewed guided by a specific outline with topics and subtopics.

Structured interview schedule: An interview that consists of precise questions and rules for follow-up and scoring as an aid to clinical diagnosis.

[a]**Subjective culture:** The totality of characteristic ways of viewing the human-made part of the environment that are prevalent or widely shared among the members of that culture. Subjective culture includes the ideas, explanations, and political, religious, scientific, aesthetic, economic, and social standards for judging events in the environment (Triandis, 1994).

Substitution: Using one variable (e.g., self-reports of smoking behavior) as a proxy for another variable (actual smoking behavior) because the latter is too difficult or intrusive to measure directly.

Support groups, self-help groups, or mutual help groups: Groups that include similar individuals who come together to provide assistance and emotional and other support for one another.

Surrogate: A person who can give consent in lieu of the subject when the subject is unable to give consent him- or herself; usually a family member. See also *Patient advocate.*

Synapse: The junction between neurons' transmitting and receiving membranes. Usually a physical gap across which neurotransmitters diffuse when released.

Systemic therapy: Therapy that treats problems via a relationship or interaction. Systems theory

[a]See references for Chapter 15.

relies on the ideas that the whole is larger than the sum of parts, that the system tends to resist change (homeostasis), and that changing one part of a system will affect other parts. All therapy should properly be considered systemic.

Tardive dyskinesia (TD): Involuntary movements associated with chronic neuroleptic therapy. Characterized by sucking or smacking of the lips, choreoathetoid movements of the tongue, and lateral jaw movements.

Test: A standardized procedure for sampling behavior and describing it with categories or scores.

Test–retest reliability: A form of reliability in which the same test is given twice to the same group of subjects to determine the stability of scores.

Therapeutic window: An aspect of therapeutic drug monitoring (TDM) in which a drug is theoretically most efficacious. Below the basal figure, often measured in nanograms/milliliter (ng/ml), the patient is not as likely to have a response. Above the ceiling figure, the patient is likely to experience more serious side effects or toxicity.

Threshold of excitation (TOE): A critical degree of excitation or depolarization at which the neuron fires in an all-or-none fashion.

Transcription: The process whereby DNA makes RNA molecules. Once transcribed, RNA participates in protein synthesis in a process known as translation.

Transference: In classical psychoanalysis, the projection of emotional feelings and wishes (often from childhood) onto the analyst, who represents important figures from the patient's past, such as parents, siblings, or teachers. Transference may be positive or negative and may occur with individuals outside of the treatment setting.

Transinstitutionalization: The notion that an individual spends his or her life moving from one institution to another.

Treatment resistance: In psychotherapy, any factor that prevents or delays therapeutic progress.

Triangulation: Refers to the triangle that occurs when both parents vie for a child's attention or loyalty.

True experiment: A research design in which the subjects are allocated by the researcher to either the experimental or the control conditions. Also called a *randomized controlled trial* (RCT).

Type I error: Erroneously concluding that statistically significant results were due to a real relationship between variables or differences between groups, when in fact they were caused by sampling error. Also called the *alpha-type error*.

Type II error: Erroneously concluding that there was no difference between groups or relationship between variables, when in fact there was one. Also called *beta-type error*.

Unconditioned response: The response elicited by an unconditioned stimulus.

Unconditioned stimulus: A stimulus that automatically elicits an unconditioned response.

Unconscious: One of Freud's three levels of awareness that refers to desires, fantasies, emotions, and ideas that prompt behavior but which occur outside of the person's perception.

Validity: The extent to which a test measures what it was intended to measure.

Veracity: The ethical rule of truth-telling.

Virtue ethics: An orientation to ethics based on ideal, desired personal characteristics.

NAME INDEX

Abbott, D., 95
Abernethy, D.R., 310
Abrami, P.C., 130
Abrams, D.B., 341
Abramson, H., 236
Achterberg, J., 4, 5
Achterberg-Lawlis, J., 263
Ackerman, D.L., 315
Ackerman, N., 173
Adam, K.S., 121
Adams, A., 337
Adams, J.F., 194
Adams, R., 337
Adler, A., 16, 140, 164
Adler, C.S., 337
Adler, L.L., 393
Adler, N.E., 339
Agras, W.S., 267, 335
Al-Issa, I., 377–378
Alazvaki, A., 297–298, 302, 318
Albee, G.W., 18
Alexander, F., 143, 144, 187, 331
Alexander, J.F., 204, 205
Alfidi, R.J., 92
Allen, R.A., 335
Alleyne, E., 130
Allonso, A., 168
Altman, D.G., 339, 342
Alvarez, W., 186, 190
Amdisen, A., 314
Anastasi, A., 57
Anderson, C.M., 268
Anderson, J., 17
Anderson, K.O., 339, 340
Andrasik, F., 334, 337, 341
Andreasen, N.C., 40, 42
Andrews, P., 413
Angell, M., 133

Anker, Korten, A., 378
Ankney, C.D., 133
Apfel, N.H., 350
Aponte, H.J., 187
Aponte, J.F., 83, 102
Appelbaum, D., 82
Appelbaum, P.S., 89, 104
Applewhaite, G., 115
Arce, A.A., 352
Archer, R.P., 197, 198, 225
Ardila, A., 390
Arena, S.C., 341
Arizmendi, T.G., 200
Arkowitz, H., 256
Arntz, A., 114
Aronoff, G.R., 307
Arpin, J., 394
Arthur, G., 95, 103
Ascher, L.M., 204, 268
Asher, S.J., 243
Asken, M.J., 332
Astin, H.S., 21
Auerbach, A., 196, 268
Austad, C.S., 186
Austin, K.M.,
Autry, J.H., 116, 118
Axline, V., 234

Babani, L., 244
Bagby, R., 34
Baird, J., 11
Bakal, D.A., 331
Baker, L., 129
Baker, R.W., 35
Baker, T.B., 71
Baldessarini, R.J., 305, 309
Ball, T.J., 339
Balla, D.A., 73, 224

Ballenger, J.C., 307, 314
Balogh, D.W., 95
Balter, M.B., 310
Baltimore, D., 342
Bandler, R., 174
Bandura, A., 148, 231, 268, 334, 339
Banis, H.T., 244
Bank, J., 341
Banks, W.P., 417
Barber, J., 156, 197
Barber, T.X., 338
Barker, P., 173
Barkham, M., 193
Barlow, D.H., 22, 34, 123, 125, 126 154, 191, 198, 336
Barnard, K.E., 350
Barnes, J.M., 102
Barrera, M., 361
Barrett, P.M., 236
Barroso, F., 393
Barry, M., 133
Basch, M.F., 199
Basco, M.R., 154
Bassos, C.A.,
Bateson, G., 173, 198, 256
Bauman, D.J., 363
Baumohl, J., 359
Baumrind, D., 86
Baxter, L.R., 297–298, 302, 318
Beardsley, R.S., 306
Beasley, C.M., 320
Beauchamp, T.L., 84, 85–86, 90, 92, 105
Beauvais, F., 385
Beck, A.T., 22, 150–151, 153, 154, 156, 195, 198
Becker, J., 361
Becker, M.H., 266
Beckham, J.C., 341
Beditz, J., 352
Bednar, R.L., 206
Beers, C., 7, 8
Beidel, D.C., 114
Beier, E.G., 200
Belar, C., 339, 342
Belcher, J.R., 357
Belissimo, A., 333
Bellack, A.S., 72
Bellack, L., 226, 232
Bellack, S.S., 226
Belsey, E., 114
Bemak, F., 393
Ben-Porath, 118, 225
Ben-Shakhar, G., 197

Benedict, J.G., 83
Benedict, R., 377
Benet, L.Z., 305
Benfield, P., 312
Bengelsdorf, J., 364
Bengen-Seltzer, B., 336
Benjamin, P., 244
Bennett, E.A., 404
Bennett, M.J., 186
Benowitz, N.L., 337
Benson, H., 334, 336, 338, 342
Benton, A.L., 62
Berg, I.K., 195, 199, 202
Bergin, A.E., 152, 189, 192, 193, 197, 199, 200
Bergman, A.B., 244
Bergman, J.S., 268
Bergman, K.S., 297–298, 302, 318
Bergman, S.S., 310
Bergstrom, R.F., 323
Berkman, A.S.,
Berla, E.P., 413
Berman, J.S., 236
Bernard, H., 172, 177
Bernard, J., 363
Berne, E, 192, 377
Bernheim, H., 11, 140
Bernstein, D.A., 334
Berrier, J., 130
Berry, J.W, 391, 394
Bershenyi, K., 103
Bersoff, D.N., 92, 106
Bertelson, A., 378
Bessel, F., 11
Beutler, L., 31
Beutler, L.E., 153, 158–159, 194, 199, 200, 341
Bielski, R.J., 316
Bilby, R., 363
Binder, J., 155, 188, 197
Binder, S.L., 190
Binet, A., 13, 51–52, 388
Birbaumer, N., 340
Bischoff, M.M., 201
Black, D.W., 40, 42
Blake, D., 34
Blakely, C.P., 355
Blakeslee, S., 175
Blanchard, E.B., 331, 334, 334, 337, 341
Blick, L.C., 243
Bloom, B., 186, 187, 190, 192, 194, 195, 196, 197, 204, 206, 215
Bloom, B.L., 350, 354

Bloom, J.R., 336
Bodkin, J.A., 316
Bohart, A.C., 146, 157
Bohm, R.M., 411
Boll, T.J., 339
Bologna, N.C.,
Bolter, K., 186, 190
Bond, G.R., 365, 366
Bongar, B., 94, 186, 192, 199, 215
Bonica, J. J., 34
Boodoo, O., 389
Booth-Kewley, S., 340
Bootzin, R.R., 359
Borduin, C.M., 197, 198
Borkovec, T.D., 334, 337
Bornemann, T.H., 393, 394
Borow, H., 102
Botterbusch, K.F., 365
Botvin, G.J., 353
Bouchard, T.J., 389
Bouhoutsos, J., 98
Bowen, M., 173
Bowlby, J., 143
Boykin, A.W., 389
Boynton, K., 103
Braaten, E.B., 90
Bradley, P., 55
Bramel, D., 118,
Brasfield, T.L., 130
Brehm, J.W., 256
Breshgold, E.,254
Bresler, C., 342
Breuer, 8, 11
Bricklin, P.M., 104
Briere, J., 416
Broadhurst, S., 363
Brock G.W., 83, 88
Broderick, C., 180, 198
Brodsky, A., 99
Brody, N., 389
Bronfenbrenner, U., 350
Bronner, A., 13
Broskowski, A., 103, 185
Brown, C., 363
Brown, D.A., 337
Brown, J.D., 354
Brownell, A., 354, 360
Brownell, K.D., 336, 337
Brubaker, R.G., 120
Bruce, M.L., 357
Bruininks, R.H., 73

Buchanan, R.W., 307
Budman, S.H., 169, 186, 187, 188, 190, 193, 195, 199, 204, 215
Budzynski, T.H., 334, 337
Buelow, G.D., 103
Bugental, J.F.T., 147–148, 254
Bulatao, E.G.,193
Bunney, W.E., 314
Burger, G.K., 358
Burgess, A.W., 242
Burgio, L., 232
Burlingame, G., 190
Burnett R., 341
Burns, B.J., 193, 194
Burns, D.D., 189, 192, 204
Burrows, G.D., 307
Butcher, J.N., 66, 118, 187, 188, 190, 194, 196, 225, 387
Butler, A.C., 22
Butler, S.F, 190
Bybee, D., 358

Cabral, R.J., 342
Cacioppo, J.T., 130
Cade, B., 198, 199
Callanan, P., 84, 87, 101
Calsyn, R.J., 358
Campbell, D.P., 55
Campbell, D.T., 114, 116, 123, 336
Campbell, M.M., 244
Camps, D., 123, 124
Caplan, G., 199, 360
Carek, D.J., 233
Carlson, C., 234
Carlson, G.A., 313
Carlson, N.R., 284,287
Carmen Luciano, M., 339
Carne, W.F., 43, 45
Carothers, J.C., 378
Carpenter, R.H.S., 278–279, 282
Carpenter, W.T., 307
Carroll, J.L., 71
Carroll, M.A., 81, 83, 91
Carse, A.L., 106
Carter, I., 337
Carter, M., 89, 90
Carter, R.T., 391
Casas, J.M., 206, 385
Cassel, J., 360
Cattell, J.McK., 7, 8, 11, 12, 51
Cattell, R.B., 69
Caudill, M., 336, 338, 342

Caudill, W., 385
Ceci, S.J., 389
Cerny, J.A., 154
Chafetz, M.D., 103
Chalmers, T.C., 130
Chambliss, D.L., 186, 192, 193, 341
Chance, N.A., 378
Chang, S.C., 381
Chapman, J.P., 39, 72
Chapman, L.J., 39, 72
Charcot, J.M., 11, 140
Cheng, S.K., 391
Cheng, T.A., 379
Chesney, M.A., 338
Cheung, F.M.C., 379
Chevron, E.S., 155, 197
Chiarello, R.J., 323
Chiauzzi, E.J., 268
Childress, J.F., 84, 85–86, 90, 92, 105
Christensen, A., 22
Christensen, L., 123
Christophersen, E.R., 236
Chuang, O., 315
Chung, R.C.Y., 393
Church, J.O., 364
Chwast, R., 244
Cicchetti, D.V., 73, 224
Claiborn, D.C., 90
Clark, D.M., 198
Clarke, G.N., 117, 118
Claver, B.G., 393
Clingempeel, W.G., 91
Cloitre, M., 34
Coccaro, E.F., 316
Cohen, E., 358
Cohen, F., 339
Cohen, H., 226
Cohen, J., 122
Cohen, P.A., 130
Colapinto, J., 174
Cole, J.O., 316, 323
Cole, N.S., 75
Collins, J.F., 116, 118
Comaty, S.B., 307
Comba, L., 394
Compton, W.M., 380
Congett, S., 390
Conners, C.K., 37
Conoley, J.C., 54, 55
Consoli, A.J., 158, 199
Constantine, L.L., 285

Constantino, G., 388, 392
Cook, D.J., 125
Cook, M.P., 369
Cook, T.D., 114, 116, 123
Cooke, G., 413, 416
Cooke, M., 416
Cooper, G.L., 319
Cooper, J., 130, 378, 403
Cooper, J.F., 185, 187, 188, 190, 192, 195, 196, 197, 198,
    199, 203, 204, 205, 207
Cooper-Lonergan, E., 169
Coppel, D.B., 36
Corey, G., 84, 87, 101, 168
Corey, M.S., 84, 87, 101
Corrigan, P., 36, 366
Corsini, R.J., 186
Costa, P.T., Jr., 67
Cotter, P.R., 350
Cowen, E.L., 349, 359
Cox, G.B., 361
Crago, M., 200
Craig, C.R., 285
Craske, M., 207
Craven, S., 193, 194
Cressler, D.L., 350
Crisp, A.H., 119
Crits-Christoph, P., 156, 197, 268
Cross, W.E., 391
Crouch, R.T., 83
Csikszentmihalyi, M., 191, 203
Cuevas, J., 337, 341
Cullari, S., 260, 266, 268
Cummings, N.A., 83, 104
Curtis, H., 273, 277, 278, 279
Cushman, P., 142, 163

Dadds, M.R., 236
Dahlstrom, W.G., 387
Damlouji, N., 320
Dana, R.H., 101, 388
d'Apollonia, S., 130
Dare, C., 252
Dasberg, H., 197
Dassel, S.W., 244
Dattiho, F.M., 198
Davanloo, H., 186, 192, 197–198
Davenport, S.L.H., 244
David, A., 115
Davidson, G., 368
Davidson, J.L., 352
Davidson, M., 307

Davidson, P.O., 263
Davidson W.B., 350
Davidson, W.S., 355
Davis, C., 125
Davis, K., 307,
Davis, R., 117
Davison G., 148–149, 150
Dawber, T.R., 337
Dawes, R., 22, 38–39
Dawes, R.M., 74
Day, J.D., 105
Day, R., 378
deGeus, E.J., 341
DeGraaf-Kaser, R., 365
de Haan, E., 121
DeHoyos, A., 379
DeHoyos, G., 379
DeJong, C.R., 336
DeLeon, P.H., 193
Derner, G., 18
DeRubeis, R., 117
de Shazer, S. 185, 186, 199, 256, 268
Desjarlais, R., 392
DeVeaugh-Geiss, J., 318
DeWit, H., 310
Dey, A., 356, 369
Diamond, P.M., 358
Diaz, L., 390
Dickens, S., 34
Dickersin, K., 122
Dickter, D., 193
DiClemente, C.C., 159, 199, 202, 261
Dies, R., 172
Diguer, L., 193
DiMatteo, M.R., 264, 265, 266
DiNardo, P., 34
Dincin, J., 365
Dinges, N., 396
DiNicola, D.D., 264, 265, 266
Dishman, R.K., 341
Dix, D., 7, 8
Dixon, W., 120
Dobson, K.S., 198
Docherty, J.P., 116, 118
Dolan, Y.M., 188
Dollard, J., 15
Donaldson, S.R., 307
Donenberg, G.R., 117, 122
Donovan, J.M., 192, 195, 196, 197
Dorner, S., 244
Dornseif, B.E., 320

Dougherty, C.J., 83
Dougherty, S., 363
Douvan E., 356
Dowd, E.T., 256
Doyne, E.S., 341
Draguns, J.G., 375, 378, 379, 382, 385, 387, 388, 394
Draine, J., 365
Drotar, D., 244
Dubbert, P.M., 338, 341
DuBois, C., 387
Dubovsky, S.L., 195
Dudek, K.J., 362
Duffy, K.G., 348, 349, 353, 356, 357, 359, 360, 369
Duffy, L., 396
Dugan, F., 123, 124
Dumont, M.P., 357
Dunbar, J.M., 265, 267
Duncan, B., 186, 189, 192, 193, 202
Dunn, L.M., 73
Dunsmore, J., 341
Dunson, K., 337
DuPont, R.L., 307
Durkheim, E., 379
Durkin, H., 171
Dvoskin, S.A., 365

Eagle, M., 117
Eber, H.W., 69
Echemendia, R.J., 390
Echtering, L.G., 364
Eckert, P., 189
Edgington, E.S., 123
Edwards, A.L., 120
Edwards, C.D., 225
Edwards, S., 340
Egan, J., 236
Egeland, J.A., 384
Ehrenwald, J., 6
Eisenberg, L., 392
Ekblad, S., 394
Elias, M.J., 393
Elkin, I., 116, 118, 197
Elliot, C.H., 244
Elliot, R., 157, 163
Ellis, A., 150–151, 198, 232, 255–256
Emmelkamp, P.M.G., 121
Emory, G., 151, 154
Emshoff, J.G., 355
Enas, C.G., 323
Engel, G.L., 339
Ensor, A., 73

Epperson, D.L.,
Epstein, L., 338
Erickson, M., 198, 256
Erickson, R.H., 310
Erikson, E.H., 216, 334
Ernherg, A.M., 378
Eshleman, S.K., 384
Essau, C.A., 114
Evans, J.H., 403
Everitt, B., 115
Everly, G.S., 334
Eversole, D., 315
Everstine, D.S., 91
Everstine, L., 91
Ewing, C.P., 199
Exner, J.E., Jr., 70, 226
Eyde, L., 45
Eysenck, H.J., 9, 114–115, 150

Fairweather, G.W., 361, 368
Falkin, S., 341
Faller, K.C., 243
Farid, N.A., 323
Farley, O.W., 366
Faust D., 38, 39, 74
Fawcett, S.B., 355
Fay, A., 255
Feighner, J.P., 320
Feldman, T.B., 422
Feldstein, S., 32
Felner, R.D., 350
Fensterheim, H., 159–160
Fenton, F.R., 378
Ferenczi, S., 187
Fernald, G., 8, 13
Feung, H.K., 297–298, 302, 318
Feurstein, M., 339
Fhagen-Smith, P., 391
Fiester, S.S., 116, 118
Filskov, S., 39
Fine, R., 253
Fine, S., 206
Finney-Owen, G.K., 191, 193
Fiore, J., 361
First, M., 34
Fisch, R., 188, 203, 198
Fischer, C.T., 45,
Fish, J., 392
Fisher, R., 95
Fishman, H.C., 198
Fitzgerald, D., 129

Fitzpatrick, M., 97, 98, 99, 100, 107
Fleming, C.M., 385
Flemming, T., 129
Fleury, F., 394
Flor, H., 340
Fogel, B.S., 295
Follette, V.M., 103
Follette, W.C., 123
Fong, K.T., 369 &
Foote, F.H., 205
Ford, M.E., 267
Fordyce, W.E., 338
Forsyth, D., 121, 392, 394
Forsythe, Q.A., 340
Forth, A., 206
Fortune, W., 30
Framo, J., 184, 334
Frank, J.D., 200, 268, 141, 152
Frank, L.K., 69
Franz, S., 13
Franzen, M., 337
Freeman, A., 154, 195, 198
Freeman, R.J., 359
French, T., 143, 144, 187
Frensch, P.A., 202
Freud, A., 142, 233
Freud, S., 8, 11, 13, 14, 16, 140, 142, 143, 187, 216, 250–252, 331
Frey, D.H., 91
Friedel, R.O., 316
Friedman, H.S., 340
Friedman, R., 336, 338, 342
Friedman, S., 188, 204, 215
Friend, R., 118
Friis, S., 72
Frishman, W.H., 307
Fromm, E., 16, 140, 142, 143
Frost, R.O., 118
Fruchter, B., 57
Fuhriman, A., 190
Fulkerson, S.C., 388
Fuller, F.B., 71

Gabbard, G.O., 96, 97, 99
Gaelick-Buys, L., 267
Galassi, J.P., 115
Galassi, N., 115
Galavotti, C., 342
Gallagher, K.M., 21
Galton, F., 8, 11–12, 51
Galvin, M.D., 90

Gamer, M.V., 117
Ganet, M., 363
Gannon, L.R., 337, 341
Gansman, D., 323
Gardner, E., 321
Gardner, R.A., 416
Gardocki, G.J., 306
Garfield, S.L., 115, 153, 187, 193, 194
Garner, D.M., 117
Gartner, A.J., 342
Gassner, S., 130
Gazzaniga, M.S., 291
Geffken, G., 244
Geisendorfer, S.,
Gelb, S., 5
Gelenberg, A.J., 314
Genest, M., 338
Gentry, W.D., 332
Giannetti, R., 34
Giannetti, V.J., 186, 192, 205, 206, 215
Gibbon, M., 34
Gibbs, W.W., 195
Gibson, C., 356, 369
Gigerenzer, G., 122
Gil, K.M., 341
Gilbert, M., 206
Giles, T.R., 201
Gilligan, C., 106
Gilmore, S.K., 236
Ginter, M., 350
Giordano, J., 86
Gitlin, M.S, 195
Glass, D.R., 116, 118
Glass, G.V., 129, 152, 194
Glenberg, A.J., 307
Glick, I.D., 197
Glickman, M., 362
Glish, M., 349
Glover, E., 252
Goddard, H., 8, 13, 14, 52
Gold, J.R., 138, 150, 153, 158, 159, 160, 163
Goldberg, A., 197
Golden, C.J., 65
Goldfried, M., 32, 148–149, 150, 158, 199, 207
Golding, S.L., 83
Goldman, H.H., 193, 194
Goldman, R., 188
Goldstein, A.P., 130, 268
Goleman, D., 200
Good, B., 392
Good, W.V., 300

Goodman, G.S., 94
Goodman, P., 146
Goodman, W., 34, 225
Goodwin, F.K., 313, 319, 320
Goodwin, J., 341
Gootnick, J., 90
Gordon, J.R., 268
Gordon, P., 323
Gorham, D., 38
Gottlieb, M.C., 100
Gottschalk, R.G., 355
Gough, H.G., 55
Gould, S.J., 11, 14, 279, 303
Grady, K., 20
Graham, J.R., 66, 225, 387
Gray, L., 94
Green, A.H., 242
Greenberg, L., 32
Greenberg, L.S., 145–146, 147, 156, 157, 163
Greenberg, M.D., 87
Greenberg, R.P., 130
Greenberg, S., 143, 144
Greenblatt, D.J.310
Greenson, R.R., 252
Greenspoon, J., 232
Greenwald, A.G., 122, 129
Gregory, R.J., 36, 42, 43, 45, 52, 56, 57, 71,
    75–76
Greist, J.H., 315
Grieger, R., 198
Griff, M.D., 234
Griggs, P., 356, 369
Grimley, D.M., 342
Grinder, J., 174
Grisso, J.T., 357
Grisso, T., 407, 408, 420
Groth-Marnet, G., 30
Guidano, V.F., 156
Guilford, J.P., 57
Guilmette, T., 39
Gulbinat, W., 378
Gumaer, J., 83
Gurman, A.S., 186, 187, 188, 190, 193, 195, 199, 204,
    215
Gustafson, J.P., 198
Gustafson, K.E., 95
Gustin, A.W., 130
Gutheil, T.G., 96, 97, 99
Guyatt, G.H., 125
Guze, B.H., 297–298, 302, 318
Gynther, M., 387

Haas, L.J., 83, 89, 104
Hadley, S.W., 116, 118
Hagen, E.P., 52, 223
Hakel, M., 20
Haley, G., 206
Haley, J., 174, 198, 234–235, 256, 257, 339
Hall, C.C.I., 21
Hall, G.S., 7–8, 13, 20, 339, 341
Hall, H.V., 413
Halpern, D.F., 389
Halstead, W., 64–65
Hamilton, J., 337, 341
Hamsher, K., 62
Han, S.S., 117, 122
Handelsman, M.M., 83, 84, 90, 91, 103
Hankin, J.R., 114
Hanlon, T.E.,
Hansen, A.M.D., 121
Hanson, R., 363
Hanston, P.D., 305
Harbeck, C, 248
Harding, A., 94
Hardman, J.G., 125
Hardy, C.J., 340
Hardy, G.E., 193
Hare-Mustin, R.T., 89, 90, 91
Harris, J., 390
Harrison, W., 321
Hart, K., 39
Hartley, D., 190, 194
Hartmann, H., 253
Hartsough, D.M., 364
Harvey, W., 6
Harwood, T., 31
Hastie, C., 363
Hawking, S.W., 172
Hawton, K., 198
Hayden, P.W., 244
Hayes, S.C., 336, 339
Haynes, R.B., 129
Haynes, S.N., 36, 334, 336, 337, 341
Hays, S., 20
Hayward, P., 115
Healey, W., 8, 13
Hecker, L., 95
Hedeker, D., 337
Hedges, L.V., 129
Hefferline, R.F., 146
Heinrichs, D.W., 307
Heinz, E., 337
Heiser, P., 337, 341

Held, B.S., 198
Heller, K., 118, 350, 356
Helzer, J.E., 380
Hendrick, S.S., 97
Hepeworth, J., 363
Herbstein, J., 320
Hernandez, P., 384
Hernstein, R., 221
Hersen, M., 72, 123, 125, 126, 232, 248, 336
Herskovits, M., 375
Hervis, O.E., 205
Hetherington, E.M., 177
Heymann, G.M., 91
Hidalgo, J., 306
Higginbotham, H.N., 121, 392, 394, 395
Hill, B.K., 73
Hirschfeld, R.M., 320
Hiskey, M.S., 73
Hodges, W.F., 350
Hodgson, A.B., 158–159
Hodgson, R.I., 338
Hoff, L., 182
Hoffart, A., 72
Hofstede, G., 381–383, 391
Hofsteter, A.M., 384
Hogan, D.B., 87
Hoiberg, A., 339
Holder, A., 252
Hollingsworth, L., 14
Hollister, L., 38
Hollon, S.D., 198
Holroyd, J.C., 99
Holstrom, L.L., 242
Holtzworth-Munroe, A., 204, 205
Holub, E.A., 97
Hoogduin, C.A.L., 121
Hopson, J.L., 273
Horn, J.L., 61
Horn, J.R., 305
Horney, K., 16, 140
Horowitz, M.J., 190
Hostetler, J.A., 383
Houts, A.C., 236
Howard, K.I., 186, 188, 194, 198, 199, 207
Hoyt, M.F., 185, 186, 188, 190, 193, 198, 204, 215
Huang, M., 194
Hubble, M., 186, 189, 192, 193, 202
Hubley, A., 35
Hudson, P.O., 204
Hug-Hellmuth, H., 232, 233
Hugenholtz, H., 63

Hughey, J., 356, 369
Hull, C., 15, 140
Humphrey, F., 180
Humphreys, K., 24
Hunt, H., 5
Hunter, J.E., 120
Hunter, M.A., 123
Hwu, H.G., 380
Hyman, S.E., 282, 285, 286–287
Hyne, S., 55

Ibrahim, F.A., 391
Imber, S.D., 116, 118
Impara, J.C., 54, 55
Ivey, A., 32
Ivey, M., 32
Iwamasca, G., 369
Iwata, B., 31

Jablensky, A., 378
Jackson, D., 173, 256
Jackson, R.W., 366
Jacobson, N.S., 22, 123, 194, 205, 334
James, M., 184
James, W., 7, 8, 339, 381
Jameson, P., 204, 205
Janet, P., 11, 140
Janicak, P.G., 307
Janis, I.L., 340
Jaremko, M.E., 232
Jason, L.A., 337
Jastak, S., 224
Javier, R.A., 392, 393
Jay, S.M., 244
Jefferson, J.W., 315
Jefferson, K.W., 130
Jenkins, R, 114
Jessell, T.M., 287
Jessup, B.A., 334
Jewell, D.P., 383
Jilek, W., 393
Joffe, R., 129
Johanson, C.E., 310
Johns, C., 307
Johnson, D.L., 352, 366
Johnson, H.G., 91
Johnson, L.D., 186, 188, 189, 191, 196, 203, 204, 205, 215
Johnson, P.W., 420
Johnson, S.B., 244
Johnsrud, C., 90

Johnston, M.B., 232
Joiner, T., 120
Jones, E.E., 197
Jones, S.R.G., 118
Jongeward, D., 184
Jordan, A.E., 105
Jorgenson, L., 98
Jumper-Thurman, P., 385
Jung, C., 16, 140
Jurich, A., 194
Jurish, S.E., 341

Kabasa, S.C., 342
Kaemmer, B., 387
Kagawa-Singer, M., 342
Kahn, H., 391
Kahn, R., 307
Kales, A., 310
Kalichman, S.C., 94
Kalous, T.D., 185
Kaltreider, N., 190
Kamin, L.J., 127
Kamphaus, R., 62, 248
Kandel, E.R., 287
Kane, J., 307
Kanfer, F.H., 232, 267, 268
Kaplan, A.G., 89, 90, 91
Kaplan, H.I., 287, 293, 295
Kaplan, S.J., 242
Karoly, P., 232
Katayama, S., 381
Katcher, A.H., 336
Katranides, M., 337, 341
Katz, R., 318
Kaufman, A.S., 62
Kaufman, N.L., 62
Kaul, T., 206
Kaye, R.A., 364
Kazdin, A.E., 232, 336
Keefe, F.J., 22, 341
Kehrer, C.A., 195
Keita, G.P., 21
Keith-Spiegel, P., 82, 83, 86, 95, 97, 99
Kelleher, J.C., 21
Kellner, R., 115
Kelly, G., 140, 150
Kelly, J., 175
Kelly, M.P., 63
Kemp, R., 115
Kemper, M.B., 90
Kems, R.D., 338

Kendall, P.C., 115, 117
Kenkel, M.B., 21
Kertay, L.,97
Kessler, L.G, 193, 194
Kesson-Craig, P., 90
Kibel, H., 168
Kiesler, C.A., 20, 114, 352
Kiesler, D.J., 155
Kilbey, M., 327
Kimball, P., 337
Kimura, B., 381
King, A.C., 339, 342
Kingsbury, S.J., 186, 192, 193, 195
Kinney, R., 366
Kirby, R.J., 194, 205
Kirk, J., 198
Kirkpatrick, B.,
Kirmayer, L., 379
Kitchener, K.S., 83, 84, 97, 99, 106
Klein, D.F., 316, 321
Klein, E., 168, 171
Klein, G.S., 142
Klein, M., 216, 233
Klein, R., 171, 210
Kleiner, R., 147–148
Kleinman, A., 379, 385, 387, 392
Kleinman, J., 379
Kleinmuntz, B., 39, 74
Klerman, G.L., 155, 197
Klesges, R.C., 337
Kluckhohn, C., 375
Klyver, N., 417
Knapp, R.H., 381
Knapp, S., 94
Kniskern, D.P., 204
Knowles, S., 323
Ko, G., 307
Kobos, J.S., 83
Koch-Weser, J., 307
Koeske, G., 361–362
Kohn, A., 189
Kohout, J.L., 21
Kohut, H., 143, 144
Koocher, G.P., 82, 86, 94, 99
Koppitz, E.M., 226
Kopta, S.M., 188, 189, 194
Korman, M., 19, 376, 396
Koss, J.D., 379
Koss, M.P., 185, 186, 187, 188, 190, 193, 194, 196, 207, 215
Kovaks, A.L., 90

Kowatch, R.A., 337
Kraemer, D.T., 361
Kraemer, H.C., 335
Kraepelin, E., 8, 11, 139, 299, 377
Krafft-Ebing, R., 11
Krause, M.S., 118, 188, 189
Krauss, L.M., 172
Kraut, A., 20
Kraxberger, B.E., 342
Kreilkamp, T., 188, 204
Kristjansson, B., 35
Kroeber, A.I., 375
Kroon, M.B., 354
Krug, S., 45
Krupnick, S., 190
Kruzich, J.M., 352
Kuczmierczyk, A.R., 339
Kulick, F.B., 413
Kulka, R.A., 356
Kumanyika, S.K., 342
Kupfer, D.J., 315
Kurtines, W.M., 205
Kurz, R.B., 244, 245

L'Abate, L., 268
Labbe, E.E., 339
Lacks, P., 337
Lah, M.I., 71
Laikan, M., 195
Lakin, M., 83
Lamal, P.A., 232
Lambert, M.J., 152, 189, 191, 192, 193, 197, 199, 200, 204
Land, J., 130
Landau, P., 318
Landrine, H., 381
Langner, T., 380
Langs, R., 253
Langtry, H.O., 312
Lankton, C.H., 198
Lankton, S.R., 198
Lannon, P.B., 358
Lansky, A., 342
Lanyon, R.I., 74
Lanza, M.L., 364
Larsen, D.B., 306
Laurent, J., 61
Lavy, E., 114
Lawson, A., 350
Lawton, S.V., 82
Lazar, S.G., 192, 197

Lazarus, A.A., 150, 158, 255
Lazarus, L.W., 195
Leader, D.S., 369
Leaf, P.J., 357
Leary, M.R., 342
Leber, W.R., 116, 118
Lebra, T.S., 385
LeDoux, J.E., 291
Ledwidge, B., 232
Lee, S.S., 97
Leenaars, A.A., 363
Leff, S., 3–4
Leff, V., 3–4
Lehman, A.K., 198
Lehmann, S., 361
Leibovich, M., 195
Lelik, D., 39
Lemburger, L., 323
Lemsky, C., 336
Leonard, B., 123, 124
Lerman, H., 102
LeShan, L., 190, 194
Lester, D., 364
Levant, R., 176, 178
Levenson, E.R., 144
Levenson, H., 186, 188, 190, 197
Levenson, J., 307
Levin, C., 350
Levin, H., 130
Levine, J., 307
Levine, M., 94, 190
Levine, R., 130
Levy, R.L., 204, 255, 339
Lewin, K., 16, 164
Lewinsohn, P.M., 36
Lewis-Fernandez, R., 380
Lex, B.W., 342
Lezak, M., 62–63, 295, 390
Liberman, B., 130
Lichtenstein, E., 336–337
Lidz, C.W., 89, 90
Liebeault, A.A., 11
Lieberman, J., 307
Lieberman, M., 170, 172
Liese, B.S., 154
Limbird, L.E., 125
Lin, T., 385
Lindemann, E., 187
Lindzey, G., 387
Linehan, M.M., 195
Lingle, D.W., 384

Linney, J.A., 369
Linskey, A.O., 101
Liotti, G., 256
Lipsey, M.W., 189
Lipsitz, N.E., 83
Lipton, M.A., 319
Liss-Levinson, N., 89, 90, 91
Litt, C., 244
Litt, M.D., 267
Locke, B.Z., 114
Locke, E.A., 232
Loehlin, J.C., 389
Loftus, E.F., 420
Logue, M.B., 202
Lonberg, S., 32, 33
Loo, C., 369
López, S.R., 379, 384
Lorion, R.P., 359
Lounsbury, J.W., 369
Loutitt, C.M., 17
Lowman, R.L., 30
Lowry, J.L., 194
Lubin, B., 356, 369
Luborsky, L., 117, 152, 155, 190, 193, 196, 268
Luchetta, T., 341
Luchins, A.S., 131, 132
Luchins, E.H., 131, 132
Lushene, R., 225
Lykken, D.T., 192, 195, 206
Lyman, R.D., 244, 245
Lynch, J.J., 336

Machado, P.P., 153
Machover, K., 72
Macias, C., 365
MacKenzie, R.,
MacKenzie, S., 323
Madanes, C., 174, 204
Maddi, S.R., 342
Maddux, J.E., 243
Maestas, D., Jr., 103
Mahler, M.S., 143
Mahoney, M.J., 187, 192, 196, 198, 232, 256
Maier, G.J., 358
Maiman, L.A., 266
Malan, D.H., 187, 190, 192, 197–198
Malgady, R., 388, 392
Malinow, K., 336
Mann, A.H., 114
Mann, J., 186, 188, 190, 197
Manning, M.M., 333

Mansky, P.A., 315
Mar, M.H., 340
Marcus, B.H., 341
Marecek, J., 89, 90, 91
Margolin, G., 88
Markides, K.S., 342
Markowitz, J.A., 197
Markus, H.R., 381
Marlan, A., 336
Marlatt, G.A., 268
Marmar, C., 32, 190
Marriotta, J.C., 297–298, 302, 318
Marsella, A.J., 378, 394
Marshall-Goodell, B.S., 130
Martin, J.E., 338, 341
Martin, W.L., Jr., 91
Martinez, D., 194
Masek, B.J., 265, 338
Maslow, A.H., 145
Mastboom, J., 362
Masters, K.S., 204
Masur, F.T., 332, 339, 340
Matarazzo, J.D., 26, 74, 87, 339
Mathews, A., 340
Matthews, W.J., 198
Maxmen, J.S., 192, 195
Maxwell, A., 206
May, R., 147–148, 254
May, R.B., 123
Mayer, J.P., 355
Maynard, H., 350
Mayne, T.J., 19
McArthur, D.S., 226
McCaughey, B.G., 364
McClellan, A.T., 196
McClelland, D.C., 381
McCrady, B.S., 195
McCrae, R., 67
McCullough, L., 195
McDonald, J.J., 413
McDowell, I., 35
McEvoy, L., 380
McGaw, B., 129
McGoldrick, M., 86
McGrath, P.J., 321
McGuire, J., 95
McIlroy, W., 125
McKibbon, K.A., 129
McLain, J., 90
McMahon, S.D., 337
McMain, S., 420

McMurray, R,G., 340
McNamara, J.R., 95
McNemar, Q., 130
McPherson, M.W., 7, 13
McSweeney, A.J., 359
Meara, N.M., 105
Meares, E.P., 369
Mechanic, D., 114, 332
Mednick, M.T., 21
Meehl, P., 38–39, 74, 201
Meichenbaum, D.H., 232, 265, 266, 267, 335, 338
Meisel, A., 89, 90
Meisel, P., 186
Meisol, P., 194
Mellinger, G.D., 310
Melton, G.B., 94
Melzack, R., 338
Mendoza, J.L., 123
Menkey, H., 334
Menninger, K.A., 253
Menzies, R., 420
Mercer, J.R., 389
Mesmer, A., 10
Messer, S., 158
Messer, S.B., 158, 187, 192, 193, 197, 198, 215
Messick, S., 57
Metraux, G.S.,
Metton, O., 404
Meyer, R.G., 313
Meyers, A., 331
Meyers, A.W., 337
Meyers, H.F., 342
Michael, S.T., 380
Milan, A.M., 403
Miles M., 170, 172
Miley, A.D., 358
Milgram, S., 132
Miller, N.E., 332
Miller, R., 90, 194, 352, 358
Miller, S, 186, 189, 192, 193, 202
Miller, S.D., 195, 196, 199, 202
Miller, T.I., 152
Millman, R.B., 353
Millon, T., 56, 68, 339
Mills, M.E., 336
Mintz, J., 268
Minuchin, S., 198
Mischel, W., 148
Mitchell, J.R., 305
Mitchell, S., 143, 144
Mobley, M.J., 418

Mohl, P.C., 194
Moline, M.E., 90
Monahan, J., 83
Monette, D.R., 336
Monroe, L.J., 337
Montagu, M., 6
Montouri, J., 225
Moore, D., 339
Moras, K., 190, 194
Moreno, J., 165
Morgan, C., 15
Morin, C.M., 337
Morishima, J., 379, 385
Morrison, J.K., 353
Morrow, B.R., 358
Morrow, G.R., 90
Morse, G.H., 358
Morton, S.G., 12
Moses, J., 340
Moss, P.A., 75
Motto, J., 29
Mount Zion Psychotherapy Research Group,
    192
Mowbray, C.T., 358, 365
Mowrer, O.H., 15
Mukherji, R.R., 393
Mullaney, D.G., 337
Mulvey, E., 91
Munford, P., 297–298, 302, 318
Munion, W.M., 138
Munjack, D.J., 255
Munoz, R., 36
Munsinger, H., 127
Muñoz, M.A., 393
Muñoz, R.F., 349
Muran, J.C., 195
Murphy, H.B.M., 378
Murray, C., 221
Murray, H., 15
Muscettola, G., 319,
Myers, D.G., 191
Myers, P., 342

Nagalingam, R., 130
Naglieri, J., 72
Nagy, L., 34
Nagy, T.F., 105
Nakano, K., 338
Nanni, C., 122
Napoli, D., 14, 15, 16
Nasrallah, H.A., 195

Nathan, T., 386, 392
Neale, M., 365
Neff, D.F., 341
Neisser, U.,389
Nelson, P.D., 87
Nelson, R.O., 336
Nelson, S.E., 300
Nester, E.J., 282, 285, 286–287
Netz, K., 337
Neufeld, R.W., 334
Neufeldt, S.A., 153
Newman, C.F., 154, 157, 186, 195, 199
Newman, R., 104
Niaura, R.S., 341
Nichols, M.P., 232
Niemeier, D.L., 192
Nieri, D., 95
Nietzel, M., 30
Nilsen, D., 55
Nolan-Hoeksema, S., 189, 192, 204
Norcross, J.C., 19, 21, 157, 186, 187, 192, 193, 199, 202,
    207
Norman, G.R., 114–115, 122, 125

O'Brien, C.P., 191, 196, 198, 199, 200, 204
O'Brien, S., 236
O'Connor, K.J., 233
O'Leary, K.D., 150
O'Leary, V., 20
O'Neal,J.H., 297, 298, 299
Oberg, K., 393
Ogles, B.M., 189, 190, 204
Ohnishi, H., 391
Olbrisch, M.E., 339
Olfson, M., 193
Oliver, J.M., 357
Olivero, J.M., 363
Olmstead, M.P., 117
Olsen, B., 72
Omer, H., 190
Opler, M.K., 380
Oriel, L.J., 255
Orley, J., 394
Orlinsky, D.E., 186, 188, 189, 198, 199, 207
Orlowski, B., 364
Orman, D.T., 120
Ots, T., 379
Otto, S., 90
Oullete Kobasa, K., 342
Overall, J.E., 38
Overdijk, W.I., 354

Overton, S., 337
Owen, S.V., 391

Packer, I.K., 410
Paleg, K.,
Palinkas, L.A.,
Pallak, M.S.,
Paniagua, F.A., 101
Paolino, T.J., 232
Papero, D., 173
Pardie, L., 341
Paredes, R., 363
Paris, J., 279
Parisi, S., 30
Parloff, M.B., 116, 118
Parmelee, W.M., 71
Partridge, K., 386
Pasteur, L., 7
Patteson, D.M., 350
Paul, S., 190
Payton, C.R.,
Peake, T.H., 197, 198
Pearce, L., 86
Pedersen, P.B., 390
Pekarik, G., 188, 191, 193, 194, 195, 195
Peller, J.E., 199
Peltzer, K., 379, 392
Peoples, C., 234
Perez-Vidal, A., 205
Perkins, D.V., 95
Perloff, R., 389
Perls, F., 146, 165, 170, 254
Perris, C., 154
Perry, N.W., 339
Persons, J.B., 117, 194, 199
Pervin, L.A., 267
Peters, T., 191
Petersen, L., 224, 248
Peterson, D.R., 18, 27
Petty, R.E., 130
Pezdek, K., 417
Pfeiffer, S., 72
Pfeiffer, W.M., 378, 391–392
Phares, E.J., 21
Phelps, L., 73
Phelps, M.E., 297–298, 302, 318
Phillips, E.L., 193
Piaget, J., 150
Piedmont, R.L., 67
Piercy, F.P., 194
Pilkonis, P.A., 116, 118

Pincus, H.A., 193
Pine, F., 143
Pinel, P., 6, 8
Pion, G.M., 21
Pisciotta, A.V., 307
Plake, B., 391
Pogrebin, M.R., 359
Polifkca, J.A., 369
Pollack, J., 195
Pollack, M.H., 311
Polster, E., 170
Polster, M., 170
Polusny, M.A., 103
Pope, K.S., 43–44, 97, 98, 99, 103
Popplestone, J.A., 7, 13
Porter, F.S., 243
Porter, N., 102
Post, R.M., 314, 315, 319
Postlewait, J.H., 273
Powles, W., 165
Prange, A.J., Jr., 319
Preston, J., 297, 298, 299
Price, K.P., 341
Price, L., 34
Price, R.H., 350, 356, 359
Prichard, D.A., 413
Prien, R.F., 315
Primavera, J., 350
Prince, M., 13
Prince, R., 378
Prochaska, J.O., 21, 159, 195, 199, 202, 261, 342
Propst, R.N., 362
Puente, A., 390
Pulos, S.M., 197

Quick, E., 196
Quitkin, F.J., 316, 321

Rabkin, J.G., 321
Rachman, S., 338
Rafferty, J.E., 71
Raimy, V.C., 18, 138
Rajab, M.H., 120
Ramirez, S.Z., 101
Ramos, D., 133
Ramsden, M.F., 129
Ramsey, T.B., 361
Randles, R., 98
Rank, O., 16, 187
Rapee, R.M., 236
Raphelson, M., 364

Rapoport, J.L, 225, 319
Rapp, S., 30
Rappaport, J., 350
Raskin, R., 145
Rasmussen, S.A., 34, 225
Raue, P.J., 150
Rauktis,M.E., 361–362
Rayner, R., 216, 230
Reding, G.R., 364
Reedy, P., 363
Rees, A., 193
Regoli, R.M., 359
Reich, W., 252
Reid, D.B., 63
Reid, W.J., 199
Reimherr, F.W., 323
Reinharz, S., 350, 356
Reiser, M., 417
Reisman, J., 7, 12, 13, 16
Reitan, R.M., 62, 64–65, 413
Reitman, D., 130
Rennie, T.A., 380
Repucci, N.D., 91
Reschly, D.J.,
Revenstorf, D., 123
Reviere, S.L., 97
Reynolds, C.R., 75, 225, 248
Reynolds, S., 193
Rheinberger, A., 123, 124
Rhode, D.L., 350
Rhodes, K., 341
Rice, L.N., 145–146, 147, 156, 157, 163
Richard, M.T., 63
Richards, P., 32, 33
Richelson, E., 319
Richmond, B.O., 225
Rickels, K., 323
Ridde, M.A., 225
Ridley, C.R., 384
Ridley-Johnson, R., 244
Riedel, S., 361
Rifkin, A., 321
Riger, S., 350, 356
Riley, G.E., 342
Riordan, M., 341
Ritzler, B.A., 388
Roberts, G.E., 226
Roberts, M.C., 243, 244, 245, 248
Roberts, S., 340
Robertson, G., 45
Robertson, I., 32

Robertson, J., 349
Rockert, W., 117
Rodichak, I.D., 341
Roesch, R., 359
Rogers, C.R., 9, 17, 32, 140, 145–146, 152, 165, 234, 253
Rogers, R., 34
Rogler, L.H., 392
Roitman, D.B., 355
Roland, A., 381
Roper, B.L., 118
Rorschach, H., 52, 69
Rosenbaum, J.F., 311
Rosenbaum, L.K., 350
Rosenbaum R., 193, 198
Rosenbeck, R.A., 365
Rosenhan, D.L., 258, 355
Rosenman, R.H., 338
Rosenthal, R., 83, 129, 133
Rosnow, R.L.,133
Rosodo, J.W, 393
Ross, L.V., 236
Rosselli, M., 390
Rossi, J.S., 341
Rossi, P.H., 358
Roth, L.H., 89, 90
Rotter, J.B., 9, 71, 140
Rounsaville, B.J, 155, 197
Routh, D.K., 11, 12, 15, 216
Rubin, D.B., 129
Rubin, S.S., 192
Rudd, M.D., 120
Rudy, T., 30
Rumberger, R.W., 350
Rush, A.J., 151, 154
Rushton, J.P., 133
Rutan S., 168
Ryan, N.C., 129
Ryburgn, M., 61

Sabin, J.E., 186
Sachs, J.S., 190, 192
Sacks, H.S., 130
Sadock, B.J., 287, 293, 295
Saeki, C., 102
Safran, J.D., 156
Saint Augustine, 139
St. Lawrence, J.S., 130
Salina, D., 337
Salkovskis, P.M., 198
Salovey, P., 198, 267,
Salter, A., 9, 148

Salzam, C., 306
Sampson, S., 192
Samstag, L.W., 195
Sanders, D.H., 350
Sandler, I.N., 361
Sandler, J., 252
Sanua,V.D., 385
Sarason, I.G., 332
Sarason, S.B., 18, 350, 352
Sartorius, N., 378
Satir, V., 174
Sattler, J.M., 52, 61, 75, 216, 221, 223, 240–242, 248
Saunders, N.L., 341
Sawyer, D., 189
Sayette, M.A., 19
Saywitz, K.J., 94
Scaglione, R., 420
Schaap, C., 121
Schaefer, C.E., 233
Schafer, R., 253
Scharfetter, C., 393
Schartzer, J.E., 362
Scheidlinger, S., 168, 204
Scher, S.J., 130
Schiffer, R.B., 298
Schlossberger, E., 94–95
Schmale, A., 90
Schmidt, F.L., 120
Schmidt K.A., 193
Schmidt, L.D., 105, 206
Schmidt, N., 355
Schmitt, N., 32
Schnable, R., 336, 338
Schnee, S.B., 358
Schneeweiss, R., 310
Schneider, H.G., 81, 83, 91
Schneider, J.A., 335
Schoenholtz-Read, J., 167
Schofield, W., 339
Schoonover, S.C., 314
Schoop, R.F., 420
Schow, M., 314
Schrader, S.S., 198
Schultz, D.F., 363
Schwankovsky, L., 122
Schwartz G.E., 331
Schwartz, J.H., 287
Schwartz, J.M., 297–298, 302, 318
Schwartz, M.S., 347
Scott, L., 83
Seaman, H., 105

Searight, H.R., 357
Sears, R., 15
Sedlmeier, P., 122
Seekins, T., 355
Seelau, E.P., 403
Segal, L., 198
Segal, S.P., 359
Segal, Z.D., 156
Seiden, R.H., 91
Seidman, E., 350
Seitz, V., 350
Selby, V.C., 341
Selekman, M.D., 194, 195, 197, 204, 205
Seligman, M.E.P., 153, 332
Selin, C.E., 297–298, 302, 318
Serpell, R., 389
Sesak, R.M., 89, 90
Sexton, T.L., 268
Sexton-Radek, K., 336, 337, 341
Seyle, H., 332
Sgroi, S.M, 243
Shader, R.I., 310
Shadish, W.R., 359
Shaffer, W.F., 201
Shakow, D., 17
Shapiro, D., 193
Shapiro, D.A., 193, 200
Shaw, B.F., 198
Shaw, J., 151, 154
Shea, T., 116, 118
Shear, M., 34
Sheffield, B.F., 115
Shefler, G., 197
Shelton, B., 341
Shelton, J.L., 204, 255
Sher, K.J., 202
Sheridan, E.P., 87, 339
Sheridan, K., 95
Sherner, L.B., 305
Sherwood, L., 285
Shiang, J., 185, 186, 187, 190, 193, 207, 215
Shiang, S., 186, 192, 199
Shinn, M., 361
Shirley, A., 130
Shlein, J.M., 146
Sholomskas, D., 34
Shriqui, C.L., 195
Shulman, K.I., 323
Shumaker, S.A., 354, 360
Shure, M.B., 349, 366
Sibulkin, A.E., 114

Siegel B.A., 407
Siegel, M., 92
Siegman, A., 32
Siever, L.J., 316
Sifneos, P.S., 192, 197
Silber, L., 355
Silver, B.V., 337
Silverman, C., 359
Sime, W.E., 354
Simek-Morgan, L., 32
Simon, T., 13, 52
Singer, B., 190, 193
Singer, D., 171
Singer, J.E., 339
Skinner, B.F., 230
Slaiku, K.A., 363
Sledge, W.H., 190, 194
Sleek, S., 97
Slovenko, R., 415
Smith, D.E., 97, 98, 99, 100, 107, 310
Smith, M.L., 129, 152, 194
Smithson, E., 310
Smyrnios, K., 194, 205
Sobel, D., 342
Sodowsky, G.R., 391, 396
Sokolov, S., 129
Solomon, P., 365
Somberg, D.R., 90
Sonne, J.L., 97
Sonnenberg, S.M., 192, 197
Soo-Hoo, T., 349
Sotsky, S.M., 116, 118
Southam-Gerow, M.A., 117
Sowell, T., 206
Sparrow, S.S., 73, 224
Speed, J.L., 186
Speer, P., 356, 369
Spence, K.W., 140
Spence, J., 20
Spiegel, D., 336
Spielberger, C.D., 225
Spitzer, R., 34
Spitznagel, E.L., 380
Spivack, G., 349, 366
Spotts, T., 323
Spreen, O., 62
Srole (Strole), L., 380
Stack, L.C., 358
Stackhaus, J., 123, 124
Staley, S., 420
Stanley, J.C., 336

Starcevic, V., 379
Stark, M., 253
Startup, M., 193
Steadman, H.J., 365
Stein, D.M., 191, 192
Stein, R., 362
Steinberg, M., 34
Steketee, O., 118
Stenmark, D.E., 369
Steptoe, A., 340
Stern, D., 143
Stern, W.L., 52, 388
Sternberg, R.J., 389
Stethem, L.L., 63
Stewart, D., 361
Stewart, E.C., 376
Stewart, J.W., 316, 321
Stewart, S., 268
Stiles, T.C., 193
Stitzel, R.E., 285
Stockton, M., 337
Stone, G.C., 339
Stone, G.L., 90
Stone, W., 168
Stoyva, J.M., 337
Strachey, J., 144
Strasburger, L.H., 98
Strean, H.S., 253
Street, W.J., 332
Streiner, D.L., 114–115, 121, 122, 125, 129, 130, 133
Stricker, G., 158, 160
Strickland, B., 20
Strupp, H.H., 118, 153, 155–156, 188, 190, 197
Stuart, R., 180
Stulman, D.A., 120
Stunkard, A.J., 337
Sturgis, B.J., 420
Sturr, J.F., 381
Stuss, D.T., 63
Sue, D.W., 91, 101–102, 395
Sue, S., 83, 206, 379, 383, 385, 387
Suissa, S., 120
Sukel, H.L., 404
Sullivan, H.S., 140, 143
Sullivan, T.J., 91, 336
Summerfelt, A.T., 307
Sundberg, W.D., 395
Svartberg, M., 193
Swanson, C.D., 95, 103
Sweet, A.A., 150
Swerdlik, M., 61

Swift, C., 350
Swonger, A.K., 285
Szpocnik, J., 205
Szuba, M.P., 297–298, 302, 318

Tabachnick, B.G., 97
Takeuchi, D.T., 357
Talaga, M., 297, 298, 299
Talbott, J.A., 357
Tallent, N., 26, 30, 43, 44, 45
Talmon, M., 187, 193, 198,
Tanaka-Matsumi, J., 378, 379, 394, 395
Tassinary, L.G., 130
Tatsuoka, M.M., 69
Taube, C.A., 193, 194
Taylor, C.B., 335
Taylor, J., 106
Taylor, S.E., 340
Tchividjian, L.R., 342
Tebes, J.K., 361
Teders, S.J., 341
Tellegen, A., 225, 387
Terman, L.M., 8, 14, 52, 61, 388
Tershko, O., 361–362
Tesar, G.E., 311
Thadani, D., 363
Theobald, D.E., 337
Thomas, S.A., 336
Thompson, C.E., 388
Thompson, S.C., 122
Thorensen, C., 339
Thorndike, R.L., 52, 223
Ticknor, C., 194
Todd, T.C., 195, 205
Tombaugh, T., 35
Topp, J.E., 380
Toro, P.A., 365
Tortu, S., 353
Tracey, T.J.G., 201
Treat, S., 203, 205
Trepanier, K.L., 118
Triandis, H.C., 376, 381, 382, 391
Tricamo, E., 321
Trimble, J.E., 385
True, R.H., 91
Trutt, S.D., 256
Trzepacz, P.T., 35
Tseng, W.S., 385
Tuke, William, 6,
Tulkin, S.R., 339
Tuma, J.M., 244

Tunks, E., 333
Turk, D.C., 30, 265, 266, 267, 338, 340
Turner, S.M., 114
Tursky, B., 341
Tymchuk, A.J., 83

Uhde, T.W., 314
Ulenhuth, E.H., 310
Urbina, S., 389
Ursano, R.J., 192, 197

Vaccarino, J.M., 91
Vachss, A., 192, 195
Vaillant, G.E., 115
Vajner, P., 244
van den Hout, M., 114, 121
van der Veer, G., 394
Van Doornen, L.J., 341
VandeCreek, L., 94
VandenBos, G.R., 193
Varney, N.R., 62
Varni, J.W., 244
Vasquez, M.J.T., 99, 103, 106, 385
Vaux, A., 361
Veroff, J., 356
Vesper, J.H., 83, 88
Vestergaard, P., 314
Vinogradov, W., 166
Visher, E., 176, 178
Visher, J., 176, 178
Voolkart, E.H., 332
Vorspan, R., 363

Wachtel, E.F., 159
Wachtel, P.L., 159, 163
Wack, J.T., 338
Wade, J.B., 337
Wade, T.C., 71
Walfish, S., 369
Walker Dilks, C.J., 129
Walker, S.E., 323
Wall, P.O., 338
Wallace, C., 30
Wallach, M.S., 153
Wallander, J.L., 244
Wallerstein, J., 175
Wallerstein, R., 190
Wallin, W., 14
Walsh, D., 30
Walsh, M.R., 5,
Walter, H.I., 236

Walter, J.L., 199
Walters, R., 148
Wandersman, A., 350, 356
Wang, J., 62
Ward, J., 106
Ward, M., 323
Ward, N.G., 192, 195
Warman, R.E.,
Warner, R., 114
Warren, C.S., 187, 192, 193, 197, 198, 215
Wasmer, D., 365
Wassef, A., 101
Waterman, R., 191
Watkins, J.T., 116, 118
Watkins, N., 123, 124
Watsky, E.J., 306
Watson, J.B., 140, 216, 230
Watzlawick, P., 198, 203
Weakland, J., 198, 256
Weakland, S.H., 188, 203
Weatherman, R.F., 73
Weathers, F., 34
Webb, J., 365
Webster, C.D., 420
Wechsler, D., 52, 59, 223
Wedding, D., 186
Wedgwood, R.J., 244
Weeks, F., 182
Weeks, G.R., 203, 205, 268
Weil, G.R., 226
Weinberg, R.B., 364
Weinberger, J., 152
Weiner, I.B., 22
Weiner-Davis, M., 191, 199
Weinstein, H.P., 67
Weishaar, M.E., 198
Weiss, B., 117, 122
Weiss, L., 339
Weiss, S.M., 331, 339
Weiss, S.R.B., 315
Weissman, M.M., 155, 197
Weisz, J.R., 117, 122
Welfel, E.R., 83
Well, G.L., 403, 420
Wells, K.C., 236
Wells, R.A., 185, 186, 190, 191, 192, 194, 205, 206, 215
Wender, P.H., 323
Wendt, H.W., 381
Wesley, G.R., 81, 83, 91
Wesson, D.R., 310
West, S.G., 121, 392, 394

Westermeyer, J., 393
Whetsel, D., 103
Whiston, S.C., 268
Whitaker, C., 173, 174
Whitley, B.E., Jr., 95
Whitman, T., 232
Wickersham, D., 120
Wiens, A.N, 31
Wilcox, K.T., 244
Wilcoxon, L.A., 232
Wiliams, G.T., 90
Wilk, J., 200, 204
Wilkinson, G.S., 224
Willan, A., 125
Williams, C.L., 66, 225
Williams, D.A., 341
Williams, J., 34
Williams, M.H., 413
Williams, R.E., 199, 388
Williamson, D.A., 337
Willner, H.S., 90
Wilner, S., 190
Wilson, C., 334, 336
Wilson, D.B., 189
Wilson, G.T., 150, 198, 336
Wilson, R.P., 391
Winegar, N., 103
Winett, R.A., 339, 342
Wing, R., 338
Winick, B.J., 409
Winnicott D.W., 144
Winston, A., 195
Winter, M.E., 305
Wissler, C., 51
Witheridge, T.F., 365
Witmer, L., 8, 11, 12–13, 24, 243
Wittchen, H-U., 114
Wittig, A.F., 95
Wittkower, E.D., 378
Wlkinson, W.H., 363
Wogan, M., 153
Wolber, G.J., 43, 45
Wolberg, L.R., 192, 198
Wolf, S.M., 104
Wolff, S.M., 342
Wolfson, D., 64, 413
Wolpe, J., 148–149, 168
Wong, F.Y., 348, 349, 353, 356, 357, 359, 360, 369
Wong, N.W., 361
Wood, D., 323
Woodcock, R.W., 51, 73

Woodring, J., 339
Woodward, C.A., 133
Woodworth, R., 52
Woody, G.E, 196
Woolen, R.L., 323
Wortman, C., 339
Wright, F.D., 154, 195
Wright, L., 20, 243, 244
Wright, T.L., 333
Wrightsman, L., 30
Wundt, W., 7, 8, 11, 51
Wysocki, T., 341

Yalom, I., 147–148, 166, 170, 172, 186, 191, 206
Yapko, M., 199

Yates, B.T., 342
Yates, D., 14
Yeh, E.K., 380, 385
Yerkes, R., 14, 17, 52
Yontef, G., 147
Young, D.M., 200
Young, K., 206
Youngren, M., 36

Zane, N., 206
Zeig, J.K., 138, 198
Zeiss, A., 36
Zerubavel, E., 89, 90
Zuniga, M.E., 392
Zuttermeister, P., 336, 338

SUBJECT INDEX

A-B-A design, 123–125, 424
Abnormal Psychology, Journal of (Prince), 13
Abreaction, 143, 233, 424
Accreditation, 14–15, 19
Acculturation, 102, 424
Achievement tests, 54, 223–224, 424
Action potential, 281, 285, 424
Actuarial judgment, 424
   in assessment, 29, 38–39
Adaptive behavior, 424
   tests for, 224–225
Adenosine triphosphate (ATP), 274, 277, 283, 424
Adjustment disorders, 412
Adrenal disorders, 301
Age-equivalent scores, 220, 424
Aggressive behavior, predictions of, 420
AIDS epidemic, 342
Akathisia, 424
Akinesia, 424
Alienation from school, 424
Alpha, 424
Alternate-form reliability, 221, 424
American Association for Applied and Preventive
      Psychology, 10, 20
American Association for Applied Psychology (AAAP),
      9, 17
American Association of Clinical Psychology (AACP),
      9, 14
American Association on Mental Retardation, 73
American Board of Examiners in Professional
      Psychology (ABPP), 9, 19, 39
American Group Psychotherapy Association, 166
American Psychiatric Association, 9
American Psychologic Association (APA), 1, 17, 20, 348
      (*see also* Name Index)
   accreditation (certification) issues and, 14–15, 19
   and child psychology, 216–217, 236
   and cultural diversity, 376
   ethical code of, 81–83, 88, 89, 93, 98, 100, 105,
   history of, 7–8, 15–16, 17, 20
   professional competence and, 87–88, 217, 305
   and psychopharmacology, 324–327
   and research guidelines, 131–132
   and social issues, 353
   structure of 10
   women in, 17
Amino-acid neurotransmitters, 286
Amnesia, 424
Antidepressants, 298–299, 302, 314, 315–319, 321–322,
      323
   side effects, 319
Antimanics/mood stabilizers, 313–315
   compliance rates and, 314
Antisocial behavior, and brief therapy, 195
Anxiolytic drugs, 306, 309–312
   addiction and, 310–311
   overdoses of, 310
Aptitude test, 424
Assertive case management (ACT), 364–366, 424
Assertive community treatment (ACT), 365–366 (*see*
      also Assertive case management)
Assessment 22 (*see also* Testing)
   behavior and, 36–38
   behavioral medicine and, 333–334
   behavioral theory and, 160
   for children, 217–229, 235
   clinical judgment and, 29, 38–39
   data collection and, 28
   definition of, 27–28, 424
   and DSM, 40–43, 201
   examples of, 45–48, 227–229
   and family therapy, 235
   and forensic psychology, 419
   history of, 26–27
   interview and, 31–35, 386–387
   legal issues and, 30, 42, 43

of minorities, 385–391
  in neuropsychology, 295–296
  phases of, 28–29
  referrals and, 29–30
  reporting of 43–48, 90
  theory and, 30–31
Assimilative psychodynamic therapy, 160
Association of Scientific and Applied Psychology
        (ASAP), 20
Asylums (*see also* Institutionalization) for the insane,
        6–7
Attention deficit disorder (ADD/ADHD), 309, 323–324,
        326
Attorney–client privilege, 424
Attrition, 120–121, 424
Autonomy, 85–86, 92, 98, 130, 348, 424
Awareness, and resistance, 262
Axon and terminal, 282, 283–285, 425

Basic Family Therapy (Barker), 173
Before–after trial, 114, 122, 425
Behavior modification, 236
Behavioral assessment, 36–38, 72, 425
Behavioral medicine, 302–303, 425 (*see also* Health
        psychology)
  education and training for, 339
  efficacy of, 336–339
  psychologists and, 333–334
  research into, 336–339
  and smoking, 336–336
  stress and, 332–334
Behavioral rating scale, 37, 331–332, 425
Behavioral therapy, 148–150, 159–160 (*see also*
        Behaviorism; Learning theory)
  for children, 229–231
  definition of, 425
Behaviorism, 140–141, 255, 258
Bell Curve, The (Herrnstein & Murray), 133
Beneficence, 84–85, 425
Best interest of the child, 425
Beta, 425
Bias 22, 116, 121, 425
Biofeedback, 24, 334–335, 337, 341–342
Biomolecules, 425
Bipolar disorder, 11
  and brief therapy, 195
  and psychopharmacology, 306, 313–315
Boulder Conference (1949), 18–19
Boundaries (in therapist–client relationship) 96–97, 425
Boundary crossings, 96–97, 425
Boundary (gestalt concept), 171

Boundary violations, 96–98, 99–100, 425
Brain (*see also* Consciousness)
  in adults, 289–293
  chemistry of, 281–287
  cognation and, 279–281
  dysfunction (minimal), 239
  emotions and, 279
  evolution of, 278–281
  injury of, 289
  in utero development of, 287–288
  mapping of (neuroimaging), 328
  metal, and effect on, 300–301
  neural transmissions in, 281–287
  and physical illness, 300–302
  postnatal development of, 288–289
  psychopathology and, 296–300
  structure of, 278–281, 289–293
Brief dynamic therapy, 425
Brief therapy (BT), 185–207
  approaches to, 196–199
  definition of, 187–188, 425
  efficacy of, 186, 193, 194
  and group therapy, 204–206
  health insurance and, 185–186, 194
  history of, 187
  limits of, 195
  models of, 190–192
  multiculturalism and, 206–207
  procedural outline of, 199–204
  shared values (general principles of), 188–190

California School of Professional Psychology, 10, 19
Caregivers, 361–362
Cells, study of (Cytology), 274–278 (*see also* Neurons)
Central nervous system (CNS), 286–287, 288, 289–291,
        301
  and psychopharmacology, 310, 311, 318, 323
  in utero development of, 287
Centrosomes, 277, 425
Cerebrospinal fluid (CSF), 295, 425
Certification, issues of, 20 (*see also* Accreditation)
Certification/decertification waiver, 409–410, 425
Child abuse, 94, 242–243, 245, 415–416, 419, 425
Child development, 14
Child psychology (*see also* Pediatric psychology)
  assessment for child psychology, 217–229
  case study of, 237–238
  cognitive-behavioral treatment in, 232
  developmental theories and, 218
  efficacy studies and, 236–237
  family approaches to, 234–236

Child psychology (*continued*)
   history of, 216–217
   learning theory and, 229–231
   measures/tests for 221–227
   and minority children, 241–242
   psychodynamic therapy in, 232–234
   psychometric issues and, 218–221
Children (*see also* Child psychology)
   abuse of, 94, 242–243, 245, 416–417, 419
   anxiety and fears in, 230
   in blended families, 175–178
   community psychology and, 366–367,
   as criminal offenders, 409–410
   custody cases, 415–416, 419
   learning disabilities in, 239–241
   medical problems and, 244–245
   and research studies, 132
Change, theories of, 143–145, 146–147
Changing with Families (Satir et al.), 174
Chlorpromazine (CPZ), 113–114
Chorea, 425
Civil commitment, 425
Civil competency, 415, 426
Class issues, 102
Classical conditioning, 230, 426
Client Centered Therapy (Rogers), 9
Client-centered (Rogerian) therapy, 145–146, 426
   for children, 234
   definition of, 426
   history of 140–141
   treatment resistance and, 253–254, 258
Clinical diagnosis (*see also* Assessment)
   definition of, 426
   and referrals, 29–30
Clinical judgment, 426
Clinical psychology
   brief therapy and, 185–207
   definition of, 1–2, 426,
   and government work, 15
   history of, 10–17
   and psychotropic drugs, 10
   trends in, 23–24
Clinical Psychology (Lowitt), 9
Clinical training, 18–19 (*see also* Psychologists)
Coefficient alpha, 57, 426
Cognitive-behavioral therapy, 140, 149, 156, 339
   and brief therapy, 195, 198–199
   cultural factors and, 394–395
   definition of, 426
   for children, 232
   group therapy and, 168–170

Cognitive therapy, 150–152, 426
   and treatment resistance, 255–256, 258
Cognitive Therapy of Depression (Beck et al.), 154
Cohort study, 114, 122 426
Collaboration, 426
Collectivism, 382–383, 426
Common (therapeutic) factors, 152, 157, 426
Communication theory, 256–256
   history of, 12–13
Community living, 357–358, 365
Community Mental Health Centers Act of 1963, 355,
   356, 363
Community psychology,
   definition of, 348–349, 426
   families and, 366–367
   future of, 369–370
   goals of, 348, 349–352
   lessons of, 368–369
   and the mentally disordered, 356–366
   and planned social change, 352–356
   and public policy, 355–356, 370
Competence, 87–88, 92
Compliance, 25, 117, 338, 426
Compliance therapy, 115–116
Computerized axial tomography (CAT) scan, 293–294
Computerized tomography (CT) scan, 62, 293–294, 299
Concurrent validity, 58, 221, 426
Conditional Reflex Therapy (Salter), 9
Conditioned response, 426
Conditioned stimulus, 426
Confidentiality, 86, 92–95, 421, 426
   and child abuse, 94
   and duty to protect, 94–95
   and group therapy, 167–168
Confucian dynamism, 426
Conjoint Family Therapy (Satir), 174
Consciousness (*see also* Brain)
   evolution of, 272–278
Construct validity, 58–59, 221, 426
Consumer perception, and psychotherapy, 153
Consumer Reports (magazine), 153
Content validity, 58, 221, 426
Continuous outcomes, 118–120
Contracts, in family therapy, 180–181
Cooperative learning groups (CLG), 123
Corrective-emotional experience, 144, 233
Countertransference, 427
Couples therapy, 175, 179–183
   and brief therapy, 204–206
Court cases:
   Canterbury v. Spence, 90

Court cases (*continued*)
 Cobbs v. Grant, 92
 Daubert v. Merrell Dow Pharmaceuticals, 405
 Dusky v. United States, 407
 Frye v. United States, 404, 405
 Jackson v. Indiana, 409
 Jenkins v. United States, 404
 Miranda v. Arizona, 409
 Tarasoff v. Board of Regents of California, 94, 414
 *White v. North Carolina State Board of Examiners of
   Practicing Psychologists,* 105
 Wickline v. State of California, 104
Craniology, 12
Criminal competency, 407–409, 427
Criminology (*see* Forensic psychology)
Crisis intervention, 199
Crisis therapy, 363–364
Criterion-referenced test, 53–54, 427
Criterion validity, 221
Cultural diversity, 83, 100–103, 350, 376–378 (*see also*
   Ethnic background; Multiculturalism)
 and American Psychologic Association, 376
 communication and, 101
 ethical issues and, 102–103
 and family therapy, 182–183
Culture, 375–377, 427 (*see also* Transcultural
   psychology)
 and mental illness, 380–381
 and psychotherapy, 141–142, 375, 390, 391–396
Culture accommodations, 427
Culture-bound syndromes, 427
Culture shock, 393–394, 427
*Cumulative Index of Nursing and Allied Health
   Literature* (CINAHL) [computerized database],
   128
Cyclical psychodynamics, 159
Cytoplasm, 274, 275–276, 282, 287, 427
Cytoskeleton, 275–276, 282, 427

Data collection, and assessment, 28
Database, computerized, 128–129
Deception, 427
Declaration of Helsinki, 130, 427
Defendant, 427
Deinstitutionalization, 355–356, 357, 427
Dendrites, 282, 283, 288, 427
Depression (major depressive episodes/MDE) 10,
   296–297, 312
 cognitive therapy and, 154–155
 in different cultures, 378–379
 health psychology and, 340–341

interpersonal therapy and, 197
 and psychopharmacology, 315, 320, 322–323, 324
Desensitization, 149
Developmental theories, 218
*Diagnostic and Statistical Manual of Mental Disorder/
   DSM* (American Psychiatric Association), 9–10,
   26–27, 34, 40–43, 379, 383, 412
 and assessment, 40–42
 and child psychology, 236–237
 and learning disabilities, 240
 legal issues and, 412
 and mental retardation, 238
 reliability of, 42–43
 and structured interview schedules, 34
 transcultural psychology and, 379–380, 383
Diathesis-stress model of illness, 303, 427
Dictionary of Behavioral Assessment Techniques
   (Hersen & Bellack), 72
Dieting, 337
Diminished capacity, 410–411, 427
Diplomate, 427
Disabilities, people with (*see* Specialized
   populations)
Discrete outcomes, 118–120
Disengagement, 235, 427
Divorce (*see also* Family therapy), 175–176
Dopamine, 286
 and psychopharmacology, 307, 318
 and schizophrenia, 299–300
Drug therapy
 and depression, 155, 312
Dual relationships, 97–100 (*see also* Boundary
   violations; Sexual relationships)
Due process, 427
Dystonia, 427

Eastern philosophies, 165
Eclectic therapy (*see* Psychotherapy integration)
Ecological perspective, 350, 427
Effectiveness, 428 (*see also* Efficacy)
Effectiveness research studies of, 113–122
Effect size (ES), 121–122, 129–130, 428
Efficacy, 122, 236, 428 (*see also* Effectiveness)
 and report writing, 44
Electroencephalography (EEG), 293, 296, 428
Emic, 377, 389, 428
Emotions, 279
Empathy, 384, 428
Empirical-criterion tests, 56
Empowerment, 349–350, 428
Enacted support, 360, 428

Endoplasmic reticulum, 276, 428
Enmeshment, 235, 428
Epidemiology, 114, 428
Epinephrine, 286
Ethical dilemma, 83, 428
Ethical guidelines, 84–86, 421, 42
Ethical imperialism, 133, 428
Ethical issues, 80–81, 130–134
Ethical Principles of Psychologists and Code of Conduct
(APA), 82, 84–86, 88, 89, 421
Ethical reasoning, 83–84, 86–87, 88, 103
Ethical Standards for Psychologists (APA), 9–10
Ethics of care, 106, 428
managed care and, 103–106, 186
Ethnic background (*see* Minorities)
Etic, 377, 428
Eugenics, 11–12, 428
Eukaryote, 274, 277, 428
European emigres, 15–16
Excitatory postsynaptic potential (EPSP), 282, 284–285,
286 428
Exercise (physical fitness), 338–339, 341
Existential psychotherapy, 147–149
definition of, 428
group therapy and, 170
history of, 140
treatment resistance and, 254, 258
Experiential psychotherapy, 140–141, 145–152 (*see also*
Client-centered psychotherapy; Humanist
psychotherapy), 428
Expert witness, 428
Exposure, 428
External validity, 116–117, 428
Extrapyramidal side effects (EPS), 428

Face validity, 221
Factor analysis, 428
False memory syndrome, 417, 428
Family therapy, 173–179
Family of origin, 429
assessment and, 235
blended families and, 176–179
brief therapy and, 204–206
and children, 234–236
and couple therapy, 179–183
divorce and, 175–176
history of, 173–175
Factor-analytic tests, 56–57, 223
Fidelity, 86, 429
Fiduciary relationship, 81, 429
Field theory, 164

File drawer problem, 429
Forensic psychology, 30, 358, 403–422 (*see also* Legal
issues)
assessment and testing in, 419
background of, 404–405
civil law and, 411–416, 419
and criminology, 406–411, 417–419
definition of, 403–404, 429
education and training for, 405–406
in legal cases, 420
in nonclinical situations, 420–421
predictions of future behavior, 420
Fourteen Ounces of Prevention (APA), 353, 366
Free consent, 429 (*see also* Informed consent)
in research studies, 130–134
Freudianism, 197–198, 331 (*see also* Psychodynamic
theory)
history of, 11
and treatment resistance, 250–253
Functional analysis, 429
Functional MRI (FMRI), 294–295, 328

General Systems Theory (GST), 171
Genetic loading, 303 and depression, 296
Gestalt therapy, 141, 146–147
definition of, 429
and group therapy, 164–165, 170
and training institutes, 170
and treatment resistance, 254, 258
Golgi bodies, 276, 282, 429
Grade equivalent scores, 220, 429
Group therapy, 166–172
and brief therapy, 204–206
history of 164–165
and inpatient therapy, 165
outpatient therapy and, 165–166
research in, 172
trends in, 172

Half-life, 429
Hawthorne effect, 429
Headaches, 337, 341
Health care reform, 833
Health insurance, 20, 185, 194
Health Maintenance Organization (HMO), 156
Health psychology, 10, 302–303 (*see also* Behavioral
medicine)
definition of, 339, 429
and minority groups, 342
research and, 339–342
Hearing impairment, testing for 73

Heart disease, 338
Heterotroph, 429
Historical controls, 113, 429
Homelessness, 358
Homework, 429
   in brief therapy, 203–204
Hormones, 286, and stress, 278
Human potential, 140
Human potential movement, 164
Humanistic psychotherapy, 140, 141, 145–152,
      155–156, 429
Hypnotic drugs, 312–313
Hypnotism, 11
Hysteria, 429

Identity, Youth and Crisis (Erikson), 216
Illusory validation, 72, 429
Immigrants, studies of, 14
Index Medicus (computerized database), 128
Individualism, 429
Individualistic self, 381–383 429
Inference, and assessment, 28
Informed consent, 43, 88–92, 428 (*see also* Free
      Consent)
   in research studies, 130–134
Inhibitions, Symptoms and Anxiety (Freud), 251
Inhibitory postsynaptic potential (IPSP), 282, 284–285,
      286, 429
Instrumental conditioning (*see* Operant theory
Intake procedure, 205
Integrative Solutions (Weeks & Hof), 182
Intelligence Quotient (IQ), 222 , 241–242
IQ Test (*see* Intelligence test)
Intelligence test, 51–52, 54, 62, 222, 239, 240–241,
      388–390 (*see* also Stanford Binet; Wechsler
      scales)
Industrial assessment, 30
Insanity, 430
Institutionalization (*see also* Asylums)
Integrative Psychotherapy (*see* Psychotherapy
      integration)
Internal validity, 116–117, 430
Interpersonal therapy (IPS), 197, 430
Interrupted time series, 125–127, 430
Interview, 430
   and assessment, 31–35, 386–387
   reliability of 32–33
Intrapsychic, 262, 430
I–Thou experience, 147

Journal of Family Psychology, 176

Jungian psychology, 140
Juvenile delinquents, 174

Language, and psychotherapy, 132–133, 242, 393 (*see*
      also Ethical imperialism)
Learning disabilities, 239–241, 430
Learning theory, 140, 229–231
Legal custody, 415, 419, 430
Legal issues (*see also* Court cases; Forensic psychology)
   in assessment, 23, 30, 42, 43, 90
   and civil law, 411–414, 419
   in criminology, 406–411, 417–419
   ethical behavior and 82–83
   of juvenile offenders, 409–410
   federal rules of evidence, 404–405
   harassment/discrimination and, 413–414
   informed consent, 88–89, 90–92
   malingering and, 414–415
   malpractice and, 414
   mental state and, 410–411
   neuropsychological damages and, 413
   Worker's Compensation/SSI and, 413
Life-skill training (LST) 353
Locus ceruleus (LC), 298–299
Long-term therapy, 188
Lysosomes, 276, 277, 430

Magnetic resonance imaging (MRI), 62, 294–295, 328,
      430
Malingering, 414–415, 430
Malpractice, 83, 105, 414
Managed care, 156, 245
   and brief therapy, 186
   definition of, 430
   ethical issues and 103–105
Manic-depression (*see* Bipolar disorder)
Manualized psychotherapies, 117, 154–156, 430
Maturation pull, 233
Measures/Scales (*see* Psychological tests)
Medical model of illness, 11, 22, 244–245, 331
Medications, over-the-counter (OTC), 301, 312, 313
      (*see also* Hypnotic drugs)
Meditation, 164
Medline (computerized database), 128
Memory, 288
Mental health, as world issue, 21
Mental health education, 353, 430
   media, use of, and, 349
Mental hospitals, 13 (*see also* Institutionalization)
Mental illness (mentally disordered):
   and community psychology, 355–362

Mental illness (*continued*)
  criminal offenders and 410–411
  intervention strategies for, 359–366
  social problems of, 357, 358–359
  and transcultural psychology, 378
Mental Measurement Yearbook, 4
Mental Research Institute, 188
Mental retardation, 430
  diagnosis of, 238
  testing for, 73
Mental status examination (MSE), 430
  in assessment, 28, 34–36
Meta-analysis, 127–130, 430
Metabolic disorders, 302
Metal, toxic affect of, 300–301
Mind That Found Itself, A (Beers), 7, 8
Minorities (ethnic and racial), 101, 385 (*see also*
      Transcultural psychology)
  and assessment procedures, 385–391
  and IQ testing, 241–242, 388–390
  problems of treatment 132–133, 358
  and psychotherapy, 390–391, 391–397
Mitochondria, 276, 277, 430
Monoamine oxidase inhibitors (MAOIs), 322–323
  side effects and, 322
Mood stabilizers/antimanics, 313–315
  compliance rates and, 314
Multiculturalism (*see also* Transcultural psychology)
  and brief therapy, 206–207
  clinical psychology and, 382–385
Multimodal therapy, 158
Multiple-baseline study, 125–126, 128, 430
Mutual help groups (*see* Support groups)
Myelin (sheath), 283, 285, 430

National Alliance for the Mentally Ill (NAMI), 354
National Council of Women Psychologists, 17
National Institutes of Health (NIH), 131
  Office for Protection from Research Risks (OPRR),
      131, 133
National Institute of Mental Health (NIMH), 17–18
National Joint Commission on Learning Disabilities
      (NJCLD), 239–240
National Mental Health Association, 7
National Register of Health Care Providers, 10, 19
Natural history, 430
Nature vs. nurture, 303, 381
Negative punishment, 231, 430
Negative reinforcement, 149, 231, 430
Networks, 431
Neurofilaments, 282, 431

Neurogenesis, 287
Neuroglia, 281, 431
Neuroimaging (brain mapping), 328
Neuroleptic drugs (tranquilizers), 306–309, 431
  side effects of, 307
Neuroleptic malignant syndrome (NMS), 307–308, 309,
      431
Neurology, 11 (*see also* Neuropsychology)
Neurons (nerve cells), 281, 282, 283–285, 287, 288, 431
Neuropeptide, 286, 431
Neuropsychological tests, 54, 62–66, 390
Neuropsychology, 23
  assessment in, 295
  definition of, 431
  and personal injury law, 413
Neuroscience, 280, 281–288
  research and diagnostic methods in, 293–296
Neurotransmitters, 281–282, 284, 285–287
  amino-acid, 26
  definition of, 431
  and psychopathology, 297
Nonequivalent control study, 114–115, 431
Nonmaleficence, 84, 85, 97, 431
Nonverbal behavior, assessment and, 32, 431
Norepinephrine, 286, 287, 298
Norm-referenced test, 53, 431
Nucleoli, 276, 277, 431
Nucleus, 276, 277, 283, 289, 431
Nuremberg Code, 130, 431

Obesity, 337
Obsessive compulsive disorder (OCD), 225, 297–298,
      302
  and psychopharmacology, 306, 311, 316, 318, 319,
      321
Odyssey (Homer), 4
Offer of proof, 431
One-group pretest/posttest study, 114–115, 431
Operant theory, 230–231
Oppositional defiant disorder (ODD), 324
Organelles, 274, 275, 277, 278, 431
Organic aggressive syndrome (OAS), 306
Organic compounds, 431
Organic model of illness (*see* Medical model)
Outcome:
  and brief therapy, 191, 201–202, 204
  comprehensiveness of, 119
  ethnic factors and, 395
  in research study, 118–120, 152–154, 182

Pain response, 338, 341, 431

Panic disorder, 298–299
    and psychopharmacology, 298–299, 309
Paradoxical techniques, 257
Parent–child relationship, 143, 366–367
Parent report measures, 226–227
    Child Behavior Checklist (CBCL), 226–227
Parent training programs, 236
Parkinson's disease, 286
Paternalism, 86, 431
Patient advocate, 431
Patient, responsibility of (see Treatment adherence)
Patient–therapist privilege, 92, 93, 431
Patient–therapist relationship, 29 32,
    in assessment, 32, 43–44
    and behaviorism, 150
    in brief therapy, 192, 193, 200–204
    and cognitive psychotherapy, 151
    confidentiality in, 86, 92–95, 421
    and ethical behavior, 81–83, 84–86, 93, 99, 106
    and humanist psychology, 147, 148, 150
    informed consent and, 88–92
    legal aspects of, 88–89, 90–91
    and psychodynamic theory, 144
    research and, 153–154
    sexual relations within, 95–96, 98, 99 (see also
        Boundaries)
    and treatment adherence/nonadherence, 268
Pavlovian conditioning, 229–230
Payments, methods of, 98–99
Pediatric psychology, 243–245, 431
Perceived social support, 360, 431
Percentile rankings, 431
Peripheral nervous system (PNS), 287
Person–environment fit, 432
Personal-construct therapy, 141
Personal injury, 419, 432
    psychological damages and, 411–416
Personality disorders, 195
Personality tests, 54, 65–72, 225–227
Personality types (Type A, etc.), 34
Persuasion and Healing (Franks), 141
Pharmacodynamics, 305, 432
Pharmacokinetics, 305, 432
Phenomenology, and treatment resistance, 253–254
Philadelphia Child Guidance Center, 174
Physical custody, 432
Physical (disorders) illness, 300–302
    and stress, 332–333, 341
Physical harm, protection from, 94–95
Physical health and clinical psychology, 23–24
Placebo, 118, 129, 432

Plaintiff, 432
Play therapy, 233–234
Polarization, 282, 283–284, 432
Police, and forensic psychology, 417
Policy science, 356, 432
Positive punishment, 432
Positive reinforcement, 230, 432
Positive self-talk, 335
Positron emission tomography (PET), 294, 296, 328,
    432
Post-traumatic stress disorder (PTSD), 412
Potentiation, 432
Power, 432
Predictive validity, 58, 432
Prescriptive brief therapy, 199
Prevention, and community psychology, 349–350
Primary prevention of, 349–350, 432
Principles of Psychology (James) 7, 8
Problem-solving, 198
Professional ethics, 80–87, 432
Professional practice standard, 89–90 432
Projective method (in assessment), 22, 69–72
    definition of, 69, 432
    drawing techniques, 226
    story telling techniques, 226
Prokaryote, 273, 432
Protoplasm, 275, 432
Pseudo-parkinsonism, 308, 432
PsychInfo (computerized database), 128
Psychoactive drugs (see also Psychopharmacology;
        Psychotropic drugs)
Psychoanalysis (see also Freudianism)
    definition of, 432
    history of, 13, 140–141
    and psychodynamic theory, 142–145
Psychodrama, 165
Psychodynamic theory, 30, 142–145, 155
    brief therapy and, 197–198
    and child psychology, 232–234
    and group therapy, 168
    patient-client relationship in, 144
Psychogenic thesis, 11
Psychological Abstracts (computerized database), 128
Psychological Bulletin (Journal), 127
Psychological Clinic, The (Witmer, editor), 8, 12
Psychological malpractice, 432
Psychological Racketeers (Yates), 14
Psychological testing, 51–79 (see also Psychological
        tests)
    abuses of, 75–76
    for achievement, 54, 223–224, 424

Psychological testing *(continued)*
  for aptitude, 54
  behavioral approaches to 72
  bias in, 74–75
  for children, 219–227
  computers and, 74, 76
  construction of, 55–57
  cultural issues and, 390–391
  definition of, 52–54, 435
  evaluation of 57–59
  and forensic psychology, 419–420
  future of, 76–77, 389–391
  guidelines for, 389–391
  intelligence, 51–52, 54, 59–62, 62, 221–223, 239, 240–241, 388–390
  neurological, 54, 62–66, 390
  origins of, 51–52
  personality, 54, 65–72, 225–227
  projective approaches to, 69–72
  scoring of, 219–221
  for specialized populations, 72–73
  types of, 53–55
Psychological tests:
  Army Alpha test, 14, 52
  Army Beta test, 14, 5
  Behavioral Avoidance Test (BAT), 72
  Behavioral rating scale, 37–38, 425
  Beck Depression Inventory, 340
  Binet-Simon intelligence test, 8, 13
  Brief Psychiatric Rating Scale (BPRS), 38
  Community Competence Scale, 357
  Counseling Topic Classification System (CTCS), 32, 33
  Differential Ability Scales
  Draw-A-Person Test (DAP), 2
  Halstead-Reitan Neuropsychological Test Battery, 64–65
  Hiskey-Nebraska Test of Learning Aptitude (H-NTLA), 73
  Inventory of Socially Supportive Behaviors (ISSB), 361
  Kaufman Assessment Battery for Children (K-ABC), 62
  Kaufmann Brief Intelligence Test (K-BIT), 62
  Luria-Nebraska Neuropsychological Battery (LNNB), 65
  McCarthy Scales of Children's Abilities
  Millon Clinical Multiaxial Inventory (MCMI-III), 68
  Minnesota Multiphasic Personality Inventory (MMPI), 9, 52, 56, 65, 66–67, 68, 220, 225,

    and minorities, 387
  NEO Personality Inventory—Revised (NEO PI-R), 66–67
  Paced Auditory Serial Addition Task (PASAT), 62–63
  Peabody Picture Vocabulary Test—Revised (PPVT-R), 73
  Personality Inventory for Children (PIC), 227
  Pleasant Events Schedule (PES), 36–37
  Revised Children's Manifest Anxiety Scale (RC-MAS), 225
  Rey Auditory Verbal Learning Test, 65
  Rorschach inkblot test, 9, 31, 52, 69–70, 226
    and minorities, 387–388
  Rotter Incomplete Sentences Blank (RISB), 71
  Scales of Independent Behavior (SIB), 73–74
  Sixteen Personality Factor Test (16PF), 57, 68–69
  Social Support Behaviors Scale, 361
  Slosson Intelligence Test
  Stanford-Binet Intelligence Scale (SB-RE), 59
    Fourth Edition, 61–62, 223
  State–Trait Anxiety Inventory for Children (STAI-C), 225, 340
  System of Multicultural Pluralistic Assessment (SOMPA), 389
  TEMAS, 388
  Thematic Apperception Test (TAT), 9, 15, 70–71
    and minorities, 387
  Themes Concerning Blacks, 288
  Vineland Adaptive Behavior Scales (VABS), 73, 224–225, 239
  Vineland Social Maturity Scale, 73
  Wechsler tests/scales, 39, 59–61, 62, 216, 222–224, 238
    Adult Intelligence Scale (WAIS-II)
    Adult Intelligence Scale—Revised (WAIS-R), 64, 65, 222
    Bellevue Intelligence Scale, 9
    Individual Achievement Test (WIAT), 223–224, 239, 240–241
    Intelligence Scale for Children (WISC-III), 216, 218–219, 220, 222, 240
    Memory Scale—Revised (WMS-R), 63–64, 65
    Preschool and Primary Scale of Intelligence—Revised (WPSSI-R), 122
  Wide Range Achievement Test (WRAT), 224
  Woodcock Johnson Tests of Achievement—Revised (WJ-R), 221, 223, 229, 239
Yale–Brown Obsessive Compulsive Scale for Children (YBOC-C) 225

Psychologists:
  and children, 245 (*see also* Child Psychology;
      Pediatric Psychology)
  clinical judgment of, 29
  competence of, 87–88, 217
  and cultural diversity, 101–103
  economic issues and, 20
  education of, 13, 15, 18–20, 21–22, 217–218, 325, 369
  ethical behavior and, 80–86, 87–100
  government work and, 15–16, 18
  and group therapy, 166
  as legal consultants (expert witnesses), 421
  and psychopharmacology, 305, 324–327
  relationship with patients, 29 32, 43–44, 81–83,
      84–86, 144
Psychology (*see also* Psychologists; Psychotherapy):
  career opportunities in, 15–16, 369–370
  future trends in, 23–34
  government and 16
  history of, 2–23
  and military, 14, 16–17, 52
  politics and, 16
  popularization of, 14
  as science, 7
  in the United States, 7–8, 13–14, 21
Psychometric issues, in child psychology, 218–221
Psychoneuroimmunology (PNI), 302–303
Psychopharmacology, 305–328
  and alcohol withdrawal, 309
  and attention deficit disorder (ADD/ADHD), 309,
      323–324, 326
  and bipolar disorder, 306, 313–315
  and depression, 315
  education and training in, 305–306, 325–327
  and insomnia, 309, 312–313
  and major depressive episodes (MDE), 315, 320,
      322–323, 324
  and mental illness, 356–357
  and obsessive-compulsive disorder, 306, 311, 316,
      318, 319, 321
  and oppositional defiant disorder (ODD), 324
  and organic aggressive syndrome (OAS), 306
  and panic disorder, 298–299, 309
  psychologists and, 324–327
  and schizophrenia, 299–300, 306–307, 309
  and Tourette's syndrome, 306, 308
Psychosocial clubs or clubhouses, 362–363, 366, 432
Psychosomatic medicine, 331
Psychostimulants, 323–324
  side effects of, 324
Psychotherapy:

cultural issues and, 141–142, 375, 390, 391–396
definition of, 138–139, 433
evaluation of 112–134
future trends in, 154–155, 395–397
history of 11, 13, 112–113, 139–141;
kinds of, 186
language and, 132–133, 242, 393
minorities and, 390–391, 391–397
research in, 152–155
Psychotherapy integration, 157–160, 171
  and brief therapy, 199
  definition of, 433
  group therapy and, 170–172
  and treatment resistance, 258–261
Psychotropic drugs, 298–300
  addiction and, 310–311
  antidepressants, 314, 315–319, 321–322, 323
  anxiolytic drugs, 306, 309–312
  compliance rates and, 314
  definition of, 433
  history of 9–10
  hypnotic drugs, 312–313
  monoamine oxidase inhibitors (MAOIs), 322–323
  mood stabilizers/antimanics, 313–315
  neuroleptic drugs (tranquilizers), 306–309
  overdoses of, 310
  psychostimulants, 323–324
  selective serotonin-reuptake inhibitors (SSRIs),
      319–321, 322
  side effects and, 307, 319, 322, 324
Public health, and AIDS epidemic, 342
Public Law (P.L.) 94–142, 239, 240
Public policy, 355–356, 370, 433

Quasi-experiment, 433

Racism, 12
Randomization of, 433
Randomized-controlled trial (RCT), 115–116, 118, 122
Rational-emotive therapy (RET), 141, 150–151, 335
  group therapy and, 169–170
  and treatment resistance, 255–256
Reactance, 256
Reasonable-person standard, 90, 433
Receptors, 282, 433
Recidivism, 357–358, 433
Referrals, 29
  and medical cases, 29–30
Reframing, 257, 433
Relational-structure theory, 143–144
Relationships, 433

Relationships *(continued)*
    parent–child, 143
Relaxation, 24, 433
    and community psychology, 349–350
    and physical illness, 336–337
    techniques for, 334–335 (*see also* Stress management)
Reliability, 220–221, 433
Religion, and psychology, 4–6
Report writing, and assessment, 43–48
Repression, Freudianism and 250–251
Research studies, 121–130 (*see also* Effectiveness)
    attrition in, 120–122
    in child psychology, 236–237
    and community psychology, 369–370
    design of 113–118, 122–127
    ethics and, 130–134
    outcome and, 118–120, 152–154
    statistical significance of, 121–130
Reversal design, 433
Ribosomes, 276–277, 433
Rogerian therapy (*see* Client-centered therapy)

Scales (*see* Psychological tests)
Schizophrenia, 9, 10, 11
    and brief therapy, 195
    and psychopharmacology, 299–300, 306–307, 309
Scientist/practitioner, 433
Second Chances (Wallerstein & Blakeslee), 175
Secondary prevention, 349–350, 433
Selective serotonin-reuptake inhibitor (SSRI), 310, 311, 313, 316, 319–321, 322, 433 (*see also* Serotonin)
    and drug–drug interactions, 320
    side effects of, 319
Self, cross-cultural concept of, 381
Self-disclosure, 96–97, 102
Self-help groups, 337 (*see also* Support groups)
Self-monitoring, 36, 265
Self-report inventories, 66–69
Self-talk, 335–336
Sense of community, 351–352, 433
Sentence completion techniques, 226
Serotonin, 286, 302 (*see also* Selective serotonin-reuptake inhibitor)
    and depression, 316
    and obsessive-compulsive disorder, 306
Sessions, number of, 117–118, 186–188
Sexual abuse (*see* Child Abuse)
Sexual dysfunction, 319
Sexual relations, 95–96, 98, 99
Short-term therapy, 155, 156, 186, 187 (*see also* Brief therapy)

Single-session therapy (SST), 198
Single-subject design, 433
Skill acquisition techniques, 335–336
    life-skill training (LST), 353
Sleep disorders (insomnia), 337
    and psychopharmacology, 309, 312–313
Smoking, 336
Social change, 352–356, 432
Social desirability, 433
Social distance, 384, 434
Social embeddedness, 356, 434
Social integration, 357, 434
Social learning theory, 231
Social support, 354, 360–363, 434
Society for the Psychological Study of Social Issues (SPSSI), 17
Sociocentric self, 434
Solution-focused brief therapy, 434
Soma, 281, 282, 434
Spearman-Brown formula (split-half test reliability), 57
Specialized populations, testing for 72, 73
Split-half test reliability (Spearman-Brown formula), 57
Standard error of measurement, 220, 434
Standard of care, 434
Standardization sample, 53, 218, 434
Statistics:
    and prediction, 22
    and research studies, 121–130
Steady state, 434
Stereotype, 384–385, 434
Strategic therapy, 198–199, 256–257, 434
Stress, as trigger for disease, 303, 332–334, 341
Stress management, 354–355 (*see also* Relaxation)
Structural therapy, 198, 434
Structured interview, 32–34, 434
Structured interview schedule, 33–34, 434
Students, as research subjects, 130–131
Studies in Hysteria (Breuer and Freud), 8
Subjective culture, 376, 434
Substance abuse, 336, 353, 362–363
    and brief therapy, 195
Substitution, 119–120, 434
Suicide, 363–364, 379
    and assessment, 29
Supplementary Security Income (SSI), 76
Support groups, 434, 434
Surrogate, 166, 434
Surviving the Breakup (Wallerstein & Kelly), 175
Symptom prescription, 257
Synapse, 282, 285, 287, 434
Systemic therapy, 158–159, 256–257, 258, 434

T-groups, 164
Tardive dyskinesia (TD), 308, 309, 318, 435
Test–retest reliability, 57, 220–221, 435
Testing (*see* Psychological testing),
Therapeutic technique, 143–144, 146–147
Therapeutic window, 435
Threshold of excitation (TOE), 282, 284–285, 435
Thyroid disorders, 301
Time-limited dynamic psychotherapy (TLDP),
    155–156, 188, 197
Time-sensitive therapy, 188 (*see also* Brief therapy)
Tomography (*see* Computerized tomography)
Tourette's syndrome, 306, 308
Toxicity, affects of, 300–301
Training groups (*see* T-groups)
Transcription, 435
Transcultural psychology, 375–397 (*see also*
    Multiculturalism)
  assessment and, 385–391
  concepts and issues of, 381–385
  history of, 377–380
  and mental disorders, 378
Transference, 435
Transinstitutionalization, 357, 435
Transtheoretical therapy, 159
Treatment adherence/nonadherence, 263–268, 338–339
Treatment resistance, 249–268 (*see also* Treatment
    adherence/nonadherence)
  behaviorism and, 254–255
  case study of, 262–263
  client's use of, 262
  cognitive therapy and, 255–256
  definition of, 249–250, 435
  and extrapersonal factors, 261
  Freudianism and, 250–253

integrated model of, 258–261
  and interpersonal factors, 261
  and intrapersonal factors, 260–261
  phenomenological approaches to, 253–254
Triangulation, 235, 435
True experiment, 115–116, 435
Type I error, 121, 435
Type II error, 118, 120, 435

Unconditioned response, 435
Unconditioned stimulus, 435
Unconscious 142–145, 435 (*see also* Psychodynamic
    theory)
  resistance and, 251–52
United States, psychology in, 7–8, 13–14, 21
University clinics, 13 (*see also* Community psychology)
Utilization review, 103–104

Validity, 57–59, 221, 435
  of evaluation studies, 116–11
Value tests, 54–55
Vanderbilt Psychotherapy Project, 155–156
Veracity, 86, 435
Veteran's Administration, assessment and, 27
  and clinical psychology, 9, 20
Virtue ethics, 105–106

Witchcraft, 5–6
Women, in psychology, 6, 17
Worker's Compensation/SSI and, 413
World Federation for Mental Health, 21
World Health Organization (WHO), 130
  and mental illness, 378
World War I, psychology and, 14, 52
World War II, psychology and, 16–17, 26–27, 130